POLITICS
OF
NURSING

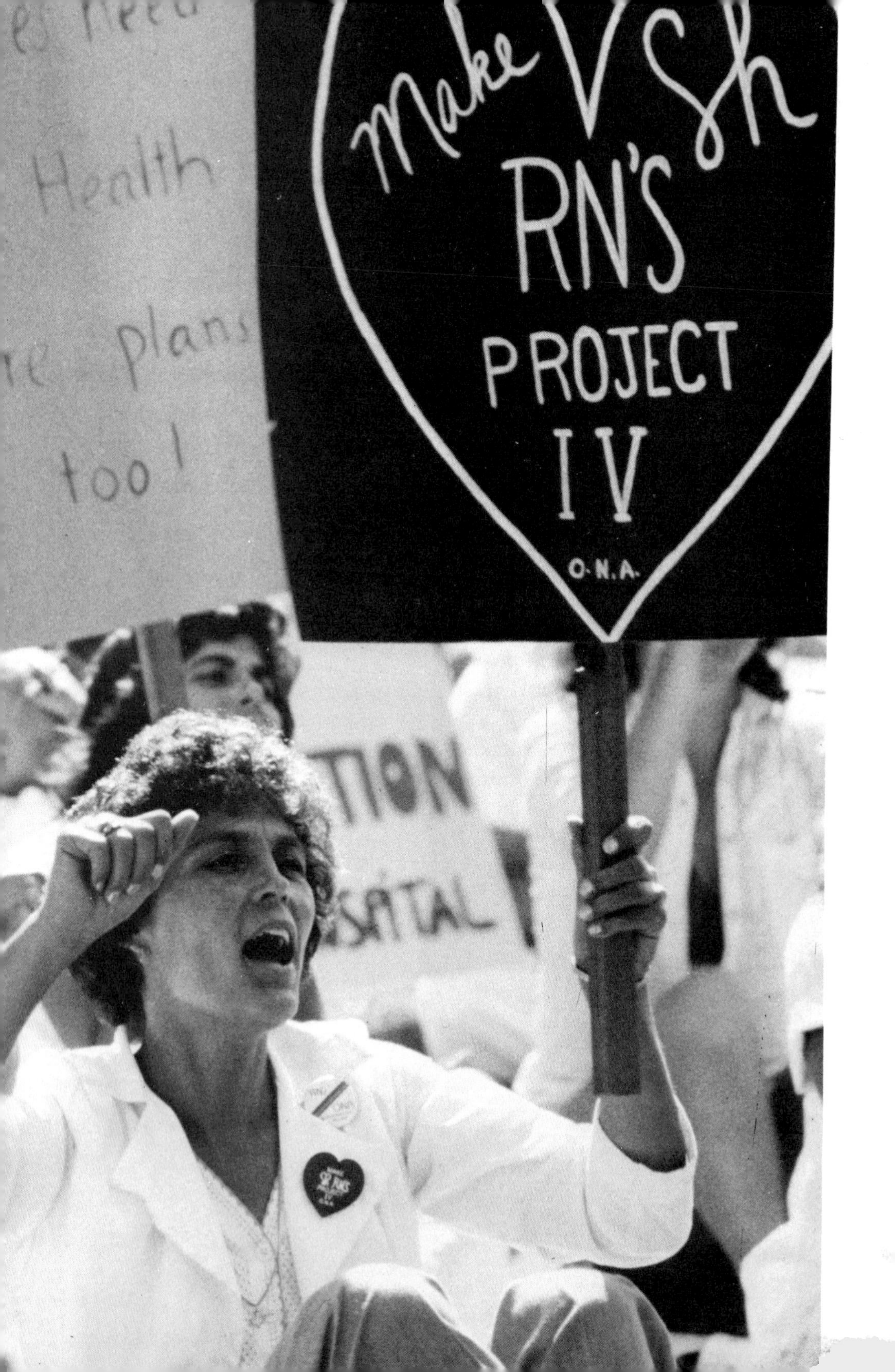
Make VSh
RN'S
PROJECT
IV
O.N.A.
Health
too!

Politics
of
Nursing

Beatrice J. Kalisch, R.N., Ed.D., F.A.A.N.

*Shirley C. Titus Distinguished Professor of Nursing
and Chairperson, Parent–Child Nursing
University of Michigan
Ann Arbor, Michigan*

Philip A. Kalisch, Ph.D.

*Professor of History and
Politics of Nursing
University of Michigan
Ann Arbor, Michigan*

Foreword by
Senator Daniel K. Inouye

J.B. Lippincott Company
Philadelphia

6 5

Library of Congress Cataloging in Publication Data

Kalisch, Beatrice J.   DATE
   Politics of nursing.

   Bibliography
   Includes index.
   1. Nursing—Political aspects—United States.
2. Nursing—Government policy—United States.
3. Medical policy—United States.   4. Nurses—United
States—Political activity.   I. Kalisch, Philip
Arthur.   II. Title.   [DNLM: 1. Delivery of health
care—United States.   2. Nursing—Trends—United
States.   3. Politics—United States.   4. United
States.   WY 16 K14p]
RT4.K33   362.1'7   81-8471
ISBN 0-397-54245-3   AACR2

Cover photo courtesy of Ladies' Home Journal.

Frontispiece photo courtesy of Register-Guard (Eugene, Oregon).

Contents

Foreword

by

Daniel K. Inouye,

United States Senator

In many ways, the publication *Politics of Nursing* is extraordinarily timely. As a nation, we are unfortunately about to commence a journey under the banners of "cost consciousness" and "balancing the budget" that I am afraid will be unlike any other that we have ever experienced in modern times. It is quite possible, if not probable, that before we are through, most of the heralded programs of the Kennedy-Johnson era, or the Great Society, will have been systematically dismantled—the good along with the bad, the effective as well as the ineffective. Even today, we know that upwards of some 18 million Americans have no health insurance coverage at all, that 19 million have health insurance that does not protect them against ordinary costs of hospitalization and physician expenses, and that an additional 46 million of our citizens have inadequate insurance against large medical bills. Further, some 51 million Americans today live in areas without sufficient access to health care, even if they could pay for it. Yet, at the same time, as a nation we spend more on health care than any other country in the world. Health care is our third largest industry, and its costs continue to escalate faster than any other segment of our economy.

For all of the rhetoric that we hear today about the inherent advantages of a competitive-oriented system, it is most unfortunate, in my judgment, that no one has really begun to address what I personally consider to be the single most important issue—the true potential contribution of our nation's alternative health care providers, and especially the nurse practitioner/clinical specialist, to our overall health care system. If we are to develop a truly competitive system, we must be consistent and actively encourage the utilization of competitive providers. If we are ever to seriously curtail our ever-escalating medical costs, and realistically we no longer have any alternative, then we must begin to think in terms of delivering comprehensive *health care*, and not merely *medical care*. To do so, we must take a serious look at enhancing "wellness," as well as responding to incidents of "sickness." We must modify our current reliance upon our traditional notions of health care. Instead, we must now systematically begin to address those barriers in our system that have hindered both the training and the autonomous practice of our nation's professional nurses. We must strive to provide appropriate regulatory flexibility to ensure that those professionals who desire to practice autonomously, whether in hospitals or birthing centers, or on an out-patient basis, can in fact do so. We must ensure that they have the legal right to admit their patients; write appropriate nursing orders, including prescriptions; and possess viable career and reimbursement mechanisms to enhance their productivity and professionalism. The approach that I have outlined is by no means fostered by our current system. However, I am confident that my objective is very definitely in the best interest of our nation, especially the consumer.

To accomplish the goals that I have suggested, it will, without question, take considerable energy and dedication. Above everything else, this will require our nation's professional nurses and perhaps more importantly, their patients, to become politically active. In essence, the nursing profession will have to enter the 20th century. *Politics of Nursing* is in a word, an excellent handbook, or a primer if you will, for political action by our nation's practitioners. It is indeed a most timely document, as we are entering a new political era. Generations to come will be directly affected by whether the nursing profession will seriously heed the lessons proffered by the Kalisches.

In reviewing this report, one can see that the authors expended considerable energy in providing a comprehensive review for the profession. I chose the term "report" purposefully, for that is exactly what this extraordinary document is. It is not only an intimate description of the history and chronology of nursing's efforts in the past in the legislative arena, but if one takes the time to look just a little behind the many described events and focus instead upon the personalities and personal orientations of the principals involved, it becomes abundantly clear why our nation's professional nurses have had such an uphill struggle. It also becomes clear what they must do in the future. As I indicated earlier, this is a handbook for political action. The authors do not purport to lead their colleagues by the hand, but through presenting distinct example after example, they clearly demonstrate not only why the nursing profession must become more actively involved in the political process, but also how they teach their colleagues to be successful. The highly concise and yet effective glimpses that are provided of the profession's advocates in action—their successes and even their frustrations—are inspiring. Yet, in my mind, one issue kept coming up: why did it always seem that either a physician or an economist was the primary spokesperson for the Administration regarding nursing issues? Why have not a sufficient number of professional nurses been promoted to nonclinical leadership positions, for example, in the area of developing health care policy on both the state and federal levels? Why hasn't the nursing profession utilized the true extent of their potential political power? Two basic but key additional questions also readily come to mind. First, do our nation's nurses really want to be true professionals—are they willing to accept and, if necessary, to demand both the responsibility and prerogatives of power and authority? A second and closely related question is whether our nation's schools of nursing are really committed to training professional nurses to be capable of accepting policy leadership roles. Is there any serious institutional support for the development of a true cadre of professional nurses?

Although from the title and a brief review of the table of contents, a reader might presume that *Politics of Nursing* focuses exclusively upon "nursing issues," in fact, everything discussed in the text is really quite pertinent to our nation's health care system as a whole. As I reviewed each chapter, I could not help but think that one could readily substitute "optometrist," "clinical psychologist," "pharmacist," or for that matter any other nonmedical discipline. The issues and arguments are essentially the same. The fundamental questions are who will control our nation's health care system: the consumer or organized medicine? As a society, are we going to continue to spend seemingly endless dollars maintaining the status quo, on fancy and admittedly highly impressive technology? Or, will we instead finally place a high priority on true preventive and psychosocial endeavors? Will we, for example, begin to finally address ways to reduce the many "bad habits" that we know are the major causes of death in our society today—smoking, poor diets, lack of sleep, lack of exercise, excessive stress, etc.? To cite a concrete example: alcoholism is the fourth largest killer in our society today. It is a major problem even in our nation's high schools. In over half of the highway accidents that result in fatalities, where young drivers are involved, someone has been drinking. It also leads to numerous incidents of family violence. Yet, the record must show that our present commitment to alcohol treatment and prevention programs is miniscule at best, and this is a target for one of the first major budget reductions proposed. Another example is that presently our nursing home expenditures alone represent 8 percent of our total health care dollar, and further, is the single fastest-growing expense item. Yet, again, what does the record show we are doing in response? In my judgment, our nation's professional nurses are without question the most appropriate discipline to address the pressing needs of our elderly. Nurse clinicians are superbly trained in both the psychosocial and the physiological aspects of care. Our elderly demonstrate major problems in both of these areas, but with appropriate intervention, we have demonstrated that they can live meaningful lives. History will unfortunately show that, once again, we have not provided sufficient financial incentives, on either the state or federal level, to our nation's schools of nursing, or to our nursing homes. Why hasn't the Health Care Financing Administration (HCFA) provided support for developing special "teaching nursing homes" on an experimental basis? These would be similar to the traditional "teaching hospitals" that have been the mainstay of our nation's medical schools. Similarly, why hasn't HCFA funded special demonstration "birthing centers" for those nursing schools that specialize in developing popular certified nurse-midwives?

Even in these days of "cost consciousness" and extreme budgetary constraints, I am confident that the vast majority of my colleagues in our state and federal legislatures would sincerely share my enthusiasm for these approaches. But as the authors vividly point out, politics is more than fancy ideas, no matter how good they might intuitively seem. Politics in a real sense is the people who take the time to participate. These are generally very dedicated individuals who are doing their best to respond to highly complex demands, often of a contradictory nature. There is no question in my mind that, especially today, we need more individuals in politics who, from their own experiences, can personally appreciate the many fine contributions that our nation's nurses can make, if only they would be given the opportunity. But again, this is exactly a major point expressed in *Politics of Nursing*. Nurses will only be accorded this "opportunity" if they begin to truly act as professionals and as a result demand the rights and responsibilities due their professional expertise. It is our nursing profession that must take the leadership and identify and then modify those aspects of the law that discriminate against them. It is they who must care enough about their patients to become politically active.

As a nation, we unfortunately have very short memories. As a people, we are especially quick to forget those who have in the past unselfishly contributed to our nation's greatness. This trait is truly one of our greatest weaknesses, and, accordingly, I was especially pleased to see the time expended by the authors in reviewing the contributions of some of the true giants of nursing. Individuals such as Pearl McIver and Lucile Petry of the Public Health Service have made major contributions to the profession that many of us have simply never been aware of before. Every day on my way to our nation's Capitol, I pass one particular federal building and marvel at the insightfulness of what is carved in stone on its face: "What is past is prologue." This is so true, yet so many of us will never appreciate its significance. I sincerely hope that our nation's nurses will learn from the lessons of their mentors.

Preface

In a nation founded on the principles of equality, more nurses are realizing that they need political expertise to overcome their second-class status in all aspects of the current health care system. For example, a disgruntled Las Vegas, Nevada, nurse, in a March 17, 1981, letter to the editor of her local newspaper, *The Sun,* observed that "when I graduated from nursing school, no one ever mentioned that I would have to have a political science degree just to make a living for my three children. I was under the impression that I was in service to patients."

It is increasingly evident that politics is important to all nurses' lives. In fact, it dominates both our own lives and the lives of our patients and clients from birth to death. The political process and resultant laws and regulations determine such realities as:

- The legitimate scope of nursing practice
- Minimum standards of nursing care
- The involvement or exclusion of nurses from health care policy-making
- The ability of nurses to independently collect fees from Medicare, Medicaid, Blue Cross and Blue Shield, and other third-party payers for providing nursing services to insured consumers
- The amount and quality of education required to become and continue licensure as a registered nurse
- The legal framework for nurse-physician professional relations
- The income ratio between nurses and physicians (1 to 2 in 1935 and 1 to 10 in 1980)
- The authority and jurisdiction of nursing within hospitals and other institutions
- The level of financial support of nursing education
- Minimum standards of community and occupational health
- Standards that regulate the quality, quantity, and prescriptions of drugs
- Who can afford health care and who cannot
- Who lives and who dies due to maldistribution of quantity and quality of health care services

As Americans continue to spend an increasingly larger percentage of their income on health care, it is the nurses' professional obligation to help ensure that they get their money's worth for the health dollars spent. Many nurses are quite aware that under a different set of federal and state laws, the public could get more health care for the money we are now spending;

or, put alternatively, they could obtain the same quantity and quality of health care currently received at a lower cost. The increased productivity (what you get out for what you put in) would come about through the more effective utilization of the professional knowledge and skills of the nation's 1.5 million active registered nurses. Artificial barriers in the form of antiquated laws and regulations that direct scarce resources heavily toward organized medicine currently inhibit or prevent the development of more cost-effective nursing services.

This book is written primarily for nurses who wish to exercise their constitutional rights and work toward changing the labyrinth of outdated laws and regulations that have placed a stranglehold on nursing's access to the scarce resources necessary to fulfill its mission in delivering quality nursing services under a biopsychosocial-oriented health care system. Every reader of this book will probably be able to recall nurse colleagues who were ideal nurses but became inactive in nursing because of the frustrations of working in a non-responsive health care setting. Organized political activity offers a solution to this needless waste of talent and promises the achievement of a higher quality of working life for the nurse and better health care at lower cost for the consumer. If this textbook encourages students in professional issues courses and active nurses to become involved in politics as a means of problem solving and to relate their everyday jobs as nurses to the political decisions that establish the framework for their nursing services, it will have fulfilled its mission.

Our enthusiasm about the potential for the political coming-of-age of nurses intensified during our work. We are indebted to the following people for their help and inspiration in the preparation of this book: United States Senators Max Baucus (Democrat, Montana); Paula Hawkins (Republican, Florida); Daniel K. Inouye (Democrat, Hawaii); Nancy Landon Kassebaum (Republican, Kansas); Edward M. Kennedy (Democrat, Massachusetts); Patrick J. Leahy (Democrat, Vermont); Carl Levin (Democrat, Michigan); Howard M. Metzenbaum (Democrat, Ohio); and Donald W. Riegle, Jr. (Democrat, Michigan). United States Representatives Lindy Boggs (Democrat, Louisiana); Marilyn Lloyd Bouquard (Democrat, Tennessee); Beverly B. Byron (Democrat, Maryland); Shirley Chisholm (Democrat, New York); Cardiss Collins (Democrat, Illinois); Silvio O. Conte (Republican, Massachusetts); John D. Dingell (Democrat, Michigan); Millicent Fenwick (Republican, New Jersey); Geraldine A. Ferraro (Democrat, New York); Bobbi Fiedler (Republican, California); Margaret M. Heckler (Republican, Massachusetts); Marjorie S. Holt (Republican, Maryland); Robert H. Michel (Republican, Illinois); Barbara A. Mikulski (Democrat, Maryland); Mary Rose Oakar (Democrat, Ohio); Carl D. Pursell (Republican, Michigan); Marge Roukema (Republican, New Jersey); Claudine Schneider (Republican, Rhode Island); Patricia Schroeder (Democrat, Colorado); Virginia Smith (Republican, Nebraska); Olympia J. Snowe (Republican, Maine); and Henry A. Waxman (Democrat, California).

The following nurses who are congressional staff members were extremely helpful: Sheila Burke, chief, Health Staff, Senate Finance Committee; Cheryl Beversdorf of the Senate Committee on Veterans Affairs; Mary Jo Dennis, legislative assistant to Representative Doug Walgren (Pennsylvania); and Debbie Hardy, legislative assistant to Representative George O'Brien (Illinois).

Nurse executives in the federal government who lent assistance included Rhetaugh Dumas, Deputy Director, National Institute of Mental Health; Carolyne K. Davis, Administrator, Health Care Financing Administration; Vernice Ferguson, Director, Veterans Administration Nursing Service; Faye G. Abdellah, Assistant Surgeon General and Chief Nurse Officer, U.S. Public Health Service; Jo Eleanor Elliott, Director, Division of Nursing, Bureau of Health Professions, U.S. Department of Health and Human Services; and Jessie M. Scott, former Director of the Division of Nursing and now Professor, School of Nursing, University of Maryland.

The following nurse state legislators were extremely helpful: Jean Moorhead (California Assemblywoman); Bonnie D. Post (Maine Representative); Rosalie Silber Abrams (Maryland Senator); Marilyn Goldwater (Maryland Delegate); Mary Elizabeth Cotton (New Hampshire Representative); Maureen E. Maigret (Rhode Island Representative); and Patricia E. Kenner (former South Dakota Representative).

Nurse lobbyists Patricia Jones, Director, Department of Government Relations, American Nurses' Association; Pamela J. Maraldo, Director of Public Affairs, National League for Nursing; and Marion Murphy, Executive Director, American Association of Colleges of Nursing generously shared their perspectives.

Special thanks are due Patrick DeLeon, health aide for Senator Daniel K. Inouye of Hawaii, and Gary G. Russell, legislative assistant for Representative Carl D. Pursell of Michigan. Edith Livesay assisted greatly in editing the manuscript. We are also indebted to David T. Miller, Managing Editor, Nursing Department, J. B. Lippincott Company, along with manuscript editors Darlene Pederson and Kathleen Dunn, for capably managing the production of this book.

Beatrice J. Kalisch, R. N., Ed. D., F.A.A.N.
Philip A. Kalisch, Ph.D.

1–Power: The Fundamental Concept

The struggle for power is a pervading feature of politics; thus, politics in general as well as the politics of nursing requires the learning of power. *Power*, like *love*, is a word used continually and intuitively in everyday speech. Defining power, however, is, at best, an elusive and complex process. Etymologically the word *power* comes from the Latin verb *potere*, meaning "to be able." Thus, in the simplest terms, *power* is the ability to affect something or to be affected by something. It can take on an almost infinite range of concrete meanings. There is a healing power, black power, woman power, Aesculapian power, economic power, divine power, the power of the government, nuclear power, the power of the press, legislative power, executive power, judicial power, the power of language, the power of positive thinking, and nursing power.

Figure 1–1. Nurse power—one of the innumerable forms of power. (Courtesy of Calgary Herald, Alberta, Canada)

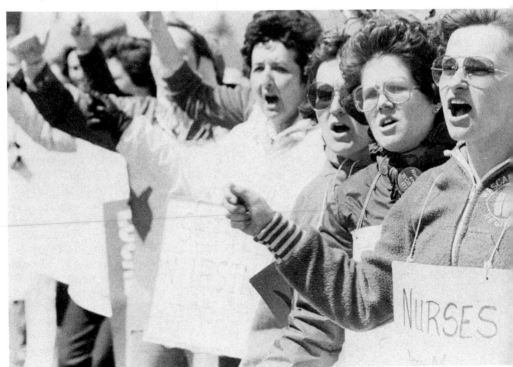

Power means the capacity to alter behavior, or to produce, in Russell's words, "intended effects."[1] Max Weber defined power as "the chance of a man [person] or a number of men [persons] to realize their own will in a social action even against the resistance of others who are participating in the action."[2] Power makes people do things that they might not otherwise do, or stops them from doing things that they might do. It can be thought of as potency or mastery, and the hallmark of power is effectiveness. It is a capacity as well as an action: one individual (A) can affect the behavior of another person (B) when and if A desires it. Power is the ability or capacity of A, the power holder, to produce (consciously or unconsciously) intended effects on the behavior of B, the power subject. The essential attribute of power is the capacity to determine or influence some aspect of the behavior of others, either individually or collectively. There are seven key elements of the concept of power as follows:[3]

1. *The base of power:* resources or assets
2. *The means of power:* the specific actions by which one can use these resources to influence the behavior of another
3. *The scope of power:* the set of specific actions one can get another to perform
4. *The amount of power:* a net increase in the probability that someone will perform some specific action as the result of the use of the means of power by one person against another
5. *The extension of power:* the number of power subjects the power holder exercises control over
6. *The cost of power:* the opportunity costs of using power
7. *The strength of power:* the opportunity costs of the one on whom power is being exerted to resist this power or the degree to which "the bidding of A can be pushed far without loss of compliance."[4]

The total of these ingredients determines the nature of a person's power in a given context.

Many nurses believe that power is essentially a negative capacity, defining it by terms such as "corrupting," "dirty," or "bad." In actuality, power is neither inherently good nor intrinsically bad. In other words, there is both "good power" (often defined as leadership) and "bad power" (often called dominance or coercion). Power, one of the fundamental aspects of all human interaction, can be used for good or bad. It is a part of every kind of relationship: parent–child, husband–wife, employer–employee, physician–nurse, politician–voter, teacher–student, and nurse–patient, just to name a few. Hawley states it well when he says, "Every social act is an exercise of power, every social relationship is a power question, and every social system is an organization of power."[5] Power is desired for purposes such as gaining respect, adding to one's knowledge, accumulating wealth, securing affection, and increasing security. Power is also used as a base for gaining more power.

A few persons have suggested that power can be overcome by altruism, and still others believe that power can be rejected completely and re-

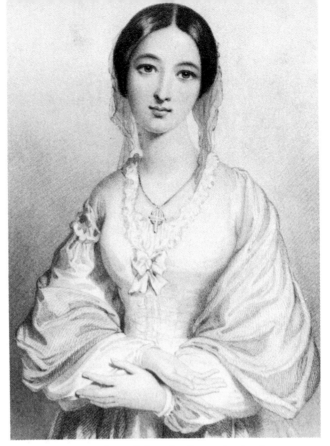

Figure 1–2. Florence Nightingale's power was derived from her humanitarian image among the British public. (Courtesy of History of Nursing Collection, University of Michigan)

placed by love or human service values. Yet our experience tells us this is merely an idealistic dream and that altruism is antithetic to human nature. Power is an inevitable part of all forms of human interaction, and those persons (including nurses) who deny this fact will only find themselves at a serious disadvantage in making change. Individuals will seldom say that their actions are motivated by a desire for power. Instead, they typically declare that ideals such as service and responsibility motivate their actions. The realization of this fact by a number of researchers in the field has led to the conclusion that power is being repressed today in the same way that sexuality was denied in the 19th century.

Perhaps the most frequent misconception about power is the notion that it is a kind of commodity, something that one can accumulate and store up to use whenever he likes. This connotation is implied when saying that someone has a great deal of power; it is as if we are saying that he has a great deal of money. Power is not a commodity as money is, but rather it is a type of *relationship* among people. It is a resource that manifests itself in fluid relationships between and among individuals and groups. In a democratic system, the basic social values associated with the possession and exercise of power are (1) that a high degree of fluidity be maintained in the relationships among the individuals and groups in society—that there be no monopoly over power—and (2) that power not be utilized in a manner that is inimical to this fluidity.

Power does not exist in a vacuum; rather, it is, in two senses, relational. In the first place, a person possesses power only in relation to another person—two or more people are necessary before it is appropriate to speak of their comparative power positions. Second, there is no fixed quantity or lump of power in a society. Power cannot be compared to a pie that can be cut into an indeterminate number of slices of varying sizes, all of which together must total the whole. On the contrary, all power is comparative. *A* may possess *more* power *than B*, but *less* power *than C*.

The fact that one person possesses power does not mean that another person lacks power. Rather, persons possess degrees of power that vary with time and circumstances. Accordingly, *A* may be more powerful than *B* in situation 1, but less powerful than *B* in situation 2. For this reason, the ability to exercise power is relative to particular contexts, to particular sets of relationships. As these relationships change, the relevant value or resources change, and, consequently, one's power changes. As with everyone else, a nurse may possess power in one area of his or her social life and not in another. For example, when a nurse recommends certain treatments or preventive measures, her patient usually accepts her advice on faith. The patient seldom questions the nurse's background, education, and motives; rather, he accepts that the nurse has the required expertise in these areas. Perhaps the nurse also will be able to sway the patient on an issue such as national health-care policy, because the patient may believe that the nurse's

Figure 1–3. The ability to exercise power is relative to particular contexts: Nurse Denise Boschen checks the blood pressure of New York Rangers' Ulf Nilsson at Lenox Hill Hospital. (Courtesy of The New York Post, New York)

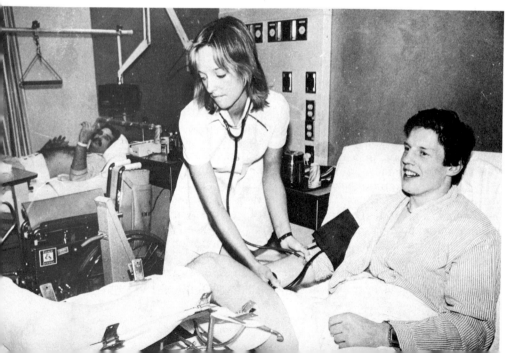

expertise carries over to this related area. If, however, the nurse begins to make recommendations on national defense policy, her opinions would most likely be challenged, because she has clearly gone beyond the usual area within which deference is granted her. Consequently the nurse has little power in this situation.

FORMS OF POWER

As a characteristic of the relationships among individuals or groups, power may occur in two forms. *Symmetrical power* occurs when each party controls a range of outcomes in relatively equal strength. In a practical sense, this occurs when both parties have essentially the same capability for affecting the outcomes of the other. *Asymmetrical power* occurs when one of the parties can control a greater range of outcomes than that controlled by the other.

AUTHORITY VERSUS INFLUENCE

There are two main subcategories of power: they are *authority*, which is based on the particular position that an individual holds, and *influence*, which is the more subtle phenomenon manifested by the willingness of others to obey those who lack formal authority. Persons in positions of authority can also exercise influence. The key element of influence is to present arguments, while the key element of authority is to give commands. In authority, B adopts A's instructions despite the logic of the orders or whether or not B wishes to comply. The "source" of the communication is the important element, whereas, in influence, B adopts A's ideas because of the "content" of the message.

Power is gained through two basic processes: They are power assertions and power inductions. *Power assertions* refer to attempts to gain voluntary compliance through direct force. This (direct force) might involve physical assault, but it is much more likely to occur in the form of threats to force an individual to carry out some action that he would find undesirable. *Power inductions*, on the other hand, are attempts to obtain voluntary compliance by using persuasion or the other forms of influence. This is made clearer in the following discussion.

The essential element in the concept of authority is legitimacy, which means that the power is based on the consensus of those affected by it. No matter how authority is defined, few people fail to see it as being bound in some way with legitimacy. Authority is said to lie in the *right* to expect and command obedience. It is the kind of power that involves the legitimized right (or obligation) to control the actions of others. In placing themselves under the authority of another, individuals set for themselves a general role, which permits the communicated decision of another to guide their own choices without deliberation on the expediency of these decisions. To accept authority, therefore, is to place one's own decision-making process (perhaps only temporarily, or perhaps only with respect to certain kinds of decisions) in the hands of someone else.

There are two ways of implementing authority: They are through coercion and inducement. *Coercion* is authority based on force. The director of nursing who dismisses a nurse because she refuses to implement a physician's order with which she disagrees is an example of this kind of authority. Both parties must believe that the capability to use coercion is present in the power holder for this approach to be viable. As long as the power subject believes that the power holder will use force, it is not necessary for the coercer to actually do so. With this kind of authority, the power holder must be informed of the power subject's behavior at all times because potential deviations are prevented only by fear of negative reprisal. This kind of relationship can also lead to hostile and distrustful interactions between power holders and power subjects. Authority by *inducement*, on the other hand, involves rewarding persons for obeying, as opposed to punishing them for not obeying. This system is less efficient, but generally yields less resistance on the part of power subjects.

Influence, on the other hand, is defined as the degree to which overt or covert pressure, not dependent on a formal authority structure, exerted by one person is successful in imposing the point of view, or desired behavior, on another. The three forms of implementing influence are force, persuasion, and manipulation. *Force* can occur in the form of physical or psychological threat. The most severe threats are those of injury, pain, or even death. Labor strikes are another example of force.

Persuasion, a symmetrical form of power, involves a process whereby A presents B with a point of view that B accepts without fear of punishment or deprivation. B is free to counter A's arguments with B's own opinions. Persuasion skills are often termed "charisma," which is defined as a certain quality of an individual personality by virtue of which he is considered extraordinary and treated as if endowed with supernatural, superhuman, or at least specifically exceptional powers or qualities. These powers, as such, are not accessible to the ordinary person, but are regarded as exemplary, and, on the basis of them, the charismatic individual is treated as a "leader" or as an "opinion molder." Charisma is not simply an attribute of the leader's personality but is a social relationship. Leaders are termed *charismatic* because they are seen as possessing a rare gift of leadership; acceptance of charismatic power is nonrational.

Manipulation is the third form of power, in which the power holder hides the intended or desired outcome from the power subject. As Easton explains, "When B is *not* aware of A's intention to influence him, but A does in fact manage to get B to follow his wishes, we can say that we have an instance of manipulation."[6] This form of influence, the "con man" being a classic example, generates considerable mistrust and suspicion. It is a form of power that cannot be openly dealt with because the intention of the power holder is unknown. Since it involves a cold calculation of desired outcomes on the part of the power holder and a deliberate implementation of actions to elicit behaviors in the power subject, it is seen as antithetic to warm, facilitative relationships. Even though a one-to-one relationship does not exist, advertising is often a form of manipulation in that it often limits information and distorts data in an effort to sell a product.

One form of manipulation is *ingratiation*, which is the technique of deliberately fostering a liking for oneself in another person to get that person to behave in the desired fashion. Among the tactics of ingratiation are

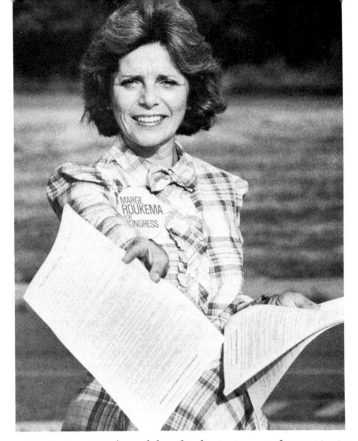

Figure 1–4. Convincing a voter to support one's candidacy for election is a use of persuasion in implementing influence. (Courtesy of Bergen Evening Record, Hackensack, New Jersey)

flattery or enhancement of the other, self-enhancing statements, and conformity ingratiation. Each of these tactics is used by a person to transmit an image of himself as kind, friendly, and intelligent. Complimenting others tends to produce the intended effect because of the general and perhaps universal norm of reciprocity, which says that one ought to return the positive acts of others. A well-known principle of interpersonal attraction is that when one likes another person it results in the development of attitudes and values similar to that person's. An ingratiator, who is intuitively aware of this relationship, may try to reap the indirect benefits from being liked by expressing attitudes similar to those of another person, without being too obvious about opinion conformity. The ingratiator may reflect back an opinion expressed by the other person without directly repeating what has already been said.

To conclude this section, it is helpful to use the example of the changing American marriage relationship to explain the concepts of authority and influence. In the past, society defined the husband as the legitimate holder of authority. He had the "right" to make decisions and direct the actions of his wife, which he did through coercion or inducement. The wife gained in power only through "influence," using the techniques of persuasion and manipulation and, to a lesser extent, force. The husband, however, did not generally need to exert influence because he had authority or "legitimate power." Today, the "power rights" of the husband have been seriously challenged, and significant changes in the social and cultural milieu surrounding husband–wife relationships have occurred. Thus, the husband's authority has been weakened or eradicated, and he must depend, as the wife always did, on influence, rather than authority, to attain his desired outcomes.

BASES OF POWER

French and Raven describe six different bases of power: reward, coercive, legitimate, referent, expert, and informational.[7] *Reward power* is based on the ability to provide rewards for desired behavioral change, while *coercive power* is based on the belief of one person that another person will administer punishment if the desired change in behavior does not occur. These are actually two sides of the same coin. Examples of these kinds of power in nursing are numerous, particularly coercive power. A staff nurse who is outspoken in her suggestions for changes not supported by the head nurse finds herself assigned to work a disproportionate number of nights and holidays. The nurse faculty member who regularly volunteers for special assignments receives the benefits of reward power when she has her way paid to the annual convention at the end of the academic year.

    Legitimate power, or authority, is the legitimate right of one person by virtue of his role to prescribe change in another's behavior. One example of this basis of power is the director of nursing giving a large salary increase to a head nurse who she feels has done a good job. The area of legitimacy, however, is often hazy. For example, is it the director of nursing's legitimate right to decide to change the organization of nursing care on a particular unit to primary care, or does the power to make this decision lie in the hands of the head nurse or the staff nurses, or should the decision include all three?

    When power is based on one person's identification with or attractiveness to another, it is called *referent power*. An example in nursing would be the ability of a respected, well-known nurse leader to mold the opinions of the House of Delegates at the American Nurses' Association convention according to her desired outcomes. Another instance would be all the nurses of a hospital signing a petition to retain the director of nursing who had just been terminated by the hospital administration for attempting to improve the working conditions and the quality of nursing care in that institution.

    Expert power is derived from the perception that the more powerful person has superior knowledge than the less powerful individual. Nurses often defer to physicians when a matter of debate involves so-called advanced medical knowledge. Nurse clinicians may have more power in clinical settings than faculty who do not engage in direct practice themselves. Nurse faculty, on the other hand, may have more power by virtue of seeming to possess greater knowledge in areas such as the scientific bases for the success or failure of certain nursing actions.

    Finally, *informational power* refers to a person's ability to use explanations or other persuasive communication to modify the behavior of others. A respected nurse faculty member who stands up in a meeting and gives an

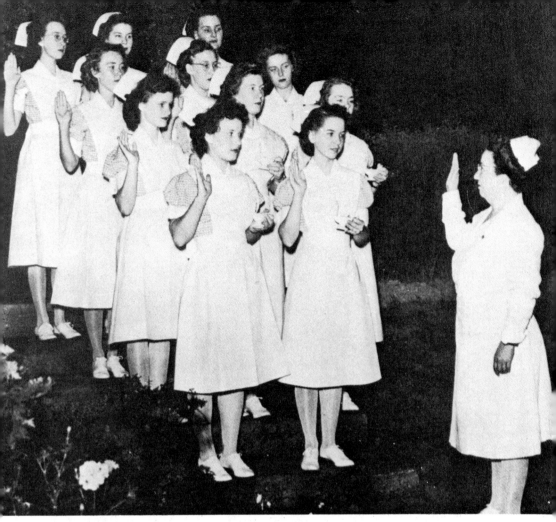

Figure 1–5. Traditionally, nurses have been subjected to a great deal of coercive power, much of which was enforced by elaborate rituals and exact codes of conflict. (Courtesy of History of Nursing Collection, University of Michigan)

eloquent speech, which sways the faculty to vote a certain way on the issue at hand, is using informational power, as is the leader of the nurses' union who speaks convincingly for going on strike at an organizing meeting.

These power bases are not mutually exclusive. Any individual can have more than one basis of power and, in fact, more than being simply additive, the sum total of several power bases is usually greater than its individual parts. A dean of a school of nursing or a director of a nursing service should have all of these power bases if she is to be a truly effective leader.

Certified nurse-midwives (CNM) have numerous difficulties in practicing their profession largely owing to the ability of obstetricians to exercise coercive, legitimate, expert, and informational power. For example, the Salt Lake City *Tribune* of April 13, 1980, carried an article entitled "Utah Nurse-Midwives Denied Opportunities." Following are some examples contained within the report:

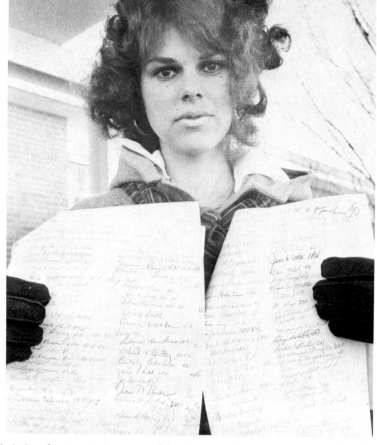

Figure 1–6. Camden, New Jersey nurse Trino Kossup holds petitions presented to Cherry Hill Medical Center administrators in support of Margaret Bergin, who was recently fired as director of nursing services without explanation. (Courtesy of The Courier-Post, Cherry Hill, New Jersey)

Example: A local certified nurse-midwife (CNM) recently asked an obstetrician if he would rent her some of his office space and provide back-up for normal gynecological care. She was told it wouldn't be politically prudent for the physician to agree since he was a junior staff member at a local hospital and the senior staff wouldn't approve.

Example: If a woman phones the University Medical Center to make an appointment with a nurse-midwife for a physical exam and Pap test, she will discover that the CNMs at the center are allowed to see only pregnant patients. They cannot provide routine gynecological care, even though this is part of their expertise and training.

Example: A recently graduated nurse-midwife applied for a position with private physicians in two separate group practices in Salt Lake City. In both instances she was turned down. One group said they already had nurses doing the same work as the CNM would be doing. The other group said they had physician's assistants so they didn't need a nurse-midwife. Neither nurses nor physician's assistants are qualified to deliver babies.

Some CNMs in Utah are ready to abandon their chosen career because, as the above examples indicate, they are tired of fighting a system that won't allow them to practice to their potential. Despite the 1971 endorsement of nurse-midwifery by the American College of Obstetricians and Gynecologists, most Utah obstetricians pay only lip service to the profession.[8]

DETERMINING WHO HAS POWER

How do we know that one person has more or less power than another; that is, how can we measure power? There are pitfalls to what would appear to be simple or obvious ways of answering this question. If one person can influence a greater number of people than another person, we might be prepared to say that he or she has more power (*i.e.*, the ability to influence 1000 people indicates more power than the ability to influence 10 people). However, if the 1000 people are average citizens and the 10 are, say, members of the Congress of the United States, influence over the 10 congressmen would probably translate into considerably greater political power.

Power relations can be understood by analyzing key elements, such as the values that are being controlled and the resources used to control them. Consider, for example, a director of nursing service's ability to determine whether a head nurse continues in her job; consider a nurse's ability to stop caring for a patient she finds is not following her suggestions for diet and exercise; or consider the nursing union leader's ability to keep nurses from going on strike. In each instance, the person who is being coerced places a value on something: a job, continued nursing care, or the avoidance of a strike. Thus, this method of influence builds on human values, and the values at stake may include not only basic considerations such as self-preservation, security, and wealth, but also less tangible values such as respect, self-esteem, and happiness. Where one person is able to control another's ability to enjoy these values, he then has the capacity to exercise power over another person. The employer can control the job and employee, the nurse can control her patients, and the union leader can control the strike and strikers. *Anyone who performs a necessary task in the productive process controls some potential power.*

The distribution of power among persons in society is distinctly uneven. Wealth or economic assets often mean that a person has more power, but wealthy people are not powerful simply because they are wealthy; it is a question of how and when they use their wealth as a power resource. Clearly, some individuals are favored by the unequal distribution of economic resources, but even the relatively powerless can shape social and political outcomes if they are able to act cohesively. A strike by nurses clearly demonstrates one kind of power resource made possible through organization.

Social interaction can be viewed as a quasi-economic process in which the participants pursue diverse ends through the manipulation and exchange of social-power resources. The unequal distribution of such resources enables some individuals or groups to have a greater impact on social outcomes than others; in this sense, they possess more power. Nurses are attempting to attack the imbalance of power in health care and gain a more equitable distribution of resources by changing their behaviors as learned through assertiveness training. One such group in Baltimore gained public exposure for their efforts in a news story under the banner "Nurses Learn to Assert Themselves into a Stronger Role on the Team":

> The nurse was obviously enjoying giving back some of what she'd been getting for years.

'Women, no wonder they're nurses,' she said contemptuously, but not succeeding at all in keeping a grin off her face. 'If something goes wrong, I'm the doctor, I'm the one who has to take the consequences, not you. You—you're just a nurse.'

The group of 90 nurses, participating in a recent assertiveness training workshop at Franklin Square Hospital, roared with laughter and heartily applauded their colleague, who was playing the role of a disgruntled physician.

Enacting little socio-dramas that go on in the hospital was just one of the ways the nurses were investigating their own assertiveness and learning how to use it in their professional lives.

'This is a time of transition,' explained Sally Sohr, the nurse who conducted the session. 'Nurses are becoming less and less passive. Doctors are very uncomfortable with it, but today's nurse is educated to the level of many GPs 35 years ago. In specialty areas, her knowledge might be as much as an intern or resident. . . .''

Nurses at the workshop agreed that the situations in which assertive behavior is usually most necessary involve doctors.

'There are occasions when you feel more like a handmaiden than part of a team,' said Donna Walker, 25, a nurse on the medical floors at Baltimore City Hospitals.

'If you have a man as a doctor and a woman as a nurse, he will degrade her and be rude to her,' said Gloria Childs, 32, a health department nurse in Charles county and the actress whose portrayal of the sexist physician had inspired such laughter. 'But it wouldn't be like that in a social situation.' ''[9]

In analyzing power, one must watch for the difference between potential power and actual power. Although a person may possess both a base of power and the means of power, the mere existence of these power possibilities is not actual power. In the case of *potential power*, the conditions and resources for power are available, but there is little or no interest or willingness to employ power; when power is used we can then refer to *actual power*. If, over the course of time, persons do not use their base of power and their means of power, which together constitute their potential power ability, and other persons are aware of this fact and, consequently, no longer feel constrained or influenced in their behavior by these persons, their actual ability to influence behavior—their power—is less than their potential ability. The presence of this psychological constraint, or influence factor, distinguishes actual power from potential power. Often, the actual power of individuals or groups may be noticeably less than their potential power, and this will result from the level of concern these individuals have for public affairs and the extent to which their interest in politics competes with family, job, religion, hobbies, and the variety of other concerns in their lives. Nurses collectively, for example, have much more potential power than actual power because they do not choose or are not able to use their power for a number of reasons, as is explored further in later chapters.

There is an ironic quality to the use of power. The actual use of power involves literally using up resources of power that cannot be used again; thus, if a leader carries through on a threat, she may weaken her own ability to exert influence in the future. Indeed, the need to carry through on a power threat may be viewed as a sign of weakness as much as a show of strength. Often the greatest effectiveness is achieved by threatening to use

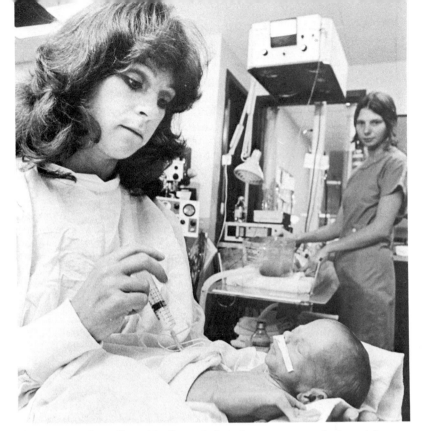

Figure 1–7. Nurses, since they offer critically needed services, possess much potential power. (Courtesy of Rochester Democrat & Chronicle, Rochester, New York)

power rather than by actually using it. The threat to use power is in itself a form of power, in that it may be sufficient to gain the compliance of the other person.

It is not always easy to recognize a powerful person because it is quite possible that a person can be successful in making his ideas and desires prevail without any public recognition of the fact. Similarly, we are not always aware of the power relationship, as such, in which we are involved. Some persons anticipate the intentions of other persons and act accordingly. These individuals may feel that they have used their free will or acted out of love or friendship, and not because of the power of the other. Yet all behavioral sequences fit into the definition of power.

The use of a covert approach, if we may call it that, is often essential with a strongly authoritative person who would easily thwart any overt attempt of influence. With this approach, the convinced individual appears to be the decision maker and perceives himself to be the powerful party. This is the basis for the "doctor–nurse game," whereby the nurse uses a variety of indirect techniques to influence the physician, that is, convincing him to order certain drugs or certain treatments or to carry out other actions the nurse sees as necessary, on the patient's behalf. The physician complies, believing it was his idea in the first place.

The complexity of determining where the power resides in any group of people, organization, or nation is underlined by the fact that one must assess the situation on several levels. Who wins in disagreements? Who decides who will win? Who determines who will decide? The powerful person in a group is the one who decides what will be done by whom and which persons will be allowed to make certain decisions. This powerful person may delegate certain tasks and decision-making authority to another because he or she finds these decisions relatively unimportant or time-consuming. The delegation of this power does not mean less power for the delegator. On the contrary, the delegating person has considerably more power than the delegatee because the delegator can orchestrate the power structure of the group according to his or her preferences. The delegatee generally does not step beyond the limits set by the person with power.

Figure 1–8. The traditional "doctor–nurse game" is an example of a covert approach to gaining power. (Courtesy of Warren Times Observer, Warren, Pennsylvania)

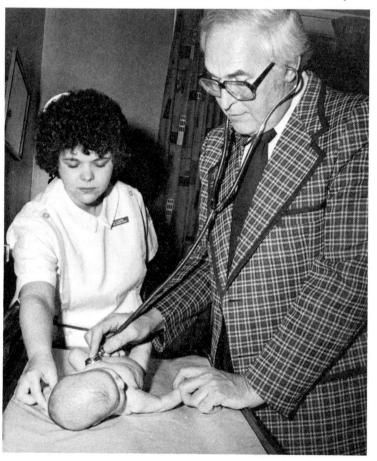

WHY ARE PERSONS POWERFUL?

There are two basic explanations for why certain persons have power: one is called *situational* and the other *personal*. The *situational* explanation states that persons with power are in the right place at the right time. For example, a nurse becomes a dean of a major university school of nursing because, at that moment, the needs of that school are for someone who can unite education and practice in that institution, and she has had a successful record of doing that same task in other institutions. In other words, this nurse happens to have the required abilities for the situation. The *personal* interpretation of power, on the other hand, says that certain persons have power because they have some special and unique characteristic; the nurse leader has a special kind of power skill just as the nurse scholar is felt to have a special cognitive ability or the nurse clinician, a special clinical ability. This way of thinking about power is close to our day-to-day experiences of power and allows us to reduce the complexities of this human interaction to a contest between persons: heroes and villains.

In actuality, both situational and personal factors play a significant part in determining who is powerful. The situation may call for a certain type of leader, but the person chosen for the power position has to be perceived only as filling this bill or meeting these needs. There is considerable room for the influence of personal factors because the question is not whether the leader actually is the person called for, but whether the members *think* that she is. These perceptions can be influenced and changed, as is true of any other judgment. Power may be created by changing the perceptions of others. Skill in defining situations, in convincing others of these definitions, and in portraying one's own role as important or indispensable to the achievement of these redefined group goals would thus permit a person to have power within the constraints of any given situation, no matter how it was originally conceived. Lukes explains it as follows:

> A may exercise power over B by getting him to do what he does not want to do, but he also exercises power over him by influencing, shaping or determining his very wants. Indeed, is it not the supreme exercise of power to get another or others to have the desires you want them to have. . . ?[10]

Research in the field has shown us that there appears to be an inherent or socially learned personality characteristic known as the *power motive*. Merei found that certain children aged 4 to 11 showed more power than other children. When these "leaders" were moved to new groups where they were unknown, they sought again to gain power through a variety of strategies including order-giving and the assumption of ownership and possession of all important objects in the room.[11] Winter studied the power motive in adults, and his results showed that strong power drives were associated with group and institutional leadership and efforts to manipulate and persuade others. These persons also sought relationships with weaker, dependent persons who would follow them.[12]

People who have a strong power motive strive for power. Lasswell says, "As such a person moves from infancy through maturity, he becomes progressively predisposed to respond to the power-shaping and power-sharing possibilities of each situation in which he finds himself."[13] These persons try to make things happen in a certain way. Their goal is power, and they want the status of having power. Every organization has at least one individual who moves in and systematically sizes up the situation, determining how he might manipulate individuals, their desires and opinions, in order to increase his power. Not only do these persons categorize all relationships around them in terms of power, they also want to feel powerful, to be more powerful than others. These persons believe that power is desirable and that the "lesser" people should defer to the "better" people. It is quite logical that individuals with a high power motive tend to move into leadership positions and cling to power, while those with low power motives move out of power positions that they have found themselves in by accident or by chance.

At the opposite end of the continuum, there are many people who do not use all of their potential power. Individuals who are "underusers" of power may be unaware of the power they have; they may lack the skills to use their power effectively; they may be afraid of power; or they may be interested in other things. Even persons with authority or legitimate power often allow it to flow through their hands and diffuse to others. Some people do not use their power resources, while others go to great lengths to increase and use them. Nurses as a group are underusers of power, perhaps owing to the fact that they have been a self-selected group with a low power motive, and nursing as a career has been seen as being less autonomous than are other professions.

POWER THEORIES

The explanations or theories for determining who has power in given social contexts are many. First there is the *resource theory*, which states that the balance of power is on the side of the person who has the greatest resources.[14] In attempting to influence Congress, physicians who have more money to contribute to campaigns wield more power, unless nurses as a group can deliver votes in sufficient quantity to offset or exceed the monetary contributions of physicians.

The *exchange theory* is a little more complicated: power is seen in terms of rewards and costs that the persons mediate for one another; the focus is on the exchange.[15] Consequently, A has power over B and can influence B's behavior to the extent that A can determine or control the rewards and punishments or costs of B's experiences. Using a nurse–physician example, a nurse will have power over a physician to the extent that she can control the rewards and costs of the physician (carrying out medical orders, assisting him with procedures, and so forth). Similarly, a physician will have power over a nurse to the extent that he can reward or punish her (reporting her to hospital administration, reprimanding her in front of others, on so on).

Decision-making theory explains power in terms of who makes the final decision. The power of A is measured in terms of the effects he has on B. The focus is on the outcome, as opposed to process, with the amount of power being expressed as the difference between the likelihood of B performing a given behavior after A intervenes and the probability of B performing the behavior anyway.[16] Pollard and Mitchell have refined this

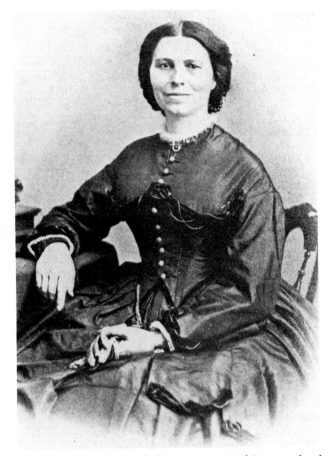

Figure 1–9. Clara Barton, the Civil War nurse who founded the American Red Cross, realized that she would have to link up with influential people to gain enough resources to permit her cause to succeed. (Courtesy of History of Nursing Collection, University of Michigan)

theory; their central question is "whether or not A is able to affect B's decisionmaking regarding some behavior A desires. Thus, the assessment of power requires the determination of *both* A's intention and the effect A has on B's decisionmaking."[17] An example would be of a staff nurse who did not want to adopt a new system of charting on the unit where she works but has to go along with the plan because her colleagues are committed to the change.

    Systems theory offers an explanation of power as a circular process of interactions between power holders and power subjects. It does not assume that there is a cause-and-effect relationship in people's interactions but that all system components are interdependent. This means that a change in one part of a system is usually followed by a compensatory change in another part of the system. This dynamic type of power relationship can be illustrated as follows: $A_1 \rightarrow B_1 \rightarrow A_2 \rightarrow B_2 \rightarrow A_3 \rightarrow B_3$. The behavior of A is part of a

function of B is essential. According to this theory, it is not possible to look at one single exchange, say $A_2 \rightarrow B_2$, and determine who is exercising power. An example would be a nurse union leader (A_1) telling a hospital administrator that if the nursing salaries are not increased by 10% for the next year, there would probably be a strike. The administrator responds with a 6% increase (B_1); the union leader responds further by reiterating that there will be a strike (A_2). The hospital administrator does not further increase the salary (B_2), a strike occurs (A_3), and after 1 day, the administrator agrees to the 10% salary increment (B_3).[18]

FEAR OF POWER

Power is feared because it can be used to cause the destruction of others. We never know how someone will react to having power. It has been likened to the influence of alcohol, with some persons getting carried away under its influence and others being able to take on a reasonable amount and still acting responsibly. Samuel Butler said, "Authority intoxicates; the fumes of it invade the brain and make men giddy, proud and vain."[19]

From as far back as Plato, it has been argued that power must be controlled or balanced with rationality or altruism if it is to be effective. Gamson explains, "Because power evokes potential without direction, we can be simultaneously excited by its possibilities for creation and alarmed by its possibilities for injury."[20] A group, a family, an organization, or a country can be destroyed if power is not used wisely and kept from undeterred exploitation by individuals using it for their own gain.

This differentiation is made more clear by comparing the "political hack" with the "statesman." Both are politicos; that is, they are persons who work to cultivate a sense of the dynamic and human relationship—the handshake, the winning smile, the listening ear. In personal dealings, these persons try to attune themselves to the personal styles of those around them, to anticipate how best to deal with these people in order to get what they want. If one individual works only for selfish reasons or personal gain, we call that person a *political hack*; if his conduct seems tempered by moral principles and aimed toward some worthy goals, we call that individual a *statesman* or *statesperson*. Similarly, if we like a person, we call power skills *charisma*, but if we do not like a person, we see the power holder as unscrupulous and as an *operator*.

Nurses in Columbia, Missouri, interacted with a "politico," Governor Joseph Teasdale, on June 25, 1980, and many wondered whether or not the governor responded in a statesmanlike manner:

> It was no party for Gov. Joseph Teasdale when he entertained opinions from more than 100 nurses Wednesday afternoon at the Hearnes Center.
>
> Teasdale seemed to trip himself more than one time when he responded to nurses' comments and questions concerning nurses. He said he did not come to 'politick.' And, although he was delayed 10 minutes by the press, Teasdale said, 'I came to speak to you (the nurses), not the press.
>
> Delivering only a few opening remarks concerning his commitment to health care in Missouri, Teasdale opened the meeting to comments from an audience of more than 100, mostly female and mostly clad in white.
>
> One nurse said one of the biggest problems facing the nursing profession is

the 'critical shortage of nurses.' In the Kansas City, Mo. area alone, there are over 400 registered nurse vacancies, she said. Another problem is the lack of educational opportunities and student loans available, she added.

'Student loans should be available,' Teasdale said. He said he signed a bill 'a few years ago.' But then, looking disconcertedly at his aide he asked, 'What have I done with the money for nursing?'

Following the audience's response of muffled laughter, Teasdale said, 'I don't know what has been done.' He said he has 'many things to tend to,' and it is impossible to know everything.

Teasdale went on to say, however, that nursing would be a new emphasis area—if he were governor for another term. 'God willing, if I am there, I will support you,' Teasdale said.

Another comment came from Gladys Courtney, dean of the University's

Figure 1–10. The abuse of power within a patient care context was vividly portrayed by Nurse Ratched in the Academy award winning film, One Flew Over the Cuckoo's Nest. (Courtesy of Nursing in the Mass Media Collection, University of Michigan)

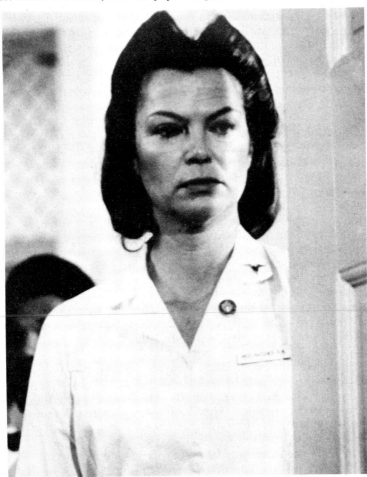

School of Nursing. 'There needs to be an appropriate recognition for nurses,' she said. 'We are on the move and our numbers are increasing, but we need more recognition.'

Teasdale suggested that nurses unite and form a nurse's lobby. 'You need clout to make politicians respond to you. Make your mind up to get together,' he said.

He told the nurses that politicians may ignore them at first but said they will eventually get their way. Explaining his certainty, Teasdale said, 'Women do know how to do it better than most.' The subsequent moans from the audience spurred the governor to add, 'I didn't come to get your votes anyway.' "[21]

WOMEN AND POWER

In the traditional pattern of female role behavior, women, and thus nurses, who are largely female, have been mostly without power, believing that power was solely in the male domain. Feminists have made the continuous plea that changes in the power structure be made so that women would have an equal share of the power and thus more control over their lives.[22] One has to question why so few women have sought power and why they have not participated in the power processes within society. Understanding the complex relationships among dependence, dominance, and power is essential in understanding the power aspects of women's behavior.

In explaining the fact that women demonstrate a much lower level of power behavior than men, several hypotheses have been offered. Lionel Tiger, a well-known anthropologist, advocates a physiologic explanation. He believes that men are programmed for leadership and decision making, while women are not likely ever to play a significant role in power and politics because they cannot elicit "followership" in subordinates. He explains, "Basically my proposition is that cultural forms result from the interaction of behavioral propensities—or inborn biological programmes—with existing social patterns and expectations in any community."[23] Tiger advances the idea that men hang together to maintain an all-male power group and that if women did dominate such powerful decision-making bodies, the status (and thus power) of such groups would diminish.

The very existence, however, of such female leaders as Golda Meir, Joan of Arc, Indira Gandhi, and Margaret Thatcher negates at least the idea that physiologic considerations are a necessary disqualifier. Cultural factors are a much more frequently espoused reason for women lacking power. As Mead wrote, "Standardized personality differences between the sexes are . . . cultural creations to which each generation, male and female, is trained to conform. . . . I have suggested that certain traits have been socially specialized as the appropriate attitudes of the behavior of only one sex, while other human traits have been specialized for the opposite sex."[24] Attribution of power to males and not females is one example of such a cultural norm. Kirkpatrick points out that "the pursuit of power [is] conceived as incompatible with feminity. . . . Simultaneously, cultural norms communicate and reinforce the expectation of women's commitment to home, family, community service."[25] Women who do seek power roles lose status because it is felt to be an inappropriate female role. Also attributed to acculturation is the fact that women often lack the essential self-confidence and autonomy to succeed in the world of power.

Sex-role stereotyping greatly influences our perceptions and behavior in all areas of life but perhaps even to a greater extent in the domain of power. The depth of these stereotypic influences is indicated in a study in which nonliberal psychotherapists of both sexes were significantly more likely to judge female clients described as left-wing political activitists as maladjusted, as compared with males who had the very same political orientation.[26]

Similarly, Dinnerstein has pointed to how pervasive the sexist double standard is and how a particular act performed by a woman carries a very different meaning from the same act performed by a man; in short, power, selfishness, and insensitivity, seen as merely unethical or wrong when present in men, become "overwhelmingly monstrous" and "wickedly unnatural" when displayed by women, and both men and women see it this way. It is possible now (and has been at times in the past) to admire female strength if such strength is seen as nurturing (*i.e.*, something that exists for others), but female wealth, power, domination, and glory are unqualifiedly

Figure 1–11. One of the stereotypical roles of the nurse is personified by Gloria Brancusi (played by Christopher Norris) in the 1981 television series "Trapper John, M.D." (Courtesy of Nursing in the Mass Media Collection, University of Michigan)

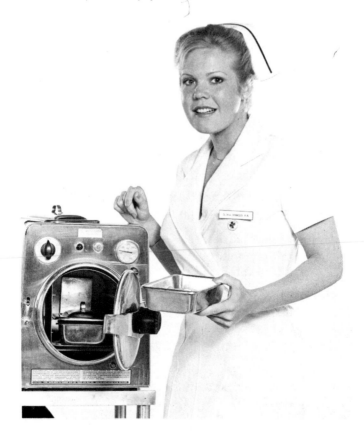

evil if nonnurturant (*i.e.*, practiced for the gratification of the woman herself), even if we immediately add honesty and competence to the list. Dinnerstein's explanations and arguments are cross-cultural here and very convincing.[27]

The use of power is associated with traditionally masculine traits. A
study by Petro and Putnam showed that the following behaviors are commonly held stereotypes attributed to men:[28]

- very realistic (not idealistic)
- almost always hides emotions
- always thinks before acting
- not at all easily influenced
- not at all excitable in a crisis
- very active
- very competitive
- feelings not easily hurt
- can make decisions easily
- never cries
- never worried
- feels very superior
- doesn't care about being in a group
- seeks out new experiences
- very assertive
- not at all able to devote self completely to others
- very blunt
- not at all kind
- not at all understanding of others
- very cold in relations with others
- very uncomfortable when people express emotions

Female behaviors, on the other hand, were found to be as follows:

- idealistic (not realistic)
- does not hide emotions at all
- never thinks before acting
- very easily influenced
- very excitable in a crisis
- very passive
- not at all competitive
- feelings easily hurt
- has difficulty making decisions
- cries very easily

- always worried
- feels very inferior
- greatly prefers being in a group
- avoids new experiences
- not at all assertive
- able to devote self completely to others
- very tactful
- very kind
- very understanding of others
- very warm in relations with others
- not at all uncomfortable when people express emotions

As Jean Baker Miller has written, it is obviously no accident that the characteristics most developed in women are the very ones that are dysfunctional for success in the world as it is. "They may, however, be the important ones for making the world different."[29]

The historic perspective offers further insight into the cultural association of men with power and women without power. In the traditional sense, men have been the norm, making women the "other," or the opposite of men. Men have been seen as strong, vigorous, competitive, and interested in money, power, and self-advancement. Women, on the other hand, have been viewed as weak, soft, intuitive, compassionate, and interested in moral, humanitarian goals. Men have cared about profits, women about people. Men have stressed peer relationships and competition, which has led to decision making along hierarchical lines. Women have emphasized cooperation in interpersonal relationships, which has led to a nonstructured, participatory, decision-making style.

Historically, males have had virtually total control over the formal and material manifestations of power; whereas, the feminine power domain has been largely informal, psychological, and interpersonal. Males have dominated females for centuries, thus leading to the development of certain personality traits and behaviors in females, which has perpetuated this dominance. Women's lack of control over, even access to, resources (*i.e.*, economic, social and political) has been most important in continuing the subordinate position. Consequently, women typically have exerted power by using the influence methods of manipulation and ingratiation, as opposed to employing the direct means of assertiveness and aggression used by males. Females have been found to rely on passive–aggressive techniques. They have also used helplessness as a source of power because men are then compelled to rescue them.

Women have been forced to employ personal means such as sex, love, and affection to gain power, because they have lacked access to the concrete power, which comes with economic independence and legal equality. In the family, for example, women have had access to and have legitimately used sexual, psychological, and interpersonal resources. These resources have led to the development of power vis-à-vis children and,

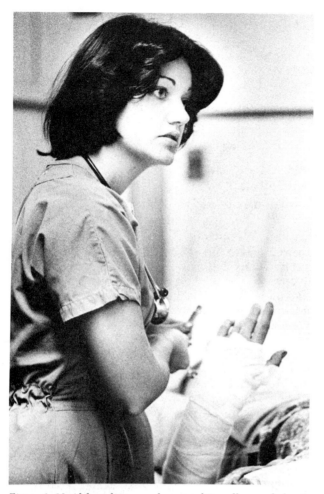

Figure 1–12. Although women have traditionally cared about people and men have tradition-ally cared about profits, there is no reason why this dichotomy cannot be blended. (Courtesy of Cleveland Plain Dealer, Cleveland, Ohio)

more rarely, husbands. Even the wife who holds a great amount of power in her relationship with her husband has not usually been able to generalize this power outside the husband–wife relationship. Many women perpetuate this situation for fear that if they lost these ways of gaining power, they would not be able to replace them with other more direct means. The purpose of assertiveness training, so popular today, is to train women to express their needs and feelings directly as opposed to employing nonasser-tive and nonaggressive techniques.

In addition to the cultural reasons for women's nonparticipation in power there are highly related role constraints. Historically, women have assumed the role of wife and mother as their "primary" role. Combining this role with a professional role has been viewed as incompatible, and trying to get a career launched in mid-life, after children are grown, is fraught with difficulties, given the competitive nature of our society.

As has been noted, women have historically lacked the resources necessary to gain and use power: education, occupational status, credit, property, and independent income. These are closely associated with the degree of employment outside the home. Today, millions of women work outside the home, but back in 1890 only 4 million women worked and only one-half million were married. A Bureau of Labor study of 17,000 women factory workers in 1887 found that only 4% were married. By and large, married women worked only if their husbands were permanently or temporarily unable to support their family. Around the turn of the century, if a married woman worked, it was usually a sign that something had gone

Figure 1–13. The value accorded to a career outside the home has soared in recent years. (Courtesy of The Daily Herald, Arlington Heights, Illinois)

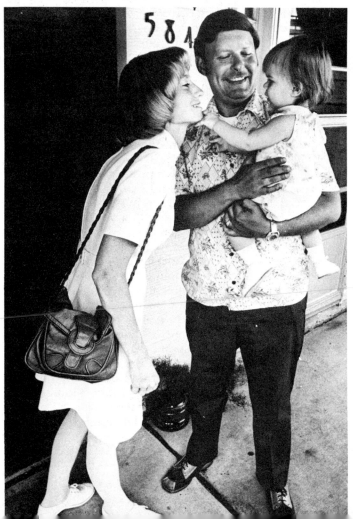

wrong. By contrast, working women today are held in high esteem. A 1979 study showed that "a majority of housewives now agree that the working woman's job is likely to bring her a richer, more active and interesting lifestyle." It further reported that "only a third of the working women gave a positive rating to the housewife's role."[30]

In general, women's work outside the home has served to increase her power. However, this is diminished by the fact that women, even with the same education and occupational experience as men, have received only a proportion of male economic rewards. Nonetheless, within marriage, women develop increased bargaining power as their earning capacity reaches a significant level. There are, however, limiting factors to married women's accretion of resources through labor market participation. The married woman's ability to use occupational opportunities may be at least partially dependent upon the cooperation (or acquiescence) of her husband, who may wish to enforce her leisure as a symbol of his affluence.

Furthermore, there are traditional holdovers even with dual-career, modern families. In one British study, for example, dual-career marriages were found to be faced with at least five areas of stress: overload dilemmas, personal norm dilemmas, identity dilemmas, social network dilemmas, and role cycling dilemmas, all of which were found to require the development of mechanisms for adjustment and stress reduction. Although these British couples emphasized egalitarian family relationships, when tensions occurred, many husbands "undercut" their wives.[31] Similarly, studies of American dual-career families have shown that in the vast majority of cases, men needed to dominate marriages. Holmstrom found that when problems arose, it generally was the wife's interests that were sacrificed. Although the wife's time, interests, and career were highly valued, the husband's were considered still more important.[32] Other studies of role conflict in married professional women describe similar results.[33] Garland's study of such families found that a wife's status as a professional did not, in itself, affect family structures. Income, however, did have an effect, particularly if the wife earned more than the husband. Despite egalitarian attitudes in some areas, these couples also maintained traditional orientations.[34]

In addition to the role conflicts, which center on the wife–mother–career woman conflict, there are other constraints that diminish power-seeking behavior in women. Lockheed and Hall, in reviewing the literature on mixed-sex small groups, found that women can work successfully as equals only when they are quiet and inconspicuous: "(1) men initiate more verbal acts than women; (2) a woman is more likely to yield to a man's opinion than vice versa; and (3) men spend a larger percentage of their interaction time making suggestions and giving orientations and opinions to the group, whereas women spend the larger percentage of their interaction time agreeing with or praising others in the group."[35] They explain this behavior in terms of group power and prestige. Male status automatically yields initial higher status and, thus, expectations for a greater level of competence. Females, on the other hand, do not feel that competence is expected of them. Lockheed and Hall also conducted an experiment in which they found that there were no differences in groups of all males or all females and that men were seven times more likely to become the group leader, unless a woman had a reputation for competence in a certain area. The implications of this study explain in part why women are seen as less powerful. Women do not seek power positions because they are expected to lack competence and thus have to overcome an initial expectation in others as well as in themselves of lesser competence.

The male conspiracy, or female oppression, explanation for the lack of power among women puts forth the idea that men maintain the balance of power in society in much the same way that the ruling class maintained its privileged position in the class/caste systems of former times. Females have been equated with the subjects, and males, with the ruling class. Men are said to work toward maintaining their power and inhibiting women from positions of power.

Similarities between women and blacks have been noted. Women, like blacks, have long constituted an oppressed group. This was recognized and explained as a caste argument most notably by Myrdal.[36] In a now famous appendix to his work on races in the United States, Myrdal discusses similarities between women and blacks. Although Myrdal never specifically calls women a caste, his discussion implies that women and blacks share the

Figure 1–14. Although Myrdal never specifically called women a caste, his 1940s analysis of their status focused on many similarities. (Courtesy of Nursing in the Mass Media Collection, University of Michigan)

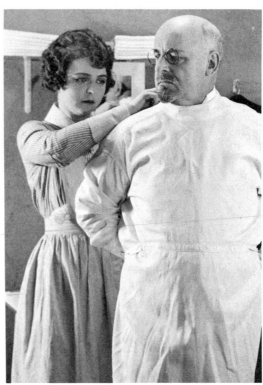

same status. Because of the high social visibility of women and blacks, and the rigidity of the caste line, both groups have been unable to transcend caste barriers (except in the rare case of the individual who can "pass" as a member of the dominant group). Both women and blacks have visible, ascribed attributes, rationalizations of status, coping mechanisms, and actual discriminatory experiences. According to Myrdal, the caste situation of women and blacks arises from similar historic context, that is, from the application of paternalistic law.

The common premise of all paternalism is that something may be done to or for persons for their own good, without their assent, or even despite their dissent. There are two main kinds of paternalism: "promotive" and "preservative." *Promotive paternalism* seeks to improve the well-being of the subjects by requiring them to perform or omit actions. *Preservative paternalism* seeks to prevent persons from harming themselves. The purpose is not to increase well-being, but to prevent diminishing it.

Thus, even while massive societal changes have occurred to allow women access to scarce resources and opportunity to influence the allocation process, certain socialization factors, which are discussed in the later chapters, have served to maintain women in a less powerful position than their male counterparts. Centuries of tradition cannot be eradicated overnight, but it is heartening to note that progress is being made in the vital area of women's power.

Power is central to change, and it is important to note that its effective use may serve as the mainspring for the advancement of the nursing profession. The present status of nursing is more clearly understood when viewed from the perspectives offered by the theories of power. The task of specifying the nature of linkages between power and politics is addressed in Chapter 2; the chapters that follow undertake the application of power through the various governmental, social, and economic institutional structures that determine the shape of nursing practice, education, and research. Illuminating the power links between the nurses and public is, after all, the principal means of building professional consciousness in our democratic society. To leave them unexamined is to negate the principles of democracy.

References

1. Russell B: Power: A New Social Analysis p 25. London, George Allen & Unwin, 1938
2. Weber M: Economy and Society Vol 2, p 926. New York, Bedminster Press, 1968
3. Harsanyi JC: Measurement of social power, opportunity costs, and the theory of two-person bargaining games. Behav Sci 7:67–80, 1962
4. de Jouvenel B: Authority: The efficient imperative. In Friedrich CJ (ed): Authority, p 160. Cambridge, Harvard University Press, 1958
5. Hawley AH: Community power and urban renewal success. Am J Sociol 68:422–431, 1968
6. Easton D: The perception of authority and political change. In Friedrich CJ (ed): Authority, p 179. Cambridge, Harvard University Press, 1958
7. French JRP, Raven B: The bases of social power. In Cartwright D (ed): Studies in Social Power, pp 150–167. Ann Arbor, University of Michigan, Institute for Social Research, 1959
8. Utah nurse-midwives denied opportunities. Salt Lake City, Utah, Salt Lake City Tribune, Apr 13, 1980
9. Nurses learn to assert themselves into a stronger role on the team. Baltimore, Md, The Baltimore Sun, Feb 26, 1980
10. Lukes S: Power: A Radical View, p 23. London, Macmillan, 1974

11. Merei F: Group leadership and institutionalization. Hum Relations 2:23–39, 1949
12. Winter DG: The Power Motive. New York, Free Press, 1973
13. Lasswell H: Power and Personality, pp 21–22. New York, WW Norton, 1948
14. Blood RO, Wolfe DM: Husbands and Wives: Dynamics of Married Living. Glencoe, Ill, Free Press, 1960; Wolfe DM: Power and authority in the family. In Cartwright D (ed): Studies in Social Power, pp 99–117. Ann Arbor, University of Michigan, Institute for Social Research, 1959
15. Harsanyi JC: Measurement of social power, opportunity costs, and the theory of two-person bargaining games, op cit; Homans GC: Social behavior as exchange. Am J Sociol 63:597–606, 1958; Blau P: Exchange and Power in Social Life. New York, John Wiley, 1964; Emerson R: Power-dependence relations. Am Sociol Rev 27:31–41, 1962; Thibaut JW, Kelley HH: The Social Psychology of Groups. New York, John Wiley, 1959
16. March JG: The power of power. In Easton D (ed): Varieties of Political Theory, pp 39–70. Englewood Cliffs, Prentice-Hall, 1966; Dahl RA: The concept of power. Behav Sci 2:201–218, 1957
17. Pollard WE, Mitchell TR: Decision theory analysis of social power. Psychol Bull 78:433–466, 1972
18. von Bertalanffy L: General Systems Theory. New York, George Braziller, 1968
19. Butler S: Miscellaneous thoughts. Quoted in Lasswell H: Power and Personality, p 7. New York, WW Norton, 1948
20. Gamson WA: Power and Discontent, p 1. Homewood, Ill, Dorsey Press, 1968
21. "Non-politicking" Teasdale addresses nurses at M.U. Columbia, Mo, Missourian, June 26, 1980
22. Kirkpatrick JJ: Political Woman, p 9. New York, Basic Books, 1974
23. Tiger L: Men in Groups, p 58. New York, Random House, 1969
24. Mead M: Sex and Temperament, p 191. New York, New American Library, 1950
25. Kirkpatrick, op cit, pp 14–15
26. Abramowitz SF, Abramowitz CV, Jackson C, Gomes B: The politics of clinical judgment: What nonliberal examiners infer about women who do not stifle themselves. J Consult Clin Psychol 41:385–391, 1973
27. Dinnerstein D: The Mermaid and the Minotaur. New York, Harper & Row, 1976
28. Petro CS, Putnam BA: Sex-role stereotypes: Issues of attitudinal changes. Sex Roles: A Journal of Research 5:29–39, 1979
29. Miller JB: Toward a New Psychology of Women. Boston, Beacon Press, 1976
30. Special report on working women. Marketing Media Decisions 14:130–131ff., 1979
31. Fogarty MP, Rapoport R, Rapoport RN: Sex, Career and Family. London, George Allen & Unwin, 1971
32. Holmstrom LL: The Two-Career Family. Cambridge, Schenkman, 1972
33. Peterson S, Richardson JM, Kreuter GV: The Two Career Family. Washington, DC, University Press of America, 1978; Staines GL, Pleck JH, Shepard L, O'Connor P: Wives' employment status and mental adjustment: Yet another look. Psychol Women Q 3:90–120, 1978; Huser W, Grant CW: A study of husbands and wives from dual career and traditional career families. Psychol Women Q 3:78–89, 1978
34. Garland TN: The better half? The male in the dual professional family. In Safilios-Rothschild C (ed): Towards a Sociology of Women. Lexington, Mass, Xerox College Publishing, 1972
35. Lockheed M, Hall K: Conceptualizing sex as a status characteristic: Applications to leadership training strategies. J Soc Issues 32, No. 1:111–124, 1976
36. Gunnar M: An American Dilemma, Vol 2, App 5: A parallel to the negro problem. New York, Harper & Row, 1944

2–Politics: The Authoritative Allocation of Scarce Resources

The word *politics* conveys different meanings and impressions to different nurses. To some, *politics* connotes the highest kind of national statesmanship and leadership. To others, the term carries overtones of graft, corruption, connivance, and manipulation. "Politics," wrote Max Weber, "means striving to share power or striving to influence the distribution of power, either among states or among groups within a state."[1] Harold Lasswell elucidated this concept of politics in his aptly entitled book, *Politics: Who Gets What, When, How.* In this volume he writes, "The study of politics is the study of influence and the influential. . . . The influential are those who get the most of what there is to get."[2] The influential seek to exercise influence for a variety of reasons. Many want prestige, economic advantages, or security. Others place principles above private gain and work for the improvement of government, for humanitarian causes, or in opposition to the selfish aims of individuals and groups.

WHAT IS POLITICS?

The basic definition of politics is the authoritative allocation of scarce resources. The three separate components of this definition are (1) scarce resources, (2) allocation, and (3) authority. *Resources* are those things that are valued by society. The most obvious one is money, because it can be used to purchase many other resources; however, health, friendship, love, votes, and prestige are some other examples of valued resources. Power and authority themselves are highly valued resources. The principle of *scarcity* is important here however. If all goods, services, and other resources were as abundant and freely available as the air we breathe (and the rise in pollution has changed even that in recent years), there would be no need for politics. Everyone would get everything he wanted without having to compete with another. Every society or group, however, has valued things that are scarce enough to be the source of potential conflict among its members. Valued scarce resources in nursing range from sufficient funding for quality nursing care to professional job opportunities that permit nurses to focus on comprehensive (biopsychosocial) patient care. For hospital administrators, the current shortage of nurses makes any nurse available for recruitment a valued and scarce resource, and many are prepared to offer a bonus to secure the services of a nurse. Under the headline, "The Issue: Tax Cut vs. Added Nurses," the *Morning News* of Wilmington, Delaware, portrayed a vivid example of conflict over scarce resources as follows:

> Capital School District taxpayers will be asked May 20 to give up a property tax cut in order to put a nurse in every elementary school and to help the district 'maintain present programs.'

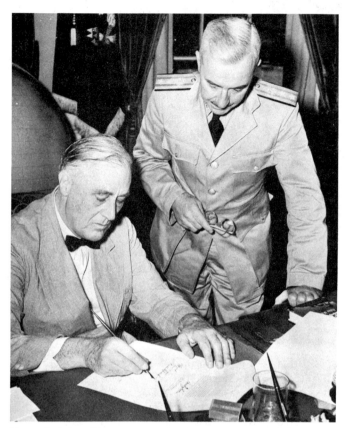

Figure 2–1. Franklin D. Roosevelt, shown here signing the bill that created the first program of federal support for nursing education, is regarded as a President who placed principles above private gain. (Courtesy of U.S. Public Health Service)

There would be no tax increase, with the present rate of $1.45 on each $100 of assessed valuation remaining intact. The referendum will ask citizens to approve the transfer of 5 cents from the district's tuition tax and 2 cents from the minor capitol levy to the general operating tax, adding about $106,400 to next year's operating budget.[3]

The next element in the definition of politics is *allocation.* If people are to resolve the question of how something of value will be distributed among them, in circumstances where there is not enough to please everyone with his ideal allocation, where ideal allocations may themselves be inherently incompatible, where flipping coins or murdering one another is not viewed as legitimate, a political process is needed. Society sets up mechanisms to make these decisions; that is, it decides on these allocations and how they will take place.

And the final component of the definition of politics is the need for *authority.* As in the discussion of power, authority refers to individuals or groups in a society with legitimate power. Another way to put it is that the authorities are those who "make binding decisions" in a system. "A decision is binding if either it is accepted as binding (for whatever reason) *or*, if it is not accepted, legitimate force can be used to implement the decision."[4] Allocations are viewed as authoritative when they follow certain rules or processes agreed upon by the group or society. As such, they are seen as "right" and "acceptable." As Easton explained, "A policy is authoritative when the people to whom it is intended to apply or who are affected by it consider that they must or ought to obey it."[5]

As individuals and groups attempt to influence these authoritative allocations of scarce resources, they are exhibiting what is called "political behavior." Political interactions are what people do that are involved in the process of making binding decisions and taking other actions that determine who gets what in a society. During this process, those in authority attempt to maintain their power and gain acceptance of their decisions for the allocation of scarce resources, and persons and groups not in authority try to make an impact on the decisions of authority through influence.

Far from being simply a question of united association for shared purposes, political experience is very much a matter of human competition and struggle of the various segments of society seeking power and authority created by the whole society, and of political values and beliefs, which are extensions of a number of purely particular and individual outlooks. This

Figure 2–2. The debate over the value of school nurses to the public, as compared to other services, has become widespread. (Courtesy of Rochester Post-Bulletin, Rochester, Minnesota)

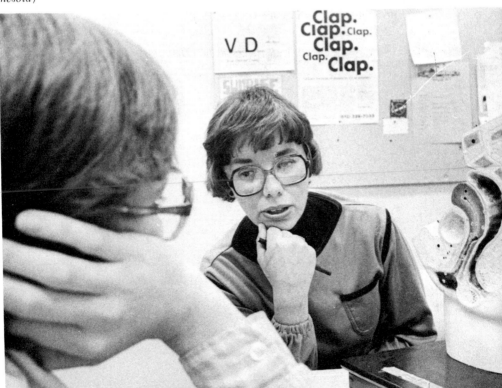

view finds its way into nurses' common language, for to say that someone is very political or is playing politics has come to describe clever opportunism and active efforts to enhance one's position of power in relation to others.

Politics, then, is an activity that human beings engage in together for the purpose of exerting control over their common affairs. The political process is a means by which the conflicting demands and aspirations of individuals and groups are reconciled. It is the method by which social needs are translated into public policies; and it is the process by which the people of a representative democracy govern themselves. It is a process that pervades the life of our nation and society, and if we are to understand modern society, then we must understand the methods and techniques of politics. It is also a process by which people bring some order to their collective life in society and try to remove some of the insecurity and unpredictability of social living.

Politics is quite different from science: in politics, the intent is to find a course of action, acceptable to various individuals espousing diverse purposes, values, and courses of action. Science, on the other hand, searches for knowledge, for "facts," and "value-free" results. Politics is value-expressive; facts are subordinate to and sustaining of values and only contribute to the delineation of an issue. Science and politics have been said to be incompatible because one trades in facts and the other in values. One example of such a clash occurred in 1979, when the Carter administration repeatedly insisted that there was no shortage of nurses and thus federal aid to nursing was not needed. The *fact* was not only that there was a shortage, but that it had reached crisis proportions throughout the country. Yet from a political point of view, the fact of a shortage was less important than the *value* of reducing federal aid to nursing, so that the money for nurses would be available to the President for more highly valued purposes.

POLITICS AS AN ASPECT OF ALL HUMAN INTERACTION

Many people use the word politics synonymously with government, but politics is an inherent part of any organized human activity. In principle, political labels may be attached to any and all human group activities because politics is an inescapable attribute of all human groups, even social groups.

If it is to survive, any group, any collection of two or more individuals, professional or otherwise, has to agree and to decide, in common, which situations or issues require common action and which do not. Failing such agreement, the group is likely to disintegrate or to be destroyed. Yet not even in the most harmonious and loving of voluntary groups, an ideal marriage, for example, can such agreement be assumed always to exist without directing considerable energy or attention to securing it. A family has to go through the process of allocating scarce resources, and thus it also becomes involved in a political process. Habit and mutual understanding will take the family or any other group part of the way, but any change in the environment, or any other new situation, will require that a fresh agreement be made. In most groups, it is impossible to build on harmony given the members' differing aims, tastes, perspectives, and interests. In its simplest form,

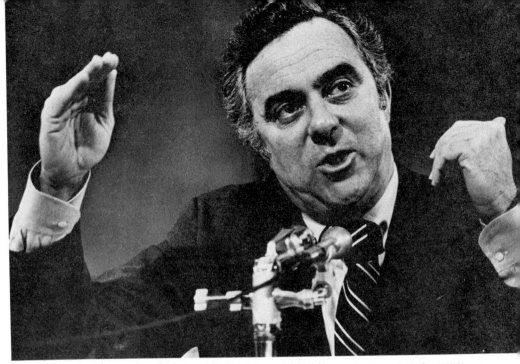

Figure 2–3. The politically created "myth" of a nurse surplus, as articulated here by HEW Secretary Joseph Califano, Jr., clashed sharply with the reality of an acute nationwide nurse shortage. (Courtesy of U.S. Department of Health and Human Services)

the human predicament, which gives birth to the pervasive activity of politics, is this: the members of a group face a situation that demands a common response but disagree as to what the response should be.

For many nurses, politics is not only remote and hard to understand, it also threatens because of the perception that it influences such things as the taxes we pay, war and peace, the quality of justice in the courts, and other burdens or benefits we enjoy in life. Like power, politics is inherently neither good nor bad. Depending upon the ability and integrity of the persons placed in public office, government can be effective or ineffective, incorruptible or corrupt; it can be characterized by efficiency and honesty, or by inefficiency and graft. Similarly an organization can be effective or ineffective, honest or dishonest, good or bad, depending on the persons who hold the power within the organization and how they use their power.

POLITICAL THEORIES

A political system, which is a type of social system, processes competing needs and wants into authoritative decisions. It is made up of interactions among individuals and institutions in a group or society. Authority and influence characterize the nature of the relationships between people in a political system; thus, a political system can be defined as one that can get persons to do what they would not otherwise want to do. There are numerous theories that attempt to explain the dynamics of political systems, several of which are now discussed briefly.

One political theory is called the *game theory*, which basically espouses the idea that politics is a great fascinating game, a game with players (people), a game with opposing sides and referees, a game with rules (laws, regulations) which are usually followed but sometimes broken, a game with goals (like winning an election), a game sometimes played with intense bitterness but often in good humor, a game with stakes so high that the victories won may vitally affect the lives of millions of people. The political game has been said to operate on the barter system where deals are made and credits and debits recorded. The simplest form of the game occurs when two players desire the same prize and it cannot be shared. These are games of "conflict," and in order to get what they want, the players have to fight. Another game is called "cooperation," where the parties involved can get what they want, or a part of what they want, by compromising. And there are "mixed" games, which have components of both conflict and cooperation. There are also more complicated games in which coalitions are formed, in which players alter their goals and change political sides in the middle. These are just a few of the games.[6]

Another theory is the *exchange theory*, which explains political behavior on the basis of a series of exchanges of one resource for another. For example, a politician votes the way his constituents desire in exchange for their votes, which keep him in office. Resources, of course, are not equally divided among persons and groups in society, which accounts in part for why persons enter the political system, when they do so, or even why they do not. According to this theory, a person has to determine where he can get what he wants, what it will cost, and whether or not he has another resource for exchange that will be of interest to the party who has what he desires.[7]

The *pluralist theory* starts with interest groups as the basic features of organized political life. The power or influence of these groups is based primarily on their effective political organization, but it also is a function of such group qualities as the political strategies and leadership abilities of party and group leaders. Competition is a key element. The competitive relationships that exist among the numerous interest groups that make up society, along with the existence of overlapping memberships (where people belong to more than one interest group yielding crosscutting allegiances), combine together to cause power to be dispersed widely. This distribution of power is essentially unstable because interests and alliances

Figure 2–4. Politics is a means by which the conflicting demands of individuals and groups are reconciled: Nurses testifying on behalf of the 1979 extension of the Nurse Training Act. (Courtesy of National League for Nursing)

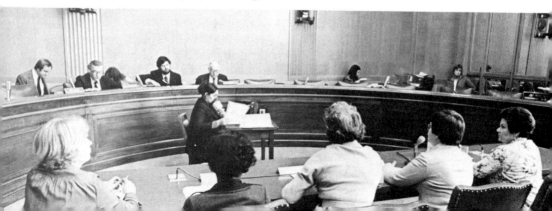

are typically short-lived, and new groups and coalitions are continually being developed as the old ones decline. There are limits to the power of any one group because of the necessity for compromises with, and, thus, dependence upon, other groups and because of the existence of a basic value consensus, which emphasizes compliance with democratic norms and values. The state is influenced by the numerous demands of the powerful interest groups but is able to achieve its own ends and gain substantial autonomy by serving as a broker or balancing agent among the competing groups.[8]

According to the *elite theory*, on the other hand, political power is said to be concentrated in the hands of elites who occupy the top positions in large and increasingly centralized institutional hierarchies. *Political elites* are small numbers of persons who appear to play an exceptionally influential part in political and social affairs and policy making. Elites hold more of the resources of power than others. They have exceptional access to "key positions" in society and appear to have control over crucial policies disproportionate to their numbers. "Nonelites" or "counterelites" refer to everyone who is not a part of the small elite group. These are the "masses." Elites tend to be unified in purpose and outlook because of their similar social backgrounds and their convergence of interests, which arise from their positions within dominant social institutions. The goals of elites are reflected directly in the actions of the state, which has little, if any, autonomy relative to elite goals and interests. Elites almost invariably get their way whenever policy decisions are made, and political conflicts are managed by elites in such a way as to produce outcomes favorable to their interests. As a consequence, there are no clearly identified limits to elite power, and the distribution of power is essentially stable.[9]

It is helpful to use such theories to observe the interactions and behaviors of any human group from the family to the Congress of the United States. Who has the power? How are decisions made? Who makes the rules? Why do people obey? Who wins? Who loses?

POLITICAL CONFLICT

Politics is an activity whereby people achieve control and regulation of their common affairs; therefore, how and what control should be exerted is a source of conflict known as *political conflict*. The study of politics can be viewed as the study of conflict because conflict is a basic fact of all political life. Political conflict between individuals or groups results from a discrepancy between preferences for the distribution of a scarce resource. Conflict is caused by differing values attached to the range of possible outcomes, different expected payoffs for the same outcome, or different vested interests in the various possible outcomes. Two or more parties become contestants when both or all are strongly motivated to achieve their most desired outcome under conditions that permit only one to be realized. To put it another way, when resources are viewed as nonshareable, and when two or more parties seek exclusive possession or use of a resource or a given part of it, political conflict occurs.

Political conflict may originate in one person, group, or nation; such conflicts are called intrapersonal, intragroup, or intranational. Or they may reflect incompatible actions of two or more persons, groups, or nations; such conflicts are called interpersonal, intergroup, and international. There are political conflicts that result from so-called "structural" inconsistencies, such as division of profits among various occupational groupings, overlapping ambitions of ethnic or religious groups, and competition between certain life-styles (class conflict). There are also conflicts that stem from personal envy and rivalry, or from family feuds and long-standing regional chauvinism. And there are in any population vague resentments and discontents that are expressed through defiance of laws, police, and bureaucratic regulation.

Conflict stimulates change, or, reversing the point, change is inevitably accompanied by conflict. Under conditions of scarcity, change usually harms some groups and helps others. The former resists and the latter advocates, producing conflict. Insofar as change is desirable, a conflict becomes not simply an unavoidable consequence that must be accepted, but also the actual stimulus of adaptation. Institutionalized forms of conflict, like party competition, are sources of continual, though moderate, change and renewal. Conflict is unavoidable. When conflict is contained, it can become a source of creative change—a vitalizing rather than a destructive force.

Vertical conflicts involve individuals or groups at different levels of the power pyramid, and they occur primarily over the distribution of power and secondarily over the use of power. An elite/nonelite conflict is one example of a vertical conflict. Physicians, and to a lesser extent, hospital administrators and health insurers, represent the elite in health care, while nurses, physical therapists, occupational therapists, nutritionists, and other health care providers constitute the nonelite. An example of the beginnings of a vertical conflict appeared in the May 22, 1980, issue of the *Houston Chronicle* under the headline "Texas Doctors, Nurses Remain at Loggerheads":

> Doctors don't want nurses telling them what to do, a doctor from the Texas Medical Association told nurses from the Texas Nurses' Association.
> During a committee hearing aimed at resolving a two-year-old controversy about the care which nurses can legally provide to patients, Dr. W. A. Godfrey said, 'You can't legislate health care.'
> And the Texas Nursing Practices Act should not contain any provisions directed at physicians' activities, Godfrey said.
> The controversy over what constitutes legal nursing care stems from an opinion issued in late 1978 by former Attorney General John Hill. In that opinion, Hill said that nurses cannot treat patients or administer medications without direct supervision by a doctor.
> During the 1979 session of the Legislature, Texas nurses proposed a bill that would have clarified the role of the advanced nurse practitioner and the types of care nurses can legally provide. The TNA warned that the attorney general's opinion placed many nurses in the state in legal jeopardy, since they were administering medications routinely in rural clinics and urban public health clinics.
> The measure was opposed by the Texas Medical Association.
> At a hearing of a special Senate subcommittee aimed at resolving the controversy, the two groups proved they are no closer to resolving their differences.
> The nurses' association proposed that the 67th Legislature consider a bill that would provide statutory recognition of advanced nurse practitioners. The nurses also proposed that nurse practitioners be allowed to provide basic health and preventive care, provide and prescribe medications, initiate changes in treatment

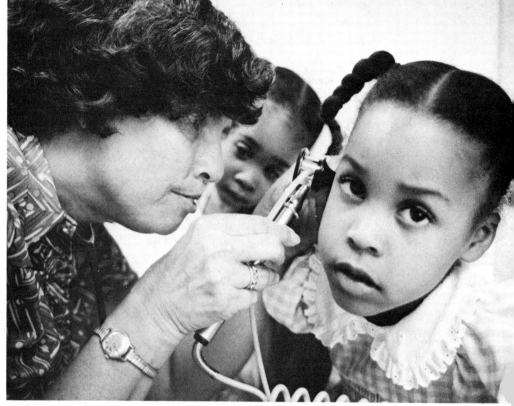

Figure 2–5. The jurisdictional dispute between nurse practitioners and physicians is a classic example of a vertical conflict. (Courtesy of Sacramento Bee, Sacramento, California)

and provide emergency medical care, if acting under 'protocols' (written policies or instructions) from a physician.

The medical association opposed those suggestions.

Godfrey told Pasadena state Sen. Chet Brooks that physicians would oppose restrictions on their activities in the Nursing Practices Act. 'I don't think they ought to put in the Nursing Practices Act what physicians should have to do. The control of medicine must be in the hands of the Board of Medical Examiners,' Godfrey said.

'You're telling me what I can do in your law,' Godfrey told Deanna Sebestyen, president of the TNA.

'We are telling the nurse what she can expect from the physician supervising her,' Ms. Sebestyen responded.[10]

Within the nursing profession, there are also political elites and nonelites, the former referring to an inner group of leaders who exert considerable influence as well as legitimate authority over the allocation of scarce resources for the profession.

Horizontal conflicts, on the other hand, involve participants in essentially the same power stratum. Nursing, unfortunately, is plagued by a high degree of horizontal conflict. Naturally, the more deeply one is involved in horizontal conflicts, the less time and energy can be devoted to vertical conflicts. Therefore, as the intensity of horizontal conflict increases, that of vertical conflict can be expected to decline. The intellectual roots of the maxim "divide and conquer" lie in this proposition. If the subjects can be set against one another, their ability to challenge the rulers is reduced. And in the case of nursing, if nurses can be set against one another, the less likely they will be able to challenge the health-care power structure.

Vertical conflict, on the other hand, may produce alliances among nurses and other groups, such as consumers, where none previously existed. The reason politics often makes "strange bedfellows" is the unifying capacity of a common enemy. A conflict involving representatives of a wider range of nursing and other groups is larger in scope than one involving fewer identifiable individuals or groups and is more likely to be successful.

One example of a horizontal political conflict in nursing concerns requirements for entry into practice. "Nursing Groups Split Over Education Bill" from an April 1980 issue of *The Herald Statesman* of Yonkers, New York, illustrates the nature of this interprofessional conflict:

> While recent attention has focused on a proposal to make teachers in the state professionals, a bill which many state nurses say would improve their professional standing seems to be stalled in legislative committee.
>
> In fact, even some proponents of the 1985 proposal, so named because of its effective date, joke now that it should be called the 1985,6,7,8 proposal.
>
> The bill, introduced in the state Legislature for the fifth consecutive year, would amend state law concerning minimum education requirements for the licensing of two categories of nurses.
>
> Persons known as registered nurses, or R.N.s, would be classified 'nurses' and have to earn at least a bachelor's degree before being licensed. (Currently R.N.s complete one of three education programs—a two-year associate degree program, a three-year diploma program or a four-year bachelor's degree program—before taking a licensing exam.)
>
> Licensed practical nurses or L.P.N.s (who now complete a one-year training program) would be called "associate nurses," and be required to earn at least an associate degree. . . . The chief proponent of the 1985 proposal is the New York State Nurses' Association, whose 28,000 members represent about one-third of the practicing licensed nurses in the state. Although the 1985 proposal would apply only to New York State, it follows closely a resolution approved by the American Nurses' Association to upgrade nursing competencies around the country. . . . While the state Nurses' Association favors the proposal, other smaller professional nurses' organizations and some individual nurses do not.[11]

Public exposure of this conflict in the mass media adds to the negative outcome of this horizontal conflict.

POLITICAL SALIENCE

A low-intensity conflict receives only divided attention, while a high-intensity one can become so obsessive that all aspects of life are interpreted in terms of it. The degree of intensity varies directly with the perceived importance of the issues involved in the conflict. The determinants of perceived importance are the salience and the number of values affected by the conflict. *Salience* refers simply to the fact that each person sees some things as being more central to his or her existence than others. Everyone possesses at least a crude hierarchy of values, and conflicts over high-ranking values are more intense than those over lower-ranking ones, other things being equal.

The salience of a particular value often depends on certain psychological dynamics, for example, the amount of effort that a person expends to reach or maintain a given value position. A reinforcing exchange may take place: a person sacrifices to attain a desired goal, which, in turn, becomes all the more valued because of the sacrifice, and thus justifies even further sacrifices. The greater the sacrifice made for a particular goal, the more salient it becomes and the more intense the conflicts triggered by challenges to it.

In any ongoing situation, the ability to get important things done is dependent upon maintaining a reservoir of goodwill. A person who fights every issue as though it were vital exhausts his or her resources including, and most especially, the patience and goodwill of those on whom he or she has to depend to get things done. Therefore, it should be considered neither surprising nor immoral that when an issue is of low salience, a sensible

Figure 2–6. In situations where issues are highly salient, intensity may be an outcome: Confrontation between security guard and a striking nurse in Providence, Rhode Island. (Courtesy of Providence Journal, Providence, Rhode Island)

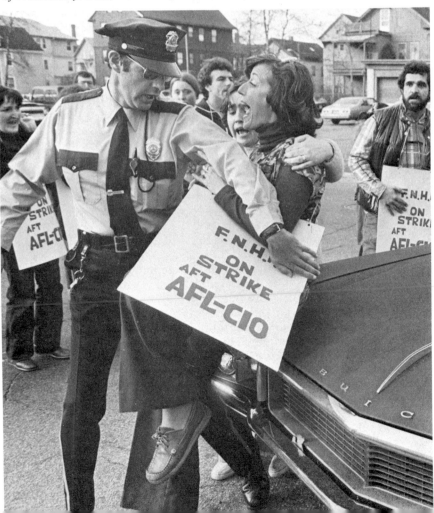

individual may use it to build goodwill for the future, or pay off past obliga-
tions, by going along with some individual for whom the issue is of high
salience. The side with far fewer allies and resources may end up winning
because of the intensity of commitment. The significance of high issue salience is that it magnifies the resources of the players. Those who feel
strongly about an issue will give more time, money, and other resources to
the cause.

RESOLVING CONFLICT: BARGAINING VERSUS COERCION

Although political conflict is inevitable because everyone cannot get everything he wants, if it gets totally out of control, politics itself breaks down. In
other words, if the wants or demands in a political system became too
numerous, the ability of the system to "produce its characteristic outputs, [and also its] authoritative decisions" will be seriously affected.[12]
Schattschneider argues, "The crucial problem in politics is the management
of conflict. No regime could endure which did not cope with this problem.
All politics, all leadership and all organization involves the management of
conflict."[13]

How then does the allocation process take place? Theft, murder, war, or
brute force are methods that could be used to allocate resources in a society,
but the disadvantages are obvious. A lottery could also be employed, but
that would not be practical either. At every point in the political system, but
particularly at the point of transforming conflict-demands into decisions, we
find conflict-management and conflict-resolution going on. Conflict-management and conflict-resolution refer to any action or process that ends
or lessens a conflict.

One method of managing conflict is to attempt to keep conflicting factions from arising in the first place. The most direct way to do this is for
whoever has substantial authority simply to prohibit certain kinds of political activity. For example, a hospital administrator might prohibit the publishing of a newsletter by nurses independent of the hospital administration, that is, a newsletter which is not controlled by administration. In this
way, using the terminology of the political system, the inputs to nursing are
being explicitly controlled by the outputs of administration. But if conflict
cannot be suppressed in this way, it will need to be managed or resolved.

There are three main approaches to conflict-resolution: *capitulation,
bargaining,* and *coercion.* In other words, when confronted with a political
conflict the individual or group has the following three choices: (1) withdraw and allow the other person or group to have just what they want
(capitulation); (2) seek conflict resolution through compromise (bargaining);
or (3) attempt to make the other person withdraw (coercion). Said another
way, if *A* does not want to give up the fight, *B* must be made to see things *A's*
way, or *A* and *B* will need to find a compromise solution to the conflict. This
definition underlines the point: in a political decision (1) some people
are prevented from getting what they want, and (2) some people end up
willing to do what they did not want to do.

Capitulation results when *A* goes along with *B's* desired outcome. This
type of solution to conflict is usually not desirable. The persons who lose
may resent the loss and will want to "get even" later, thus causing the con-

flict to re-emerge. Thus in politics, every effort is made to make capitulations look like compromises so that the losers do not feel humiliated. This can happen in the following ways: (1) the losers pretend they desired the winning outcome and wanted to lose all along; (2) the losers leave, escaping the situation; (3) the winners confer an award on the loser or provide other benefits; (4) the winners claim that they barely won; or (5) the losers join the winners.

Bargaining, a process of communication between *A* and *B* aimed at resolving initial differences in preference, is the second approach to dealing with political conflict. To bargain, you have to have something to exchange, to find someone who wants what you have and who, in return, has something you want, and then you have to have the opportunity to make the exchange. The problem is that some groups, primarily resource-poor groups, are left out of the bargaining process because they don't have anything to exchange. Bargaining always involves joint consideration of two or more "options" or potential agreements. Some options are more productive than others in the sense of providing greater joint utility to the bargainers when taken collectively. Productive bargaining includes processes by which bargainers locate and adopt such options. One process is considered to be more satisfactory than another to the extent that it is more capable of locating the best option among the options available to the bargainers.

Bargainers can often discover productive potential in a situation if they are willing to engage in *logrolling*, which involves the development of tradeoffs or exchanges of concessions on issues of differing importance to the bargainers. Bargainers get their way on one issue in exchange for making a concession on another of lesser importance to them. A difference in priorities often facilitates logrolling. Bargaining is best served if each bargainer can distinguish clearly between issues of greater and lesser importance. This allows them to adopt the strategy of holding firm on high-priority issues while conceding on low-priority issues. It encourages the development of tradeoffs; it also contributes to valid information exchange. Unfortunately, some nurses often have difficulty gaining insight into their own priorities.

An example of a group of nurses who effectually negotiated their differences and achieved more for nursing was reported in the February 15, 1980, issue of the Denver *Post*, under the headline "Senate Committee Backs New Nurse Act":

> Colorado nurses won an initial victory Thursday in the state Legislature, when a Senate committee unanimously approved a modernized state nurse-practice act despite strong opposition from state medical, hospital and nursing-home groups.
> Controversial clauses that would have outlawed nurses' strikes and closed nurses' pools weren't included in the proposed bill. And the proposed act contains an expanded definition of the duties of professional nurses and new authority for the State Board of Nursing to establish lists of 'advanced practitioners of nursing' working in the state.
> Pat Uris, lobbyist for the Colorado Nurses' Association, said that if the full Legislature approves the bill as it stands, it will be one of the most up-to-date in the country. 'It will be a model law, as was the 1973 Colorado act when it was passed,' Uris said of the proposed act that would replace the 1973 law.
> After being sent away from the Legislature in 1979 and told 'to get their act together,' Uris said nurses did exactly that.

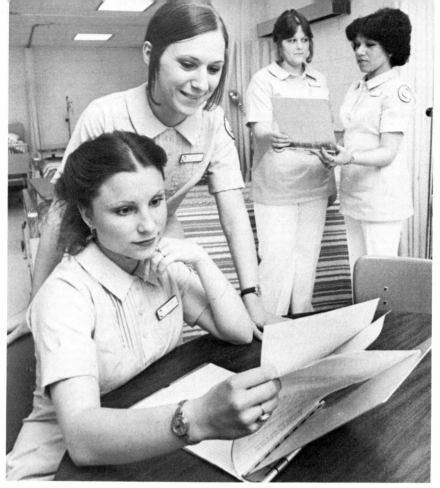

Figure 2-7. *Development of skills in bargaining and negotiation in the course of nursing education may yield nurses who are more effective patient advocates. (Courtesy of Norman Transcript, Norman Oklahoma)*

Contending that unity permitted nurses to ward off the attacks against the proposed act, Uris said, 'We decided that no longer were our opponents going to be able to divide us and conquer us.'

As a result, the Colorado Federation of Nursing Organizations was formed last summer to draft a bill with which all involved nursing groups could agree.

In 1979, when the Colorado Nurse Practice Act originally was up for its regular sunset review, various factions of the nursing profession fought each other as well as the other opposing groups.[14]

Reciprocity is a desire to repay the other party for a past favor or favors and can contribute to the development of a solution in a sequential agenda if one party makes an initial concession. The other may feel some obligation to reciprocate this favor with a return concession, which may elicit a further concession from the first, and so on. Of course such a chain of concessions often involves one party's "trust" that the other will concede at a later time.

Prospects for successful bargaining are enhanced by:

· the ability and willingness of each participant to state the position of the opponent to the opponent's satisfaction (exchange of roles)

- the ability and willingness of each participant to state the conditions under which the opponent's position is valid or has merit
- the ability and willingness of each opponent to assume that in many respects the opponent is like himself or herself, that is, that a common ground exists where the opponents share common values, and each is aware of this common ground and perhaps of the circumstances that have led the opponent to the position he or she holds (empathy).

Bargaining usually does not occur unless each of the parties believes he can gain something from making an agreement. If one of the parties believes he or she is much more powerful than the other, he or she may try to *coerce* the weaker party into giving up resources without receiving anything in return. This is the third approach to dealing with political conflict. Hence, the bargaining situation requires that the parties not be too asym-

Figure 2–8. Sister Elizabeth Kenny, the Australian nurse whose treatment of polio ran counter to that of organized medicine, was the object of coercion as she was denounced as a quack and charlatan. (Here portrayed by Rosalind Russell in the film Sister Kenny.) (*Courtesy of Nursing in the Mass Media Collection, University of Michigan*)

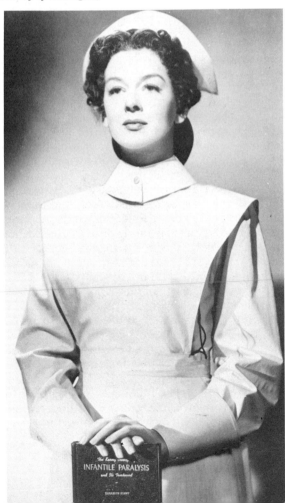

INFANTILE PARALYSIS

metrical in power. However, the lower limits of this necessary equivalence between persons or groups involved are not clear. Even when a strong legitimate authority confronts relatively weak protestors, bargaining can still take place if the latter can offer cessation of physical disruptions of institutional processes in return for something the authority is willing to concede. When bargaining parties are about equal in their relative strengths regarding an issue, coercion and escalation of conflict become counter-productive for both, because the similar resources of the other means probable retaliation and, hence, high costs.

While not all coercive acts are labeled as aggressive by observers, labeling has consequences for both the actor and the observer. The process of labeling an actor as aggressive is associated with assigning responsibility to that person and evaluating him or her negatively, and it implies a willingness by the observer to support retributive actions. Bargainers who use coercion are usually aware that being labeled as aggressive is associated with retribution, and so they try to justify their use of coercion to prevent observers from labeling them as aggressive. The anticipation of being so labeled is probably a powerful inhibitor of the use of coercive power, because such a label implies that the actor will incur costs involving negative evaluations, as well as the reactions of others. Yet the gains may outweigh the costs.

Coercion is usually not a preferred mode of influence because of the obvious dangers of escalation. It is introduced only when it appears that something of great value will be lost by failure to gain an agreement when there is great disparity in power between the bargainers (for example, when "bargaining" is simply a cover-up for a more unequal interaction mode). The use of coercive power is usually the influence mode of last resort.

The course of conflict will be greatly affected by whether a coercive action is perceived as offensive or defensive in character. To some extent, the way a threat is phrased indicates whether the source is taking an offensive or a defensive action. One must distinguish between *compellable threats*, which require that a target person or group perform specific actions to avoid a threatened punishment, and *deterrent threats*, which order the target not to do something. Compellable threats are usually perceived as more offensive, hostile, and constraining because the threatened party must make one particular response and forego all other responses; deterrent threats forbid only one particular behavior and by omission allow the target to do anything else he or she wishes.

An escalation of conflict is usually likely to occur when one party punishes the other. By failing to retaliate against a threat, individuals may leave the impression that they are weak and compliant, thereby inviting further attacks. Even if the targets are subjectively willing to accede to a powerful adversary's demands, they may still openly defy the threatener for fear of encouraging even greater demands in the future. Appeasement consists of yielding to a threatener's demands for a change in the status quo. Resistance not only is a matter of monetary defense, but may also serve to deter future attempts to coerce the person. Although one cannot out-muscle a more powerful opponent, a target may threaten at so great a cost that it would not be worthwhile for the opponent to pursue his objectives through coercive means. Allowing a threat to go unchallenged also causes the target to lose self-esteem; most people are willing to pay a price to save face. All these considerations work against excessive coercion.

The more intense the conflict, the more likely that threats and punishments will be used. An advertised desire and willingness to fight is a way to promote a tough image. The aggressive promoter acts to provoke others into fighting him or her. It is not necessary for these persons to win all of the fights; the important thing is to show that they have "guts." The reputation gained by the aggressive promotor may cause others to defer to his demands; even the very assertive may back down before the fury of a stronger person unless the stakes are clearly worth it. These tough self-image promoters build a reputation that lends credibility to their threats and enhances the effectiveness of their course-of-influence attempts.

Possession of an abundance of relevant resources enhances the believability of a source's threats and, hence, contributes to success. Experts are superior to nonexperts in getting conformity to their persuasive communications. Expertise enhances the effectiveness of warnings and recommendations. A person's reputation for a certain expertise apparently leads others to

Figure 2–9. The epitome of the arrogant physician, who appeared "tough" and therefore gained a more favorable power exchange rate in his interaction with others, was Dr. Ben Casey, the hero of the early 1960s television world. (Courtesy Nursing in the Mass Media Collection, University of Michigan)

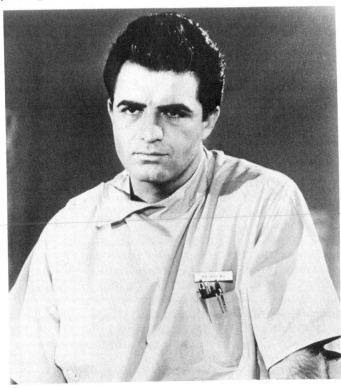

assume that his or her credibility is high because it would be difficult to acquire such a reputation if the recommendations and predictions were almost always wrong. The scope of influence of an expert is usually assumed to be confined to the area of special competence. High self-esteemed persons generally believe they will be accepted, approved of, and rewarded by others, while low self-esteemed persons expect to be rejected, disapproved of, and punished. These expectations affect behavioral styles in that high self-esteemed persons are active in self-defense, in anticipation of the harm others are apt to do them.

Persons who appear "tough" (bad and potent) may gain a more favorable exchange rate than those who appear "soft" (good and impotent). Observers tend to use the valuative (good–bad) potency (strong–weak) dimensions in forming impressions of others. A person who is consistently cooperative and rewarding is perceived as good and impotent, while a person who frequently attempts exploitation and administers punishment is perceived as bad, but potent. A bargainer who yields the most is viewed by the opponent as good, but weak, while a bargainer who yields the least is perceived as bad, but strong. Similar reactions to persons who use threats and promises have been found. A threatener who consistently punishes defiance is perceived as bad and potent, but viewed as good and impotent if defiance is seldom punished. A case in point was the conflict at Wright State University School of Nursing.

The dispute at Wright State University (WSU) began in November 1979 when the president of the University, Robert J. Kegerreis, and the university trustees recommended to Dean Gertrude Torres and the faculty of WSU's School of Nursing that a 2-year baccalaureate program for registered nurses who had degrees from associate degree and 3-year programs be instituted. The proposal essentially gathered dust, at least at the School of Nursing, until mid-January 1980 when suddenly the trustees and President Kegerreis began to talk about the establishment of the program as if it had already been approved. They further stated that the new program would not be under the School of Nursing, but instead, it would be placed under Dr. John R. Beljan, dean of Health Affairs, who also headed up the University's medical school.

The reasons put forth by the university trustees and the president for instituting the new program were numerous. First, it was claimed that there was a "growing desire of working nurses and graduates of two and three-year nursing programs for a college diploma."[15] Second, it was claimed that as the current Dayton-area nursing shortage was mainly in hospitals and inasmuch as the WSU School of Nursing was preparing nurses to work in community settings, a program was needed that would provide more hospital expertise. In this context, the "high failure rate" of WSU nursing students on the state licensing examination was touted as an important issue. The chairman of the board of trustees said, "My quarrel is with their performance. . . . They [the nursing school] are not teaching nurses how to perform clinically or how to pass the state examinations."[16]

Another reason given for the proposed new program centered on the school's causative role in the area's nurse shortage. Dayton, university administrators claimed, was "losing some nurses with associate degrees to other areas which don't make it so difficult as WSU does for them to obtain a four-year college degree."[17] And finally, the new program was justified on the basis that the WSU School of Nursing had made its transfer policy unusually difficult. President Kegerreis commented to an interviewer,

> Some registered nurses in the area had enrolled at other Ohio universities or at institutions in other states . . . because of the 'perception' that their 'previous education and training are denigrated' and that they face 'rigidities of requirements at the school of nursing.'[18]

The faculty, staff, and students of the WSU School of Nursing hotly disputed most of the arguments made in support of the proposed 2-year baccalaureate program by President Keggereis and the trustees. Faculty pointed out that a program established for registered nurses should not be different from the generic program in terms of its emphasis on hospital as compared to a community focus of care. One perplexed Dayton newspaper reporter wrote,

> In the January 17 article, Dr. Beljan was quoted as saying the program under the Medical School would be put in his division because it would focus on clinical and hospital work. But aren't these people quoted as coming from hospital and clinical conditions already? How much clinical training is needed by nurses working for a number of years in hospitals?[19]

Refuting another point, School of Nursing supporters emphasized that the majority of WSU's graduates were doing clinical nursing in area hospitals and that area hospitals were reasonably well satisfied with the nursing competencies of WSU's graduates. Faculty of the nursing school also noted that "the failure rate [of WSU's nursing students on the state exam] has no

Figure 2–10. Who should be in charge of nursing education: Physicians or nurses? The Wright State University clash was over this age old question. (Courtesy of History of Nursing Collection, University of Michigan)

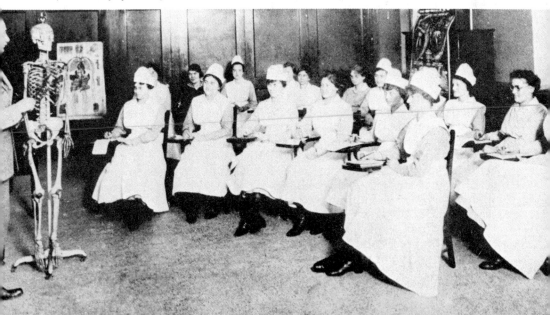

bearing on the proposed program because the program is aimed at registered nurses, who already have passed the state board examination."[20]

An additional aspect of the conflict centered on the fact that the School of Nursing had been asked in December, 1979 to accept a funding cut of 17%, twice that given to any other division of the university, owing to financial problems at WSU. This reduction would necessitate the elimination of eight faculty positions, thus making it impossible to adequately staff the proposed new program. Wrote one WSU student,

> Granted, the Dayton area is short of nurses, but we at Wright State did not create this shortage. Neither can one program alone solve the problem. If Dr. Robert Kegerreis is really concerned about nursing in the community, why hasn't he helped the School of Nursing obtain the classroom space, the budget and the additional faculty needed so that more people could be accepted into the program?[21]

In response to charges that the School of Nursing made it too difficult for R.N.s to enter WSU's existing program for a 4-year degree,

> Ms. George [assistant professor of nursing at WSU] said registered nurses made up 13 percent of the nursing students. Last fall, after Miami University moved a degree program designed for registered nurses to a location farther from Dayton, she said Dean Torres had told administrators that the Wright State nursing faculty would look at ways to increase access for such students. She added that the state's student nurses organization had concluded that Wright State's nursing school was the most flexible in Ohio in allowing registered nurses to take examinations that make it possible for them to earn advanced standing.[22]

The dean and faculty of the WSU School of Nursing were particularly concerned about what the proposed new program would do to the School of Nursing's accreditation. It was charged that allowing the new program to be set up outside of the School of Nursing would violate National League for Nursing guidelines which prohibit accrediting two separately run programs at the same school. Furthermore, Dean Torres explained,

> The new program's emphasis on hospital training could violate League guidelines that require a bachelor's degree program to provide training in areas such as public health clinics and nursing homes. And she said the failure of the medical school and Wright State trustees to involve the nursing school faculty in planning the new program also goes against the guidelines.[23]

The first move the School of Nursing faculty made in protest against the proposed 2-year program was to vote to call for the resignation of President Kegerreis. At the time, they said that the "faculty was forced to pass the resignation resolution after being unable to arrange a meeting with the trustees."[24] However, when the resolution went up before the faculty of the entire university it failed to achieve a majority of votes. In response, the chairman of the trustees "declined to meet with nursing school officials unless there is 'compelling new evidence' why the program should not be set up under Beljan's division."[25]

The direction of the dispute continued on a losing course. The resignations of the dean and associate dean were tendered and accepted. The University chose an acting dean from another University who did not meet with the faculty prior to accepting the position. The assistant dean for the undergraduate nursing program was quoted as saying, "I just can't believe this, because the nursing school faculty was not involved in the selection process in any way, shape, or form. . . ."[26] Twenty-five of the thirty-seven faculty members, including all of the graduate faculty, all professors and associate professors, and all tenured assistant professors, then indicated in writing that they would resign June 30th in protest. Picket lines were manned by nursing students at the university. Some were quoted as saying that they were thinking of transferring if the dispute were not resolved in the School of Nursing's favor. Attempts were made to widen the arena of the dispute and thus gain support for their fight. At an Ohio Nurses' Association meeting, for example, led by members of the WSU faculty, nurses "voted to purchase a newspaper ad to call a meeting of all Dayton-area nurses to dispense information about the controversy."[27] They also attempted to send out a newsletter (with national distribution) that explained the nature of the dispute, but the university confiscated the newsletter and only released it under extreme pressure, sending it out along with a separate letter to accompany the newsletter stating the university's side of the dispute.

The eventual result of this effort was a loss for nursing as reported in the Dayton *Journal Herald* editorial of May 22, 1980, under the headline, "Nurses' Philosophy Suffers in Agreement":

> The atmosphere at Wright State University will be more peaceful now that a 'compromise' has been reached in the nursing school–medical school controversy. There's also going to be something artificial about it.
>
> The faculty committee that was formed to make recommendations about the need and feasibility of creating a second nursing program has reached an agreement with trustees to move the nursing school into the medical school division. The faculty correctly scrapped the proposal of creating a second program, but unwisely sacrificed the independence of the nursing school for some written assurances that the medical school division won't try to swallow the nursing program.
>
> It's not much of a compromise. In effect, the medical school and Dr. John Beljan got what they wanted, but refused to acknowledge all along. Repeatedly Beljan and WSU President Robert Kegerreis denied the goal was to put the nursing program under the medical school division. What they wanted was to get the nursing school to respond to the needs of the community's registered nurses who want baccalaureate degrees, they said.
>
> The statistics clearly show the nursing school was becoming more responsive to area nurses. That and even the resignation of the feisty nursing dean, Gertrude Torres, was not enough.
>
> The significance of this brouhaha is that WSU's emphasis on nurses as health professionals, rather than doctor assistants, is likely to be undermined. Opponents said this was going to happen. It's too bad they were right.[28]

The loss for nurses at Wright State bespeaks the underlying presumption that, again, nursing's role is thought by policy makers to be one of thoughtless action and subservience to medicine. Upon reflection it is clear how pervasive the sexist double standard has been and how a particular act, done by a nurse, still carries a very different meaning from the same act done by a physician. Such perceptions are the result of political socialization.

THE PROCESS OF POLITICAL SOCIALIZATION

Political socialization refers to the way in which individuals acquire political orientations, that is, norms, beliefs, values, and attitudes toward all matters of politics. The socialization process ensures a transmission of the political culture from generation to generation. For any social system to remain differentiated it must meet two requirements: it must create the condition for differential allocation of people to political roles, and it must socialize, that is educate in the broadest sense, the people for the performance of these political roles. Socialization is used to ensure voluntary compliance with role assignment and with expected types of performance.

Political socialization should not be thought of narrowly, meaning government classes in high school, but instead broadly, meaning all political learning. Socialization is a process that continues throughout the life of the individual. The first agent of socialization is the family; but in later years, the influences of school, peers, the media, and one's profession or occupation are added to the pressures the family creates for certain political behavior. Political socialization involves both direct and indirect learning. Direct learning includes: (1) imitating the behavior of others; (2) direct education; (3) direct experience; and (4) predicting what other persons expect in given situations (such as when nursing students are socialized into acting and behaving like graduate nurses). Indirect learning or socialization, on the other hand, does not involve direct experience with other persons but instead with symbols and roles such as those conveyed in the mass media.

Figure 2–11. Socialization is the way in which children acquire political norms, values, and attitudes about nursing and all other aspects of life. (Courtesy of Blackfoot News, Blackfoot, Idaho)

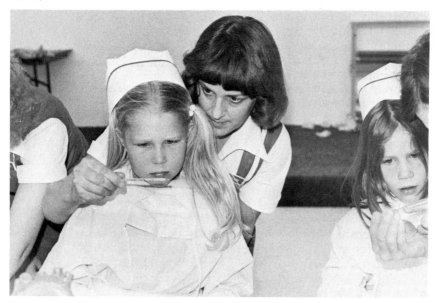

What family and other socializing agents tend to produce (or not produce) is political participation, political attitudes, and political efficacy. The experience of *political participation*, from voting to running for office, builds on the original socialization patterns. *Political attitudes* range the continuum from liberal to conservative, from idealistic to realistic, and formulate the basic political orientation of the individual. *Political efficacy* refers to the feeling of being able to do something about what goes on in politics, or the feeling that politics is a meaningful or possible area for personal involvement. Renshon defined it as "the belief that one has sufficient control over political processes to satisfy the need for control in relevant life areas."[29] People who feel that political matters bear heavily on their lives are more likely to participate in certain political activities than people who don't feel so. A person with a low sense of efficacy may hardly be inclined to bother with political matters at all. This sense of efficacy is developed through the process of political socialization. It forms the personal self-confidence and positive feelings about oneself, which are essential for political involvement.

POLITICAL SOCIALIZATION THROUGHOUT THE LIFE CYCLE

When does political socialization begin? Political ideas begin to form early in childhood. In fact, today there is a tendency to identify "political socialization" exclusively with the study of the political behavior of the preadult, or even of the preschool-aged child. This, of course, is a reaction against an earlier assumption that the citizen blossoms completely upon entry into the electorate, because children were believed to have no political thoughts. Consequently the vast amount of research on political development in recent years has focused on children and adolescents, although some political socialization scholars have urged that socialization be investigated as a lifelong process and that research take greater note of life-cycle effects. As Brim has pointed out in his study of socialization after childhood, investigation of developments during all phases of the life cycle is particularly important in societies undergoing structural change or with persons whose status is changing.[30] This is particularly relevant to American society today because the role of nurses and women is experiencing considerable upheaval.

Political attitudes and behavior continue to change throughout the life cycle. These attitudes start with aloofness, then move to engagement, and finally to disengagement. Children are not born political animals; they must learn about politics. They must learn its scope, its functions, and its processes. They must learn to identify the expected roles of all those who are a part of the process, as well as the appropriate behaviors involved. In addition to acquiring this knowledge, children develop emotional reactions to politics, and acquire political behaviors appropriate to their own interests and capabilities. All this political development, or political socialization, takes place as children simultaneously form their basic personalities and acquire a mass of nonpolitical knowledge, attitudes, and behaviors.

Indirect political learning begins long before children know anything about politics as such. The evidence supports the idea that "*lifelong* patterns of social and political interaction are established before a child leaves home."[31] In the first year of life, children learn that parents, and, by extension, other adults on whom they depend, can generally be trusted or else should be viewed with distrust. As parents begin to impose behavioral limits, children acquire feelings of comfort or discomfort in connection with these external regulations, feelings which develop into beginning attitudes toward what adults call "law and order." As children learn to walk, talk, and engage in social activities, they also acquire different feelings of confidence in their ability to interact with the world beyond the family. Although direct relationships between these early patterns of personality development and adult political behavior are not readily demonstrable, and such relationships can be altered to some extent by a great variety of later experiences, political behavior plainly emerges from the context of the child's total experience of life. Davies has pointed out that the early patterns established "will either prevent or seriously damage [the child's] ability to make political choices as an adult."[32]

Research has shed light on how children acquire political beliefs, values, and attitudes relative to candidate orientation, party identification, and issue orientation. The first of these to develop is candidate evaluation. Children become aware of the existence of the President and view him in idealized and very positive terms. They also see all other public officials in a very favorable light. The President is seen as extremely powerful and benevolent. As the child develops, however, this view changes to one of valuing personal and role qualities such as morality, kindliness, and intelligence. The older child also becomes more aware of other players in the policy-making process, such as Congress and the law, and these come to be regarded more positively than the President. All of this shows a growing realism from childhood to adolescence as the cognitive ability to differentiate roles develops.[33]

Party identification is widely evident among children. Greenstein showed that 60% of children identified themselves with one or another of the major parties by the age of ten. This party identification has been found to persist through adulthood and to be greatly influenced by parental preference. Greenstein noted that "only a handful of children in the entire sample indicated that their own party preferences differed from those of their parents."[34] Persons whose parents were both Democrats rarely identified themselves as Republicans, and those whose parents were both Republicans were rarely traitorous enough to become Democrats. Similarly, Jennings and Niemi, by interviewing high school seniors and their parents separately, assessed parent and child agreement relative to political participation, attitudes, and knowledge. They found close agreement between parents and adolescents relative to basic partisan orientations (*i.e.*, party affiliation), although only minimal agreement on specific attitudes and political participation.[35]

Issue orientation does not appear until later in a child's life. Even though Greenstein found that 10-year-olds engaged in party identification, only a "little more than a third . . . could name even one [leader] of either of the two major parties."[36] It is not until the eighth grade that children have any idea about political issues, and even then, one study found that only 6% were found to be able to distinguish any difference between political par-

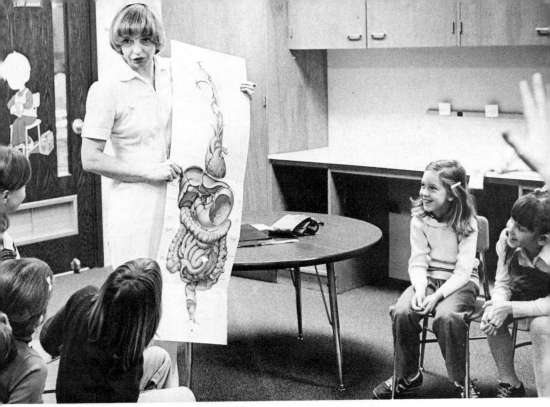

Figure 2–12. Children acquire socialization about nursing from subject matter as well as from role models. (Courtesy of Naperville Sun, Naperville, Illinois

ties. On the other hand, sixth graders have been found to understand that public policy and laws can be altered to make change. But they do not understand or comprehend political conflict. To them, politics occurs without conflict.[37] By the end of high school, however, adolescents are able to take different positions on issues. They can and do attend to issues and accept conflict as an inevitable part of politics.[38] Knowledge of political and governmental matters expands markedly during the high-school years.

Piaget, and other developmentalists, explain the basis for this delay in acquiring advanced political understanding by pointing to the fact that the reasoning ability of the child, or abstract thought processes necessary for political thought, do not mature until adolescence. Thus, it is not until late adolescence that political orientations begin to include true insight into allocation of scarce resources issues, and understanding of the complexity of this concept takes a number of years to fully comprehend.[39]

Although the political socialization that occurs in childhood and during the adolescent years is of great importance, as noted earlier, socialization is a continuous process throughout life. Jaros points out that "early socialization may be displaced or overriden by later socialization, nullified by adult experiences or even by deliberate countersocialization."[40] He points to the impact of generational change, referring to expected alterations in political beliefs, norms, values, and attitudes from one generation to another, and of maturational change, referring to the inevitable developmental changes

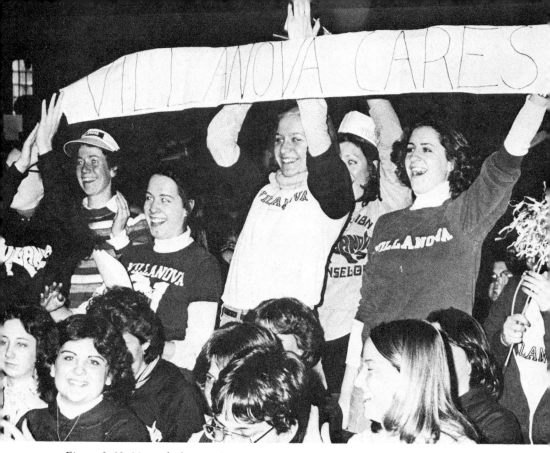

Figure 2–13. More idealistic political pursuits are followed by young adults. Here nursing students rally against President Carter's 1979 veto of the Nurse Training Act. (Courtesy of Philadelphia Bulletin, Philadelphia, Pennsylvania)

that occur as a person grows older. Both of these factors impact on the course of adult political socialization.

Looking first at young adults aged 18 to 25, studies have found that they are less interested in conventional politics than are older persons, perhaps because of competing demands on their time and energy during this time in their lives. For example, they have been found to vote considerably less than older adults. On the other hand, young adults do develop distinct political attitudes, usually idealistic and oriented toward reform, and tend to make up the majority of those involved in such political movements as the civil rights movement or the anti-Vietnam War movement. They tend to be more radical, and their views are usually more liberal than their parents'. Persons in this age bracket are also more likely to demonstrate and protest.[41]

Between 25 and 30 years of age, these more extreme views diminish, and political participation in the traditional sense increases (i.e., voting). As compared to adolescents, adults as they grow older have been found to have a greater knowledge of political matters and have a more cynical attitude toward political office holders. They also exhibit greater interest in politics, exposing themselves to political stimuli in the form of television and newspapers, to a much greater extent than adolescents. Adult responsibilities and the pressures of such things as taxes, purchasing a home, and getting one's children an education shed a new light on political matters and greatly alter political outlooks, usually toward more conservative viewpoints.[42]

In seeking to explain the political activism of many adolescents and young adults who challenged the political system during the 1960s, Easton and Dennis speculated that the attitude of "diffuse respect" for authority characteristic of young children declines during the teens and early twenties. Although data were limited to attitudes toward police, they nonetheless suggest that this might extend to all objects of authority. With increased age and responsibility, with the acquisition of "additional stakes in life," the curve of respect ascends again. The adult returns to his earlier and more deferential views.[43]

During the age period between 30 and 50 years, political attitudes are

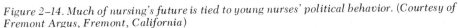

Figure 2–14. Much of nursing's future is tied to young nurses' political behavior. (Courtesy of Fremont Argus, Fremont, California)

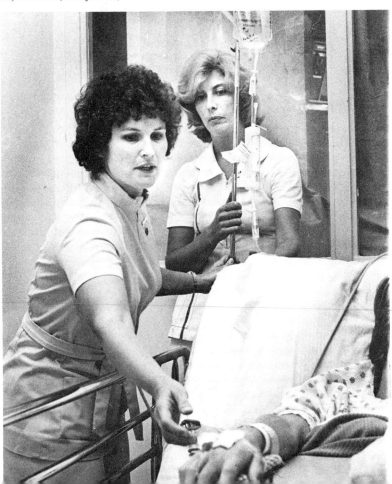

said to become more and more inflexible with little change occurring. The research evidence is sketchy and inconclusive in this area, however. It appears that conservatism increases relative to previously learned social norms, but where a vested interest is the issue, more liberal attitudes may be in evidence (*e.g.*, an economic problem that affects the person directly).

A gradual disengagement in political participation has been shown to take place after the age of 50. It has been explained in terms of the normal aging process, in terms of expected role behavior ("older persons are not supposed to be politically active"), in terms of the natural withdrawal that takes place as a person ages, and in terms of a growing sense of powerlessness, which leads to a loss of political efficacy.[44] These findings have been challenged by Neugarten who has found that persons between 55 and 75 years of age are actually becoming more involved politically, and he attributes this development to the fact that levels of education are rising.[45]

Added to the usual agents of socialization in adulthood is that of one's profession or occupation. That persons belonging to the same professional group tend to have similar political views underlines the importance of this influence. Ziegler found that colleges that primarily educated teachers inculcated respect for political authority to a greater extent than did liberal arts colleges.[46] Similarly, Becker found that persons who had entered medical or law schools changed their more liberal altruistic outlooks to the more conservative ones held by members of their professions by the time they had graduated.[47] The interconnection between one's profession and social status is close, and this has an automatic impact on political power and attitudes. Persons in high prestige professions are more apt to be involved in politics, and the more active a person, the more chance he or she will have to influence political decisions. Furthermore, the higher the status, the more conservative the individual and the higher the degree of political efficacy experienced. Lower-status persons tend to be more liberal, but at the same time experience a low level of political efficacy.

The primary purpose of this chapter has been to present the concept of politics and to illustrate effects, sometimes adverse, which politics has on nurses' work and morale. In so doing, we have deliberately attempted to highlight what we see as a resource deficiency for nurses, arising from the fact that the apolitical tradition inherent in the political socialization of nurses and women, in general, has placed them at an initial disadvantage in the conflict-resolution that inevitably accompanies reallocation of scarce resources.

References

1. Weber M: Miscellaneous thoughts. Quoted in Lasswell H: Power and Personality, p 7. New York, WW Norton, 1948
2. Lasswell H: Politics: Who Gets What, When, How, p 3. New York, Meridian Books, 1958
3. The issue: Tax cut vs. added nurses. Wilmington, Del, Morning News, Mar 27, 1980
4. Gamson WA: Power and Discontent, p 22. Homewood, Ill, Dorsey Press, 1968
5. Easton D: The Political System, p 132. New York, Alfred A Knopf, 1953
6. Brams SJ: Game Theory and Politics. New York, Free Press, 1975; Miller N: Logrolling, vote trading, and the paradox of voting: A game theoretical overview. Public Choice 30:51–73, 1977; Kuhn HW, Tuckers AW (eds): Contributions to the Theories of Game, Vol

2, Annals of Mathematic Studies, No. 28. Princeton, Princeton University Press, 1953; Rapoport A: Two Person Game Theory. Ann Arbor, University of Michigan Press, 1966

7. Harsanyi JC: Measurement of social power, opportunity, costs and the theory of two-person bargaining games. Behav Sci 7:67–80, 1962; Homans GC: Social Behavior: Its Elementary Forms. New York, Harcourt, Brace & World, 1961; Blau P: Exchange and Power in Social Life. New York, John Wiley, 1964

8. Dahl RA: Who Governs? Democracy and Power in an American City. New Haven, Yale University Press, 1961

9. Wright Mills C: The Power Elite. New York, Oxford University Press, 1956

10. Texas doctors, nurses remain at loggerheads. Houston, Tex, Houston Chronicle, May 22, 1980

11. Nursing groups split over education bill. Yonkers, NY, The Herald Statesman, Apr 27, 1980

12. Easton D: A Systems Analysis of Political Life, p 57. New York, John Wiley & Sons, 1965

13. Schattschneider EE: The Semi-Sovereign People, p 56. New York, Holt, Rinehart & Winston, 1960

14. Senate committee backs new nursing act. Denver, Colo, Denver Post, Feb 15, 1980

15. Roth M: Nursing school debate heats up. Dayton, Oh, Journal Herald, Jan 19, 1980

16. Roth M: WSU board chief gives Kegerreis his full backing. Dayton, Oh, Journal Herald, Jan 26, 1980

17. Hill DJ: Nursing rating lowered at WSU. Dayton, Oh, Dayton Daily News, Jan 29, 1980

18. Fields CM: 2 nursing deans quit in Wright State dispute. Washington, DC, Chronicle of Higher Education, Feb 19, 1980

19. Blackwell B, Eilers K: Wright State conflict a clash of two approaches. Dayton, Oh, Journal Herald, Jan 26, 1980

20. Ray K: WSU nursing grads last among four-year schools on test. Dayton, Oh, Dayton Daily News, Jan 31, 1980

21. WSU nursing school plans draw mixed reactions. Dayton, Oh, Dayton Daily News, Feb 3, 1980

22. Fields CM, Chronicles of Higher Education, op cit

23. Roth M: WSU dean of nursing resigns. Dayton, Oh, Journal Herald, Jan 22, 1980

24. WSU nurses want president to resign. Springfield, Oh, The Sun, Jan 19, 1980

25. Nursing school debate heats up, op cit

26. Pagano T: WSU nursing faculty unhappy with naming of acting dean. Dayton, Oh, Beavercreek Daily, Feb 7, 1980

27. Ray K: Nursing faculty at WSU seeks no-confidence vote. Dayton, Oh, Dayton Daily News, Jan 30, 1980

28. Nurses' philosophy suffers in agreement. Dayton, Oh, Journal Herald, May 22, 1980

29. Renshon SA: Psychological Needs and Political Behavior: A Theory of Personality and Political Efficacy, p 75. New York, Free Press, 1974

30. Brim OG: Socialization through the life cycle. In Brim OG, Wheeler S (eds): Socialization After Childhood: Two Essays. New York, John Wiley, 1966

31. Davies JC: Political socialization: From womb to childhood. In Renshon S (ed): Handbook of Political Socialization, p 170. New York, Free Press, 1977

32. Ibid, p 170

33. Easton D, Dennis J: Children in the Political System: Origins of Political Legitimacy. New York, McGraw-Hill, 1969; Hess RD, Torney JV: The Development of Political Attitudes in Children. Chicago, Aldine, 1967

34. Greenstein FI: Children and Politics, p 72. New Haven, Yale University Press, 1965

35. Jennings MK, Niemi RG: The Political Character of Adolescence: The Influence of Families and Schools. Princeton, Princeton University Press, 1974

36. Greenstein FI, op cit, p 71

37. Ibid, p 67

38. Jennings MK, Niemi RG: Family structure and the transmission of political values. Am Polit Sci Rev 62: 169–184, 1968

39. Inhelder B, Piaget J: The Growth of Logical Thinking from Childhood to Adolescence. New York, Basic Books, 1958

40. Jaras D: Socialization to Politics, p 57. New York, Praeger, 1973

41. Merelman KM: The development of policy thinking in adolescence. Am Polit Sci Rev 65:1033–1047, 1971; Merelman RM: Political Socialization and Educational Climates.

New York, Holt, Rinehart & Winston, 1971; Flacks R: The liberated generation: An exploration of the roots of student protest. J Soc Issues 23, No. 1:52–75, 1969; Feuer L: The Conflict of Generations. New York, Basic Books, 1969; Roszak T: The Making of a Counterculture. Garden City, NY, Doubleday, Anchor Books, 1968

42. Verba S, Nie NH: Participation in America. New York, Harper & Row, 1972; Milbrath LM: Political Participation. Chicago, Rand-McNally, 1965; Glenn ND, Grimes M: Aging, voting and political interest. Am Sociol Rev 33:563–575, 1968

43. Easton D, Dennis J, op cit

44. Cumming E: Further thoughts on the theory of disengagement. Int Soc Sci 15, No. 3:377–393, 1963; Agnello T: Aging and the sense of political powerlessness. Public Opinion Q 37:251–259, 1973; Culter NE: Aging and generations in politics: The conflict of explanations and inference. In Wilcox AR (ed): Public Opinion and Political Attitudes. New York, John Wiley & Sons, 1974; Foner A: Age stratification and age conflict in political life. Am Sociol Rev 39:187–196, 1974; Riley MW, Foner A, Hess B, Toby ML: Socialization for the middle and later years. In Goslin DA (ed): Handbook of Socialization Theory and Research. Chicago, Rand-McNally, 1969

45. Neugarten B: Age groups in American society and the rise of the young–old. Ann Polit Soc Sci 415:187–198, 1974

46. Ziegler LH: The Political World of the High School Teacher. Eugene, Ore, University of Oregon Center for the Advanced Study of Educational Administration, 1966

47. Becker H, Hughes EC, Greer EC, Strauss AL: Boys in White. Chicago, University of Chicago Press, 1961

3–The Policy Process

One of the most distinctive features of American society is that most people have opportunities for expressing their views on issues. Our system with its fairly widespread openness of institutions allows for the raising of demands with relative ease and thus fosters the involvement of its citizenry in political activities. If, on the other hand, the raising of issues were strictly and narrowly limited, as in many other nations, the bulk of the people would necessarily accept the notion that politics was not an activity for them. Because of the large number of different participants, however, the American policy process, whether it be at the federal, state, local, or institutional level, often appears to be indecisive and cumbersome, and yet decisions do get made, and policies get adopted and implemented.

A *policy* is a consciously chosen course of action (or inaction) directed toward some end. If this course of action is chosen by government, it is a public policy; if selected by a nongovernmental organization, it is an institutional or business policy. Policy is what governments or institutions do, or do not do; it represents the goals or purposes of government or institutional programs and may be either stated explicitly, for example, in laws or in the statement of administrators, or implied in programs and actions. Policy may be apparent only to those who are intimately familiar with the specifics of programs and able to discern patterns and the sum total of what is being done. Indeed, some policies exist in a lack of action and may be especially hard to discern if officials or leaders wish to conceal their real purposes. For example, on July 1, 1980, nurses at University Hospital in Louisville, Kentucky, attacked what they perceived as a poor nursing standards policy in a story with the headline, "Nurses Charge University Hospital Couldn't Pass Accreditation Check:"

> If the Joint Commission on Hospital Accreditation inspected University Hospital by surprise, they'd close it, staff nurse Vera Harper, spokeswoman for a group of hospital nurses, said yesterday. That belief was the basis of the nurses' decision yesterday to continue their work slowdown while accepting the wage-benefit package offered by the hospital and the University of Louisville. About 35 members of the University Staff Nurse Organization voted to continue the job action, now in its second week.
>
> The nurses said they will continue to refuse to work overtime until hospital and university officials talk with them about working conditions and patient care. The hospital meets nursing standards once a year—when the accreditation team comes, Ms. Harper said, and then only after a lot of spit and polish and everything's perfect. We spend weeks getting things ready. She said every nurse on the staff must work those days, making it appear there are plenty of nurses.[1]

The *policy makers* in society are generally those with authority of legitimate power to allocate scarce resources (legislators, administrators,

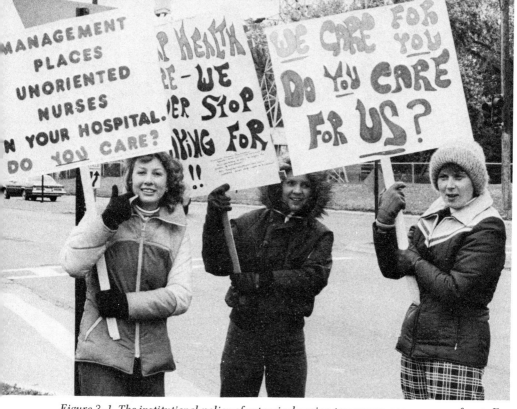

Figure 3–1. The institutional policy of extensively using temporary agency nurses for staffing was protested by these regularly hired nurses. (Courtesy of St. Louis Park Sun, Edina, Minnesota)

and various officials). The policy-making process has many points of access, however, and interest groups and other constituents can and do impact on policy-makers' decisions through the process of influence.

The process whereby wants and needs are converted into policies is called the *policy process*. The policy process refers to all the specific decisions and events that are required for a policy to be proposed, considered, and finally either enacted and implemented or set aside. Policy outputs of the system are predicated on a few issues that comprise numerous demands. Policy outputs are in some way a function of the inputs prescribed. Figure 3-2 illustrates the process.

As will be noted, from a large number of unarticulated needs and wants, a smaller number of articulated demands emerge, which are communicated to policy makers. The reduced demands are only a fraction of the total number of demands expressed in a system, and the expressed demands are an even smaller fraction of the vast number of unarticulated wants and needs. The conversion of some demands to issues represents the next distinct stage in the process. Finally, the issue-conversion process occurs when packages of issues are acted on as policy outputs. The whole process is one in which the system strives to cope with demand inputs by reduction, aggregation, and resolution. The policy process applies not only to government but also to institutions, families, and any other group involved in the process of allocating scarce resources. The primary focus of this chapter, however, will be on the policy process as applied primarily to governmental or public policy.

In the analysis of public policy, electoral activities should be distinguished from governmental activities. The failure to recognize the existence of this dichotomy goes to the heart of the ambiguity of the political and

Figure 3–2. The process whereby "wants" and "needs" are converted into policies. (Adapted from Easton D: A Systems Analysis of Political Life, Diagram 3, pp 74–80. New York, Wiley, 1965)

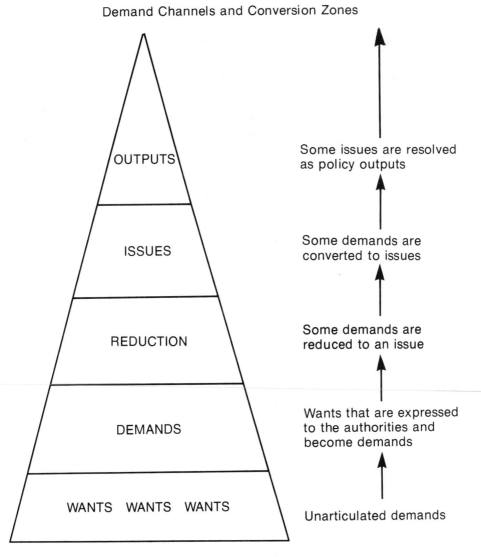

Demand Channels and Conversion Zones

OUTPUTS — Some issues are resolved as policy outputs

ISSUES — Some demands are converted to issues

REDUCTION — Some demands are reduced to an issue

DEMANDS — Wants that are expressed to the authorities and become demands

WANTS WANTS WANTS — Unarticulated demands

policy process. *Electoral politics* includes activities related directly to the selection and support, financial and otherwise, of candidates or issues to be decided upon by the public. *Governmental politics* includes political involvement (normally associated with interest groups) directed toward the formulation, implementation, and enforcement of policy by legislative, executive, administrative, or judicial bodies. Also included in this category are activities intended to influence public opinion concerning such matters as the operations of government, the behavior of opposing interests, and the needs and goals of the political participant.

The policy-making process involves four overall stages: (1) problem formation; (2) policy formation and adoption; (3) policy implementation; and (4) policy evaluation (Table 3-1).

PROBLEM FORMATION

During the problem formation phase of the policy process, demands are converted into issues. Of the hundreds of thousands of wants for which people seek governmental action, only a small number receive serious attention. Only those wants that move policy makers to action and are articulated into recognized demands become policy problems. *Issue recognition* is a process whereby a problem gains the attention of policy makers and is determined to be a potential area for action. An issue emanates from a demand, which is a human need or dissatisfaction, self-identified or identified by others, for which a solution is sought. It is no simple task to articulate a demand and turn it into an issue. That something is wrong may be clear to all, but exactly what is wrong and what can be done to solve the problem is not always clear. While almost anyone may conceive of a solution for some social injustice, the mere origination of an idea (even a good one) is far from a guarantee that it will ever receive serious consideration by policy makers.

Just as in people's personal lives, issues come up because people raise them or because events impose them upon us in such a way that they must be confronted. Issues frequently involve redefinition of values and reassessment of "reality." Generally, there are four situations in which issues

Table 3–1.   *The Stages of the Policy Process*

STAGE	DEFINITION
I. Problem Formation	
A. Issue recognition	An issue is recognized as a potential area for action
B. Issue adoption	An issue gets placed on the policy agenda
C. Issue prioritizing	The existing agenda is reordered to include the new issue
II. Policy Formation and Adoption	Development of policy for dealing with an issue and adoption of a law, rule or order to implement the policy
III. Policy Implementation	Implementation of the authoritative policy directive
IV. Policy Evaluation	Determination of whether or not the policy was effective

are created. Most common is the development of an issue by one or more contending groups who are directly affected by the issue or for whom it has considerable relevance. *Issue relevance* reflects the degree to which public-policy decisions on an issue can alter the customary behavior patterns of an individual. Persons vary greatly in their relationships to a given issue, and obviously different issues impinge on persons to varying degrees. For example, a nurse can speak of the relevance of a given issue for a given nurse and compare the relevance of a single issue for various nurses. An issue is relevant to an individual nurse to the extent that it can potentially modify the status quo in areas significant to her. The greater the potential effect of a public policy on an individual's life, the more likely that he or she will be motivated to affect the outcome of this policy. People also live in networks of affective ties. If persons realize that an issue affects not only themselves but those to whom they are personally tied, their reaction to the issue may be much more extreme.

One important characteristic of a problem that helps determine the likelihood of its exposure to an enlarged audience and subsequent recognition as an issue is its social significance. The more socially significant an issue is defined to be, the greater the likelihood that it will be extended to a large public. For example, issues that are concerned with the health of a substantial segment of the population have much greater potential than those concerned only with the health of a small group of persons. Thus, the larger the public to which an issue is expanded, the greater the likelihood of the matter being recognized as highly important. Issues that are limited to a small group of dissatisfied persons are going to have much greater difficulty attaining the attention of decision makers than disputes that can attain mass visibility.

Another assessment of an issue that is made by a policy maker is its *political feasibility,* or chances for resolution, in the political arena. For both raising an issue and successfully advancing a point of view on an issue, it is necessary to gain the support of other people. One of the surprises to newcomers in politics is discovering the limited range of decision making available to contemporary policy makers, and no matter how rational the policy, their options are severely restricted. Policy makers need each other to make policy and can rarely act unilaterally. Because they must bargain and negotiate to reach deicisions, political feasibility is an essential element of policy making. Political support must be tailored to circumstances in full recognition that for an individual or group of individuals to raise an issue requires the use of political resources and available opportunities, and these resources and opportunities may be susceptible to control by people who may not want to see the issue raised at all or may want to control who raises the issue.

As an example of issue recognition and its drive for expansion by the relevant group, in late 1979, some Tennessee nurses launched an effort to gain recognition for an issue under the newspaper headline, "Nurses Seeking Right to Write Prescriptions:"

> Tennessee nurses will again ask the upcoming session of the General Assembly for the legal right to prescribe medicines. Voting to seek prescription rights came last week at the group's annual meeting here. The nurses, representing 2,700

registered nurses in the state, voted to propose legislation that would amend Tennessee's Nurse Practice Act. The proposal would allow a nurse practitioner who has taken specific pharmacology courses, who meets certain educational requirements and who is in joint practice with a physician licensed to practice medicine in Tennessee to prescribe medicine.

There are now 200 nurse practitioners in Tennessee living in both urban and rural areas, said Rosemary Bowman, executive director of the Tennessee Nurses' Association. Passage of this legislation would insure that a nurse practitioner would be authorized to prescribe medicine if they meet the requirements, Mrs. Bowman said. 'This measure would assure that nurses prescribing know what they are doing and would assure the continued delivery of services in both rural and urban areas of the state,' she added.

There are a number of different locations where a nurse practitioner may be practicing. They may be practicing in a hospital setting, working in a primary care clinic, involved in a private practice with a physician or working in an occupational health program. A proposal to allow nurses to prescribe medicine failed during the last legislative session, but 'this proposal is more specific with the requirements,' Mrs. Bowman said. The proposal has not yet received support from the state's doctors association, the Tennessee Medical Association.

Although state law has never been changed, physician assistants and nurse practitioners across the state are now writing prescriptions. A hearing is pending in a suit brought by the Tennessee Board of Pharmacy to get a clarification on who has the right to prescribe a medicine in the state.[2]

ISSUE ADOPTION: GETTING AN ISSUE ON THE POLICY AGENDA

The next phase of policy formation is issue adoption or getting an issue placed on the policy agenda. If an issue is to receive action, it must achieve agenda status. *Policy agenda* refers to the problems receiving active and serious consideration by important policy makers. The men and women who must take responsibility for policy setting are faced with hundreds of issues that compete for their time, energy, and attention. These issues involve interests and values that must be traded off against the other interests and values involved in any particular policy decision. Some events, which might normally have low priority in a given policy maker's scheme of values, may have the capacity to grab and hold his or her attention and command resources.

There are three essential prerequisites for an issue to obtain access to the political agenda: (1) widespread attention or at least awareness; (2) shared concern of a sizeable portion of the public that some type of action is required; and (3) a shared perception that the matter is an appropriate concern for a policy-making body and falls within the bounds of its authority. The terms *shared concern* and *shared perception* refer to the prevailing climate of opinion, which is conditioned by the dominant norms, values, and etiology of an institution, a community, a state, or the nation. An issue requires the recognition of only a major portion of the polity, not the entire organization or citizenry. In addition to gaining popular recognition, the problem must be perceived by a large number of significant people as being important as well as subject to solution. To foster such popular conviction, the mobilization of a sufficient number of groups or persons is required.

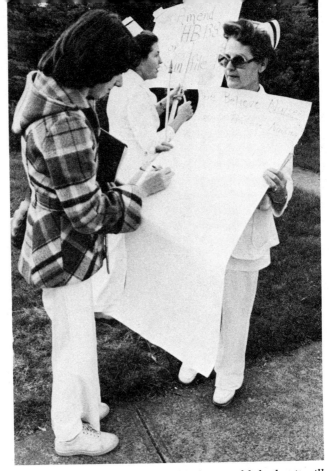

Figure 3–3. The larger the public to which an issue is expanded, the more likely that it will become recognized as highly important: Gaining public support against a threat to dilute the Colorado nurse practice act. (Courtesy of Canon City Record, Canon City, Colorado)

Depending upon the power, status, and number of people in the group, policy makers may even be forced to put a problem on the agenda.

The mass media often play a crucial role in getting an issue added to the agenda. Sometimes members of the media themselves initiate discussions of a problem. Examples include the Watergate affair, the Billy Carter case, and the Presidential qualifications (or lack thereof) of Edward Kennedy. The media, however, ordinarily are not the initiators of arousal; an issue must be recognized by a visible group of people before the media will focus on an issue. The mass media serve as a conduit for policy makers and interest groups who wish to bring problems to the public's attention. Once the media take an interest in a controversy, however, they will often play an important role in reinforcing or altering the prevailing definition of a conflict.

Political leadership is another important factor in issue adoption. Political leaders are active participants, not simply impartial arbiters, in the issue-adoption process. For a variety of reasons (its usefulness in winning

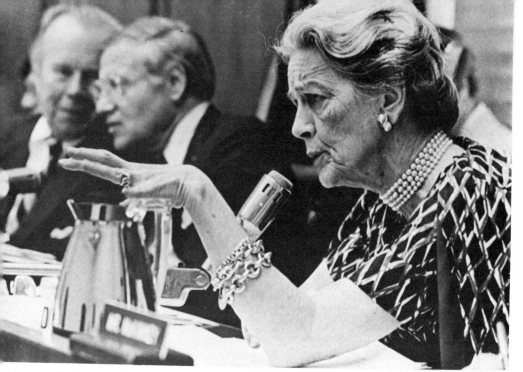

Figure 3–4. *The men and women who set public policy are faced with hundreds of issues that compete for their time and attention. (Courtesy of New York Times, New York, New York)*

votes for election, wide citizen interest in the policy area, officials' concern for the public interest, and so on), leaders may take a problem to heart, publicize it, and propose solutions. The President of the United States is the most important agenda setter because of his position. The problem of the poor in Appalachia was placed on the agenda after John F. Kennedy became President, because of his deep interest in and commitment to providing assistance for the region. Similarly, a separate Department of Education was established because of the desires of President Jimmy Carter. Congress is another major institution for initiating and creating political issues and projecting them onto the policy agenda.

The strategic location of political leaders assures them of media visibility when they want to promote an issue and places them in an excellent position to bargain with other decision makers over agenda content. Because they have almost direct control over what appears on the policy agenda and considerable freedom to choose among the plethora of issues competing for attention, leaders can insist that an issue of concern to them be considered in return for agreement to consider an issue that is salient to another decision maker or group of decision makers. An example of an issue that was championed by a nurse and also successful in gaining a position on the New Hampshire policy agenda in 1979 was elaborated in *The Lebanon Valley News* under the banner, "N.H. Solons Grapple with Nurse Practitioner Bill:"

When does a nurse cross that invisible line and start practicing medicine, a duty reserved solely for physicians? This is the question now before the New

Hampshire Legislature as it grapples with a bill considered essential in some rural parts of the state where doctors are few and far between. The House has passed and sent to the Senate a bill that could allow *Advanced Registered Nurse Practitioners* to prescribe certain drugs under controlled conditions. The ARNPs are a select group of nurses who have considerable work experience and advanced educational backgrounds as well. They are licensed and monitored by the New Hampshire Board of Nursing and today there are 80 of the specialized nurses working in the state. Many work in clinics throughout the state specializing in home health care services.

The ARNPs now want to be allowed to prescribe certain drugs from a list, or protocol, that would be jointly agreed upon by the Board of Nursing and the Board of Medicine. The nurses say they want this added authority so that they may be allowed to prescribe commonly used drugs to treat common medical problems. However, while some doctors believe the plan is sound, other doctors and many pharmacists in the state are opposed to the proposal, saying it would violate state law which restricts the practicing of medicine to physicians only.

The bill's sponsor, Rep. Eugene Daniell, D-Franklin, told a Senate commit-

Figure 3–5. Policy questions about expanded roles for nurses in rural settings have achieved a place on the agendas of several state legislators. (Courtesy of Wilmington Morning News, Wilmington, Delaware)

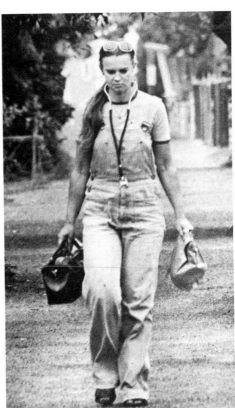

tee studying the bill, 'We have excellent doctors in New Hampshire, but they are expensive and hard to come by sometimes. There are times when an ARNP would be a gift from the gods.' The bill, Daniell said, would allow the ARNPs to provide better health care for their patients. Rep. Gertrude Butler, R-Freemont, told the same committee she had been a nurse during World War II. 'I had to be convinced that a nurse should be allowed to prescribe drugs,' she told the committee. 'I have been convinced.'[3]

In addition to asking why and how some issues achieve a place on the policy agenda, it is necessary to ascertain why some issues do not. Some aspects of the policy-making process suppress certain issues. If policy makers can kill an issue before it gets on the agenda, they and those of their constituents who oppose the change necessary to resolve the problem will not have to worry about the issue reaching a broader public and sympathetic policy makers. Attempts to limit the agenda are particularly likely to occur on issues that challenge values of high priority to powerful persons.

Delaying tactics can also be used to keep certain issues from the agenda. Officials can deflect weakly organized groups (who find it difficult to sustain pressure on policy makers) by assigning their demands to committees for study, by sending them through the labyrinth of routines that characterize most policy-making systems, by postponing consideration of the matter, by making token changes in established programs, by apparently showing cooperation (to decrease political pressure) and then reverting to previous stances, and by pointing to perennial constraints such as a tight budget.

There are several specific strategies that an opponent can use to keep an issue off the agenda. Perhaps the most prominent kind of direct attack is *discrediting the group;* a second tactic of attack is *discrediting the leaders of the group.* Opponents may whittle away at a group's base of support, indirectly preventing expansion. A third direct tactic is to *co-opt the group's leaders.* This common strategy involves "buying out" dissidents and bringing them into the existing power structure as "window dressing" to create the impression among the public, and those vying for change, that progress has been achieved and that the issue is satisfactorily resolved.

Symbolic techniques can be used to keep an issue off the agenda. One of the most successful symbolic techniques is to create an enemy that evokes an irate public response. One of the reasons the American Medical Association was able to keep Medicare off the formal policy agenda for such a long time despite widespread public support was its effective use of the loaded word, "socialized medicine." This conjured up all kinds of emotional feelings, anxieties, and hatreds among the public, and stymied federal participation in health programs for more than fifteen years.

The problem confronted by any newly formed group is often how to legitimize the group and the interest represented, rather than how to legitimize a particular issue position. The legitimacy of the group is greatly determined by the status and community standing of its leaders and the affluence of its members. Members of groups without ample resources have greater difficulty attaining legitimacy than their higher-income counterparts.

ISSUE PRIORITIZING AND MAINTENANCE

Even when an issue is adopted for the agenda, there are difficulties in getting the issue sufficiently high enough on the agenda to receive action. There is a limited amount of time, money, and personnel to handle policy problems as well as limited resources with which to try to solve problems. The policy agenda is clogged with issues, and therefore they must compete for agenda rank. When one issue gains in prominence, it will tend to reduce attention to others. The resources of the United States have become more and more constrained over the past several decades. For example, in 1950, the United States, with only 6% of the world population, enjoyed almost half of the world gross national product. Then, as Western Europe and Japan prospered in the 1950s and 1960s, gradually the United States' share dropped to 40%, to 30%, and now in the early 1980s, it is less than 25%. By the end of the century our share may be below 20%. As a consequence, it is more and more difficult for new social issues to achieve high agenda status because of the shrinking gross national product and concommitant economic decline.

Perhaps one of the most important elements in elevating an issue to a prominent position on the policy-making agenda and maintaining its position is the urgency of the problem. To obtain immediate consideration, issues must strike policy makers as pressing and in need of urgent attention. The perceptions of policy makers and the public as to the urgency of problems may be much more important than actual events. For example, if many people believe there are insufficient resources allocated to an issue of pressing concern, policy makers will act to address the situation, whatever the "truth" of the matter.

The mass media can be particularly important in impacting on people's perceptions of the urgency of an issue. As noted earlier, when the media take an interest in a situation, they usually follow up on it, generating greater and greater attention and concern and acting to perpetuate an issue once it has been adopted by them. The larger the public to which an issue is expanded, the greater the likelihood of the problem being placed high on the policy-making docket. It is worth reiterating that issues that are not positively covered by mass media and are limited to the initially dissatisfied persons are going to have greater difficulty getting an issue prioritized high upon the agenda. For example, favorable media coverage was of great assistance to California nurses in trying to defeat a bill that would have "deprofessionalized" nurses in that state. A December 15, 1979, *San Diego Union* editorial made an appeal to the public by pleading, "Professionalism First:"

A well-intentioned proposal before the Legislature would allow persons to qualify as registered nurses through an apprenticeship. We fear it would result in an erosion of the quality of nursing care. Senate Bill 666 by State Sen. Diane Watson, D-Los Angeles, is proposed as a means by which those working at the lowest level of health care could climb to the rank of registered nurse through on-the-job training. It is opposed by the California Nurses Association on the grounds that it would lower the standards not only of registered nurses but of licensed vocational nurses, a conclusion with which we agree.

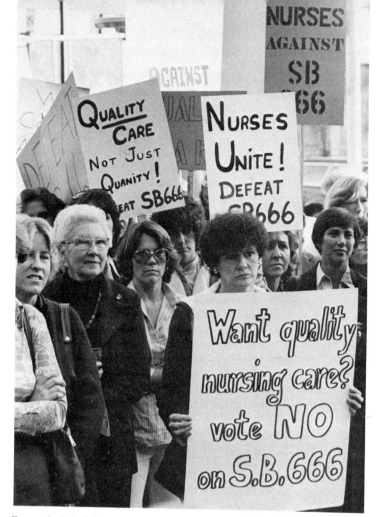

Figure 3–6. California nurses effectively utilized the mass media in defeating a proposal to deprofessionalize the status of registered nurses. (Courtesy of Times-Advocate, Escondido, California)

The idea of allowing health care workers to advance in rank through a clinical apprenticeship has a false attraction. The formal education now required at an accredited school of nursing is essential training for a registered nurse facing the complex demands of modern medicine. Such education can be curtailed or detoured only at a risk to patients and we think this is a mistake, even in the name of opening the profession to deserving and underprivileged persons.

It is true that there are not enough nurses to go around in California, the other argument advanced by advocates of SB 666. It does not reasonably follow, however, that the shortage should be eased by a lowering of standards. SB 666 should not be allowed to undermine the hard-won professionalism of registered nurses, whether in the name of providing career opportunities for underprivileged or in the name of easing a shortage of trained nurses.[4]

POLICY FORMATION AND ADOPTION

Agenda status does not necessarily imply remedial or corrective action; it simply means that decision makers will officially recognize and consider an issue. Often a problem appears on the agenda many years before corrective action is taken. This is particularly true when the issue is salient to a great number of people, but is not sufficiently urgent to overcome the objections of an entrenched, vocal minority or to justify the potential disruption that its resolution might create. For example, the question of Medicare for the aged was on the formal agenda for decades before decision makers adopted a corrective program.

Policy formation involves the development of a politically acceptable approach to dealing with a problem and adoption refers to the passage of a law or decision of some type to implement the plan of attack. Public policy proposals come from the executive branch (the President, his advisers, Presidential commissions, advisory committees, and more rarely career governmental officials), the legislative branch (senators, congressmen, their aides), and interest groups (who have their proposals introduced and promoted by elected officials).

A part of the policy-formation and adoption process involves determining whether or not a policy can gain the acceptance of those persons who have to decide on its legitimization; in other words, how can the policy be assured of passage? Through this process certain aspects of a proposed solution for a problem may be altered in an effort to pick up necessary support.

POLICY IMPLEMENTATION

Once the policy has been formulated and adopted, it is turned over to an administrative agency for implementation. This signifies the execution of a selected option, and the law or decision that has been adopted is now public policy. The kind of implementing mechanism adopted influences the character and formulation of the policy. The gap between ambition and accomplishment, legislation and execution, promise and performance, often rests with the effectiveness of implementation. The major source of policy implementation is the executive branch assigned to administer the legislation. In the case of most laws pertaining to nursing education and research, it is the Division of Nursing of the U.S. Public Health Service. Usually executive agencies have a considerable degree of latitude in implementing policy as most laws are not highly detailed and purposely leave some flexibility for the agency that must apply them.

The intent and nature of a policy, however, can be altered a great deal during the implementation process. In some cases, the original intent of the policy is lost. Thus, policy makers may continue in an overseer's role by monitoring the direction of program implementation and by suggesting means for redirecting legislated programs toward their intended goals. Congress occasionally affects the implementation process by passing legislation in appropriations bills, which limits the discretion of the implementing

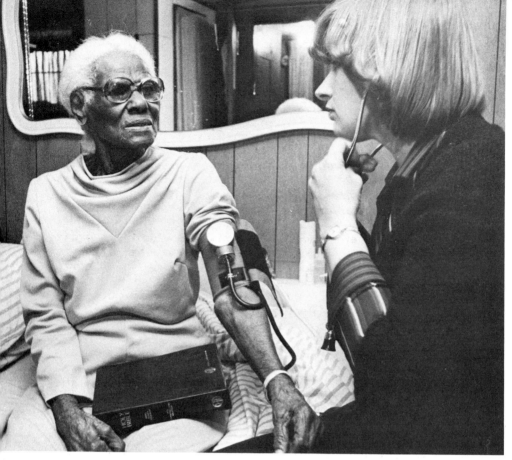

Figure 3–7. Much of the potential of home health care has been thwarted by restrictive implementation regulations. Courtesy of Fairbanks News-Miner, (Fairbanks, Alaska)

agency as in the case of payments for abortions by Medicaid. The courts also become involved in policy implementation by rendering judicial interpretations of the meaning of policies and by interpreting rules and regulations.

POLICY EVALUATION

The final stage in the policy process is policy evaluation. In contrast to the previous phase, it is mostly retrospective. Policy formation is anticipatory, implementation stresses the present, and evaluation asks: Has the policy been successful or unsuccessful? How can the outcome be assessed and measured? This final stage includes:

- observation of the consequences of the adopted policy
- comparison of actual outcomes with predicted outcomes and appraisal of the significance of any unanticipated consequences
- identification of new problems that have arisen as a result of applying the policy

There are two kinds of policy evaluation: (1) nonsystematic (which tends to be political) and (2) systematic. *Nonsystematic policy evaluation* is derived primarily from subjective and global impressions; evidence is disjointed and fragmentary at best and is usually reflective of the biases of the vested interests involved. *Systematic policy evaluation* seeks to make a more scientific or objective assessment of the policy's impact. Evaluation can lead to additional policy, initiating the policy cycle again.

AN EXAMPLE OF THE POLICY PROCESS: CHILD ABUSE

The policy-making process in terms of child abuse, provides an excellent example of how an issue develops into policy. Back in the early 1870s, a child named Mary Ellen was being beaten routinely and was found to be seriously malnourished, but church workers were unable to gain the attention of the local authorities to take action. Thus, they appealed to the Society for the Prevention of Cruelty to Animals, who promptly removed Mary Ellen from her home. Primarily as a result of this occurrence, the Society for the Prevention of Cruelty to Children was established in New York City in 1871. There were some other parts of the country that followed suit. This agency was privately supported, as was true of the vast majority of human assistance programs available in that era because the government had not yet involved itself in health and welfare programs.[5] Despite this early recognition of the problem of child abuse, it was 80 years later before issue recognition and agenda status were achieved, first within the executive branch of the federal government, then later within state legislatures, and finally in Congress.

The process of achieving agenda status for child abuse in the executive or administrative branch of the federal government occurred as follows:[6]

- The American Humane Association conducted the first nationwide survey on child abuse in 1954, which served to spark the Children's Bureau (CB) into recognizing the issues as a problem.

- The Children's Bureau began considering policy options, leading to the 1957 publication of *Proposals for Drafting Principles and Suggested Language for Legislation on Public Welfare and Youth Services* and to the support of research on the subject by C. Henry Kempe. At this point, it can be said that child abuse was clearly on the CB agenda.

- Kempe reported the results of his research in 1961 at a meeting of the American Academy of Pediatrics, labeling it the "Battered Child Syndrome." He also published it in *JAMA* in 1962.

- This well-titled article in a prestigious journal gave the problem professional legitimacy and served to innervate health professions and initiate national media attention.

- In 1962, the Children's Bureau held a conference where a model child-abuse-reporting statute was recommended.

- This law was published in 1963 in the booklet, *The Abused Child: Principles and Suggested Language for Legislation on Reporting on the Physically Abused Child*, and distributed to the states.

- The Children's Bureau continued support of research on child abuse. David Gil of Brandeis University, for example, was given funds to do a large demographic study, which was widely read by both professionals and lay people, legitimizing the call for legislation.

- In 1969, Secretary of HEW, looking for a home for the Head Start program, created the Office of Child Development to house Head Start and child abuse research as well. This created a federal focus for the child abuse problem.

Meanwhile, child abuse was also emerging as an issue on the agenda of state legislatures:

- Using the model law provided by the CB, in 1963 alone, 18 states introduced legislation. Thirteen states passed laws, ten of which were reporting laws.

- Four years later every state had passed some form of legislation acknowledging child abuse as a public problem. This adoption rate was five times faster than the average for other innovations between 1933 and 1966.

And finally Congress's attention was drawn to the problem of child abuse:

- In 1969, Congressman Mario Biaggi (Democrat, New York) introduced legislation to deal with the increasing epidemic of child abuse. He periodically reintroduced his legislation and spoke about it on the floor of the House. However, all of these bills failed and eventually died in the House Ways and Means Committee.

- Senate interest was first marked by the Subcommittee on Children and Youth's 1972 publication of a book of readings on the topic. (This followed failure of Senator Walter Mondale's [Democrat, Minnesota] Comprehensive Child Development Act.)

- In February, 1973, Senator Mondale, having chosen to concentrate on child abuse as opposed to his earlier wide-ranging efforts on behalf of children and introduced legislation, instructed his committee staff to begin to prepare for hearings. Mondale's decision to proceed indicated that the issue had been adopted, and the speed with which legislation was introduced and hearings were scheduled indicated its high priority.

- Hearings were held in the Senate pointing out the most extreme cases of child abuse. National press coverage was achieved.

- Somewhat more sedate House hearings were also held.

- House legislation was introduced by Congresswoman Pat Schroeder (Democrat, Colorado). (Kempe was her constituent.)

- The Child Abuse Prevention and Treatment Act (CAPTA) moved from subcommittee to committee to the floor of both Houses of Congress. The vote was 57 yeas, 7 nays in the Senate and 354 yeas, 36 nays in the House.

- In April, 1978, CAPTA was reenacted with the title of Child Abuse Treatment and Adoption Reform Act.

- The child abuse legislation later led to government recognition and remedies for related problems: battered women, sexual abuse of children, child pornography, and so forth.

As can readily be seen from this depiction of the policy process, many steps and a great amount of time and effort are needed for success to be achieved. The final policy outcome in 1973 and 1978 had its genesis in the work of the Children's Bureau, some twenty years earlier.

THE ROLE OF THE MEDIA

The key role of the media in the policy process is best described by Cobb and Elder who emphasize that "the underlying proposition is that the greater the size of the audience to which an issue can be enlarged, the greater the likelihood that it will attain systemic agenda standing and thus acceptance to a formal agenda."[7] Audiences react to the media in a way that underlines their adoption of the circular belief that if something matters, it will be the focus of mass media attention, and if something is the focus of mass media attention, then it must really matter.[8] As Lazarsfeld and Merton have noted, "The mass media bestow prestige and enhance the authority of individuals and groups by legitimizing their status. Recognition by the press testifies that one has arrived."[9] This is also true of an issue or problem that has emerged in the media and subsequently receives considerable attention and, more importantly, agenda status.

The issue of child abuse can be used as an example of how the media assisted in the process of policy formation:[10]

- The 1962 *JAMA* article by C. H. Kempe, "Battered Child Syndrome," set the stage for issue recognition by the mass media.

- *Time* magazine published an article on the battered child syndrome two weeks after Kempe's article appeared in July, 1962.

- Four other mass-media journal articles appeared in 1962 and 1963, and an additional 12 were published between 1963 and 1967. There were three entertainment television programs featuring child abuse (an episode of "Ben Casey," of "Dragnet," and of "The Nurses"), which reached millions of viewers. During this same period of time, 51 articles on the subject appeared in the *New York Times*.

• This media attention yielded an increased awareness on the part of the public and state legislatures.

• Professional media demonstrated the growing awareness and interest in child abuse; 137 articles were listed in professional indexes between 1961 and 1967.

• As noted earlier, between 1962 and 1967, every state passed a child abuse reporting law.

• In 1973, Congress (the Subcommittee on Children and Youth) actively encouraged media coverage:

  The year federal legislation was introduced, the *New York Times* published 43 articles on child abuse.

  In 1974, the year when federal legislation became effective, the *New York Times* carried 34 articles, and the *Readers' Guide* indexed 11 stories, its all-time high on the subject of child abuse.

• In March, 1973, the *Washington Post* (a key publication in terms of national political communication) reported a case where parents were found guilty of beating their 2-year-old to death. Several members of Congress reported that the article brought home to them the problem of child abuse.

It is difficult to determine whether or not the issue of child abuse would have achieved agenda status without the intense interest of the media. It certainly served to generate considerable interest in the problem among the public and the profession.

LEVELS OF POLICY MAKING

The scope, the visibility of an issue, and the number of participants determine what level of policy making is appropriate. When a small number of people are involved and the policy or governmental action has limited impact, one has a situation called *micropolitics*. It involves the efforts of individuals, communities, or local institutions to gain favorable governmental action for something important to them. A larger arena occurs in *subsystem politics*, which centers on a broader policy. The people and groups involved in subsystem politics are particular congressional committees or subcommittees, one or two administrative agencies, and the appropriate interest group. For example, the subsystem focusing on nurse training funds is composed of the House and Senate health subcommittees, the Division of Nursing, and the nursing interest groups (ANA, NLN, AACN, AANA, ACNM, and so on). These political subsystems exist because not all policy makers are interested in every area of policy and because it would be impossible for them to find the time to deal with the full range of possible areas. Thus, the policy maker with a great interest in nursing may have little interest in commercial air transportation. Subsystems have a relatively large amount of independence in developing and implementing policy. When the approval of the larger political system is required, there is a tendency to

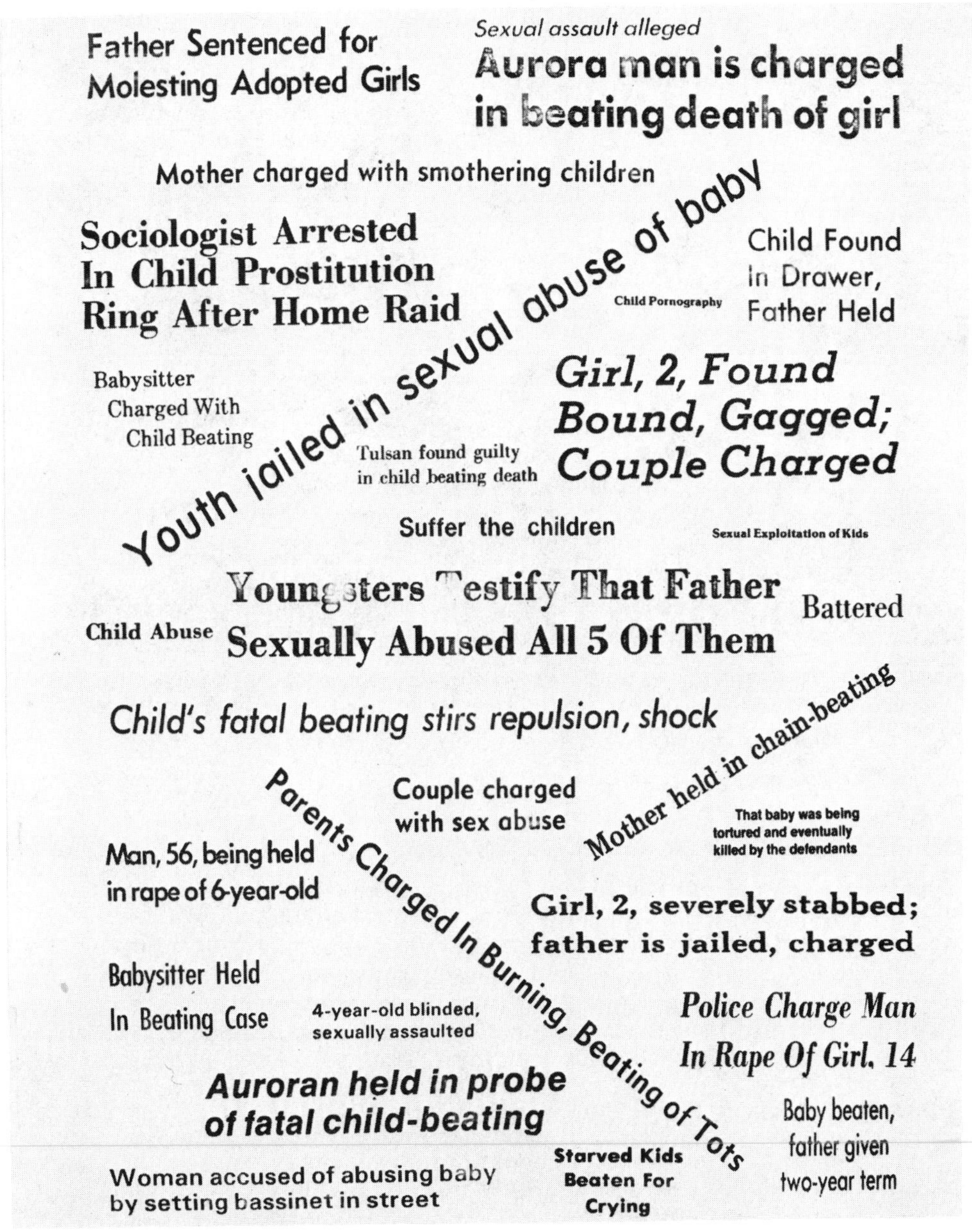

Father Sentenced for
Molesting Adopted Girls

Sexual assault alleged

Aurora man is charged
in beating death of girl

Mother charged with smothering children

Sociologist Arrested
In Child Prostitution
Ring After Home Raid

Child Pornography

Child Found
In Drawer,
Father Held

Youth jailed in sexual abuse of baby

Babysitter
Charged With
Child Beating

Girl, 2, Found
Bound, Gagged;
Couple Charged

Tulsan found guilty
in child beating death

Suffer the children

Sexual Exploitation of Kids

Child Abuse

Youngsters Testify That Father
Sexually Abused All 5 Of Them

Battered

Child's fatal beating stirs repulsion, shock

Mother held in chain-beating

Parents Charged In Burning, Beating of Tots

Couple charged
with sex abuse

Man, 56, being held
in rape of 6-year-old

That baby was being
tortured and eventually
killed by the defendants

Girl, 2, severely stabbed;
father is jailed, charged

Babysitter Held
In Beating Case

4-year-old blinded,
sexually assaulted

Police Charge Man
In Rape Of Girl, 14

Auroran held in probe
of fatal child-beating

Baby beaten,
father given
two-year term

Woman accused of abusing baby
by setting bassinet in street

Starved Kids
Beaten For
Crying

Figure 3–8. Child abuse became a matter of public concern after widespread publicity by the mass media. (Headlines arranged by Carolyn Hohnke, Nursing in the Mass Media Research Project, University of Michigan)

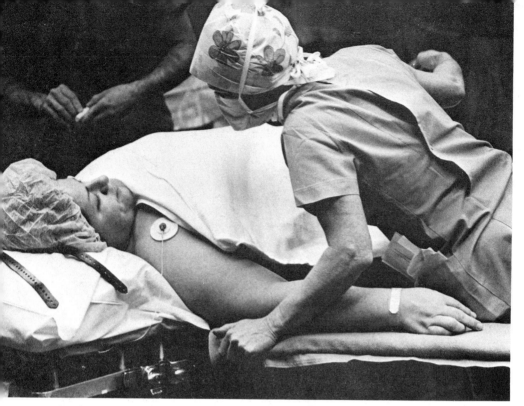

Figure 3–9. Decisions pertaining to U.S. health policy have recently moved to the macropolitical level and involve a broad range of policy participants. (Courtesy of Denver Post, Denver, Colorado)

go along with those who are considered the specialists in the area. *Macropolitics* involves an even broader range of policy participants: the President, executive departments, Congress, the mass media, and others. The policies of macropolitics are very visible and have broad public interest. Decisions pertaining to U.S. health policy have gradually moved into a macropolitical arena over the past thirty years. Limited modifications in health policy still take place on the subsystem level, but major developments in health policy are dealt with at the macropolitical level.

DISTRIBUTIVE, REGULATORY, AND REDISTRIBUTIVE POLICIES

Governmental policies designed as *distributive* are those that are broadly dispensed to numerous beneficiaries. There is no direct connection between those who benefit and those who pay. As a consequence, there is no direct political confrontation either among the groups who secure benefits or between these groups and those who do not gain from the policy. While in the long run it seems evident that those receiving benefits are depriving others of possible benefits, in the immediate political context, the politics of distributive policies resemble a noncontroversial policy situation. The immediate allocative decisions are made by Congress without regard to limited resources. Distributive policies are often labeled "pork barrel," "patronage," or "subsidy" policies and politically are characterized by accommodation, noninterference, and logrolling. The important decisions with respect to distributive policies involve small, homogeneous groups, each acting without serious opposition in its own particular area of interest. Congressional subcommittees and committees are generally the centers of decision making on distributive policies. Such politics are also highly stable, because the best way to create majority coalitions that ensure enactment is through pacts of mutual noninterference. Part of that agreement is the assurance of support of each other's pet project. The capitation provisions of the Health Manpower Act and the Nurse Training Act are examples of a distributive policy as funds are distributed by formula and the benefits are widespread. President Carter's effort to slash funding for nursing ran into difficulty because of the broadly based congressional support for this distributive program. The *Baltimore Sun* on March 7, 1979, told the story as follows:

Caught between an intense lobbying effort by nurses and growing public pressure to cut federal spending, the House yesterday devised a mechanism to satisfy both interests. The nurses, who have been trooping into congressional offices for more than a week, won restoration of $37 million for a variety of health scholarship and training programs that had been severely cut by President Carter. Acutely conscious that the expenditure would be interpreted as defiance of the public senti-

Figure 3–10. These participants in the 1979 Washington lobbying effort to restore nursing funds found nearly all congressmen receptive because the distributional nature of the program benefited schools and students in all districts and states. (Courtesy of History of Nursing Collection, University of Michigan)

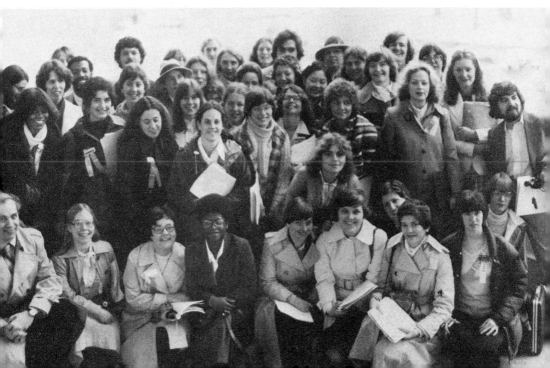

ment for fiscal conservatism, the House then compensated by cutting $37 million for the construction of a child health research center in Bethesda, Md. And, to insure that no one could accuse them of excessive spending, House members topped off the cuts with an additional reduction of $2.4 million that had been set aside for the purchase of a jet airplane for the National Aeronautics and Space Administration. Although the figures are tiny compared to the entire federal budget of more than $500 billion, the measure before the House had been billed as the first test of fiscal restraint at a time when 28 states have passed resolutions calling for a constitutional convention to require a balanced federal budget. Instead, the maneuvers over the bill became a case study of congressional compromise. The restoration of $37 million was a major victory for nurses and other health professionals because it serves as a signal of congressional intent to the President. Mr. Carter, who has argued that there is now adequate health manpower in the country, had been prepared to eliminate altogether major federal aid programs for nursing scholarships, grants, traineeships and advanced training in his 1980 budget.[11]

Because of the expanded nature of this political conflict, the important decision making occurred, not in congressional committees and administrative agencies, but on the floor of Congress. Political conflict is expanded in scope and is, therefore, less stable. The political visibility of the policy is also enhanced.

Regulatory policies govern specific standards and activities and include such examples as antitrust legislation and the regulatory programs of the Occupational Safety and Health Administration. A regulatory policy of a civil rights nature was applied in the assignment of a male nurse to a female patient. In a news story bearing the headline, "Patient's Prerogatives Versus Civil Rights" in the *Washington Post* of May 26, 1980, the individualized impact of the regulatory policy in question was highlighted:

> The afternoon at the hospital was tense. A white-haired man and his wife saw their daughter, 19, wheeled off for gynecological surgery, then rode the elevator down to double check on the private duty nurse they'd engaged for the evening. 'We've assigned Mr. Ron Jones,' a secretary began matter-of-factly. The parents looked at each other and gasped. Their teen-aged daughter had been assigned a male private duty nurse to help her recuperate from ovarian surgery. The lobby of the hospital bustled with elevators disgorging patients on stretchers and clusters of interns and yellow-frocked women pushing food carts around. The couple sat and tried to explain to the private duty nursing supervisor.
>
> They did not feel a male nurse was appropriate for a teen-ager who had just had gynecological surgery. Could she be assigned a female nurse? 'Absolutely not,' they were told. Equal opportunity laws and anti-discrimination laws forbade such sex discrimination. The girl's mother was still a 95-pound bundle of fury when I talked to her a few hours later. 'The average person doesn't have any rights; the patient in the hospital doesn't have any rights,' she said. What a splendid test for a defender of civil and equal rights, an advocate of nondiscrimination. At first, I saw her point. I felt their daughter deserved to make the choice in advance, not in the hospital, in a somewhat alien world where wondrous-frightening events occur, and at a time when a patient is vulnerable. But it would be just as discriminatory to require that subscribers to a nursing service be informed that a male nurse might be assigned.
>
> Later, the father said, 'I just came to see my daughter through a difficult time period. I didn't expect to get involved in a civil rights matter.' The girl's male

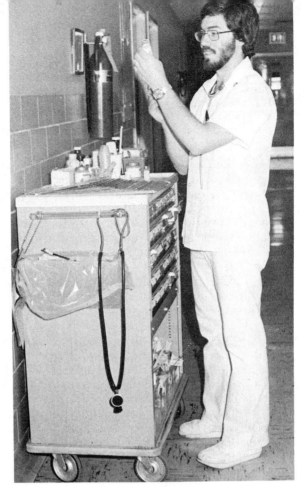

Figure 3–11. Questions about the legitimate roles of male nurses have, on occasion, involved regulatory policies related to equal rights. (Courtesy of Waynesboro News-Virginian, Waynesboro, Virginia)

gynecologist thought nothing of it when the couple told him of the experience. 'It's equal rights for men,' he said. 'She had a male doctor, didn't she? Besides, there are male nurses in the obstetrics ward.' When the young woman was wheeled from the recovery room, she mumbled before dropping off to sleep, 'Where's my nurse, Mom?' 'You don't have one,' the mother responded, having canceled the private service when she was refused a female nurse.

That night I raised the question with my husband. He thought it was discriminatory, period. A male nurse is as good as a female one, he said. The hospital's floor nurses naturally gave the young woman excellent care through the night. Returning the next day, the parents popped the question: Would she have wanted a male nurse? 'No way,' the patient, a college junior, responded. 'The nurses just gave me a bath and I was stark naked. I couldn't have handled it if it had been, say, a 25-year-old man.' Another 17-year-old I casually asked said flippantly, 'Not me.'

I understand their feelings. But the new freedoms and guarantees against discrimination mean many old values must be cast aside by all of us. Ultimately, the incident showed that one person's freedom may be another's momentary or long-term discomfort. But what is important is that non-discrimination laws exist and are enforced; the law is the law. Resisting intimate care by a male nurse may be only a hold-over from the prudish puritan past. Like the song says: 'In this modern world we're living in, the rules ain't like they've ever been.' To that I say, like singer Ray Charles, 'Amen for the rules.'[12]

Redistributive policies involve allocation of benefits to different groups in disproportion to the amounts those groups pay in. Governmental resource allocation decisions affecting racial minorities versus whites, physicians versus nurses, the middle class versus the poor, one region of the nation versus another, and big business versus small business, are examples of redistributive policies. The effect of redistributive policies is usually characterized by long-term impacts on the allocation or reallocation of resources among broad classes. Issues that involve redistribution tend to reflect ideological and class conflict. This brand of political activity most nearly resembles the view of politics that defines it as a struggle between the haves and the have-nots. Group involvement centers on major associations (groups that speak for broad sectors of society such as the AFL-CIO and the Chambers of Commerce). Redistributive issues usually polarize those who are concerned into two sides. Because of the centralization of conflict, the role of the President is great. Examples of redistributive policies include the Social Security program, the progressive federal income tax, and the proposals for a government-operated national health insurance system that would transfer health resources from private medicine to government control. Redistributive policies are at state, local, and institutional levels also. For instance, nurses challenged a hospital's redistribution policies concerning reallocation of institutional resources, as was reported in a July 30, 1980, news article in the Dallas *Morning News* entitled "Nurses Quit in Protest at Parkland":

> Six nursing supervisors at Parkland Memorial Hospital have resigned this week to protest to hospital officials what the women call 'the crisis in nursing' at the county facility. The resignations—with more promised in the next few weeks—resulted from a disagreement between the professional nursing staff and the hospital administration over budget cuts and personnel policies said Carol Lubbers, one of the nurses who resigned. Ms. Lubbers, 27, a 5-year veteran at the hospital, and four other nurses resigned Monday to protest a budget-minded cutback last week of nursing personnel. They said the cutback endangered patients' lives. A sixth nurse resigned Tuesday.
>
> All six nurses volunteered to stay until Aug. 22 to train their replacements, but they were asked by administrators to leave immediately. 'We didn't want to compromise our professional ethics,' said Ms. Lubbers, one of only two nurses willing to give their names. The others said they were afraid they would be unable to find jobs at other Dallas hospitals if they revealed their identities. 'We could not condone non-professionals giving non-professional nursing care at Parkland Hospital,' Ms. Lubbers explained. 'The patients deserve better.' Ms. Lubbers and the other nurses spoke at a meeting of about 50 nurses Tuesday evening to show support for the six women.
>
> 'For every one of us here, there are 10 others who feel the same way but were afraid to come,' one woman said. Parkland, which has been plagued by nurse shortages the past year, employs 700 nurses. Hospital spokesman Gregory Graze said the nurses who quit 'are basically people who've had long-standing differences with the hospital. They're blowing the situation all out of proportion,' Graze said. 'They've been replaced by highly qualified personnel.'

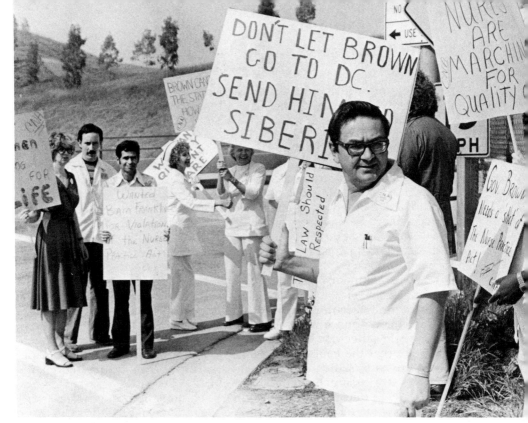

Figure 3–12. Governor Jerry Brown's plan to cut costs at California state mental hospitals by reallocating patient care responsibilities from registered nurses to nurse's aides drew angry protests from RNs. (Courtesy of San Gabriel Valley Daily Tribune, Covina, California)

The nurses and administration have been fighting over the presence of 'agency nurses' hired from private firms to make up staff shortages at salaries higher than those paid staff nurses. In a budget-cutting move, hospital officials told nursing supervisors last Wednesday to eliminate agency nurses from all floors. The nurses' request that agency nurses be retained was denied so the nurses resigned in protest.

'On my floor, 90 percent of the nurses were agency nurses,' said one of the nurses who quit. 'We were already critically short. When they left, that meant that only two nurses were left on a floor for 40 patients who needed total patient care.' 'Most of us are afraid,' said another nurse who has not quit. 'I've been told that my job is on the line. We're mainly worried about our patients. The Dallas public hears how great things are from the administration, but they don't hear from the nurses.'

Graze said Parkland has more nurses on staff now than at any time in the hospital's history. 'We have 700 nurses on staff, and having five quit isn't going to cause a big problem'[13]

INCREMENTALISM IN THE POLICY PROCESS

Incrementalism is the term most commonly used to describe public policy making in the United States. Each new generation of decision makers does not tackle policy starting with a fresh slate, able to make decisions at will.

Even assuming a relatively affluent economy, permissive public opinion, and cooperative colleagues, there are a limited number of options open to policy makers. The past is a major constraint. Former commitments cannot be nullified without upsetting the clients of the terminated program as well as the government employees who anticipate that their jobs will be discontinued. In addition, judges and administrators consider themselves bound by the precedents of past cases and actions. These historical restraints are reinforced by habitual modes of behavior inherent in human nature and a constitutionally based governmental structure and political party system that make sharp departures from the past difficult and unlikely.

Therefore, most policy decisions prescribe change in small increments, and the focus of the decision is on these increments, that is, on the difference between a proposed policy change and the status quo. *Incrementalism* is the practice of making relatively small changes which affect only the edges or margins of existing activities. Policy makers consider a restricted number of alternatives, usually concentrating on options whose known or anticipated consequences differ only slightly or moderately from those of existing policy. Because policy makers do not consider the full range of possible alternatives for achieving a goal, there is less of a need for developing revolutionary change options, and gathering and analyzing information that is not politically achievable.

Most new policies simply provide for incremental changes from existing policies; some decisions generate incremental change. Policy in a given area is not made once and for all; rather, it is made and remade continuously in a chain of incremental steps, as in the annual budgetary reviews of executive departments by appropriations committees. This has several advantages for policy makers. By taking one small step at a time, they can deal with the familiar; they can understand the probable consequences of a marginal departure from past experience. They can estimate which incremental results follow from which incremental changes in policy. Later decisions modify earlier ones as the consequences of the immediate-past steps become the new concerns of policy. Moreover, the consequences of an incremental change in policy are usually fewer and less controversial than those of a major change; thus, incremental changes require less understanding of comprehensive relationships and less effort to achieve.

Reliance on precedence and options restricted to incremental policy changes means that many potential solutions to problems are unexamined. If policy makers opened up the entire area of a policy for debate each time they wanted to make a change, policy making would be chaotic. Incrementalism allows past commitments to remain in effect so that clients, employees, contractors, and recipients of governmental action do not continually face the threat of a possible interruption of existing arrangements. Moreover, these policymakers who compromised and bargained in the past to establish present policy need not go through the entire process again. They can save for other agenda items the time, energy, and goodwill such repetition would consume.

Unlike incremental policies, highly innovative or revolutionary *nonincremental policies* are unstable. They seem to be in a state of either rapid growth or rapid decay. They require strong public commitments to reach their productive threshold and are not able to maintain equilibrium once public support wanes. Examples include some of the antipoverty programs of President Johnson's Great Society. Another difficulty faced by nonincremental policies is that it takes a major commitment of public support and mass media focus to initiate them. Advocates frequently oversell policies to obtain the necessary support, and opponents spotlight their subsequent weaknesses. This in turn may rigidify policy making by locking policy makers into an unyielding "all-or-nothing" commitment, which inhibits them from making incremental adjustments to new political coalitions or policy needs.

Even when there is substantial policy innovation, it is likely to face severe problems. Much of the time, innovation takes place in spurts; re-

Figure 3–13. Many of the innovative anti-poverty health care programs of the "Great Society" were unstable as their funding base rapidly expanded and then rapidly contracted. (Courtesy of Alabama Journal, Montgomery, Alabama)

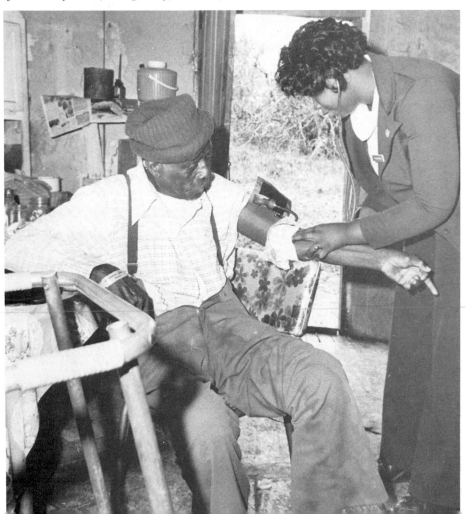

sources do not expand consistently. Rapidly expanding bureaucratic units need a chance to consolidate, to hire trained personnel with the appropriate skills, and to make the necessary organizational adjustments to their new programs. Moreover, the political problems of continued innovation increase geometrically as each new controversial policy alienates additional interest groups and members of the executive and legislative branches. Larger policy questions involve dilemmas and trade-offs virtually by definition: if a problem is clear and uncontested, it does not ordinarily emerge at high levels of political debate; it is merely a technical problem. Its solution is debated and resolved through technical and bureaucratic institutions away from the central policy-making arenas of government.

Political factors limit the choices available to officials. Some alternatives are not politically feasible because they violate important public values and beliefs, and others require bargaining and compromise. History also has a conservative impact on policy making: the constitutionally determined structure of government, inherited disputes among politicians, and the traditional procedures of policy making circumscribe the possibility for substantially changing the status quo or rejecting tradition. Previous decisions create policy predispositions and commit scarce resources in ways that are difficult to alter. Finally, the fragmented nature of government precludes a comprehensive approach that is absolutely required for the effective resolution of some complex problems.

The theory of "disjointed incrementalism" is presented by Charles Lindblom and David Braybrooke in their book, *A Strategy of Decision: Policy Evaluation as a Social Process.* The disjointed feature of disjointed incrementalism calls attention to the many disparate and relatively uncoordinated influences and phases that characterize most policy decisions. Thus, disjointed incrementalism stresses the haphazard interaction through which most policy decisions come to affect relatively small parts of the problem situation. Lindblom and Braybrooke discuss disjointed incrementalism in terms of eight characteristic features, which are outlined as follows:

- *Marginal calculation.* Decisions in disjointed incrementalism are always related to an existing base and propose only relatively small changes in that base.
- *Consideration of limited alternatives.* Only a few alternative courses are explored before a selection or choice is made.
- *Consideration of limited consequences.* Not only do decision makers look at only a few alternative courses of action, they will also consider only a few consequences of any given alternative.
- *Goals adjusted to means.* This feature of disjointed incrementalism reverses the traditional priority, which begins with goal selection and then finds the means to realize the goals.
- *Reconstructive treatment of data.* All data, all interpretations of those data, and all recommendations based on these interpretations are changeable; calculation is never finished.
- *Serial analysis.* Problems are approached piecemeal and over time.

- *Social fragmentation of analysis.* A great many people in institutions share the work of policy decision making.
- *Remedial orientations.* The objectives of most programs of action are not to "solve" a problem in the sense of eradicating it, but rather simply to make the problem situation somewhat better.[14]

POLICY STUDIES

It is widely accepted that knowledge is power, and producing knowledge can play a role in the bid for power. *Public policy studies* is the name given to research that relates to determining the causes or effects of alternative public policies. A generation ago, when events moved more slowly, the corrective effects of past experience played a very much larger role than they do today. Through trial and error and political give and take, it was possible for public officials to develop policies that took into account the objectives, estimates, and values of everybody in society, or at least the few groups who were making their influences felt. This is no longer the case: technology, events, and the impact of many powerful interest groups create such a volatile social environment that natural trial-and-error and give-and-take processes can become too catastrophe-prone for comfort before the process approaches completion.

Public policy is a complex field that lends itself to numerous analytical approaches. Some studies examine the details of individual policies, showing what policy makers intended to accomplish and what actually was accomplished (and sometimes what ought to have been accomplished). Others seek to extrapolate society's needs into the future in an effort to identify emerging problems that require the attention of policy makers. Still other research is in the form of case studies that focus on policy making in substantive fields like education, welfare, transportation, or health care; such research identifies the key people responsible for formulating and implementing policies in those fields and shows how officials receive demands and make their choices amidst political conflict.

COST-BENEFIT ANALYSIS

Cost-benefit analysis is perhaps the best known of the numerous methods or techniques designed to evaluate and then rationalize or improve the kinds of policy decisions made by government. Examples of other such techniques are zero-based budgeting, planning–programming–budgeting (PPB), systems analysis, cost-effectiveness analysis, and environmental impact analysis. Of these, however, cost-benefit analysis is perhaps the most sophisticated; it also has the most agreement over its essential elements. In addition, it has a long track record from which one can judge its effects.

Put simply, the aim of cost-benefit analysis is to choose from the array of potential governmental investments or programs by constructing a ratio of benefits to costs for each project. Because both benefits and costs of each project occur at various points in the future, both are reduced to their *present values* by use of a *discount rate* (which is similar to an interest rate).

Theoretically, in order to obtain the maximum efficiency from governmental investment, the potential projects should be ranked according to their cost-benefit ratios. They should be selected in order of the highest to the lowest ratio until available current or long-term resources are exhausted, with the proviso that no projects should be undertaken whose ratio of benefits to costs is less than one (*i.e.*, the value of the expected benefits is at least equal to the anticipated costs).

Figure 3–14. A major problem in figuring the costs of many health care problems involves difficulties of estimating future benefits in relation to the amount of money spent today. (Courtesy of Robert Stockfield, Monroe, Louisiana)

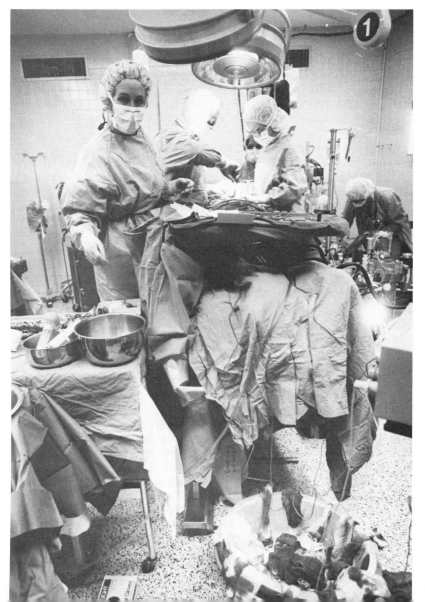

The major problem encountered in figuring the costs of many long-term projects is with the use of *discounting*. Because recipients prefer immediate benefits and value them less the longer they take to occur, and because of inflation, the amount of money that must be spent on a program in the future does not have the same value as an equal amount of money spent in the present. The process of discounting involves multiplying future expenditures (or benefits) by the fraction of the current cost (or benefits) the expenditures represent. However, because there is seldom consensus on what rate of discount to apply, policy makers can manipulate the appearance of a program's total cost by their choice of discount rates. The calculations can also be altered by assumptions about the length of projects. Because costs generally are incurred disproportionately at the beginning of projects and benefits occur after the project has been completed, the longer the assumed life of a project, the greater the benefits are likely to be in relation to costs.

The experience with Medicaid and Medicare programs illustrates the difficulties in estimating the future costs of policies. The costs of these programs were difficult to estimate initially because no one knew exactly how many people would make use of services made virtually free by public subsidies or how the level of use would affect the cost of services. An increase in demand generally increases costs; this seems especially true for hospitals and physicians. Increased demand for health care also increases both the demand for and the cost of the more elastic components of health care such as drugs, laboratory tests, radiographs, and special medical technology as more services and more expensive services are provided.

Many policies impose indirect or *spillover costs* on society by increasing the prices people have to pay for goods and services. Medicare and Medicaid increased the cost of health care by increasing demands for services and by authorizing payment of inflated prices for the health care received by Medicaid and Medicare beneficiaries.

There are also *opportunity costs*. Because the government does not have sufficient resources to carry out all proposed programs, every expenditure of resources (including money and manpower) precludes the opportunity of carrying out another worthy policy, the benefits of which therefore cannot be received. Resources spent on President Reagan's national defense buildup are resources that are not available for national health insurance, child care, or the space program. The cost of a policy thus includes lost benefits that would have resulted from alternative policies. It is not easy to measure those foregone benefits, first, because they have not occurred and, second, because there is no assurance that the "lost" programs would have been enacted in the absence of those actually chosen.

Public-policy studies are valuable because they can help decision makers by providing information through research and analysis, by isolating and clarifying the issues, by revealing inconsistencies in aims and efforts, by generating new alternatives, and by suggesting ways to translate ideas into feasible and realizable policies. Their major contribution may be to yield insights, particularly with regard to what is possible in the way of solutions, and to serve as a resource, a powerful one, to the judgment, intuition, and experience of decision makers. By making information available and exposing hidden assumptions and value preferences, public-policy analyses can widen the area of informed judgment and counter the purely subjective approaches of program advocates by forcing them to defend their line of argument and to talk about the specifics of the situation. This prevents the mere expression of personal opinions with general statements, thereby raising the quality of public discussion.

References

1. Flagler E: Nurses charge university hospital couldn't pass accreditation check. Louisville, Ky, The Louisville Times, July 1, 1980
2. David E: Nurses seeking right to write prescriptions. Nashville, Tenn, Nashville Banner, Oct 15, 1979
3. Nichols H: N. H. solons grapple with nurse practitioner bill. Lebanon, NH, Lebanon Valley News, May 29, 1979
4. Editor: Professionalism first. San Diego, Calif, The San Diego Union, Dec 15, 1979
5. Helfer RE, Kempe CH: The Battered Child. Chicago, University of Chicago Press, 1968
6. Hoffman E: Policy and politics: The Child Abuse Prevention and Treatment Act. Public Policy 26:71–88, 1978
7. Cobb R, Elder C: Participation in American Politics: The Dynamics of Agenda-Building. Boston, Allyn & Bacon, 1972
8. Kalisch P, Kalisch B: Perspectives on improving nursing's public image. Nurs Health Care 1:10–15, 1980
9. Lazarsfeld P, Merton R: Mass communication, popular taste, and organized social action. In Schramm W, Roberts D (eds): The Process and Effects of Mass Communication. Urbana, University of Illinois Press, 1971
10. Hoffman, op cit
11. Edsall TB: House solves a problem despite opposing pressures. Baltimore, Md, Baltimore Morning Sun, Mar 7, 1979
12. Gilliam D: Patients' prerogatives versus civil rights. Washington, DC, The Washington Post, May 26, 1980
13. Kenny S: Nurses quit in protest at Parkland. Dallas, Tex, The Dallas Morning News, July 30, 1980
14. Lindblom C, Braybrooke D: A Strategy of Decision: Policy Evaluation as a Social Policy. New York, Free Press, 1963

4–The Nation's Health Care System

America's health care crisis has been hitting the headlines for the last decade. The 1960s crisis of equity and access became the health care cost crisis of the 1970s, and this crisis continues unabated in the early 1980s. Economists who have watched the national health bill soar over $245 billion annually fight in vain to control costs; contemporary social critics, such as Ivan Illich, claim that health care has little to do with health and lament the insidious effects of professional control over medicine. Some of the dimensions of today's health care system are as follows:

· *The health care industry.* At $245 billion annually, it is the nation's third largest industry and includes 6% of the labor force. Forty percent of the payments go to hospitals, 20% to physicians, 8% to drugs, 8% to nursing homes, and the remaining 4% to a variety of vendors.

· *Health care usage.* Sixteen percent of the population are hospitalized yearly for an average stay of 7.7 days. Seventy-five percent of Americans visit a physician at least once during the year, and the average number of visits per year per person is 5.1. There are 1.5 billion prescriptions filled annually.

· *Health care payments.* The nation's $245 billion health care bill is paid in four ways—through private health insurance premiums ($68 billion), government programs ($102 billion), out-of-pocket payments ($66 billion), and philanthropy ($9 million).

· *Health insurance coverage.* In terms of types of insurance coverage, 132 million persons have group insurance, 20 million have individual insurance, and 52 million use Medicare and Medicaid. More than 18 million of these people have inadequate insurance, which fails to cover basic hospital bills and physicians' services. An additional 24 million Americans have no health insurance coverage whatsoever.

· *Protection against catastrophic illnesses.* About 40% of Americans have no protection against very large medical bills. Seven million families pay out-of-pocket catastrophic medical expenses that exceed 15% of their incomes.

· *Gaps in government programs.* Medicare and Medicaid fail to cover at least 10% of disabled and chronically ill patients under age 65. One-third of the poor are excluded from Medicaid coverage.

· *Rising health care costs.* Health costs are almost doubling every five years and are outstripping other price increases. From $43 billion in 1965, health care expenditures are expected to grow to $758 billion in 1990, unless more cost-effective forms of care are established.

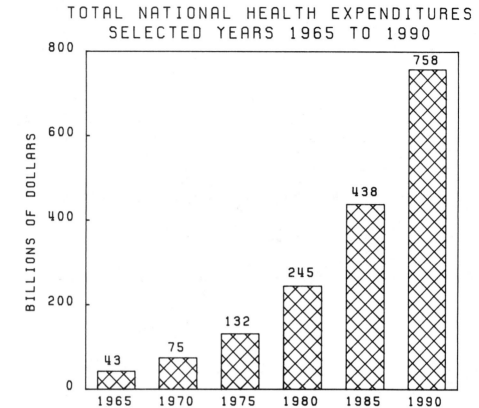

Figure 4–1. (*Courtesy of History and Politics of Nursing, University of Michigan*)

• *Gross national product (GNP) expenditures.* The percent of the GNP spent on health has grown from 6.2% in 1975 to 9.5% in 1980 and is expected to jump to 11.5% by 1990.

• *Individual costs.* A family of four spent $533 in 1963, $1138 in 1973, and $2500 in 1980 on health care.

• *The existing health care system.* Fifty-one million Americans live in areas with insufficient health care services. While there are more than 600 physicians for 100,000 people in San Francisco and in Boston, in Mississippi and in South Dakota there are fewer than 100. The current system also provides for two-class care, with the health of minorities and the poor ranking lower than that of the rest of the population on every indicator of health status.

    The advance of nursing and the reform of the health system runs headlong into the entrenched interests of a great number of powerful constituencies, including physicians, hospitals, health insurance agencies, and the pharmaceutical industry. Most state and local governments have demonstrated little capacity for effective planning in the provision of health services; the real power still resides in the nongovernmental spheres just mentioned.

HEALTH CARE ISSUES

The key issue in government health policy of the 1980s is what role the federal government should play in seeking to provide health care for all persons regardless of income. One choice is a laissez-faire policy of allowing the medical profession, the drug industry, and the medical insurance companies to handle the problem by charging in accordance with ability of individuals to pay, with some free services to the indigent. At the other extreme would be a national health insurance program in which physicians, nurses, and other providers would mainly work for the government and provide services to patients without charge because the taxpayers would in effect be paying the health fees. In the middle are various government programs designed either to subsidize private health insurance or to incorporate health insurance into a social insurance system such as Social Security. Subissues of the insurance alternative relate to: (1) whether all people should be covered or mainly the aged and the poor; (2) whether all health problems should be covered or mainly medical catastrophes; (3) whether premiums should be paid by employers, employees, or general taxpayers, and at what levels; and (4) to what extent should the government show concern for the quality of the health services for which it is paying.

Figure 4–2. Rising health care costs are a matter of much concern. (Courtesy of Morning Sentinel, Waterville, Maine)

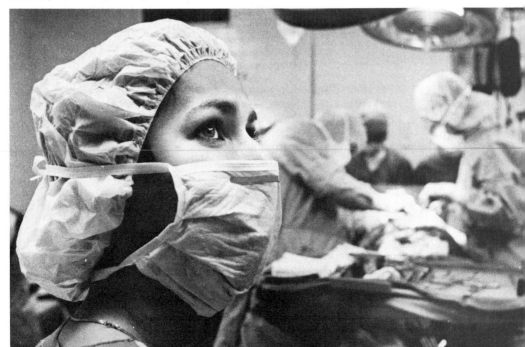

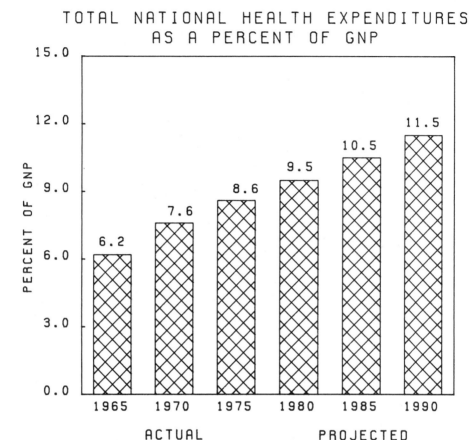

Figure 4–3. (*Courtesy History and Politics of Nursing, University of Michigan*)

In addition to health care financing problems, other health policy issues include: (1) regulation of the drug industry with regard to prices and quality of products; (2) subsidizing nursing and medical education and education of other health care providers to generate more providers, especially in underserved geographic areas; (3) subsidizing health care facilities and requiring as part of the subsidy some consideration for the health problems of the poor; (4) disease prevention and control; (5) health promotion; (6) enhancing environmental health; (7) promoting occupational health; (8) subsidizing nursing and medical research; and (9) special provisions for mental health problems, although all of the issues mentioned relate to both mental and physical health.

All citizens receive the benefits and pay the costs of health policy. The costs, however, often outweigh the benefits for they include not only the direct burden of taxation, but also the disappointments, frustrations, and losses of life resulting from policies that are poorly conceived or improperly implemented. At the April 25, 1980, convention of the National Student Nurses' Association, Jean Steel charged that the nation did not yet actually have a national health policy as reported under the headline, "U.S. Health Care Called Political Jousting Contest" in the Salt Lake City *Deseret News:*

> 'Health care in America has become a political popularity contest, with the federal government providing only shortlived 'Band-Aid' programs to meet the nation's needs. . . . The federal government has attempted to respond to the nation's health care needs with Band-Aid programs, forceful but brief, whose life span is often directly related to current politics or politicians,' said Jean E. Steel, assistant professor of nursing at Boston University.
>
> Ms. Steel, also an independent nurse practitioner at Boston City Hospital . . . [and] director of the primary care program in Boston University's Graduate School of Nursing, said America has no national health care policy. Consequently, emphasis on health care often depends on political expediency.
>
> 'When the politicians hit the campaign trail and especially during a year of national elections, health care becomes popular again, with promises of major reform. Without a national plan for health care, a kind of popularity contest begins,' she said.
>
> She said nurses and nursing students should be concerned because without a national health care policy, there is little direction for development and support for the nursing profession.[1]

COST-CONTAINMENT PROBLEMS

There are many difficulties in constraining health care costs; a number of problems converge to reinforce each other. Physicians have a monopoly on

Figure 4–4. High health care costs are seen as endangering the financial health of both patients and taxpayers. (Courtesy Sam Rawls, Atlanta Journal-Constitution, Atlanta, Georgia)

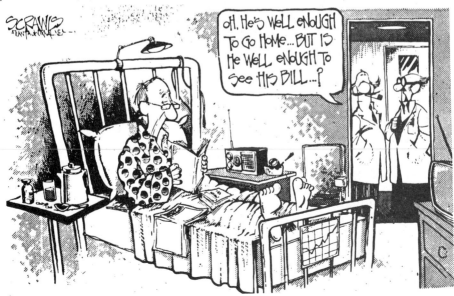

price setting. Hospital-based practice drives up costs and assists in a third-party payment in which neither physician, patient, nor hospital has much incentive to save money for the government or the insurance companies. There is weak professional peer review in regard to excessive cost. American physicians are entrepreneurs who favor solo practice and high-priced specialties and resist group practices that might reduce costs. Hospitals compete for prestige in an entrepreneurial way and pass cost pressures along to third-party payers.

The North American continent has had the highest per capita health care expenditures of any region in the world. Even though the United States contains only about 6% of the world's population, our nation spent over one-third of the estimated $800 billion that was expended on health care throughout the entire world in 1980. In the years after World War II, $1 out of every $22 that Americans spent went for health care. In 1980 that figure was $1 out of every $12, which means that the average American now works an entire month a year—one-twelfth of his time—to pay his share of the national health bill. A large part of the bill is paid in taxes. About 40% of this year's $240 billion in national health care costs will be met with public funds; health care costs are now about one-eighth of the federal budget.

Until very recently the great equation—elaborate health care equals health—held fast, but now the price of that care has become so unhealthy that every segment of the economy, from industry and labor to government and consumer groups, is struggling to contain health care costs. Put simply, health care expenditures reflect the following five variables:

· The nature and extent of consumer expectations
· The nature and extent of medical technology
· The number and behavior of physicians
· The number and organizational character of hospitals
· The structure and scope of third-party payment mechanisms

These variables interact with one another at the "micro" level, that is, at the point of service delivery in local areas; they also interact with one another at the "macro" level, or at the point of policy formation in the federal government. In addition to this horizontal interaction at each level, there is interaction vertically between the two levels. These variables encapsulate the rapidly changing dimensions of the American emphasis on individual rights to access to health services. These are:

· Higher health expectations among larger numbers of consumers
· Greater demand for a growing number of medical techniques and procedures
· A greater willingness on the part of a growing number of health care providers to give each patient the most and the best
· Increased expansion of beds, facilities, and services by hospitals seeking organizational prestige
· A tendency for third-party payers to reimburse uncritically for health care services

Much of the inflation in health costs simply reflects expanded services. Far more sophisticated, and expensive, health care is provided now than was twenty years ago. In addition, the nation's high health bill reflects a steadily growing demand for more and improved health care, expanded private and public-health insurance coverage, rising costs per unit of service, a continuing intensification of services related to the expansion of medical technology and drug use, and rising physician fees and hospital costs.

RISING PHYSICIAN COSTS

Physicians are the keystone of the health care delivery system in the United States. In other words, for better or for worse, the function of the whole system revolves around what physicians do, regardless of the fact that they make up less than 10% of the health-care work force. A number of non-physician health care professionals give certain kinds of carefully defined

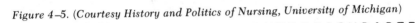

Figure 4–5. (Courtesy History and Politics of Nursing, University of Michigan)

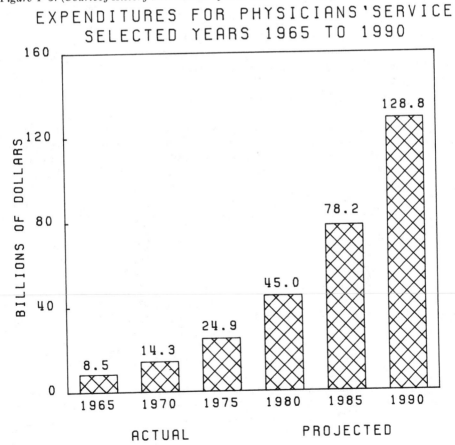

and restricted services to patients: nurses, optometrists, podiatrists, speech pathologists, clinical psychologists, chiropractors, and physical and occupational therapists. The largest group, of course, is nurses, who constitute over 50% of all health care personnel. Although in most states nurses are allowed by law to provide certain services to patients independent of physicians' orders, in many cases, in order for the services to be reimbursed under insurance policies, patients must receive these services only on physicians' orders. Physicians admit patients to hospitals and order much of the care that is to be done to them. The fact that *admit* and *order* are words of command is not an accident.

Current methods of paying physicians play a major role in the kinds of services delivered and in the rising costs of health care. There is growing recognition that decisions made by physicians are an important determinant of health resource use. Hospitals unashamedly court physicians, offer them cut-rate office space and adjacent office buildings, for example, or buy them equipment they say they need, because physicians are the source of patients. According to a government estimate, America's practicing physicians collected some $40 billion for their work in the fiscal year that ended September 30, 1980. Physicians are among the highest paid Americans. The latest survey figures and estimates showed the median 1980 net income (after expenses) for all private, office physicians was over $80,000. Only 1% of the U.S. population earns that much, and this figure may actually understate the situation. Dr. Zachary Dyckman of the Council on Wage and Price Stability has expressed his belief that the highest earners among physicians probably do not answer income surveys.

Forty years ago physicians made approximately twice as much as other professional–technical workers, the rest of the educated population, and almost three times as much as the average wage earner. Today physicians average more than four times as much as all other professional–technical persons, twice as much as lawyers, and more than five times as much as all wage earners. It is certain that thousands of physicians earn $100,000 and more before taxes, and many are in the $200,000 and higher bracket. Physicians defend these incomes by arguing that a high income is a necessary incentive to offset the years of education, high stress, and long hours that go with the job.

The practice of modern medicine in the United States received its start in the early part of this century and is still tied to the dominant pattern of professional behavior initiated in those early days: fee for service, independent private and solo practice, and very few public restraints (or the doctor-knows-best policy). That kind of medical system encouraged the seller (the physician) to tell the buyer (the patient) how much the buyer would have to buy, and it also set many of the prices. Gross abuse from severe exploitation of this essentially monopolistic system was limited by the integrity of physicians, compassion for patients, and the fact that high prices would drive the patient to another physician or to no physician at all. Current medical practice, in many respects, preserves this earlier character, especially the fee-for-service principle under which the profit motive continues to control costs. Also, there exists within the medical profession many physicians who insist that they must be in control of their own destiny. The

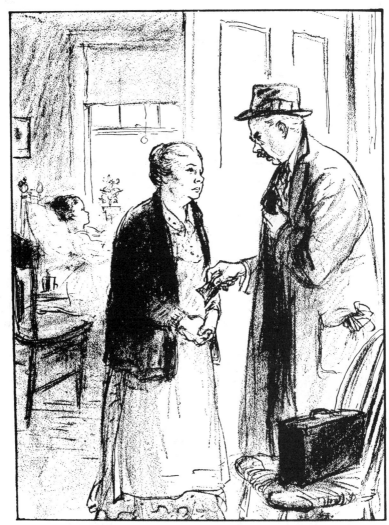

"Nonsense! Put this in your purse.

It's worth something to me to know

that my patient gets the proper food."

Figure 4–6. Today's public image of the physician sharply contrasts with that manifested 40 years ago. (Courtesy of History of Nursing Collection, University of Michigan)

argument is that government or any other outside regulation stands contrary to good health care delivery.

From a political perspective, physicians often tend to act more in accordance with their own self-interests than the public service ideals that they proclaim. The pull of self-interest leads them not only to oppose changes threatening to the status quo, but also to sometimes oversell services of dubious value and services which, in certain cases, may actually harm patients. To maintain a division of labor to its advantage, organized medicine acts through a variety of industry-wide organizations, including such bodies as the American Medical Association, the American Hospital Association, the Joint Commission on Accreditation of Hospitals, the Council on Medical Education, the American Association of Medical Colleges, and Blue Shield.

Most of the huge sums that the nation spends each year on health services is spent, directly or indirectly, at the direction of physicians. Patients buy health insurance, but physicians decide how the patient should spend his health insurance benefits. Pharmaceutical companies make drugs and pharmacists sell them. But, with rare exceptions, only a physician (or dentist) can prescribe what are considered the more powerful or more potentially dangerous drugs, not classified by the government as over-the-counter. A patient chooses to visit a physician's office, but the physician recommends how many return visits the patient will make and if the patient will see other physicians.

Physicians, not patients, decide when surgery is in order. Physicians have these powers of determining expenditure levels not only in private practice, but also in government-operated direct service programs, in county hospitals, state mental hospitals, Veterans' Administration programs, and local health department services. Physicians are in a position to generate their own income when they diagnose and prescribe. In effect, they can control the demand for the very services they supply. The physician is a combined salesman, buyer, and deliverer of health care. And the kind of health care he chooses to deliver cannot help but affect his income.

EXCESSIVE SURGERY

One example of the problem of rising health care costs based on physician-generated expenditures is excessive surgery. A condition suggesting unnecessary surgery is being increasingly documented. For example, the number of hysterectomies rose 25% between 1970 and 1975, an increase labeled "staggering" and clearly excessive by Dr. Kenneth Ryan of Harvard. A 1977 Baltimore study found that one hysterectomy in every six was unnecessary.

A congressional investigation estimated that there were two million unnecessary surgical operations wasting more than $4 billion and costing ten thousand lives in 1977. The chief finding of the congressional investigators was that unnecessary surgery is "a major national problem." It said that the claims by organized medicine that such surgery cannot be defined are "diversions and obfuscations." The House subcommittee found wide variations in the quality of surgery, based on studies by the National Academy of Sciences and the surgical community. An individual may have

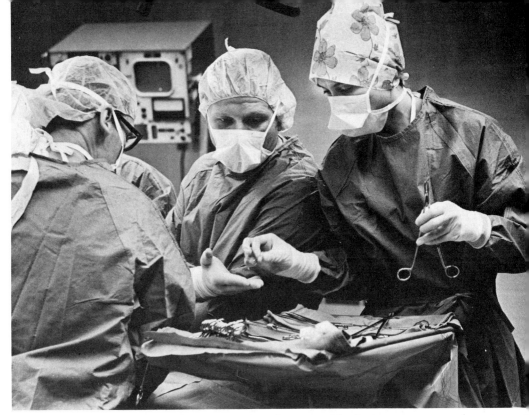

Figure 4–7. Questions about excessive surgery have been raised by both congressmen and leaders in the medical profession. (Courtesy of Denver Post, Denver, Colorado)

twice the chance of dying simply by having an operation at one hospital rather than another. For example, one study by medical specialists show that 49% of open heart operations at Malden Hospital in Massachusetts from 1968 to 1975 resulted in patient deaths. In nearby Mount Auburn Hospital in Cambridge, the mortality rates were about 22%. Open heart surgery at other major medical centers in Boston showed mortality rates in the 10% range. The subcommittee also found that many surgeries ended in what are called "misadventures" or, delicately put, "unexpected adverse results." One-third of the misadventures were preventable, and a majority of these were found to be surgeon related. The subcommittee also reported that a majority of tonsillectomies performed in 1977 were unnecessary. The study of a federal employee program showed the probability of having a tonsillectomy varied from 41.3% for Blue Cross subscribers to 10.5% for prepaid group practice subscribers. A medical expert testified that national data showed the rate of surgical operations per 100,000 of the population ranged from 84.6 in the South to 137.5 in the North Central region.

The subcommittee report also criticized state licensing agencies and medical societies for failing to control unnecessary or incompetent surgery. One physician in Chicago made a practice of performing multiple tonsillectomies for families on welfare. In one case, on the same day, a family of five brothers had their tonsils and adenoids removed. They also had three circumcisions, an umbilical hernia repaired, and a cyst removed. This enterprising physician, in preparing the children for the tonsillectomies, gave them electrocardiograms in order to accrue more patient charges. This physician received $119,000 from the Medicaid program in 1976 alone.

The House subcommittee concluded that second opinions would sharply reduce unnecessary surgery and asked the Department of Health, Education and Welfare (HEW) to promptly create a program to require mandatory independent second opinions on highly elective procedures such as hysterectomies and tonsillectomies paid for by the federal government. The panel also urged legislation to require minimum competency standards and rapped HEW for negligence in overseeing professional standards.[2]

Additionally, more than 12% of all childbirth deliveries are now done by cesarean section, a doubling in 10 years, and the rate has reached 25% in some hospitals. Obstetricians claim the procedure produces many healthier babies. But many also concede that there are added risks to the mother, and the rate is up partly because physicians fear a malpractice suit if they fail to "do everything possible." The following is from a 1979 study by the staff of the U.S. General Accounting Office entitled, *A Review of Research Literature and Federal Involvement Relating to Selected Obstetric Practices*:

> There was general agreement in the research literature we reviewed that cesarean section is a valuable obstetric tool which has increased in safety over the years and that the frequency of use of cesarean section has increased. However, we also found in reviewing the research literature that:
>
> - The scope of the studies we reviewed was limited, and only two looked at long-term effects on the infant.
> - Although various reasons were given for the increasing incidence of cesarean sections, it is still unclear whether they are excessive.
> - There was a controversy in the literature over whether a repeat section is always necessary when the previous indication no longer exists.
> - There is a difference of opinion on the effects of cesarean section on the infant, but prematurity is often cited in the research literature as an effect of an incorrectly timed cesarean section.[3]

THE NURSE-MIDWIFE AS AN ALTERNATIVE PROVIDER

The American College of Nurse-Midwives (ACNM) defines nurse-midwifery as "the independent management and care of essentially normal newborns and women antepartally, intrapartally, postpartally, and/or gynecologically, occurring within a health care system that provides for medical consultation, collaborative management, or referral."[4] In normal pregnancies, care provided by the nurse-midwife is being viewed increasingly as an improvement over that provided by obstetricians in terms of emotional and psychological well-being and in terms of long-term health. Nurse-midwifery is also being depicted as an alternative, which should be available to women as a way of giving birth. The competition between the nurse-midwife and the obstetrician may be construed as an ongoing struggle between opposing philosophies of health care: the one being a surgical, technologic approach, and the other being a more natural, personal approach. The medical profession has largely maintained the myth that birth is a private

BY THE COMPTROLLER GENERAL

Report To The Congress

OF THE UNITED STATES

Evaluating Benefits And Risks Of Obstetric Practices--More Coordinated Federal And Private Efforts Needed

The Federal Government, through the Department of Health, Education, and Welfare, has a number of responsibilities relating to U.S. obstetric practices, including

--ensuring the safety and effectiveness of drugs and medical devices,

--funding medical research and Professional Standards Review Organizations,

--educating the public on health care, and

--paying for deliveries under some federally funded programs.

HEW needs to better coordinate these responsibilities, better educate the public on the benefits and risks of various childbirth practices, and do more to help minimize incorrect use of obstetric practices.

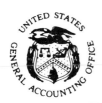

HRD-79-85
SEPTEMBER 24, 1979

Figure 4–8. The federal government has created doubt about U.S. obstetric practices through investigations by the General Accounting Office. (Courtesy of U.S. General Accounting Office)

entrepreneurial matter between physician and patient. Such materialistic overtones are evidenced by a report in the March 27, 1980 Newark *Star-Ledger* headlined, "Dozens Fault Regulations on Midwives:"

Several dozen witnesses at a Newark public hearing yesterday criticized proposed State Board of Medical Examiners' rules regulating nurse-midwives.

An audience of Essex County College of about 200 nurse-midwives, physicians, nurses, mothers in various stages of pregnancy, fathers, children and health administrators clearly favored rejection of the board's proposal.

Opponents of the recommended regulations received sustained applause after their speeches while the few speakers favoring the regulations were greeted with silence.

The public hearing was part of the board's attempt to address the confusion surrounding nurse-midwives. . . . The state has a 1910 law that governs lay midwives who have less training and fewer responsibilities than nurse-midwives. The board contends that its proposed regulations would expand nurse-midwife duties, but these health care workers charge the regulations are restrictive.

With the cries, squeals and screams of young children periodically punctuating yesterday's testimony, critics said the board's proposal would handcuff properly trained nurse-midwives, limit parents' childbirth choices, create a monopoly for doctors and boost the cost of medical care.

The critics are backing a bill . . . that would overrule some of the limits proposed by the Board of Medical Examiners.

'This would permit them to practice within the scope of their training and education,' said Representative Kern, whose bill is a revision of a measure that died in committee during the previous legislative session.

'The board is using the [existing] statue as an excuse,' he said. 'We need a new statute.'

Supporters of the board's proposal say the recommended rules guard against possible complications before, during and after birth. They say nurse-midwives should be allowed to assist in caring for pregnant women—but only under a doctor's supervision.

The major controversial issues include the following:

- The board wants pregnant women under nurse-midwife care to be examined at least twice by a physician. Critics, including some state agencies involved in health care, say a doctor's examination of a "normal" pregnant woman is unnecessary.

- The board says all pregnant women must deliver their children in a hospital. Nurse-midwives and their backers say free-standing birthing centers under strict state Department of Health guidelines can offer safe and less expensive deliveries for normal pregnant women. There is one birthing center in the state.

- The proposed regulations call for direct physician supervision of all deliveries. The critics say nurse-midwives have ample training to manage normal pregnancies without a doctor's assistance and have sufficient knowledge to know when to refer women with complicated pregnancies to physicians.

- The board says post-delivery care by nurse-midwives should be halted after three months. Its opponents say there should be no limit to post-partum care. They maintain the rule would restrict the nurse-midwives' family planning and contraception activities.

- The proposed rules prohibit nurse-midwives from inserting intrauterine devices (IUDs). Nurse-midwives and their supporters say this procedure should not be restricted to medical school graduates.[5]

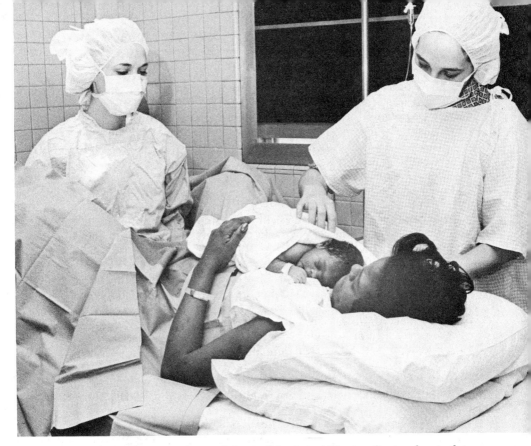

Figure 4–9. Nurses are increasingly struck by medicine's inability to adjust and assimilate more autonomous roles such as nurse-midwifery. (Courtesy of The Tennessean, Nashville, Tennessee)

Nurses are increasingly struck by medicine's seeming inability to adjust and assimilate nursing practice innovations. Given this fact of resistance, the kind of health care provided is predetermined along certain rather narrowly prescribed lines of reasoning. By predetermining the kind of care that is legitimate, modern medicine establishes the criteria for the evaluation of that care as well as any alternative forms of health care. New approaches to health care, or even an expansion of old approaches such as nurse-midwifery, which was first established in this country in the 1930s, are forced to adopt the criteria used for evaluation that has been developed in accordance with the existing medical care system. Needless to say, these criteria are often based on the existing medical care rationality, which, by definition, excludes or devalues alternative forms from viable consideration.

HEALTH INSURANCE ARRANGEMENTS

Most health care bills are paid through insurance systems that were created in the 1930s to spread out the costs of health care and in effect anesthetize policy holders against them. Most health costs are directly paid for by someone other than the patient or by what is referred to as third-party payers: Blue Cross, Medicare, Medicaid, or other insurance carriers and public programs. Few patients even know the cost of their hospital stay or other insurance-covered health care.

There are two basic methods of payment: the fee-for-service and the capitation payment, or prepayment. Under the *fee-for-service plan*, a fee is charged to a patient for each service that he receives. Fees differ according to the length and difficulty of the service. Under the *capitation system*, a fixed amount of money for a specified time period is paid to the party or parties responsible for health care, regardless of the amount of care that a patient receives. Over 95% of all payments are currently handled on a fee-for-service basis.

These third-party payments finance about 70% of the nation's personal health care bill. Almost 95% of all hospital bills and about 60% of physicians' fees are paid by private health insurers or from public funds. Although public spending on health services continues upward as the number of individuals eligible for Medicare benefits increases, private health insurance benefits and out-of-pocket expenses by consumers continue to account for almost 60% of all personal health care expenditures. Consumers pay directly for about 80% of their dentist fees, 83% of expenditures on prescription drugs, and more than 90% of all spending on eyeglasses and other appliances. These, of course, are in addition to rising health insurance premiums.

Two major kinds of health insurance institutions exist in the United States today: the nonprofit, tax-exempt Blue Cross and Blue Shield company and the commercial insurance company. Although insurance companies had begun to insure people against sickness in the 19th century, private health insurance only became a major industry during the Depression in the 1930s. At that time, people had little money to pay for hospital services, which resulted in empty beds and unpaid bills and created financial trouble for hospitals. To solve the problem, hospitals joined together to organize a prepayment-plan system called Blue Cross, to which patients paid a certain amount each month, and Blue Cross paid their hospital bills. Blue Shield also began at this time, when physicians noticed that many people were too poor to seek care and of those patients who did often many could not pay. State medical associations sponsored the Blue Shield plans to which patients would pay monthly sums so that Blue Shield could reimburse physicians for services.

In their present form, the 110 separate Blue Cross and Blue Shield plans in the United States function as individual organizations, each of which offers hospital insurance for a specific geographic area, usually a state or part of a state. There are actually 74 Blue Cross and 71 Blue Shield plans, but in many cases they function as a single unit. Of these 110 plans, then, 35 are joint, 39 are Blue Cross only, and 36 are Blue Shield only. In addition to the home office of each geographic unit, there are 400 district and field offices to ensure close contact with local subscribers and government beneficiaries. The Blue Cross and Blue Shield plans are administered by a staff of 73,000 employees, including specialists in such fields as electronic data processing, claims administration, actuarial science, subscriber relations, provider relations, marketing, communications, benefit design, statistical analysis, corporate planning, cost containment, research, and training.

A total of 85 million people are direct subscribers of the Blue Cross–Blue Shield plans, or approximately one out of every two-and-one-half persons in the United States. These 85 million subscribers are enrolled as groups, as individuals, as student members, or as family dependents. Seventy-two million members in an estimated 650,000 groups receive group coverage, while an additional 13 million are subscribers of the individual (nongroup) coverage available to all persons. Among the latter are 7.9 million elderly persons provided by Blue Cross and Blue Shield plans with complementary insurance for costs not covered by Medicare.

In addition to their primary role as direct insurers, Blue Cross and Blue Shield organizations assist in the administration of state and federal health programs such as Medicare for the aged, Medicaid for the poor, and the Civilian Health and Medical Program of the Uniformed Services (CHAMPUS) for retired members of the armed forces and for dependents of military personnel. Another 30 million people are insured by these government-sponsored programs: 28 million by Medicare, 11.5 million by Medicaid, and 5.7 million by CHAMPUS.

Under their own plans and those they administer for the government, Blue Cross and Blue Shield now pay almost 40% of the physician and hospital bills in this country. At the same time, the boards of directors of most of the Blue Cross and Blue Shield insuring organizations around the country are controlled by physicians and hospital administrators, who often hold the majority or set percentage of seats on the board by law. The staff of the Federal Trade Commission has investigated this arrangement to study its price-fixing implications. In short, the nation's physicians and hospitals have had an advantage over most other providers of services. To a large extent, they or people close to them have sat in judgment on their own incomes, because these insurers decide which fees and rates to accept and to pay; in other words, they have been their own bankers. In several states this practice has started to change. Some states, like Maryland, are developing strong hospital rate-control bodies. Several Blue Shield plans have come into conflict with the physicians who created these plans over the control and extent of physicians' fees.

Since patients can afford to spend more for health care when they are insured, more services have been used, physicians' fees have increased, and extra charges have multiplied. Evidence indicates that persons enrolled in prepaid group plans are hospitalized about only one-half as many days as those enrolled in other health insurance plans, primarily because the former discourage overuse of hospital facilities and encourage office visits and outpatient care.

Methods of third-party reimbursement may work more to the detriment of the patient than to his benefit. For example, the exclusion of certain outpatient diagnostic services from insurance coverage forces physicians to admit patients to hospitals so that these same services, although more costly on an inpatient basis, can be covered. Similarly, the refusal to cover most preventive services, although an economical short-term measure, may in the long run result in either the patient's or the insurer's having to pay for more

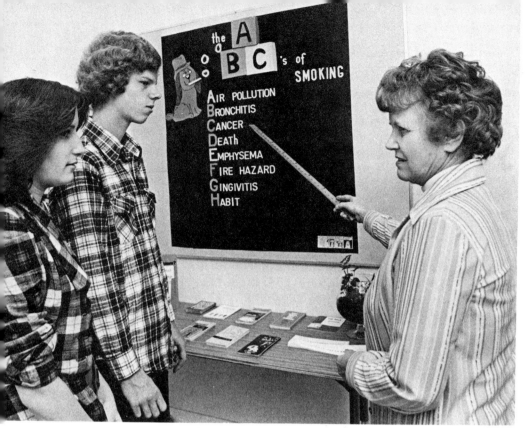

Figure 4–10. The lack of third party reimbursement for preventive health services may lead to much more expensive long term costs. (Courtesy of Daily News, Van Nuys, California)

expensive acute services. Such patchwork coverage, which inflicts overhospitalization and unnecessary surgery upon the health care consumer, but fails to include such basic and cost-effective benefits as diagnostic care, immunization, and well-baby care, seriously undermines the development of a rational health care system.

The second kind of insurance is provided by commercial insurance companies. This did not become important in the health field until after World War II when Blue Cross and Blue Shield were already well-established. Labor unions, as part of their negotiations with management over wages, began to demand health benefits for workers, and, as these benefits were fought for and won, employers started to pay part of the employees' wages into health and welfare funds, which were used to buy private health insurance at group rates. Commercial companies were successful in capturing a large share of the union health insurance market because of the way they could set premium rates. They have a choice of setting the amount of premium by either community rating or experience rating, the first being to charge the entire population one rate, and the latter to charge a lower rate to healthier people. Under community rating, the system traditionally used by Blue Cross/Blue Shield, sick people were subsidized by well people, while experience rating actually allowed insurance companies to appear benevolent to healthy people, by enabling them to charge less. Thus, commercial companies offered better deals to young, healthy workers than Blue Cross/Blue Shield could offer them. And partly because they were able to obtain so much of the labor union population, commercial companies grew enormously during the 1950s, and combined they now sell slightly more health insurance than Blue Cross/Blue Shield.

DRUG INDUSTRY PROBLEMS

The pharmaceutical industry also plays a role in escalating health-care costs. Twenty years ago people took drugs only when they became acutely ill. Today, the top 20 drugs are taken by relatively healthy people who want to alter a basic circumstance—prevent conception, alter a mood (tranquilizers), treat hypertension. Drugstores filled 1.38 billion prescriptions in 1979. In addition, 70% of Americans used nonprescription drugs, 40% on a daily basis. Drug industry sales have grown at an annual rate of more than 10% since 1967, and this trend is expected to continue through the 1980s. Sales in 1981 are estimated to climb to over $20 billion, a 13.7% increase over 1980; and drug industry sales are estimated to reach $47 billion by 1985.

At a Senate hearing on October 1, 1979, Sidney M. Wolfe, M.D., testified to the problem of excessive drug use, especially among women:

> Last year doctors wrote about 900 million prescriptions for drugs in the United States. Altogether there were far more prescriptions written for women than for men—536 million for women and 363 million for men, or 1½ times as much. When we get down into the 20- to 39-year-old age bracket, where most people are by and large healthy, we have two times more prescriptions, 2.1 times more prescriptions for women than for men—65 million for men and 137 million for women.
>
> As you mentioned in your introductory remarks, one of the categories this is clearly seen in is minor tranquilizers such as Valium. In this group the ratio is even higher than overall. You quoted figures for men and women of all ages but in the 20 to 39 age group there were 5.3 million prescriptions of minor tranquilizers for women and 2.4 million for men, which is 2.2 times more for women.
>
> Other classes of prescription drugs widely prescribed to women in this age range, and some older women, include the estrogen and progesterone hormones, virtually never used on men except in the case of estrogens in the treatment of cancer. Whether tranquilizers or hormones, a large portion of the drugs prescribed to the 20- to 39-year-old women—and in the case of the menopausal estrogens to older women—have the potential to and actually succeed in making healthy women sick.
>
> The way healthy women become victims of this gross overuse and misuse of drugs is that the drug companies, through drug-oriented practicing doctors, make women feel that the drug option is the only viable one. Do you want to be anxious or take a transquilizer? Do you want to become pregnant or take the pill? Do you want to lose your baby, have a miscarriage, or take DES or, more recently, progestins? Do you want to lose your femininity or take menopausal estrogens?[6]

THE HOSPITAL EMPIRE

In economic terms the hospital may be thought of as a plant whose inputs consist of labor of various grades and skills, fixed capital (land, buildings, beds and equipment) and circulating capital (food, bandages, bedding, drugs and so forth) with their associated costs. It is the function primarily of the administrative and provider staff to combine these inputs so that they achieve a maximum impact in terms of improved functioning on the consumer end of the product—the patient. In proprietary institutions, the administrators or owners would seek to keep the cost of production at a minimum and attempt to obtain maximum revenues so that the rate of profit per capita invested would be maximized. The management of nonprofit hospitals, governmental or otherwise, however, is not similarly motivated because there are no "owners" who seek to maximize the return on their investment.

The 7099 hospitals in the United States constitute the major capital component in the nation's supply of health resources. In 1977, these hospitals had a total capacity of 1.4 million beds and overall assets of over $72 billion. They handled some 37 million admissions and nearly 254 million outpatient visits at a total cost of more than $63.6 billion. They employed more than 3.2 million full-time equivalent employees with a total payroll of more than $33.7 million. Short-stay and long-stay hospitals are distinguished by the average length of stay of the patient's discharge from them. In short-stay hospitals, the average length of stay is less than 30 days; in long-stay hospitals, the average length of stay is 30 days or more. Most hospitals in the United States are defined as short-stay. The number of beds in short-stay hospitals increased from 1,004,854 in 1972 to 1,088,348 in 1977, a rate of growth of 1.6% per year. Short-stay hospitals accounted for 80% of all hospital beds in 1977, compared with about 69% in 1972. About 90% of short-stay hospitals are community hospitals. These community hospitals account for approximately 90% of the beds and 94% of the discharges from all short-stay hospitals. Furthermore, 56% of the community hospitals are nonprofit institutions, 30% are run by state and local governments, and the remainder are proprietary. The nonprofit hospitals account for 70% of all community hospital beds and 71% of all community hospital discharges. The average length of stay in community hospitals in 1977 was 7.6 days, a figure reflecting a continuing decline from 8.4 days in 1968, when the impact of Medicare on length of stay reached its peak. Nationwide hospital occupancy rates for 1977 were around 73.8%, down from 78.2% in 1968.[7]

It is significant that actual costs of nursing services are generally subsumed under other entities and are rarely broken out separately in hospital accounting or on the patient's bill. This practice prevents nurses from identifying the costs of nursing services and, in turn, how they might be made more cost-and-quality effective. Overall, dollar outlays for hospital care, which account for 40% of all health expenditures, represent the largest service expenditure category. Perhaps the most basic fact about American hospitals is that for well over 30 years they have had more beds than necessary. Medical economists figure that an efficient hospital should have an average of 85% of its beds occupied, the other 15% serving as a reserve for victims of epidemics and for seasonal fluctuations in illness. In 1946, the actual hospital bed occupancy rate was a mere 72%; 30 years later, it had increased only to 74%, although hospitalization had doubled. That is, the

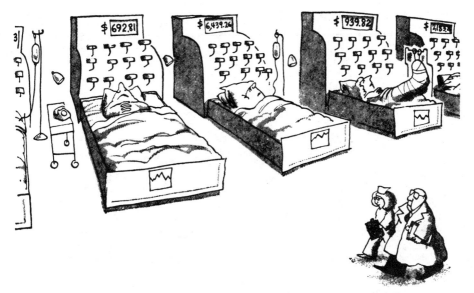

Figure 4–11. Actual costs of nursing services are generally subsumed under other entities in hospital accounting. (Courtesy of Robert Auth, Philadelphia Inquirer, Philadelphia, Pennsylvania)

already underoccupied hospitals had added new beds almost as fast as their patient loads had increased. A hospital is like a hotel, in that empty rooms mean less income, which must be made up by increasing the charge for occupied rooms. Experts estimate that maintaining an unoccupied hospital bed costs between one-half and two-thirds as much as maintaining an occupied one; taking the lower figure, it turns out that excess hospital capacity is increasing hospital costs by some 7%—nearly $5 billion in 1980.

Recently, a prestigious committee of the Institute of Medicine, an affiliate of the National Academy of Sciences, issued a comprehensive report on the subject entitled, "Controlling the Supply of Hospital Beds." As a major reason for hospital overcapacity, the committee cited, "powerful community influences" to build new hospitals, expand old ones, and resist the closing of unneeded ones, "regardless of their efficiency or even their financial viability." These influences included "community pride," "influential sponsors," and the economic lure of hospital payrolls. Another influence that the committee might well have cited is the political clout of local business interests that handle hospital funds and make construction loans and employ local contractors and building trade unions in hospital construction projects.

Against these powerful incentives to expand, the committee found essentially no incentives not to expand. Hospitals (as we have already noted) get nearly all their revenue from third-party payers, and "these revenues are provided primarily on the basis of costs incurred." In simple

TABLE 4-1.   *Prices Paid by Hospitals in Six Cities for 250 mg Penicillin VK Tablets*

CITY	HIGHEST PRICE	MEDIAN PRICE	LOWEST PRICE	PERCENT DIFFERENCE BETWEEN HIGHEST PRICE AND LOWEST PRICE
Cincinnati	$2.39	$1.95	$1.95	23
Columbus	8.90	8.02	1.95	356
Atlanta	3.75	—	1.59	136
Miami	4.50	—	2.79	61
Seattle	8.90	2.85	1.90	368
Pittsburgh	9.13	7.33	1.85	394

Source: *Comptroller General. U.S. General Accounting Office. Hospitals In the Same Area Often Pay Widely Different Prices for Comparable Supply Items, p 5. Report to the Chairman, Subcommittee on Health, Committee on Finance, U.S. Senate, Washington DC, U.S. General Accounting Office, Jan 21, 1980*

language, the more hospitals spend, the more they get. Thus, said the committee, when a hospital invests money in expansion, the risk is "largely transferred to the federal government and other third-party payers." In short, the forces that shape decisions in the hospital business "virtually guarantee the widespread development of excess hospital bed capacity."[8]

Another reason for excess hospital costs that has been recently uncovered is the varying costs of routinely purchased supply items. The U.S. General Accounting Office conducted a study of the procurement practices of certain hospitals in January, 1980, at the request of the Senate Committee on Finance. Investigating 37 hospitals in six large cities (Atlanta, Cincinnati, Columbus, Miami, Pittsburgh, and Seattle), they found that hospitals within the same cities are paying significantly different prices for the same routine supply item. Some hospitals were found to be paying double or triple the amount for a given item than that paid by other hospitals. Furthermore, the same vendor was found to sell the same item to different hospitals in the same city at different prices.[9] Table 4-1 contains the disparate findings relative to the purchase of penicillin VK.

EXPANSION OF MEDICAL TECHNOLOGY

Rapid changes in medical technology have fostered the development of expensive new equipment and of new diagnostic and therapeutic techniques, all of which have improved the quality of health care but have also significantly increased costs. Over one-half of the income of the typical hospital goes out in labor costs. Health care is a labor intensive activity, and labor is a hospital's largest expense, although labor costs as a percentage of the total hospital budget have been decreasing in the past 15 years. Significantly, hospitals also spend billions each year for technology and medical devices and supplies, and costs for these are rising at a much greater rate than labor costs. Since the early 1970s, a large share of the health care dollar has been spent on manufactured goods of all kinds ranging from furniture, bed linens, and disposables for use in hospitals and nursing homes to costly computer-linked diagnostic scanners that reduce the need for exploratory surgery, to computerized systems for medical record keeping, drug dispensing, and patient billings. In some communities, electronic monitoring systems in hospitals allow specialists at leading medical centers to monitor patients at neighborhood hospitals and advise on treatment procedures.

Figure 4–12. More and more nurses are aware that labor costs are a declining portion of hospital expenditures, and they are seeking a more equitable share of the hospital dollar. (Courtesy of New York Times, New York)

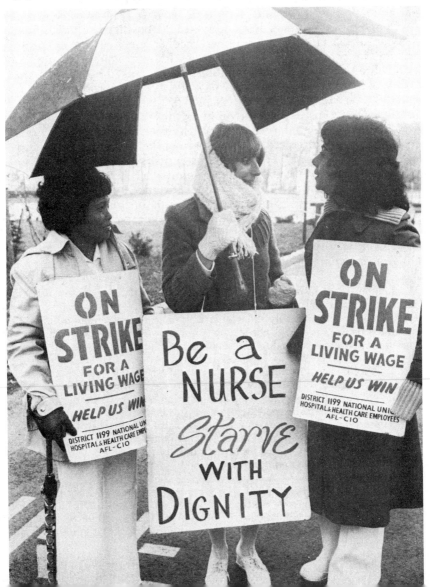

A typical battery of hospital equipment today would include a $400,000 radiation therapy unit for cobalt treatments, a $250,000 continuous-flow blood analyzer, a $75,000 gamma camera and computer, and a $200,000 ultrasound scanner, a $350,000 radio nuclear scanner, and a computerized tomography scanner priced at $300,000 to $600,000. The technology explosion has also permitted hospitals to install specialized services, such as intensive care and cardiac care units. On the average, to equip them, it costs $100,000 per bed. The number of intensive care units increased 130% between 1970 and 1975, and the nursing hours per patient day in these units rose from 14.2 to 15.5 in the same period (factors which added substantially to hospital costs). One of these sophisticated pieces of equipment, the computerized tomography (CT) scanner, has an annual operating cost of $400,000 to $500,000. Each CT scanner can perform over 2000 scans per year at about $225 per scan.

Over the past 15 years, less and less of the hospital dollar has been spent on labor costs. This trend is remarkable in view of the ever-increasing demands for more and better skilled health care workers throughout this period of time. Yet, despite tremendous increments in both the quantity and quality of hospital labor, hospital payrolls as a proportion of total hospital expenses have steadily declined from 66.5% in 1962 to 50% in 1980. While total labor costs in the hospital industry now constitute about one-half of operating costs, the salaries of administrative and supervisory personnel account for a proportionately larger share of the labor-cost bill compared to their numbers, because of their higher salary levels. Supervisory employees make up approximately 15% of the hospital work force, but earn about 30% of the compensation paid in a hospital. For nurses, the largest category in numbers, but quite low on the pay scale, it is becoming increasingly frustrating to be underpaid in comparison with other workers. This problem has been directly attacked by nurses in Denver, as reported in a syndicated story in the Wilmington, Delaware, *Evening Journal* under the headline, "Do Women Nurses Get Heavenly Recognition?":

Washington—Increasingly rare is the judge who will concede sex discrimination in employment, but at the same time will decide that to correct it would disrupt the economy. Yet, precisely this ruling is at issue in a case now pending before a federal appeals court. And because it is nurses who are the plaintiffs, and nurses are about 98 percent female, the outcome could profoundly affect the future care of the sick.

By way of background, nurses employed by the city and county of Denver filed the original suit because—as is true in municipalities throughout the nation—such traditionally male job classifications as sign painter, tree trimmer and parking meter repairman get higher starting salaries.

These jobs, of course, do not require education beyond high school. Nor do they entail life-and-death responsibilities. No matter, said Judge Fred Winner of the U.S. 10th District Court. The Denver nurses' gripe would be legitimate only if what they were earning compared unfavorably with what private-sector nurses as a whole were being paid.

And what does the typical nurse earn in hospitals, where most R.N.s are employed? For staff nurses, the top is generally $12,000 to $14,000 a year. For head nurses, no more than $20,000—this despite the fact that they often supervise at least 30 people and annually make decisions that involve hundreds of thousands of dollars worth of expenditures.

Unlike sign painters, tree trimmers and parking meter repairmen, furthermore, nurses are like doctors in that they constantly keep abreast of complex and changing technology.

The galloping advance of that technology and the increasing use of it in treatment of a rapidly aging population might seem to point to a fairer economic shake for nurses, even without a women's movement to act as impetus. Not so. A new category of health professionals, known as physicians' assistants, is just part of the evidence that the reverse is true.

His duties and responsibilities—physicians' assistants are about 98 percent male—are, if anything, less onerous than those of the so-called "clinical nurse." But the P.A. qualifies for his title by having been a military medical corpsman, or having had equivalent on-the-job experience, whereas she must usually have, in addition to more experience, at least a B.S. in nursing degree. And not only does his entry salary (after brief apprenticeship training) start thousands of dollars above hers, but her maximum compensation never equals his.

Strictly speaking, none of this is coincidence. Rather, it is a vestige of the past when the only jobs open to most women were teaching and nursing and when female careers smacked heavily of what the American Nurses' Association calls the 'you'll get your reward in heaven' philosophy. The question is does historical precedent serve either nurses or society?[10]

PRESIDENT'S HOSPITAL COST-CONTAINMENT PROPOSAL

Hospital costs grew rapidly during the 1970s. From 1968 to 1978, costs grew at an average annual rate of 15%. This growth increased the burden of health care costs on individuals, employers who paid health insurance premiums, state and local governments, and the federal government. In response to this problem, the Carter administration proposed hospital cost-containment legislation in 1977. Although this bill was not passed by the Congress, the hospital industry implemented a voluntary cost-containment program in 1978. In 1979 the Congress again considered hospital cost-containment legislation proposed by the administration. On March 6, 1979, the administration sent the Hospital Cost Containment Act of 1979 to the Congress, an act which would have specified guidelines for increases in hospital expenditures and imposed revenue control on hospitals that failed to keep within them. The guidelines—based on the inflation rate for goods and services purchased by hospitals, population growth, and intensity-of-service factors—would have allowed hospitals to increase their expenditures by about 11.3% in 1979. If implemented, the proposal was supposed to generate substantial savings for those who paid for hospital care and reduce the increase in the Consumer Price Index (CPI).

According to the Carter administration spokespersons, there were many reasons for the rampant inflation in hospital costs. Demand for health and hospital services had of course risen since the passage of Medicare and Medicaid in the mid-sixties. And hospitals, like other institutions, were affected by general inflation in the economy. But the extraordinary inflation in the hospital sector was primarily due to inflationary pressures that were built right into the system, pressures that cost-containment legislation would forcefully counter. Ninety percent of all hospital bills were paid by

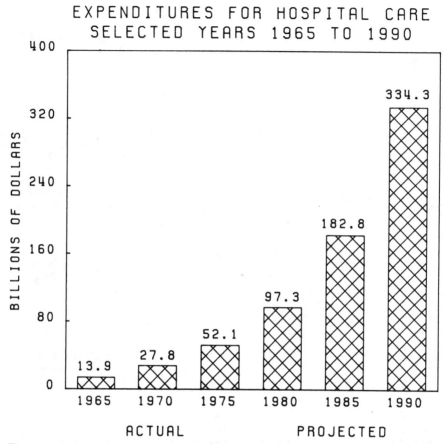

Figure 4–13. (*Courtesy of History and Politics of Nursing, University of Michigan*)

third parties. Thus, neither the consumer (the patient) nor the provider (the physician in the hospital) felt the pinch of rising costs. Payments to hospitals were primarily cost-plus payments; that is, most payments were based on cost and insurance coverage, whatever service had been provided. There were few incentives in such a system to hold down costs, and the more hospitals spent the more they received.

Carter administration officials insisted that examples of waste and inefficiency in the hospital industry were plentiful. Literally billions of dollars could be saved each year in the industry by cost-effective management, and without affecting the quality of care. Increased productivity and efficiency were thus the critical area in which savings from hospital cost containment could be realized. Historically, hospitals had expanded services and introduced new technology with little effort to offset these additional costs. Major reforms could yield savings such as the following:

A. *Hospital control savings—potential sources of annual savings in the hospital industry.*

Eliminating 130,000 excess beds	$4 billion
Replacing inefficient supply purchasing practices	$1⅓ billion
Eliminating excess CT scanners	$200 million
Eliminating energy waste	$1¼ billion

B. *Joint hospital and medical staff control savings—potential sources of annual savings in the hospital industry.*

Eliminating unnecessary weekend admissions	$1½ billion
Eliminating routine admission diagnostic tests for nonsurgical patients	$300 million
Decreasing average lengths of stay nationwide to the average in West Coast hospitals	$2½ billion
Eliminating unnecessary roentgenograms	$435 million[11]

Hospital administrators repeatedly argued that hospital cost increases were primarily the result of changes in the following cost components: the inflation in the general economy; the imposition of government-mandated programs; the introduction of and changing amount and type of services and technology; patient utilization patterns; and the hospital's increase in complexity and its coordination needs. A cost-containment program to reduce hospital costs without disrupting necessary health services would have to be designed with full recognition of the hospital's limited ability to influence or control many of its cost components. This was especially true of the inflation level present in the economy and the requirements of government-mandated programs. These cost-increase factors were beyond the control of hospitals, individually and collectively. Also beyond the control of hospitals were the following unclear and inconsistent policies and priorities that confronting them:

- Practitioners were encouraged to "optimize" the use of hospital services to contain costs while large malpractice awards to patients with adverse outcomes encouraged practitioners to request more professional consultations and ancillary services and dramatically increased malpractice premiums.
- Regionalization of health services, which concentrated expensive services in a few hospitals, was sought while reimbursement programs applied uniform payment levels without recognition of case differences.
- Health-planning regulations for capital expenditures in institutions were undertaken while similar expenditures in physicians' offices were excluded from review and approval.
- Free-care and below-cost care were mandated for public patients while third-party payers and consumer groups pressured the hospital to prevent charges from exceeding costs for paying patients.
- Certification and licensure were sought and frequently legislated for non-physician health care professionals and technical personnel while hospitals were encouraged to use fewer but more flexible personnel.

- Primary care emphasizing ambulatory and preventive services was sought while outpatient clinics lost money, and special program funds for catastrophic illness care were more easily obtainable and abundant.
- Utilization controls to optimize the use of hospital services were sought while fully insured patients wanted to remain in the hospital through complete recovery and while chronic patients had to remain until a long-term bed was available.
- Optimum standards for care were sought while high costs were opposed.
- Expanded health benefit programs were incorporated in collective bargaining agreements while consumer and industrial groups opposed increases in health insurance premiums.

In short, a day of hospital care in 1979 was a product that had been continually changing. The rising cost of hospital care was therefore not comparable to price increases for other goods and services that consumers purchased. Moreover, the changing character of the product indicated that cost increases should not be interpreted as evidence of inefficiency or a low rate of technical progress.

With these two opposing viewpoints, hospital cost control legislation was difficult to sell because its benefits were relatively remote, and because most members of Congress were sympathetic to its target—hospitals. The administration claimed overall savings of more than $40 billion dollars over 5 years from the plan, but because so many Americans were shielded from

Figure 4–14. Hospital administrators stress that today's hospital care is far different from the hospital care delivered 10 or 20 years ago, and this difference must cost more. (Courtesy of Robert Stockfield, Monroe, Louisiana)

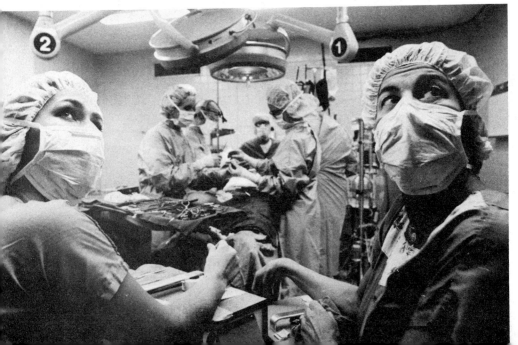

massive hospital bills by health insurance, the payoff was hard to dramatize. By casting the bill as a prime anti-inflation measure, President Carter had hoped to give it a broader appeal than in 1977, when he had pushed the measure as a prerequisite to national health insurance.

Lobbying against the bill was led by the two major industry associations, the Federation of American Hospitals and the American Hospital Association, along with the American Medical Association. They argued that Carter's proposal would be a regulatory burden, putting an excessive costly record-keeping burden on hospitals, would unfairly single out the hospital industry for price controls, and was unnecessary because the industry's "voluntary effort" campaign was already bringing down the rate of hospital cost inflation. They also suggested the bill would harm health care in the United States by forcing hospitals to curtail services in order to keep down costs. According to hospital spokespersons, the hospitals' voluntary effort had lowered the rate of the increase in hospital costs to 12.8% in 1978 and 13.3% in 1979. Opponents also insisted that Carter wanted the bill for political reasons and that any potential savings would be far outweighed by the bill's two major defects: it was more government regulation, and it would freeze medical technology at its present status, closing off future growth and development.

The House on November 15, 1979, emphatically rejected President Carter's hospital cost-containment bill, adopting instead a very weak substitute measure. The House turned down cost controls entirely by a 234 to 166 vote and, with 99 Democrats voting against the President, adopted a substitute that simply created a national study commission on hospital costs and authorized some funds for state cost control programs. The White House called the November 15th vote to reject mandatory cost controls "a blow to the fight against inflation."[12]

HEALTH-PLANNING EFFORTS

On another front, the federal government had embarked on a series of programs in the 1960s to support and integrate health-planning activities at the regional, state, and local levels, including the regional, or areawide, voluntary health-facilities planning agencies (1964), the Regional Medical Programs (1965), and the Comprehensive Health Planning Program (1966). Although many of these programs had made impressive contributions, their efforts had also been marked by austere financing, overlap and duplication of responsibilities, and absence of a sufficient mandate for implementation of their plans. In addition, there had been inadequate coordination of maintenance organizations from capital expenditure review. The legislation continued to emphasize three primary goals as follows: (1) to curb rising health care costs, (2) to improve health care quality, and (3) to increase access to health care services, particularly for underserved populations.

The Health Systems Agencies, established in 1975, are funded through grants on the basis of the latest census population of their health service areas. Direct grants have averaged 45¢ to 48¢ per capita. Minimum funding is prescribed by statute and has been raised over the past few years from $175,000 in 1979 to $225,000 in 1980 and $240,000 in 1981. In addition to the per capita funding, agencies may earn up to an additional 25¢ per capita in federal funds to equal state and local funds collected during the previous budget year. At the present time, 199 of the 205 local Health Planning Agencies have achieved full approval by the federal government.

The primary responsibility of State Health Planning and Development Agencies is twofold: (1) to develop a statewide health plan which is based on and incorporates provisions of each local health systems plan, and (2) to certify the genuine need for the services, facility, or equipment requested and to issue certificates-of-need. Determination of appropriate levels of cost, quality, necessity, accessibility, and continuity of institutional health care services are the explicit responsibilities of these agencies. They attempt to link health planning with health regulation. By 1980 there were 57 State Health Planning and Development Agencies, including all of the states and territories of the United States, and 35 of these state agencies had achieved full designation. The major obstacles to achieving full designation at the state level included the lack of a federally acceptable certificate-of-need program, the absence of a statewide health coordinating council and the inadequacy of a preliminary state health plan. Most states, however, were moving rapidly to meet these requirements.

The Health Planning program was created to improve the delivery of health services, contain costs, and improve the health of the nation through the establishment of a nationwide network of Health Systems Agencies (HSAs) and State Health Planning and Development Agenices (SHPDAs) responsible for health planning in their respective areas. Legislation for the Health Planning and Resources Development Program (PL 93-641) was signed in January, 1975. Much of the program's first five years was spent in helping to establish the nationwide network of Health Systems Agencies and State Health Planning and Development Agencies, which were to carry the principal responsibility for health planning and resources development for their areas. During this time, Health Systems Agencies were established in 205 geographic regions in 57 states, including 8 low-population states and territories which, were to carry out both HSA and SHPDA functions.[13]

In October 1979, the health-planning legislation was extended for an additional three years and amended to improve the functioning of the program (PL 96-79). Major changes in the legislation included: (1) highlighting the role of competition and the allocation of health services; (2) requiring coordination of state health plans with other planning, most particularly in the area of mental health, drug abuse, and alcoholism; (3) strengthening the role of the governor; and (4) revising the certificate-of-need program, which governed large expenditures for new buildings and equipment. Each state receives a minimum of 1.25% and each territory .5% of the total appropriation. Any state may receive up to 75% of its total operating budget. The remaining portion of the budget is funded through direct state or territorial funds. In 1981, the average grant to states was approximately $877,000.

A major focus of the planning agencies is on reducing the rapid increase in health care costs. By influencing the number and kinds of capital investments made and the kinds of health facilities built, they contribute to the control of the rapid rise in health care expenditures. The most singular piece of evidence showing that Health Systems Agencies and State Health Planning and Development Agencies have been effective in reducing the growth rate of health care costs appeared in the results of a 1979 American Health Planning Association survey, which showed that over the previous two-year period, Health Planning Agencies had denied or disapproved of $2.3 billion out of a total of $10.6 billion in proposed hospital and nursing-home projects formally reviewed.

In addition, over $1 billion in proposed capital expenditures had been discouraged, projects for which applicants never submitted certificate-of-need requests because there was a clear indication they were unlikely to be approved. As a result, some 3700 hospital and 20,000 nursing-home beds were not added or replaced from 1979 to 1980. (From a program cost-effectiveness standpoint, the rate of return had been $8 in capital expenditures denied by health-planning agencies for each federal dollar granted them.) The $2.3 billion in capital investments denied or discouraged, and their associated debt service costs, would of course have added to the nation's and average patient's hospital charges, had they been made. This $2.3 billion figure also excluded the estimated annual operating expenses of projects denied, which, within a few years, would have far exceeded the proposed capital outlays.

PROGRAMS FOR UNDERSERVED POPULATIONS

There are significant disparities in the use of certain health services by persons living in urban areas and those living in rural areas. In 1980, more than 51 million people lived in approximately 7743 urban and rural underserved areas, of which 23.6 million persons were in urban and 27.6 million in rural locations. The disparity in health care has been attributed in part to the fact that rural people have far fewer health providers available to attend to their needs than do people in urban areas. Data for the mid-1970s on physician office visits, for example, showed that metropolitan people visited physicians 5.2 times a year whereas people in non-metropolitan areas visited physicians 4.5 times a year. Inner city residents also have limited access to private physicians. A major share of their care is provided through hospital outpatient departments, with these departments becoming a major source of care as outpatient visits increased from 125 million visits in 1964 to over 250 million visits in 1979.

One program designed to alleviate this problem was the Community Health Centers (CHC) program, established in 1962. The purpose of this program is to provide persons in rural and urban medically underserved areas with comprehensive high-quality health care in a community-based setting, regardless of ability to pay. The program develops health-services-delivery capacity by awarding project grants to public and nonprofit entities to fund ambulatory health care projects. These projects provide primary health care services, including diagnostic, treatment, consultative, referral and other services rendered by a physician, nurse practitioner, or physician-extender; preventive health services including nutritional as-

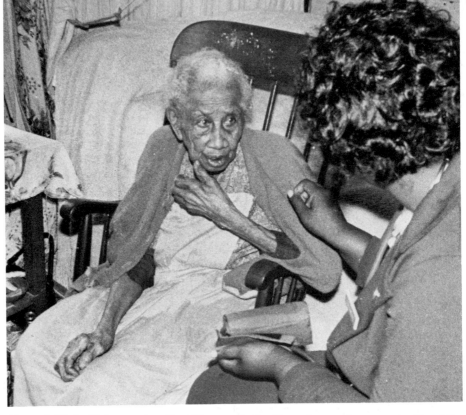

Figure 4–15. In 1980, more than 51 million people lived in underserved areas and suffered the results of less adequate health care. (Courtesy of Alabama Journal, Montgomery, Alabama)

sessment, diagnostic laboratory services, and emergency medical services; and supplemental services including home health care, dental treatment, health education, and vision screening.

The Area Health Education Center (AHEC) program was also created to address problems of geographic maldistribution and overspecialization of health professionals by fostering changes in the pattern of education and the educational environment. The original ten AHECs were started in 1972 and, as of 1980, they were in their ninth year of support; another eleven AHECs are in their third to fifth year of support. Of the twenty-one supported AHECs, six are rural, three are urban, four are rural/urban and eight are statewide and a combination of rural and/or urban. Altogether a population of approximately 58 million people are or have been served by this program. Through this effort, federal funds are provided to medical and osteopathic schools for the purpose of decentralizing education for medical and other health professions. Funds are also given to primary health-manpower shortage areas to improve the coordination and use of existing resources. Primary care training in graduate, undergraduate, and continuing-education offerings in medicine, dentistry, nursing, and other health professions is emphasized in this federal program.

The purpose of the Migrant Health Program, established in 1965, is to provide an adequate level of health care services for migrant and seasonal farm workers and their families. The migrant and seasonal farm workers population in 1980 is estimated to be 2,700,000 persons, of whom 700,000 are migrants and 2,000,000 are seasonal farm workers. Financial assistance is provided through project grants to public and nonprofit private entities to establish and support health services for migrants, such as physician services, diagnostic, laboratory, and radiologic services, preventive health services, emergency medical services, and transportation services, as well as outreach and environmental health services. Also, supplemental services, such as home health, dental health, and inpatient and outpatient hospital services are provided as appropriate. Priority is given to applicants in areas heavily populated with migrant and seasonal farm workers.

A much larger program aimed at underserved populations is the National Health Service Corps (NHSC), established in 1970. Its goal is to improve the delivery of health services in health shortage areas and to reduce the number of such areas by the appropriate placement of health professionals and resources. The NHSC budget provides salaries and related payroll costs for federally employed health professionals and support costs required to assist communities in developing NHSC sites in shortage areas. Monies from the budget are also used for recruiting and assigning NHSC health professionals to these areas and maintaining health care delivery systems in these locations.

The National Health Service Corps can assist only those areas that are federally designated as health manpower shortage areas. Designations can be given to geographic areas, population groups (such as American Indians, Alaskan natives, and migrant populations) or facilities (such as correctional institutions and public or nonprofit medical facilities). At present most designations are for geographic areas. A geographic area is designated as having a shortage of primary health care providers if the following two criteria are met: (1) the area is a rational area for the delivery of primary health care services; that is, either the area has a population to primary-care physician ratio of at least 3500 to 1, or the area has a population to primary-care physician ratio better than 3500 to 1, but worse than 3000 to 1, and has either unusually high needs for primary care services or insufficient capacity of existing primary care providers; and (2) primary care providers in contiguous areas are overutilized, excessively distant, or inaccessible to the population of the area under consideration.

Criteria for the designation of population groups and facilities are similar to those for geographic areas; however, the criteria are based on factors that are specific, such as access barriers preventing certain kinds of population groups, for example Medicaid patients, from using an area's primary care providers, or the number of inmates in a correctional institution in relation to the number of primary care providers.

When the Corps started in the early 1970s, physicians often were assigned by themselves to isolated rural areas. This was done to meet the pressing need for health professionals in a number of areas. However, it soon became apparent that the reasons that there were no physicians in such areas were the same as those that resulted in the loss of the Corps assignees placed alone in these areas—professional isolation, family pressures, constant overwork, and no opportunities for professional education or stimulation. Professional dissatisfaction with these demands contributed to the poor retention of Corps assignees upon completion of these assignments; only 3% of such assignees chose to remain on site. The general approach, thereafter, was to develop sites in a way that would assure that some of the initial problems were minimized. In many instances, this required assigning more than one provider to a site. Ultimately, this approach was also discarded. What was perceived as needed for the retention of professionals and the effective delivery of services was the organization of systems of care with an adequate supply of corps physicians, nurses, dentists, and others and the infusion of grant dollars. This approach then became the first priority in placing corps assignees.

The NHSC Scholarship Program, established in 1972, two years after the corps began functioning with volunteers, was intended to influence a more effective distribution of nurses, physicians, dentists, and certain other health professional personnel practicing in rural or inner-city shortage areas. It achieves this end by requiring one year of full-time clinical practice in a health manpower shortage area in return for each year of scholarship support received. A minimum of two years of service is required and can be met either by serving as a salaried member of the National Health Service Corps or by practicing privately in a shortage area. Nurses and physicians and other providers fill the service requirement by either becoming commissioned officers in the U.S. Public Health Service or working under the

Figure 4–16. The National Health Service Corps places nurses, physicians, dentists, and other health providers in acutely underserved areas such as Indian reservations. (Courtesy of U.S. Public Health Service)

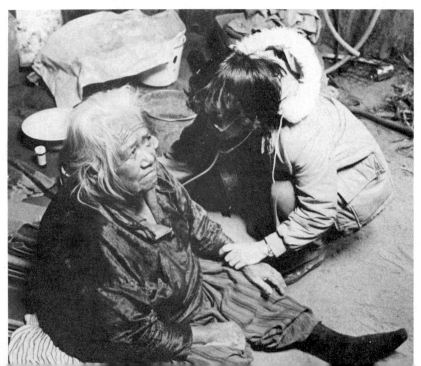

Civil Service Personnel System. In 1980, nurses who become commissioned officers receive anywhere from $12,486 to $14,498 per year whereas those entering the National Health Service Corps under the Civil Service System receive anywhere between $10,507 to $15,920, depending on educational degree and continuing education. Scholarship benefits provide payment to the school of all tuition and required fees, plus twelve monthly stipends of $485 (adjusted annually to federal salary changes) for the student's living expenses, and an additional amount to cover all reasonable educational expenses, including fees, books, equipment, and laboratory expenses.

In 1976, the first NHSC scholarship recipients were assigned to shortage areas in repayment for their scholarship awards. The number of NHSC scholarship recipients serving in shortage areas increased from 17 in 1976 to 696 in 1979. Using both the voluntary recruitment and the scholarship placement programs, the NHSC field strength grew from 596 in 1976 to 1824 in 1979. In 1979, these 1824 health professionals were providing services to 818,025 people in 875 sites with a federal program funding level of $63 million. By May 1979, there had been 1407 primary care shortage areas, designated along with 676 dental shortage areas, and 90 psychiatric shortage areas. During 1979, under the expanded definition of shortage areas, six NHSC health professionals were assigned to correctional institutions to provide health care services to incarcerated populations.

Nurses recruited for National Health Service Corps scholarships are provided advanced education to enhance their primary care skills and are used in primary care shortage areas. Most of the other nurses employed by corps sites are readily available within the area and are recruited from within the community and employed directly by the community organization sponsoring the National Health Service Corps primary care site. The Corps has a goal to expand the use of nurse practitioners, nurse-midwives, and public health nurses in providing health care services. Initiatives that have been undertaken to achieve this end include supplementing the skills of nurses from rural communities with preparation for primary health care. By 1980, the corps had sponsored education for over 170 registered nurses in nurse practitioner programs since 1972. In addition, corps scholarships were increasingly being provided to master's degree students as can be noted in the following breakdown of National Health Service Corp scholarship recipients as of September 30, 1979, by discipline:

Medicine and Osteopathy	9,978
Dentistry	769
Nursing (B.S.)	279
Public Health Nursing (M.S.)	34
Nurse-Midwifery (M.S.)	29
Nurse Practitioner (M.S.)	74
Public Health Nutrition (M.S.)	72
Medical Social Work	57
Speech/Audiology (M.S.)	35
Veterinary Medicine	4
Optometry	3
Podiatry	106
Pharmacy	6
TOTAL	11,446

Nursing's lack of access to direct third-party payments for services rendered has been a major deterrent acting to keep nurses from providing the kind of care they are prepared to offer. If a nurse, for example, wishes to set up an immunization clinic or a nurse-midwife a maternity practice, she cannot collect payment for this service directly from an insurance company or from federal health programs as a physician does, unless a physician is present and in essence acts as if he is the provider. Consequently, the patient or client is forced to choose between paying for the nursing service out-of-pocket or seeking reimbursable service from a physician instead. Many poor people have no choice because they have no money whatsoever to pay for health services.

One significant exception to this rule was created by the Rural Health Services Act of 1977 (PL 95-210). This law made it possible for nurses and physicians' assistants to receive payment through Medicare and Medicaid for services provided in a certified rural health clinic. This legislation represents a landmark first step in an incremental process, but the provisions of the Rural Health Clinic Services Act are relatively limited; for one thing, only rural clinics are included. During House hearings on the Rural Health Clinic Services Act, some witnesses also recommended that reimbursement be extended to clinics staffed in medically underserved urban areas. The act did provide for the initiation of a Physician-Extender Reimbursement Study of urban practices to be completed by 1981, but reimbursement of nonphysician services in urban clinics will require further legislation. Another drawback is that only clinics without a full-time physician are included in this program, which is severely self-limiting because only 12% of nurse practitioners and 16% of physicians' assistants practice in settings where physician supervision is indirect. In addition, clinics staffed by only nurse-midwives are not considered eligible.

Still another major shortcoming of the program is the regulation that reimbursement for nurse practitioner services be cost-related rather than charge-related. Nonphysician services under Medicare and Medicaid are reimbursed on the basis of the "reasonable cost" of the service whereas physician services are reimbursed on the basis of the "prevailing charge" for the service. Reimbursement based on government defined criteria of reasonable cost of the service is significantly lower than reimbursement based on the physician-established principle of the prevailing charge.

Health care is not found within a single system in the United States; it comprises many different professions, agencies, corporations, and branches of government. One might suggest that there exists a leadership crisis in the health field because there is no private intergroup leadership with recognized authority to coordinate roles between groups. The setting of health priorities must be primarily concerned with the equitable distribution of resources. The federal government, with its huge outflow of tax dollars for Medicare, Medicaid, and other programs, is increasingly called upon to develop health policy that optimizes services for all geographic areas, various social-class groups, as well as the numerous disease and dependent groups. In providing these health services, it must choose between kinds of care (for example, outpatient or inpatient care), between different forms of intervention (for example, prevention, cure, or care), and between different health care providers (for example, physicians, nurses or physicians' assistants). Of course, there is the possibility of avoiding a systematic approach and continuing to place considerable reliance on the "muddling-through" processes of health policy making that, as we show in Chapter 5, have characterized national health efforts up until now.

References

1. U.S. health care called political jousting contest. Salt Lake City, Utah, Salt Lake City Deseret News, Apr 25, 1980
2. U.S. Congress. House. Committee on Interstate and Foreign Commerce, Subcommittee on Oversight and Investigations: Quality of Surgical Care, Vol 2. Hearings before the Subcommittee. Washington, DC, United States Government Printing Office, 1978; U.S. Congress. House. Committee on Interstate and Foreign Commerce, Subcommittee on Oversight and Investigations: Getting Ready for National Health Insurance: Unnecessary Surgery. Hearings before the Subcommittee. Washington DC, United States Government Printing Office, 1975; U.S. Congress. House. Committee on Interstate and Foreign Commerce, Subcommittee on Oversight and Investigations: Cost and Quality of Health Care: Unnecessary Surgery. Hearings before the Committee. Washington, DC, United States Government Printing Office, 1977; U.S. Congress. House. Committee on Interstate and Foreign Commerce, Subcommittee on Oversight and Investigations: Quality of Surgical Care. Hearings before the Subcommittee. Washington, DC, United States Government Printing Office, 1979
3. U.S. General Accounting Office: A Review of Research Literature and Federal Involvement Relating to Selected Obstetric Practices, p 63. Washington, DC, United States General Accounting Office, 1979
4. What is nurse-midwifery practice? J Nurse-Midwifery 25:39, 1980
5. Stayer R: Dozens fault regulations on midwives. Newark, NJ, Newark Star-Ledger, Mar 27, 1980
6. U.S. Congress. Senate. Committee on Labor and Human Resources, Subcommittee on Health and Scientific Research: Women in Science and Technology Equal Opportunity Act, 1979, pp 55–56. Hearings before the Subcommittee. Washington, DC, United States Government Printing Office, 1979
7. U.S. National Center for Health Statistics: Utilization of Short-Stay Hospitals: Annual Summary for the United States, 1978. Washington, DC, United States Government Printing Office, 1980
8. National Academy of Sciences, Institute of Medicine: Controlling the Supply of Hospital Beds, pp 7–16. Washington, DC, National Academy of Sciences, 1976
9. Comptroller General. U.S. General Accounting Office. Hospitals In the Same Area Often Pay Widely Different Prices for Comparable Supply Items, p 5. Report to the Chairman, Subcommittee on Health, Committee on Finance, U.S. Senate. Washington, DC, United States General Accounting Office, 1980
10. Randel J: Do women nurses get heavenly recognition? Wilmington, Del, Evening Journal, June 2, 1980
11. U.S. Congress. House. Committee on Ways and Means, Subcommittee on Health and the Environment: President's Hospital Cost Containment Proposal, p 16. Hearings before the Subcommittee. Washington, DC, United States Government Printing Office, 1979
12. Roberts SV: Hospital Cost Bill defeat: Elements in the decision. New York, NY, New York Times, Nov 20, 1979
13. Kalisch PA, Kalisch BJ: Nursing Involvement in the Health Planning Process. Washington, DC, United States Government Printing Office, 1978

5–Toward a National Health Policy

The federal government is extensively involved in health through its programs in biomedical research, health provider education, the provision of facilities, and the delivery of services. The degree of federal involvement varies, with each federal agency undertaking such activities as are essential for the accomplishment of its goals. In a crude sense, the federal program in health is simply the sum of all federal agency activities. But only the Department of Health and Human Services has a mission that is specifically concerned with the overall health of the nation. It is significant that, on the whole, the systems for the actual delivery of health services to the general population are privately based, although their underpinning—through research, education, and the provision of facilities and services—is a mixed responsibility of federal, state, and local governments as well as the private sector.

Any statement of problems in the health-services delivery system must encompass the generally accepted, though somewhat ambiguous, national commitment to provide competent health services to all, regardless of socioeconomic status. Viewed in this light, as we have seen in the previous chapter, problems are apparent in the rapid and continuing rise in the cost of services, the poor distribution of services, particularly to the urban and rural poor, the less than optimal quality of the services available to the general population, and the difficult access to nonphysician services for most people. All these are accompanied by the sense of an impending catastrophic breakdown of an obviously overloaded system, and the accompanying impetus for reform.

ORIGINS OF HEALTH CARE REFORM

The history of 20th century attempts at health care reform in the United States began with the origins of the state governments' health-insurance movement about the time of World War I. This movement was primarily set off by the passage in 1911 of the British national health-insurance law. Similar health insurance bills were introduced in a dozen American state legislatures, and some of them appointed legislative commissions to investigate the proposals. Several commissions gave a favorable report, but no bill was passed, although New York came within a few votes of enactment. By 1921, interest had died down. One of the main causes for the failure to enact any state law was the inclusion of a small funeral benefit in these bills. This clause brought on the powerful opposition of the industrial insurance companies, whose business was recognized as being essentially burial insurance. The American Medical Association did not officially either oppose or approve the legislation; some of the component state and county medical

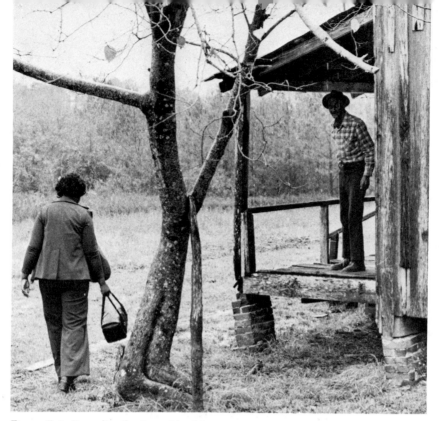

Figure 5-1. *Poor distribution of health services constitutes one of the major gaps in the current health care systems (Courtesy of Montgomery Journal, Montgomery, Alabama)*

societies vigorously opposed it, but others approved the proposal. The American Hospital Association and the National Organization for Public Health Nursing endorsed compulsory health insurance at this time.

Interest was also shown in federal grants for public health work in the states during this period. The Chamberlain-Kahn Act, passed in 1918, set up a system of federal grants for state venereal disease programs. Senator Joseph France of Maryland, a Republican and a physician, introduced in 1919 a bill that provided for federal public-health grants-in-aid of $15 million and federal grants of $48 million for hospital construction. That same year, Representative James R. Mann of Illinois introduced a bill providing federal grants of $1 million a year for rural public health work. The social climate of the 1920s, however, was not favorable for a consideration of federal involvement in health issues and little was heard of legislative reforms. The American Medical Association in 1921 formally denounced compulsory health insurance. Congress permitted the federal program of venereal disease grants to lapse, but in 1921, after several years of strong public agitation and the efforts of such organizations as the National Organization for Public Health Nursing, it enacted the Sheppard-Towner Bill for federal grants to support state infant and maternal hygiene programs. The decade was marked by a development of interest in health on the part of several major private foundations such as the Commonwealth Fund, the

Milbank Memorial Fund, and the Rockefeller Foundation, all of whose health care demonstrations showed, by actual practice, the lifesaving possibilities of organized interventions to supply health care.

COMMITTEE ON THE COSTS OF MEDICAL CARE

The next important event in the history of efforts to develop a national health policy occurred in 1932 when the Committee on the Costs of Medical Care was formed. This group's recommendations attempted to resolve the problems resulting from rising costs and unequal distribution of medi-

Figure 5–2. Efforts to establish a national health insurance plan prior to 1920 centered on the concept of the patient as the center of the system. (Courtesy of History of Nursing Collection, University of Michigan)

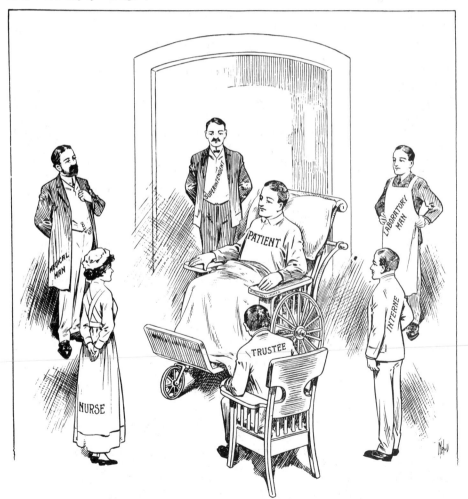

cal care before and during the Depression years. The committee's recommendations sound progressive even today:

- Health care should be provided by organized groups of providers (physicians, dentists, nurses, pharmacists, and other associated personnel).
- Health care costs should be placed on a group prepayment basis.
- Health care should be made available—through governmental or nongovernmental means—to the entire population according to need.
- Health services should be studied, evaluated, and coordinated by agencies in every state and every local community.

An editorial in the *Journal of the American Medical Association*, appearing in December 1932 after the committee had disbanded, attacked the majority report as a plan that would turn physicians into hirelings who would treat sick people like robots. This was said despite the fact that in addition to nearly all the economists, the public health officials, and the other nonmedical members of the committee, sixteen physicians had signed the report, including a past president of the American Medical Association, who was a member of President Hoover's cabinet. The editorial specifically denounced the plan as "socialism and communism—inciting to revolution," contrasting as its alternative, "the organized medical profession of this country urging an orderly evolution guided by controlled experimentation."[1]

During early 1936, the U.S. Public Health Service, assisted by hundreds of unemployed nurses under a Works Progress Administration grant, conducted a "nationwide family canvass of sickness in relation to its social and economic setting." The survey of 740,000 households included some 2,650,000 individuals from 83 cities and 23 rural areas located in 18 states, a representative sample of the total urban population and a significant group of the rural sections.

This study showed that on an average winter day at least 6 million people in the United States (exclusive of certain institutional groups, some with high disability rates) were unable to pursue their usual activities because of illness or injury. Of these, 42%, or 2,500,000, were suffering from chronic diseases. For every death reported during a year, there occurred on the average sixteen cases of illness, which disabled the sick person for a week or longer. A minimum of two and one-half billion days of incapacitating illness was suffered yearly. This meant that, on a per capita basis, each person in the United States suffered an average of at least 10 days of incapacitation a year. As applied to wage earners, it meant a potential wage loss of about one and one-half billion dollars a year.[2]

The relationship between sickness and economic status displayed a sharp contrast. Two persons on relief were disabled for a week or more for every one person in the middle-to higher-income groups ($3000 and over). The nonrelief population with incomes under $1000 had a volume of disability over twice that of the highest-income groups; that is, the incidence of illness was 100% higher among the poor than among the moderately well-to-do and the wealthy. Similarly, the relative frequency of chronic disabling disease was 87% higher among relief clients than among families with annual incomes in excess of $3000. In terms of annual days of chronic disabil-

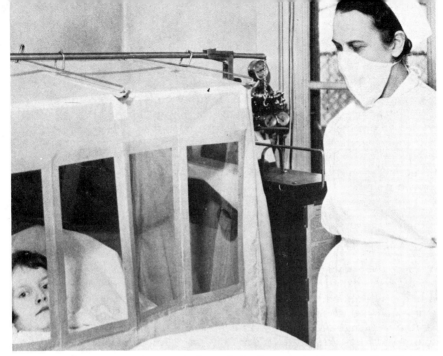

Figure 5–3. In 1936, each person averaged ten days of incapacitation annually. (Courtesy History of Nursing Collection, University of Michigan)

ity, an even sharper contrast existed between persons in the relief group and their more fortunate neighbors, the ratio being 3:1. Thus sickness was found to be not only more frequent but also more severe among relief and low-income families than it was among those in the upper-income brackets.

The survey showed that, despite the greater volume of illness among the poor, they received less adequate medical care than their more fortunate neighbors: 21% of the sick among the relief and low-income group were *not* attended by a physician; the corresponding figure for families with incomes of $3000 and over was 12%. Among cases that were attended by a physician the number of calls per case was less for the relief and low-income groups than for the highest-income group. Bedside nursing care from a private duty nurse was similarly maldistributed: 1% of the relief population received this care as contrasted with 12% in the upper-income groups.

There was no shortage of hospital beds during this time as records of the American Medical Association on general-hospital bed occupancy for the previous ten years showed the following occupancy statistics:[3]

YEAR	PERCENTAGE OF OCCUPANCY
1927	66.1
1928	66.0
1929	65.5
1930	64.7
1931	64.4
1932	63.3
1933	59.9
1934	60.3
1935	64.3
1936	67.4

In 1936, the best year of the decade, out of a total of 402,604 beds in 4207 general hospitals, 130,947 remained empty on the average day.

The nature of this problem and the nature of the risks involved suggested an application of the health insurance principle to replace the variable and uncertain costs for individuals with fixed and predictable costs for large groups of individuals. Health insurance was still variously defined. Perhaps the simplest inclusive definition was that health insurance was a procedure whereby the individual, aided sometimes by his employer or the government, paid in advance a stipulated sum of money to guarantee payment of the costs of medical and hospital care in the event of illness.

NATIONAL HEALTH CONFERENCE, 1938

In 1935, the Social Security Act was passed into law and several sections of the act established a federal–state partnership in public health that provided some funds to the state for basic programs in environmental services, communicable disease control, training of public health professionals, and limited maternal and child health services. Three years later, at the suggestion of President Franklin D. Roosevelt, the Interdepartmental Committee to Coordinate Health and Welfare Activities called a National Health Conference in Washington, July 18th to the 20th, in 1938. About 170 delegates attended this conference, and some 200 observers were invited, including persons from large, organized public groups (labor, farming, industry, women's organizations, civic bodies, social work, and public welfare) and from the leading professional bodies concerned with furnishing health services, including physicians, dentists, hospital administrators, and nurses.

The Technical Committee on Medical Care (a subcommittee of the Interdepartmental Committee), composed of officers of the U.S. Public Health Service, the U.S. Children's Bureau, and the Social Security Board, had been at work for many months studying health needs and programs for discussion at the conference. The committee's report cited deficiencies in existing health services, which they divided into four broad categories: (1) preventive health services for the nation as a whole were grossly insufficient; (2) hospital and other institutional facilities were inadequate in many communities, especially in rural areas, while financial support for hospital care and for professional services in hospitals was both insufficient and precarious, especially for services to persons who could not afford the costs of the care that they needed; (3) one-third of the population, including persons with and without income, were receiving inadequate or no medical service; and (4) an even larger fraction of the population suffered from the economic burdens created by illness.

Strongly divergent points of view were expressed at the National Health Conference. The dangers of unnecessary delay were outlined by Dr. Thomas Parran, surgeon general of the U.S. Public Health Service, who declared that "the care of the public health may well be the next great social advance in this country." Michael M. Davis of Boston urged that liberal and conservative groups in the medical profession work together on a democratic basis to formulate a program of national health insurance of the United States. Dr. S. S. Goldwater of New York City made a plea for caution

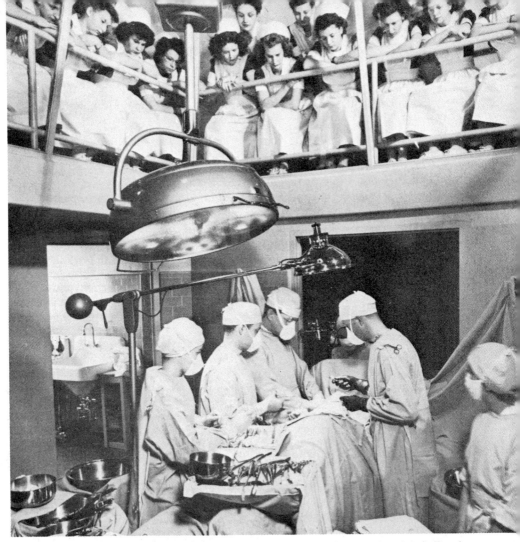

Figure 5-4. *Many communities across the nation did not have the benefit of modern hospital facilities such as this operating room at the University of Oregon (Courtesy of University of Oregon Medical School, Portland, Oregon)*

in starting federal programs and for the continuation of voluntary efforts in the health field. Federal aid should be requested only after all possibilities of local and voluntary help have been fully explored and exhausted, he declared.

One of the most positive notes regarding health planning was struck by nurse Annie W. Goodrich, former dean of the School of Nursing at Yale University, when she said,

If the family is accepted as the strategic point of attack, and it should be, what is needed is: (1) an organized, integrated program of care and prevention of illness, and of health education, based on the needs of a given area or unit of population and carried out through institutions equipped with adequate diagnostic facilities;

(2) care for all forms of illness, mental and physical; and (3) complete maternity services and health instruction. Such provision should imply hospitalization, dispensary service, and home care as needed, by a qualified personnel, regardless of the financial status of the patient.[4]

Miss Goodrich stated that the strongest agent in a national health program was the nurse. "If the complete mobilization of the nursing resources of the country could be encompassed for the service of preventive medicine one might predict as remarkable an influence upon the community." She added,

> The opportunity of the nurse in the fields of curative and preventive medicine is illustrated by the following estimate of contacts that could be made by the 180,000 plus nurses—20,000 plus in the public health field, 60,000 plus in institutions, and 100,000 plus serving as private duty nurses. One hundred eighty thousand would make in one year approximately 18,000,000 contacts with the people of the country. Multiplying these figures by 10 [years], we find that a population of 180,000,000 would have been contacted. . . .[5]

Figure 5–5. Annie Goodrich stated nursing's case for a national health program at the 1938 National Health Conference. (Courtesy History of Nursing Collection, University of Michigan)

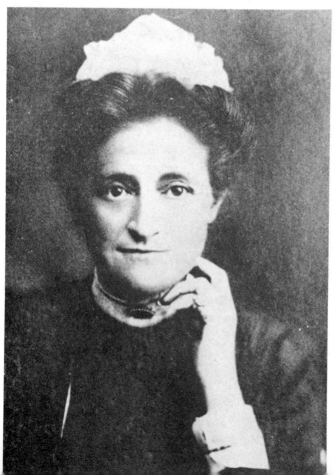

Miss Goodrich ended on this note: "An army of unemployed youth, unemployed nurses and teachers, physicians and dentists who cannot collect their bills, an ever-shortening span of working years on the one hand, and on the other, understaffed and over-crowded institutions for the mentally and physically ill and uncared for needs in the home—all this leaves no question of the social responsibility involved. . . . Cooperation rather than competition is the keynote in achieving the results we are here to further."[6]

Delegates to the conference were asked to discuss the proposed recommendations and to report facts and findings to the organizations that they represented. No attempt was made to pass resolutions or plan legislative action. The conference was noteworthy because of the active participation of the general public, the indications of a vast ground swell of public interest in matters of health, the agreement of all but a small minority with the statement of national health needs, and the potential benefits of long-range health planning by federal authorities. The specific form of the legislative action to implement the recommendations and the scope of the health plan put into effect depended upon the degree of public interest in the whole problem.

EARLY ATTEMPTS TO ENACT A NATIONAL HEALTH PROGRAM

Public interest in national health insurance developed to an unprecedented level following the National Health Conference. The Interdepartmental Committee made its report to the President on January 12, 1939, and he transmitted this report with a special message to Congress. On February 28, 1939, Senator Robert Wagner of New York introduced a bill designed to implement the broad recommendations of the Interdepartmental Committee. The hearings on this bill were the most extensive and exhaustive inquiry ever made by a congressional committee on the state of the nation's health and on the need for measures to make more adequate health services available to the population. A preliminary report was made to the Senate by Senator James Murray, of Montana, chairman of the subcommittee, which had conducted the hearings, indicating the lines along which the committee was pursuing its study of the proposals.

In December 1939, President Roosevelt announced a special interest in seeing at least a beginning made toward implementing the national health program through the construction of hospitals in the poorest areas where the need was greatest. This proposal was outlined in a special message to Congress on January 31, 1940, and was submitted soon thereafter in definitive form in a bill (S 3230) introduced by Senators Wagner and Walter George and by Representative Clarence Lea. After special hearings and considerable amendment, this bill was favorably reported out of committee and passed by the Senate in May 1940. This bill would have authorized annual appropriations of $10 million for each of six years for the construction of needed hospitals, especially in rural and economically depressed areas. During the first year, the construction program would have been wholly federal; in the following five years, it would have provided for federal grants-in-aid to the states. It also would have provided temporary grants on a diminishing scale to help cover the first five years of operating

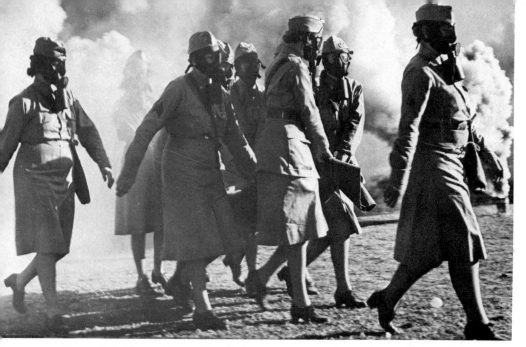

Figure 5–6. The outbreak of World War II interrupted consideration of a national health program. Nurses donned gas masks on December 7, 1941 following news of the Pearl Harbor attack. (Courtesy of History of Nursing Collection, University of Michigan)

costs of the new hospitals. The Wagner bill, however, could not gain sufficient support in the House of Representatives, and died in committee as World War II intervened.

A STRONGER FEDERAL FOCUS FOR HEALTH

Although a program of national health insurance was not enacted, the 1930s did bring about profound changes in the concept of the role of the federal government. Among these was the idea that the government had a responsibility to act in major problems affecting the national health. It was in such a context that the National Cancer Act was passed in 1937, establishing the National Cancer Institute as a division of the U.S. Public Health Service. This agency had wide duties covering investigation and research on cancer as well as treatment and providing assistance to other institutions, public and private. It was the purpose of the act to extend current knowledge of the cancer problem for the benefit of future cancer patients and to secure a more complete application of existing knowledge for the benefit of present cancer patients. An appropriation of $570,000 was made for the work of the Institute for FY 1940. (Forty years later, in 1980, the annual appropriation had grown to $1 billion.) The National Cancer Act represented the first instance in which grants-in-aid for medical research were authorized to private institutions.

President Roosevelt on July 1, 1939, consolidated the principal agencies of the federal government concerned with health, education, and welfare into the new Federal Security Agency. He appointed former Indiana Governor, Paul V. McNutt as its administrator. The Federal Security Agency was named *Security* instead of *Welfare* because the vice-president, John Nance Garner, told President Roosevelt that there was a great objection in Congress to the terms welfare, social welfare, public welfare, and so forth. It was feared that its use might lead to a continuation of the Depression-era welfare activities of the government, which they hoped to stop as soon as possible. There was no objection, however, to the word security because it looked as if the Social Security program had gained wide acceptance from the public.

As set forth in its authorization, the purpose of the Federal Security Agency was to provide social and economic security, educational opportunity, and better health for the citizens of the nation. The activities of the Federal Security Agency were placed under the direction and supervision of a federal security administrator. The five agencies principally concerned with health that were transferred to the FSA were: (1) the U.S. Public Health Service; (2) the U.S. Children's Bureau; (3) the Social Security Administration; (4) the Office of Vocational Rehabilitation; and (5) the Food and Drug Administration.

In speaking before the 1940 annual conference of State and Territorial Health Officers, Surgeon General Thomas Parran of the U.S. Public Health Service pointed to the changing initiative for new advances in public health. Hitherto, it had been the professional groups, such as the American Medical Association, who had assumed the major burden for advancing the nation's health movement and for determining the content of the program. At last, Dr. Parran pointed out, the general public had become informed on such matters and was beginning to assert its views. Popular notions as to what should be done and the methods for doing the job were apt to be at variance with those of professionals. As yet popular opinion had not become particularly definitive in matters pertaining to individual and community health, but a clear-cut public policy, he felt, was almost certain to grow out of awakening interests.

PRESIDENT TRUMAN'S HEALTH CRUSADE

Following the war, President Harry Truman in a pioneer effort carefully prepared a special health message, which he submitted to Congress on November 19, 1945, asking for enactment of legislation with the following provisions:

- Prepayment of medical costs through compulsory insurance premiums and the general revenues
- Protection against loss of wages from sickness and disability
- Expansion of public health, and maternal and child health services
- Federal aid to medical schools and for research purposes
- Stepped-up construction of hospitals, clinics, and medical institutions under local administration

During extensive congressional hearings in 1946, the American Nurses' Association, the National League of Nursing Education, and the National Organization for Public Health Nursing supported President Truman's health program. On the other hand, the American Medical Association was bitterly opposed, denouncing the proposal as communism and socialism.

Only the last of these proposals was enacted into law. The Hospital Survey and Construction Act of 1946, commonly known as the Hill-Burton program, became one of the landmark federal health programs of the post-World War II period. During the following 27 years nearly $4.5 billion worth of grants would be distributed under the program. These grants provided for the construction of 488,000 hospital and nursing home beds as well as 3,330 other health facilities, including clinics and public health and rehabilitation centers. The Hill-Burton program also presented the nation with its first hospital planning bodies with technical guidelines for hospital architecture, construction, and equipment.

In an attempt to have the bulk of his health program enacted into law, Truman, on May 19, 1947, sent a special message to the Congress on Health and Disability Insurance in order to ensure, as he pointed out, ". . . the ultimate strength from the vigor of our people." The president appealed for a fair chance for a healthy life for everyone through the efforts of "a great and free Nation to bring health care within the reach of all its people." This significant and far-reaching recommendation for improved health care emphasized the need for more physicians, hospitals, and increased medical research for preventive medicine and for the cure of disease. Truman suggested that a national health insurance program be made part of the Social Security Act. He further stated that, "a national health insurance program is a logical extension of the present social security system which is so firmly entrenched in our American Democracy," and emphasized that until national health insurance was established in our health care system, "we shall be wasting our most precious national resource."

After several unsuccessful efforts to obtain congressional approval of proposed appropriative measures, President Truman renewed his struggle by sending another health message to the Congress in April 1949. His premise was the same as that of his original proposal of November 1945. He appealed again to good sense in order to provide (1) a nationwide system of health insurance; (2) congressional support for the expansion of medical and nursing schools; (3) government aid for the construction of medical facilities; and (4) consolidation of existing grants with provision of state matching funds to adjust financial resources. The President said with characteristic candor, "the real cost of medical services and the need for them cannot be measured merely by doctors' bills and medical bills. The real cost to society is in unnecessary human suffering and the yearly loss of hundreds of millions of working days." He directed congressional attention to the "shattering of family budgets, disruption of family life, the suffering of disabilities, the permanent impairments left by crippling disease, and the death of tens of thousands of persons who might live." This is the price, Truman warned, that America pays for inadequate health care.[7]

In May of 1948, President Truman convened a National Health Assembly, which was attended by 800 professional and community leaders, including several prominent nurses. Using the assembly as a publicity springboard, Federal Security Administrator Oscar Ewing prepared a report to the President entitled, *The Nation's Health: A Ten Year Program,*

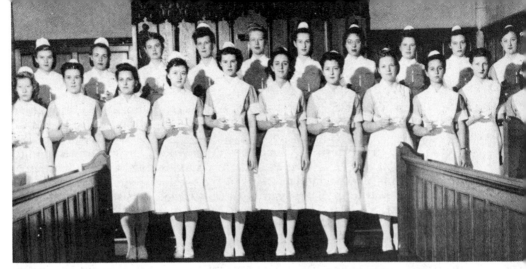

Figure 5-7. Few nursing students of the late 1940s were aware that President Truman was engaged in a bitter fight for a national health program which would also have provided funds to advance nursing. (Courtesy History of Nursing Collection, University of Michigan)

outlining a plan for comprehensive, federally sponsored, compulsory health insurance. This report was regarded as a signal of danger by the leaders of the American Medical Association (AMA). They were frightened by its attractive format almost as much as by its content. They decided that a grave danger had arrived, and arrived for good, when Truman won his second term.

In December 1948, shortly after the election, the AMA assessed its members $25 each for a nationwide plan of education, and during the next 3½ years it spent over $4.5 million [12 million 1980 dollars] in informing the American people about the hazards of socialized medicine. The AMA asked, "Does the Report on *The Nation's Health* give a factual picture of the people's health in America?" And then it answered, "No. This widely publicized *Report* is a hoax. It is a propagandist treatment of a subject far too important for such loose handling by political experimenters." The AMA went on and asked, "Who is for Compulsory Health Insurance?" and it answered, "The Federal Security Administration. The President. All who seriously believe in a Socialistic State. Every left-wing organization in America. . . . The Communist Party." The plan to improve the nation's health was dismissed as part of a trend toward complete socialization of American life: "The Government proposes to assume control not only of the medical profession, but of hospitals—both public and private—the drug and appliance industries, dentistry, pharmacy, nursing and allied professions."[8]

Frustrated by the lack of congressional action on his health program proposals, Truman created in December, 1951, the President's Commission on the Health Needs of the Nation, which included Marion W. Sheahan, R.N., director of the National Committee for the Improvement of Nursing Services. It was his hope to produce a critical study of the Nation's immediate and long-range health requirements and thus provide useful data for comprehensive action, but by the time the commission distributed its report, Dwight Eisenhower was President, and federal action in the health care field had ceased.

SLOW ADVANCE IN THE 1950s

After Truman's efforts in the 1940s to establish a national health program failed, the next incremental gain came in 1950 when the Public Assistance Title of the Social Security Act was amended so the federal government would share in the costs of vendor health payments for welfare recipients. Between 1950 and 1965 there was a gradual broadening of federal participation in paying for the medical care of the welfare population, while the debate on some form of national health insurance persisted. By 1955, the tactical effort to achieve a consensus on health insurance narrowed to focus on the plight of the elderly. In 1960, Congress passed a compromise: the Kerr-Mills Bill (PL 86-778). It provided more generous coverage from federal sources for aged persons on the welfare rolls and also established the precedent of federal participation in paying for the care of a new category of persons, the medically indigent aged, who were not on welfare but whose income was insufficient to pay the full cost of illness. State participation in the program was optional, and, most important, each state was allowed to determine its own standards of indigency.

MEDICARE AND MEDICAID PROGRAMS ENACTED

The idea of national health insurance simmered through the 1950s, only to boil up again in John F. Kennedy's march on the New Frontier and in Lyndon Johnson's dream of a Great Society. In 1965, some thirty years after health insurance emerged as a topic of national political concern, Congress took a significant step, creating Medicare and Medicaid to fund health care for the elderly and the poor. Medicare and Medicaid fell far short of national health insurance, yet they soon became the most costly health care financing programs ever undertaken by any nation in the world and would, by 1980, consume more than 10% of the entire federal budget.

Medicare provided all persons over age 65 in all parts of the country with insurance to cover the costs of hospital and related care to be chiefly financed by employer–employee contributions to the Social Security Trust Fund. It also initiated a system of elected participation in supplemental insurance covering physicians' fees and certain other health services. The Medicare program, a 100% federally financed health-care insurance program, is available to anyone 65 years of age or over who is eligible for Social Security payments or Railroad Workers' Insurance. Medicare provides payments for traditional forms of health care, including up to 100 days of care in a nursing home that qualifies as a skilled nursing facility under federal regulations. Although the Medicare program is financed and administered by the Social Security administration, insurance companies act as the fiscal intermediaries between patients, skilled nursing facilities, and the government. Using Social Security administration guidelines, insurance companies determine the rights of patients to Medicare benefits. The health care facilities providing the services are paid on a cost-plus basis, that is, for costs plus a reasonable profit. A state agency, usually the department of health, determines the rate of repayment.

Medicare's benefit package stresses the acute, episodic form of health services to the elderly. This is borne out by such examples as finding that

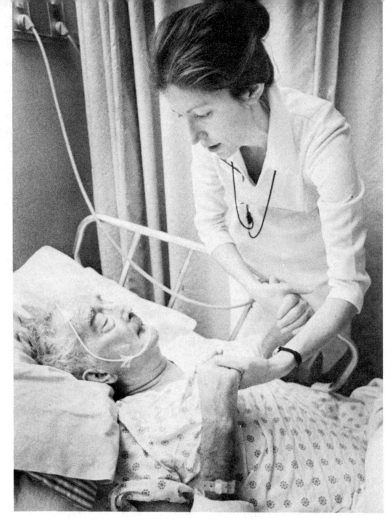

Figure 5–8. *Social concern for the plight of the elderly in need of health care and unable to afford it led to the establishment of Medicare.* (*Courtesy of Grand Rapids Press, Grand Rapids, Michigan*)

nursing home expenses of the aged were scarcely affected by Medicare. In 1980, nursing homes accounted for only about 4% of the total costs because Medicare covered skilled nursing services only when ordered by a physician and only when provided by a skilled nursing facility after a specified hospital stay; time limitations and co-payments were also imposed. Likewise, potential use of home health services was seriously undercut owing to strict interpretation of the scope of and eligibility for such services.

HOW MEDICAID OPERATES

Enacted at the same time as Medicare was Medicaid, a cooperative federal–state medical care program operated under state direction. The *Medicaid program* is a medical-care payment system for the medically in-

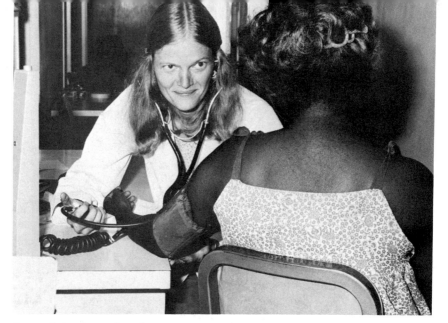

Figure 5–9. The Medicaid program finances health care for needy families. (Courtesy of Madison County Herald, Canton, Mississippi)

digent. Its purpose is to enable states to provide a more effective medical assistance program for welfare recipients and to offer medical care of high quality to additional persons with low income who are unable to pay for care in whole or in part. In administering the Medicaid program, states are expected to make such health services readily available to all eligible persons. The states are further expected to set appropriate standards ensuring the high quality of these services and their administration in a sympathetic and dignified manner. Subject to broad federal regulations, each state decides who is eligible for its program, to which services they are entitled, the manner in which providers of health care are reimbursed, and the way in which the program operates.

Medicaid operates as a matching state and federal program. The amount of federal assistance is based on the per capita income of each state and ranges from 50% to 78%. Medicaid payments for nursing home care are made to those skilled nursing facilities and intermediate care facilities that qualify as nursing care facilities for the aged or infirmed under the federal regulations. The Department of Health and Human Services (HHS) administers the Medicaid program and sets the standards for participating facilities. But HHS has delegated most of the regulatory power of the program to the states, including responsibility for determining who is eligible for Medicaid payments and the amount of money to be paid to facilities for each patient. Generally the state Welfare Department makes these determinations, and the Department of Health, under contract with HHS, licenses and inspects facilities to be sure of compliance with the federal regulations and standards. Every state in the union except Arizona has some form of Medicaid in operation. The provisions vary widely from state to state, as does the proportion of federal funds available for financing Medicaid services, which are based on a formula inversely related to state per capita income.

While the states were initially given considerable flexibility in the administration of Medicaid, the federal state-sharing formula was conceived so as to offer an incentive for poorer states to initiate a program. This formula permitted federal sharing of up to 80% of the program costs for the poorer states and 50% for the more prosperous states. These currently range from 50% matching in New York to 78% in Mississippi. The effect of this formula was, of course, that most states did move fairly swiftly to enact a Medicaid program, although some programs were more limited in their scope of benefits and groups covered than those prescribed by federal statute. In spite of the formula, by 1980 the five more affluent states of California, Michigan, Illinois, Pennsylvania, and New York were consuming over half of the total Medicaid expenditures.

While Medicaid's purpose had been to relieve the financial burden of health care of millions of poor Americans, both rural and urban, several structural problems prevented fulfillment of this goal. Medicaid was to guarantee the quality of health care and services by eliminating the differences in treatment for people of different social and economic status. The needy and the medically underserved were to be treated in identical fashion under the law. Neither Medicare nor Medicaid were designed to finance or encourage new forms of primary health care delivery. Instead, both programs sustained and supported the patterns and traditions of health care that existed in 1965.

SENATOR INOUYE'S CRUSADE FOR NURSES

During his service in the Senate, Senator Daniel K. Inouye has focused much of his attention on reforms that would result in more innovative provi- 97th Congress and in several previous Congresses, the Senator from Hawaii introduced legislation that would broaden Medicare and Medicaid reimbursement along with other federal health benefits programs to include services provided by professional nurses, nurse midwives, psychiatric nurses, and gerontological nurse practitioners. An advocate of improved use of health care personnel, Inouye has repeatedly pointed out that professional nurses are being used increasingly to provide health care services in areas of physician shortages; nurses are health care professionals in their own right and not simply handmaidens to physicians, the Senator has stated. "It is ironic that our present health care system and methods of reimbursement militate against utilization of nurses in a way that would make health services more widely available and at the same time contribute to the containment of health care costs," Senator Inouye has said.

The Inouye legislation would provide Medicare and Medicaid reimbursement for services provided by nurses in all settings, including hospitals, nursing homes, rural clinics, and ambulatory care centers. Inouye has noted that his bills would keep pace with new trends in health care. For instance, the trend in professional nursing education, which has "changed drastically" over the past decade, is producing nurses who are more "assertive and accountable." But, according to Inouye, many of the services

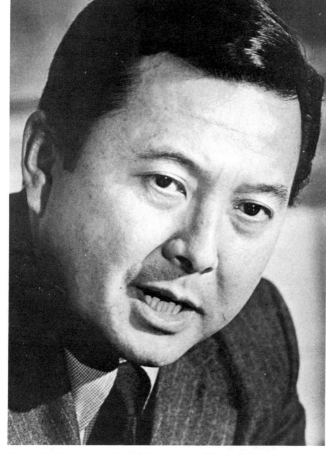

Figure 5–10. Senator Daniel K. Inouye of Hawaii has pushed for legislation to directly reimburse nurses for various services under Medicare and Medicaid. (Courtesy of Daniel K. Inouye)

these nurses are qualified to deliver are not reimbursable by insurance carriers unless performed under the direct supervision of a physician. Another trend, Inouye said, is toward patient care in a "community setting," and home health services by nurses could "prevent the need for costly hospitalization." Inouye also noted that people with chronic diseases are living longer than before owing to "sophistication of treatment," adding, "one way to meet this need for high-quality care at reasonable cost is the services of registered nurses."[9]

As Senator Inouye and other congressmen have observed, costs have emerged as the major inhibitor to broadened access to health care. In fiscal 1981, according to the President's budget, combined federal spending for the government's two largest health care programs, Medicare for the elderly and Medicaid for the poor, will total $54.6 billion, an astonishing 13.7% increase over the 1980 fiscal year. Outlays for Medicare alone will have thus soared by nearly $10 billion in two years, from $29.3 billion in fiscal 1979 to $39.1 billion in fiscal 1981. With the dramatic growth of these public programs—Medicare and Medicaid in 1980 accounted for 40% of total hospital spending compared with 30% just a decade earlier—the federal government is increasingly taking a closer look at how and where the money is being spent.

PROFESSIONAL STANDARDS REVIEW ORGANIZATIONS AND NURSES

One of the chief approaches toward evaluation of health care programs was initiated in the early 1970s. The Social Security Amendments of 1972 required the establishment of Professional Standards Review Organizations (PSROs) to "promote the effective, efficient, and economical delivery of health care services of proper quality" by assuring that services for which payment was made under Medicare and Medicaid are medically necessary and rendered in the most appropriate setting and time periods. The PSRO statute requires PSROs to review care provided in hospitals, in skilled nursing facilities, and in those intermediate care facilities where the state requests the PSRO to perform the review or the state was found to be performing reviews ineffectively. Ambulatory care review was also authorized in the PSRO act. Statewide PSRO Councils were required, in states with three or more PSROs, to coordinate PSRO activities and to review reconsiderations of PSRO decisions.

PSROs accomplish these objectives through the application of sophisticated concepts of peer review, including concurrent review, quality review studies, and profile analysis. About 200,000 physicians are members of PSROs, and there are 195 designated PSRO areas nationwide. By 1980, PSROs had been established in all but three of the 195 PSRO areas. A majority of these PSROs had fully implemented their hospital review systems. In addition, 55 PSROs were performing long-term care reviews, and 6 PSROs were carrying out ambulatory care reviews, on a demonstrations basis. In 1980, an estimated 14.5 million of the total 16 million annual Medicare and Medicaid hospital admissions were subject to PSRO review. About $130 million was spent for PSRO hospital-review activities.

Although nurses are excluded from PSRO membership, Senator Inouye has sponsored a bill whereby registered nurses would be given full voting membership on local Professional Standards Review Organizations as well as on statewide and national Professional Standards Review Councils. "It would seem to me," he explained, "that if we are to provide for effective review of health care, the present law must be amended to include participation of registered nurses—the largest single group of health practitioners in the country." According to Inouye, his bill would in no way distort, interfere with, or "appreciably" add to the costs of the PSRO program. He noted PSROs have limited their membership to licensed physicians of medicine or osteopathy even though the services of other health professionals, such as dentists, psychologists and registered nurses, have been subject to the PSRO review process.[10]

Exclusion of nonphysician health care professionals is "clearly discriminatory and wholly contrary to any rational understanding of the prime objective of the PSRO program," Inouye maintained, pointing out that his bill would:

- allow nonphysician health professionals to review health care services already being provided by them under the Medicare, Medicaid, and maternal and child health programs
- include a dentist and a psychologist on the statewide PSRO councils and a registered nurse on the advisory groups to the statewide PSRO councils
- expand the National Professional Standards Review Council to include a registered nurse, a dentist, and a psychologist
- establish an advisory committee to the National Professional Standards Review Council composed of nonphysician health professionals who were not represented on the national council.[11]

HEALTH MAINTENANCE ORGANIZATIONS

Another federal effort to control health care costs has been to foster the widespread growth of Health Maintenance Organizations (HMOs) as a cost-effective alternative to the traditional fee-for-service health-care system. HMOs are organizations that assume responsibility for both the financing and delivery of health care. They provide a comprehensive range of

Figure 5–11. HMOs provide a comprehensive range of health services in exchange for annual payments which are set in advance. (Courtesy of Wheeling News Register, Wheeling, West Virginia)

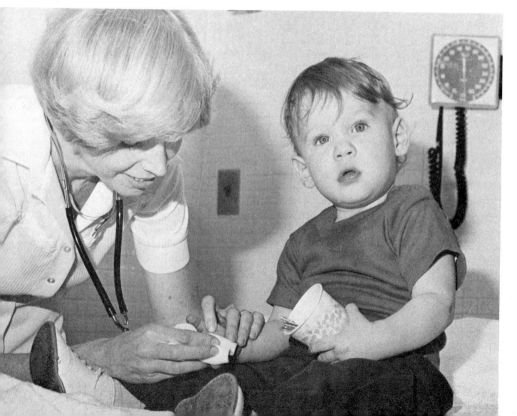

health services to voluntarily enrolled members in exchange for annual payments, which are set in advance.

The Health Maintenance Organization (HMO) concept is not a recent innovation in the United States. The first prepaid health plan was established in Los Angeles in 1929. The HMO concept calls for the delivery of specified health services to the members of an HMO, either directly or through arrangements with others, in return for compensation at predetermined, prepaid rates. The prepayment approach differentiates the HMO from the more common fee-for-service concept, whereby health care providers are reimbursed for each service provided.

Ten years ago, in response to the rapid escalation of health care costs, President Richard Nixon in February 1971 announced in a health message to Congress the administration's intention to stimulate the development of HMOs as an alternative health care delivery system intended to reduce the costs and enhance the quality of health care. Among other things, Nixon advocated development by the end of the 1970s of 1700 HMOs to enroll 40 million people. His ultimate goal was to enroll 90% of the population—"if they (so) desire"—in the prepaid health plans. By the 1972 election, however, Nixon had backed off from his original broad endorsement, reportedly at the insistence of the American Medical Association and his personal physician. The AMA continued to regard any payment system other than fee-for-service to be unethical.[12]

Another early advocate of an extensive HMO system was Edward M. Kennedy, who gained Senate approval in 1972 of his wide-ranging $5.1 billion HMO bill. By the time the House version of an HMO bill passed that chamber, however, it had shrunk to a much scaled down $375 million experimental program that effectively limited the number of federally assisted HMOs over a five-year period to about 100.

The Health Maintenance Organization Act of 1973 (PL 93-222) amended the Public Health Service Act and called for DHEW to establish a federal demonstration program to develop alternatives to traditional forms of health care delivery and financing by assisting and encouraging the establishment and expansion of HMOs. For the five-year demonstration program, the act authorized federal financial assistance consisting of grants and contracts to public or private nonprofit organizations for HMO feasibility studies and for planning and initial development costs, loans to public or private nonprofit organizations for initial operating assistance, and loan guarantees for nonfederal lenders on loans made to private profit-making organizations for planning, initial development, and initial operating assistance for HMOs serving the medically underserved.

The act defined an HMO and its operating requirements in considerable detail and among other things specified the basic and supplemental health services to be provided for the HMO members, the basis for fixing the rate of prepayment, the organizational structure of an HMO, and the requirement for open enrollment periods during which individuals may join without restrictions (such as preexisting medical conditions). The act authorized $325 million in grants and loans for HMO development. Of this amount, $250 million constituted grants for feasibility studies and for the planning and development of HMOs, and $75 million was used to capitalize a loan fund to cover initial operating deficits of HMOs.

Dissatisfaction with the act and the slow progress in implementing the program led to the passage of the HMO Amendments of 1976 (PL 94-460), which were signed into law on October 8, 1976. PL 94-460 modified some restrictive elements in the HMO act of 1973, which had been cited as reasons for the failure to implement the act as rapidly as had been expected. Among other changes, the amendments reduced the services that HMOs were required to offer and, provided they did not incur a deficit in the most recent fiscal year, exempted HMOs from the open enrollment provisions until they had enrolled 50,000 members or until they had been in operation for five years. The amendments also provided a grace period of forty-eight months for an established HMO to meet the requirement that its contracts be community rated and changed the requirements for medical group practices, including a provision that medical groups would be required to provide at least 35% of their services, rather than a majority of their services, to HMO members.

Under the act, as amended, federal financial support is available to HMO applicants in the form of grants, loans, and loan guarantees. The only requirement is that the group be a legal entity showing fiscal responsibility and the capacity to carry out HMO development to comply with the HMO application requirements. The amendments increased the grant limits from $50,000 to $75,000 for feasibility studies; from $125,000 to $200,000 for planning studies; and from $1.0 million to $1.6 million for HMO expansion activities. The amendments extended the HMO program for two additional years through 1980, authorizing grants of $45 million for FY 1978 and $50 million for FY 1979. Loan and loan guarantee authority was extended through September 30, 1980.

From the inception of the federal HMO program, the number of HMOs increased by 1980 from 50 programs in 20 states to over 220 HMOs in 37 states. In addition, HMO enrollment had nearly doubled since 1972. Numerous studies documented that HMOs provided significant economic benefits to consumers, employers, and the government. For example, the total cost of health care for HMO members was 10% to 40% less than for people with comparable health insurance. The state of Michigan estimated that it saved $4.7 million in 1976 because some Medicare recipients received their care through HMOs. A Federal Trade Commission study of the competitive impact of HMOs indicated that the greater the percentage of a state's population belonging to HMOs, the lower the Blue Cross hospitalization rate and the greater the Blue Cross benefit plan. The 1975 Health Interview Survey conducted by the National Center for Health Statistics showed that in contrast to the fee-for-service sector, HMO members tended to be younger, to have a higher proportion of males, to have a higher proportion of blacks and other minorities, to have more educated heads of households and, hence, higher family incomes, to be concentrated in metropolitan areas and in the western part of the country, and to have a higher proportion of families with five or more persons.

The *New England Journal of Medicine* published a special article by Dr. Harold F. Luft in June 1978 entitled, "How do Health Maintenance Organizations Achieve Their Savings?" Dr. Luft undertook a comprehensive review of all studies published since 1950 and presented virtually all of the evidence of the last 25 years on cost and utilization differences; he also examined how such savings were achieved. Luft, who identified 47 sources of data in his references, employed the number of inpatient days per 1000 enrollees per year as the overall measure of hospital use and summarized findings for 51 comparisons of HMO and non-HMO enrollees. In 41 of the 51 pairs, enrollees in HMOs had fewer hospital days than the comparison groups, and the admission rate was lower in 42 instances. Luft's findings indicated that individual practice associations are "less likely to demonstrate lower rates of hospitalization." Hospital days were found to be 25% to 45% lower in prepaid group practices and 0% to 25% lower in the individual-practice association (IPA) model. With respect to hospital admis-

Figure 5–12. Health maintenance organizations offer a more cost-effective form of health care. (Courtesy of Providence Journal, Providence, Rhode Island)

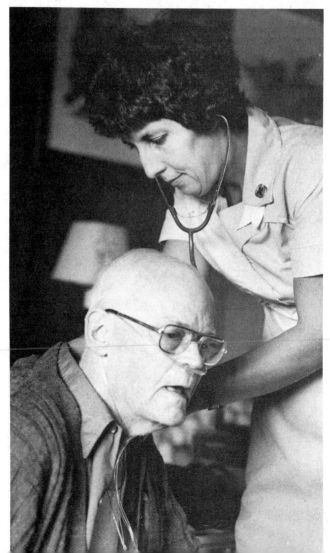

sion rates, group-practice HMOs had lower rates of 15% to 40% and IPA rates were 0% to 25%. On the basis of available data, Luft generalized that most of the cost differences are attributable to hospitalization rates that are about 30% lower than those of conventionally insured populations. His findings conclusively pointed to large savings in hospitalization utilization.

The federal HMO program continues to implement a 10-year National HMO Development Strategy, which targets 61 priority cities as candidates for HMO growth. The number of people enrolled in health maintenance organizations is expected to triple in the next 10 years and, according to a 1980 study by the New York marketing firm of Frost, Sullivan and Company, HMO purchases of medical products and services will reach $3.5 billion in 1990. Although the HMO concept faltered in the 1970s because of physician opposition and public apathy, according to the Frost, Sullivan and Co. investigators, soaring medical costs have caused a turnaround in the HMO movement. These researchers predict the 1980 level of 8 million HMO members will reach 24 million by 1990, and the 50 HMO-owned hospitals will reach 150 by that time.

REBIRTH OF NATIONAL HEALTH INSURANCE DEBATE

National health insurance (NHI) proposals began to again receive serious consideration in the late 1970s. When presidential candidate Jimmy Carter addressed the Platform Committee of the Democratic Party on June 16, 1976, he declared, "We need a national health insurance program . . . which is universal and mandatory." Urging preventive medicine and early detection, Carter continued, "Our major cripplers and killers are cancer, heart disease, stroke, respiratory diseases, hypertension and six others of decreasing incidence within the population. Almost every one of these afflictions can be prevented, to a degree, by regular physical examinations and routine medical care." On the maldistribution of health care, Carter was also clear when he said, "In the county where I live, there is not a doctor, dentist, pharmacist, or hospital bed," and there are nearly 300 areas with similar shortages elsewhere in the nation. On runaway costs, Carter also grasped the facts and trends. In his most famous speech on health policy, Carter in April 1976 pointed out that Americans spent $39 billion on health care in 1965. By 1976, that total had tripled. The total cost would double again in five years and triple in a decade, Carter warned, unless costs were controlled.[13]

After being elected, President Carter began to see complications for a national health-insurance program. First, the federal price tag would be too high—$25 to $40 billion. It was difficult for Carter to advocate increased federal spending for NHI when he had promised to balance the budget by decreasing federal spending. Second, his economic advisers kept reminding him that the biggest problem was inflation, and nothing was more inflationary than health costs. Thus, moving the federal government deeper into the health care business was asking for open-ended fiscal trouble. In January 1978, President Carter had HEW secretary Joseph Califano float a "trial balloon" about the prospects of delaying national health insurance; this set off angry reactions from Senator Edward Kennedy and several labor groups, which had long been backing such legislation. Thus, in March 1978, the President sought a compromise plan.

Carter's advisors sat down with Senator Kennedy and labor representatives who made important concessions on a proposed administration bill. Private insurance companies were to be given a much bigger role in the plan. To keep down the price tag, patients would pay part of their bills. The whole program would be put off for several years and then phased in, one part at a time. The progress of these negotiations was deceptive. When the breakdown came, it seemed to be on a fairly technical point. President Carter refused to commit himself to the entire program in one bill; he would back only one phase at a time. Incredulous, Senator Kennedy went to see the President and received the decision directly from him: no advance commitment would be made by the President to the whole package, given the inflationary perils. Kennedy's argument that commitment to reform of the system was the only way to get control of health care inflation fell on deaf ears.

In December 1978, launching a battle for a National Health Program independent of Carter, Senator Kennedy, as chairman of the Senate Human Resources Health Subcommittee, opened three days of hearings on his universal national health insurance plan with the assertion that no other

Figure 5–13. The place of the nurse in the various national health insurance plans was uniformly vague. (Courtesy of San Antonio Express-News, San Antonio, Texas)

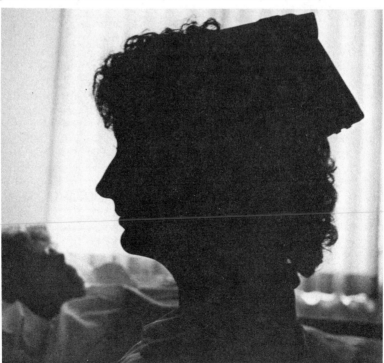

program could guarantee the comprehensive benefits with costs less than his proposal. Calling the economics of the situation "truly frightening," Kennedy told a packed hearing-room that "everyone agrees that health care costs are out of control. National health insurance is the last, best chance to halt the staggering economic waste," he warned. "Cost containment is at the very heart of the health insurance debate." Advocating his Health Care for All Americans Act (S 1720, HR 5191), Senator Kennedy said that "once cost containment takes effect, the nation will pay less for health care under national health insurance than if the current non-system is left unchecked. The choice is not . . . between an expensive new program and no program at all," he said. "The choice is between comprehensive benefits for all Americans in a system with cost controls at every level, or a continuation of the patchwork system, with millions and millions of Americans denied care and costs continuing out of control."[14]

With charts to illustrate health care costs comparisons between the United States and Canada, Senator Kennedy said that Canada, which had in place a national health insurance for the previous ten years, "has been able to effectively stabilize health care costs as a percentage of its gross national product since 1968." Comparing health care costs of the U.S. and Canada as a percentage of the gross national product, he noted that in 1963, U.S. health-care costs were 5.6% of the GNP, and in Canada, 6%; in 1968, U.S. costs were 6.5%, Canada's 6.8%; in 1973, the U.S., 7.7%, Canada's 6.7%; and in 1978, the U.S., 8.8%, Canada, 7%.[15]

To compare experiences of citizens from both countries under their current systems of health care, Senator Kennedy asked six American and six Canadian families to tell about the health care they and their families had received. Witnesses represented various categories of age and income. Some were poor; some were middle class; some had had catastrophic medical expenses; some of the patients described were children, and some were elderly. Their testimonies spoke effectively of the differences in health-care costs and services in Canada under the national health insurance system and in the United States. Among them was Mrs. Daniel Corbett of Newton, Massachusetts who told of severe physical illnesses of her children that cost thousands of dollars. "My husband makes good money," she said. "But we can't enjoy it. Most of it goes for doctor bills."[16]

Organized medicine quickly came out in opposition to the Kennedy bill. "Senator Edward Kennedy's latest proposal for national health insurance is a slap in the taxpayer's face," charged Dr. Nicholas Krikes of the California Medical Association. "Evidently Kennedy doesn't understand—or refuses to accept—the message that the people have sent to government through Proposition 13 (California Initiative Limiting Property Taxes) and similar initiatives in other states. That message is simply 'cut government spending.'"[17]

Noting that the Kennedy proposal would add $22 billion per year to federal health expenditures, Dr. Krikes said, "It appears that this additional tax load would cover benefits, ignoring the huge cost of a new federal bureaucracy to regulate and administer the plan." As an example of the impact of government regulations on health costs, Dr. Krikes cited a study by the Hospital Association of New York State that found that 25% of the operating expenses of hospitals in that state is incurred to comply with government regulations—"many of them redundant, nonproductive, or in conflict with other regulations," he charged.

"Inevitably," noted Dr. Krikes, "NHI would add heavily to the national debt, increasing inflation and boosting health costs even further, just as the Medicare and Medicaid programs have done. Kennedy's proposal certainly isn't cost effective, and it is ill advised, especially now with people clamoring for tax relief, with polls showing that the majority of people are satisfied with their health care, and with the realization that 90 percent of all Americans already have some kind of health insurance." Krikes concluded that, "instead of expensive, unneeded NHI, Senator Kennedy could constructively serve the needs of Americans if he would focus on health insurance for the 10 percent who are not covered and catastrophic insurance to protect everyone from potential bankruptcy that can be caused by catastrophic illness or injury."[18]

On the second day of the hearings, the Massachusetts senator directly took on the American Medical Association, whose executive secretary and representative, Dr. James Sammons, said the AMA did not feel Kennedy's NHI plan was in the best interests of the American people. When Sammons began telling Kennedy that, although there were some problems with the American health care system, "it is the finest in the world," Kennedy interrupted and said, "Just a moment, doctor, I can't let that statement go by without commenting. It may be the finest for those who can afford it, but it's not the finest for the 26 million Americans who have no health insurance." He added, "It's not the finest for 51 million Americans living in the underserved areas."[19]

The position of the American Nurses' Association on National Health Insurance was given at this series of hearings by Barbara Nichols:

Ms. Nichols. 'I am Barbara Nichols, president of American Nurses' Association.'

Senator Kennedy. 'We are very glad to have you here. [*Applause*] That ought to warm you up a little bit on a cold day.

'We have heard your organization speak for years on matters affecting nurses. We have worked very closely with your association in the past and look forward to that association in the future.

'We are very mindful that you speak for a very important and significant element in the whole health care system. The nurses in many respects are closest to the patients. They have a very professional perspective on these issues. We are particularly grateful. I want to hear from you.'

Ms. Nichols. 'Mr. Chairman, my remarks today will speak in support of the national health insurance principles you recently outlined.

'As nurses, we see and experience in our daily work the results of the lack of an adequate health care system. This is why as an organization we support the concept that the goal of public health policy must be to make adequate health care available to all.' [*Applause*]

Ms. Nichols. 'As you know, and as you stated yourself, but I will reiterate, approximately 25 percent of the poor and near poor are not covered by any Medicare or Medicaid. The unemployed and newly employed often are without health insurance. Health services for many rural and inner-city residents are minimal, or nonexistent, and some of the testimony of the witnesses here today bore that out.

'Other groups are discriminated against in various ways under the present insurance plan.

'Divorced women, for example, frequently must pay disproportionately high premiums for their own health insurance, as so many divorced women stay at home with young children or work part time in one of the many places that offer no fringe benefits as such to employees.

'Many health insurance plans do not cover newborn infants. We heard that over and over today, particularly during the first 1 or 2 weeks after birth which, in fact, is the most critical time for the newborn. This fact can result and does result in astronomical bills if the child should require intensive care or special procedures of any kind.

'The American Nurses' Association believes that a national health insurance program is essential in order to guarantee that all U.S. residents will in fact have access to full comprehensive health services.

'Mr. Chairman, we refer to a health care system, but the system we have is not a health care system. It is a medical care system, an acute care system which focuses on trying to cure people after they become ill or patch them up after they have been injured or, God forbid, if you are old, relegate you to a nursing home. In other words, our present delivery system is focused on acute and chronic care, which relies primarily on the most expensive health care setting, the institution, and the expensive health care practitioner, the physician.

'We believe that no national health insurance plan can be successful that does not make substantial changes in the present system. This would include changes in reimbursement policies to encourage alternative care settings. I am glad to hear Mr. McMahon say he believes that as well. We believe there must be much greater use of registered nurses and other nonphysician health care personnel.

'We are pleased to note, Senator Kennedy, that the outline you have provided on national health insurance specifies comprehensive health service, including inpatient services, physicians' services, in and out of hospital, home health services, x-rays, lab tests and specified mental health benefits. We urge that the plan also include coverage for the following additional services:

'Twenty-four-hour emergency care, rehabilitative care, full mental health benefits, dental care, nutrition services and supportive care—health teaching, counseling and health education, maintenance care.' [Applause]

Ms. Nichols. 'These services, for the most part, are not medical services, but are integral to the delivery of comprehensive preventive health care.

'Additionally, the Kennedy plan, as outlined, makes no reference to nursing services as a covered benefit. You have said, and we agree, that nursing care is a key element in the delivery of health care in all settings. We believe that any comprehensive national health insurance plan must recognize registered, professional nurses as providers and must include nursing services as a benefit, regardless of the setting for that service; that is, home, clinic, hospital, school, nursing home, et cetera.' [Applause][20]

In contrast to the Kennedy proposal, catastrophic insurance was the core of Carter's "first-phase" national health plan, and in 1979 administration officials worked closely with Senate Finance Committee Chairman Russell B. Long (Democrat, Louisiana) and other key committee members on the legislation. Kennedy and his allies, principally organized labor, opposed the plan for catastrophic coverage for fear it would reduce pressure for a more comprehensive national health program. Catastrophic insurance would cover only "catastrophically" high medical bills, those remaining after a family had already paid several thousand dollars out of its own

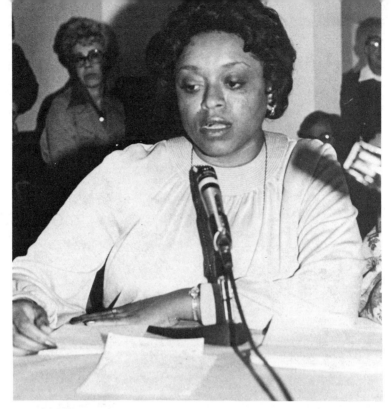

Figure 5–14. Barbara Nichols, ANA president, testified before the Senate health subcommittee. (Courtesy of American Nurses' Association, Kansas City, Missouri)

pocket in a year, or after private insurance coverage had been exhausted. But many members of Congress and the Carter administration believed the country could not afford a comprehensive health plan and opted to work for "fifty percent of something," rather than hold out for "one hundred percent of nothing."[21]

During the 96th Congress (1979–1980) more than a dozen different plans for some kind of national health insurance were introduced. These included:

- *S 1720, HR 5191—Health Care for All Americans Act.* Introduced by Senator Edward Kennedy and seven others in the Senate, by Representative Henry Waxman (Democrat, California) and 59 others in the House, this bill would set up a national health insurance program for the entire population, administered primarily by certified private health insurers and health maintenance organizations, with the federal government continuing to run Medicare. It would set a national budget for all services covered under the program with increases limited to rates of growth in the Gross National Product. A heavily regulated insurance industry would administer much of the plan. Insurance would be mandatory, with all individuals required to be insured for basic health services. Employees would have to pay up to 35% of the cost of their premiums, but would not have to meet any deductibles or make copayments. Assuming enactment

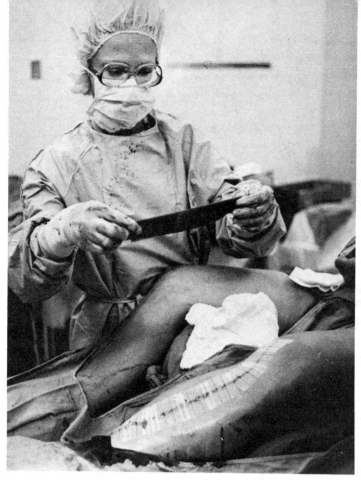

Figure 5-15. Concern over the costs of a national health insurance program made some congressmen favor a plan for catastrophic coverage only. (Courtesy of Robert Stockfield, Monroe, Louisiana)

in 1980, benefits would be phased in over an unspecified period of time, after a two-year lag to put cost control mechanisms in place. In the first year of benefits, the plan would add $28.6 billion to the federal budget and $11.4 billion to expenditures by business and workers for the mandatory coverage. According to Kennedy, costs would climb above those of existing programs for the first four years, but then there would be a "crossover," and after that point, total U.S. spending for health care would be less each year than if the existing system were to continue.

• *S 1812, HR 5400—National Health Plan Act.* The Carter administration proposal, introduced by Senator Abraham Ribicoff in the Senate and Representatives Charles Rangel (Democrat, New York), James Corman (Democrat, California), and Harley Staggers (Democrat, West Virginia) in the House, would set up a federal insurance program called Health Care to provide comprehensive coverage for the aged, disabled, and poor and coverage for everyone for catastrophic health care costs. It would also require employers to provide insurance for workers and their families through private plans. But except for the poor and disabled, and workers, who could receive full coverage from employers, Americans would have to pay up to $2500 a year in medical bills, plus part of the cost of their health insurance. This strategy was popular with economists who thought it would discourage overuse of physicians and hospitals and save money. Organized labor and well-paid professionals who had generous "first dollar" and major medical coverage for all or most health care bills would notice little difference in their coverage or out-of-pocket expenses, but there would be a dramatic cut in the tax deductions they could take in figuring their annual taxes. Agricultural and retail trade workers and others in poorly insured occupations would, for the first time, be covered for a package of basic benefits, because their employers would have to buy insurance for them or face tax penalties. But unless they developed enough clout to get employers to provide more than the minimum requirements, these workers would face new expenses as well.

- *S 350, HR 3277—Catastrophic Health Insurance and Medical Assistance Reform Act.* This bill, introduced by Senator Russell Long and Senator Abraham Ribicoff along with seven others, would provide insurance against catastrophic illness for the entire population through a federally run plan for the poor and aged and through private plans for the employed. It would also replace Medicaid.
- *S 351, HR 3276—Catastrophic Health Insurance Act.* This bill, introduced by Senator Russell Long and ten others, was similar to S 350, but it would not federalize Medicaid. It would authorize employers to provide catastrophic coverage for workers, covering physician bills over $2000 and hospital bills after 60 days of hospitalization. Persons not covered by employer plans would be covered by the federal government through a trust fund supported by a 1% payroll tax on employers. Employers could subtract premium costs from their payroll tax bill and get a tax credit. The cost of the bill was estimated at $5 billion to $7 billion a year.
- *S 760—Catastrophic Illness Insurance Act.* Another bill introduced by Senator Russell Long would require employers to provide workers and their families with catastrophic health insurance, would give tax credits to individuals who bought their own coverage, and would replace Medicaid with a federal program. Drafted to the specifications of a major insurance company, it made these major changes from his earlier bills: eliminated the 1% payroll tax; made it mandatory for employers to provide catastrophic insurance; provided tax rebates for half their premium expenses for employers and individuals buying their own coverage; imposed a tax penalty on employers failing to provide catastrophic coverage (150% of the premiums they would have paid); and required plans to cover employees' dependents up to age 26 and workers for up to 6 months after they left a job.
- *S 748—Catastrophic Health Insurance and Medicare Improvements Act of 1979.* This legislation was introduced by Senators Robert Dole (Republican, Kansas), John Danforth (Republican, Missouri), and Pete Domenici, (Republican, New Mexico). It would provide catastrophic health insurance coverage by improving Medicare, setting up employer-based private

plans, establishing a program for those with no other coverage, and requiring states to upgrade Medicaid.

- *S 1590—Comprehensive Health Care Reform Act.* Introduced July 26 by Senator Richard Schweiker (Republican, Pennsylvania), this bill would provide a minimum level of catastrophic coverage through a combination of tax incentives, state-run insurance pooling arrangements, and increased Medicare benefits.

- *S 1485—Health Incentives Reform Act of 1979.* Introduced by Senator David Durenberger (Republican, Minnesota) and three others, this legislation would make changes in the tax code and the Social Security law to encourage competition in the health insurance industry and to encourage employers to provide catastrophic coverage.

- *S 1014—Maternal and Child Health Protection Benefits and Catastrophic Medical Expense and Reimbursement Act.* This bill, introduced by Senator Gary Hart (Democrat, Colorado), would provide comprehensive health services for children and pregnant women and catastrophic insurance coverage for others.

- *HR 21—The Health Security Act.* Introduced by Representative James Corman and twenty-four others, this was the latest version of the all-federal government plan once sponsored by Senator Edward Kennedy. It would set up a national system to provide comprehensive health services for everyone.

- *HR 2969—Health Service Act.* Introduced by Representative Ronald Dellums (Democrat, California) and eight others, this bill would create a United States Health Service through which salaried health care workers would provide free comprehensive health services to all citizens.

- *HR 1804—National Health Care Act of 1979.* Introduced by Representative Ray Roberts (Democrat, Texas), this legislation would strengthen the health planning program and set up a national system of comprehensive health benefits.

- *HR 7528—Consumer Health Expense Control Act.* Introduced by Representative James Jones (Democrat, Oklahoma), this bill would set up a catastrophic national health insurance program to protect those otherwise not covered and would attempt to discourage "over-insuring" by limiting an employer's tax-exempt contribution to his or her employee's health care plan to $100 a month for family coverage.

- *HR 7527—The National Health Care Reform Act of 1980.* This bill, introduced by Representative Richard Gephardt (Democrat, Missouri) and Representative David Stockman (Republican, Michigan), would abolish much of the nation's existing health regulatory mechanisms and set up a system of tax credits and vouchers to enable consumers to shop for their own health insurance coverage. Under the bill, every American would receive, in one form or another, a federal Health Care contribution, which he or she could use to buy coverage from a qualified health care plan. Qualified health care plans could be sponsored by hospitals, physicians, Blue Cross and Blue Shield plans, commercial insurance companies, or any other private organization or government agency. HR 7527 would

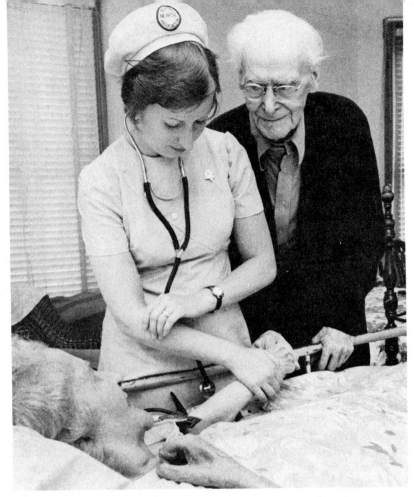

Figure 5–16. A serious omission from many national health insurance proposals is provision for the payment of nursing services in the home. (Courtesy of Indianapolis Star Indianapolis, Indiana)

abolish the health planning structure, with its network of health systems agencies and its certificate-of-need laws. It would abolish tax deductions for health care expenses. It would gradually phase out the Medicare and Medicaid programs and, with them, professional standards review organizations and the cost-based reimbursement system that has taken much of the blame for running up health care costs. The bill would also preempt any state laws, such as hospital rate regulations, that were inconsistent with its purposes. Gephardt said that he estimated the revenue costs of the bill to the federal government would be $10 billion in the first year, increasing to $14 billion the second. Between the fifth and the tenth year, the new system would pass the break-even point and begin to save money.

National health insurance will sooner or later become a reality in the United States, and the proposal most likely to be accepted by Americans will not rely solely on either government or private sector control, according to Wilbur J. Cohen, former HEW secretary and a leader in the development of the Medicare program. Cohen, in a December 1979 speech before a conference of the Blue Cross and Blue Shield associations, said he believed the NHI program that is likely to evolve will be a "mixed system" of public and private entities. While the details of any future national health insurance program remain "shrouded in mystery," Cohen said, public policy is likely to reject "exclusive continued reliance on the private voluntary insurance mechanism [and] . . . the complete reliance on a public medical service approach—such as that in Great Britain and the Soviet Union." How national health insurance is paid for and who controls the cost are two of the unresolved questions about a national policy. Cohen noted that the major plans proposed in Congress assumed that funding would come from either employers, employee contributions, federal revenues, or state, and possibly local, monies. But how much should come from each source and who should collect these funds remain unanswered questions which are likely to cause debate. With these remarks Cohen set the tone for debate on the most massive health issue facing Americans in the 1980s—the adoption of a real national health policy with the enactment of some form of national health insurance.[22]

In the next several years, new approaches intended to stabilize health care prices and provide quality care will continue to be forthcoming from legislators, health care providers, insurers, the business community, and organized labor. Gradual changes in the financing and delivery of health services are already emerging. In order to develop more efficient and improved health delivery services for the nation's 230 million citizens, many financial and structural problems are yet to be resolved, and nursing input is vital. What should be the appropriate mix of public and private financing? What portion of public spending should be for preventive care and how much for treating illness? Who should provide the care? What would be the most efficient type of administrative structure to regulate public spending on health care? Should incentives in the form of reimbursement practices or tax benefits be provided to hospitals, physicians, nurses, and insurers who cut costs and improve services? Can efficient reimbursement mechanisms be developed? These and other questions will need to be answered in the near future if the health care crisis we are now experiencing is not to become a catastrophe.

References

1. Editorial: JAMA Dec, 1932
2. National Health Survey, 1935–1936, Preliminary Reports, Sickness and Medical Care Series, Bulletin No. 9: Disability from Specific Causes in Relation to Economic Status. Washington, DC, National Institutes of Health, 1938
3. Hospital service in the United States. Annual issues of JAMA, 1928–1937
4. U.S. President. Interdepartmental Committee to Coordinate Health and Welfare Activities: Proceedings of the National Health Conference, p 70. Washington, DC, United States Government Printing Office, 1938
5. Ibid, pp 71–72
6. Ibid, p 72
7. Special message to the Congress on health and disability insurance, May 19, 1947. In Public Papers of the Presidents of the United States: Harry S. Truman, 1947, pp 250–252. Washington, DC, Office of the Federal Register, National Archives & Records Service,

1963; Special message to the Congress on the nation's health needs, April 22, 1949. In Public Papers of the Presidents of the United States: Harry S. Truman, 1949, pp 226–230. Washington, DC, Office of the Federal Register, National Archives & Records Service, 1964

8. Burrow JG: AMA: Voice of American Medicine, pp 368–369. Baltimore, Johns Hopkins University Press, 1963
9. Congressional Record. Jan 10, 1977, p S-303, S 104: To amend the Social Security Act to provide for inclusion of the services of licensed registered nurses under medicare and medicaid.
10. Congressional Record. Jan 14, 1977, p S-615, S 223: To amend part B of Title XI of the Social Security Act to assure appropriate participation by professional registered nurses in peer review, and related activities authorized thereunder.
11. Ibid
12. U.S. General Accounting Office: Factors That Impede Progress in Implementing the Health Maintenance Organization Act of 1973. Report to the Congress. Washington, DC, United States General Accounting Office, Report #HRD-76-128, Sept 3, 1976
13. New York, NY, New York Times, June 17, 1976
14. U.S. Congress. Senate. Committee on Human Resources, Subcommittee on Health and Scientific Research: National Health Insurance, 1978, p 793. Hearings before the Subcommittee. Washington, DC, United States Government Printing Office, 1979
15. Ibid, pp 795–796
16. Ibid
17. Ibid, pp 892–898
18. Los Angeles, Calif, Los Angeles Times, Dec 16, 1978
19. Ibid
20. U.S. Congress. Senate. Committee on Human Resources, Subcommittee on Health and Scientific Research: National Health Insurance, 1978, pp 638–664. Hearings before the Subcommittee. Washington, DC, United States Government Printing Office, 1979
21. U.S. Congress. Senate. Committee on Finance: Catastrophic Health Insurance and Medical Assistance Reform. Hearings before the Committee. Washington, DC, United States Government Printing Office, 1979
22. National Health Insurance Reports, Jan, 1980

6–Development of Federal Nursing Education Policy

Federal policy making for nursing is conducted in a policy arena characterized by charter legislation, by executive, congressional, and lobbying institutions, and by a political culture. One of the most evident characteristics of federal nursing programs is that there is no comprehensive policy in the sense of an integrated, coordinated, and comprehensive blueprint of where the federal government is going and why with respect to the profession. While the programs in this policy arena have substantive coherence because they all deal with federal support for nursing and the financing of nursing services through military, Veterans Administration, Medicare, Medicaid, and other health programs, a coherent, intellectual, and philosophical approach has not characterized the federal government's nursing activities. The federal government has, without a doubt, had a profound influence on the development of nursing in the United States. But this influence has come about through a complex of federal activities lacking in a sufficient concentration of authority.

The absence of a comprehensive federal nursing policy is seen in how the federal institutional structure deals with nursing education. The nursing education policy arena can perhaps be thought of as a truncated policy arena because all the programs of the federal government that affect nursing are clearly not included within it. The basic legislative charter of nursing education policy is the Nurse Training Act of 1964, though this is not the first piece of federal nursing education legislation. One can trace the roots of the federal focus of nursing education as far back as the establishment of the Public Health Service (PHS) in 1798.

It was nearly 190 years ago that the second president of the United States, John Adams, signed a bill to provide "for the relief of sick and disabled seamen," paving the way for the evolution of the U.S. Public Health Service and the eventual emergence of its Division of Nursing. Back in that era the word *health* was rarely used by the fledgling federal government, but disease and sickness existed to such an extent that the Congress on April 3, 1794, passed an act that authorized the President of the United States to alter in certain cases the meeting place of Congress. It read,

> That whenever the Congress shall be about to convene, and from the prevalence of contagious sickness, or the existence of other circumstances, it would, in the opinion of the President of the United States, be hazardous to the lives or health of the members to meet at the place to which the Congress shall then stand adjourned, . . . the President shall be . . . authorized . . . to convene the Congress at such other place as he may judge proper.[1]

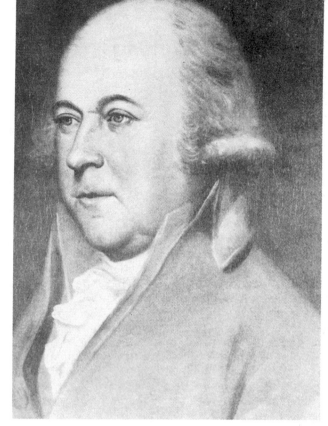

Figure 6–1. President John Adams signed the law that created the U.S. Public Health Service in 1798. (Courtesy of Library of Congress)

ORIGINS OF THE U.S. PUBLIC HEALTH SERVICE

In the 1790s, practically the entire population of the United States resided upon the Eastern seaboard or closely adjacent to it, and transportation was by water whenever possible. Because a well-developed merchant marine was an essential factor in promoting the economic development and stability of the new nation, it was natural that ways would be sought to foster and encourage the development of trade. One possible means was to provide for the medical care of merchant sailors who became sick or injured. This idea was probably borrowed from the English, who, after the defeat of the Spanish Armada in 1588, established at Chatham what was called a "chest" to which sailors could contribute a monthly stipend. As a result, the British government erected a hospital at Greenwich and later, in 1750, another at Liverpool, for the care of sailors who had contributed to this fund.

The desirability of establishing similar protection for American sailors was discussed in Congress at various times between the years 1790 and 1798. The proponents of such bills argued that, in addition to humanitarian considerations, the national defense and the promotion of commerce demanded a nationwide system of direct medical and hospital care for the seamen. Thus the concept was born that where national health needs were not being met—because of the complexity of the problems, the insistence of the need, or the magnitude of the resources required—the federal government was under an obligation to help.

Several developments led to serious consideration of such measures. The mortality rate among merchant seamen was high. Sick or injured sailors were often dropped ashore at the nearest port where they became dependent on well-meaning housewives and families to nurse them back to health. Towns along the East Coast were soon receiving so many disabled seamen that they could no longer find nurses for them. In 1787, the Commonwealth of Virginia built a marine hospital at Norfolk and appropriated state funds for its operation. No other state followed this example, however, as the financial resources of the other states were slender.

The federal government soon swung into action. On February 28, 1798, Robert Livingston, a representative from New York, reported a bill from the Committee on Commerce and Manufacturers for the relief of sick and disabled seamen. The report stated,

> the committee finds that numbers of seamen, as well as foreigners and natives, arrive at the different ports of the United States in such a disabled situation that they either become a great burden to the public hospitals, where any such are established, or are left to perish for want of proper attention. They are of the opinion that a sufficient fund might be raised for the support and relief of sick and disabled American seamen, as well in foreign ports as in the United States, either by an additional tonnage duty on all vessels entering the ports of the United States, or by a charge on the wages of all seamen shipped within the United States, proportioned to the length of the voyage, to be paid or secured by the master and deducted from the wages of his crew.[2]

After a good deal of debate the bill passed the House of Representatives on April 9, 1798, the Senate on July 14, 1798, and was signed into law the following day.

More than a century later, in 1902, Congress passed an act entitled, "To Increase the Efficiency and Change the Name of the U.S. Marine Hospital Service." During the preceding 104 years, a small number of professionals who constituted the Marine Hospital Service had worked so earnestly and consistently for public health protection from the prevention standpoint that Congress changed the name of the U.S. Marine Hospital Service to that of the U.S. Public Health and Marine Hospital Service. Public health, characterized by prevention, now took precedence over the marine hospitals, which represented an earlier, custodial focus.

EMERGENCE OF TRAINED NURSES IN THE PUBLIC HEALTH SERVICE

During the first 120 years of the Public Health Service (PHS), nurses were used only in a very limited way. World War I changed this, marking the first extensive deployment of nurses by the PHS. When special zones were established around military camps to safeguard the health of the adjacent civilian population, more than 120 nurses were assigned to carry out the sanitary measures designed by the PHS. In this effort, the services of local health organizations were enlisted, along with the assistance of the Red Cross.[3]

The nurses of the U.S. Public Health Service were responsible for investigating cases of communicable diseases, instructing families of patients about proper care and sanitation, and assisting in the health inspection of school children. In these endeavors, Supervising Nurse Mary E. Lent coordinated various local nursing forces, which had traditionally been independent of each other; the activity of Miss Lent therefore helped to build up a wholly new, well-organized system of local public health nursing in this country. And by the time the extracantonment (special) zones were closed and the federal officers withdrawn at the war's end, the work of the nurses employed by the PHS had created a public demand for public health nursing, and marked the real emergence of trained nurses in the U.S. Public Health Service.

Following the war, the initial federal stimulus to public health nursing at the state level came with the Maternity and Infancy Act of 1921 (Sheppard-Towner Act), which allocated more than $1 million annually to those states that would establish agencies to improve the health protection of mothers and babies. The Maternity and Infancy Act achieved considerable impact in a number of areas as birth and death statistics improved throughout the country. A number of new state agencies and child health centers were created, and states increased their own health appropriations.

In general, the public health expenditures of the 1920s proved that public health nursing could be a purchasable commodity: the effective public health nursing programs, which had grown up in the first quarter of the 20th century, had helped to lower the mortality rate, to increase life expectancy, and to reduce significantly the morbidity rate from tuberculosis, typhoid fever, smallpox, malaria, and most infant diseases. However, much of this progress was threatened by the Great Depression, which worsened the health of many Americans while frightening the government into economizing on public health nursing activities. As a means of limiting government expenditure in the face of a shrinking national economy, public health expenditures were cut sharply between 1929 and 1933.

The advent of President Franklin Roosevelt's New Deal in 1933 produced a dramatic turnabout in fiscal policy, which meant an unprecedented expansion of the federal involvement in the social welfare of the American people, and so nursing was not neglected. In the spring of 1933, with one-quarter of the labor force out of work, Congress created the Federal Emergency Relief Administration (FERA) to aid the states in alleviating the hardships caused by the Depression. Under FERA, relief funds were available for nursing services, and Pearl McIver of the Division of Domestic Quarantine (States Relations) of the PHS was consulted by FERA and many states in planning such programs. Shortly thereafter, the Civil Works Administration temporarily hired over 10,000 unemployed nurses in various health institutions, public health campaigns, and other services. And the most influential relief program in the Depression, the Works Progress Administration, helped the states to support various health projects and hire nurses as supplements to the regular staffs of their overburdened state and local public health departments. It was recognized that the traditional federal delegation of responsibility for public health facilities to local and state authorities had resulted in a very uneven and inadequate development of health service from state to state.

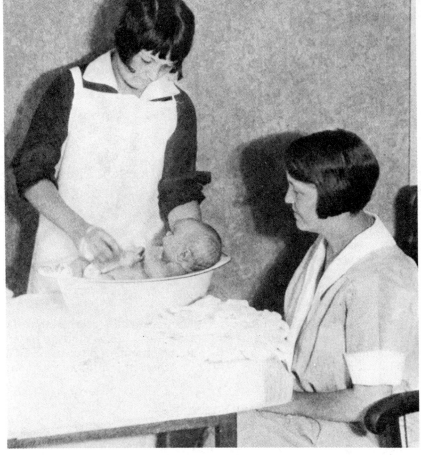

Figure 6–2. The Sheppard–Towner Act supported state infant and maternal hygiene programs. (Courtesy of History of Nursing Collection, University of Michigan)

The first Roosevelt administration embarked upon a number of other health initiatives, the most significant of which was the Social Security Act of 1935, which provided for old-age benefits, the health care of mothers and children, and grants for state and local public health services, largely carried out by nurses. This act imposed on the PHS the duties of assisting states and districts in establishing health organizations and facilitating the training of public health personnel, representing the federal government's very first acknowledgment of a responsibility to train nursing personnel. In order to meet immediate needs, the state health departments could designate nurses to undertake short-term training at colleges or universities that taught public health programs that met the standards of the National Organization for Public Health Nursing.

During the late 1930s, the combination of federal funds with state and local appropriations brought about an impressive expansion of basic health services on the local level, among these being the provision of facilities for the diagnosis and treatment of cancer, pneumonia, dental defects, and crippling conditions, and the establishment of programs for industrial hygiene, mental health, and venereal disease. The federal involvement with nursing—largely providing support for postgraduate training for public

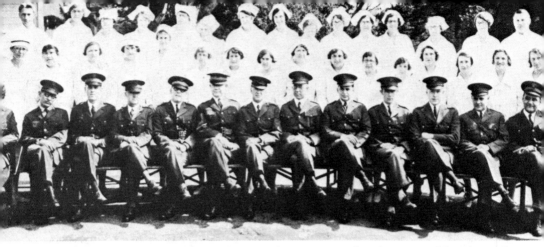

Figure 6–3. The nurses of the U.S. Public Health Service saw their focus expand from hospital care to broader public health activities during the mid-1930s. (Courtesy of U.S. Public Health Service)

health nurses for state and local health departments—increased as the federal health programs grew and multiplied. But federal funding for nursing remained on a small scale until the nursing shortages of the Second World War threatened the war effort. And even then, the full-scale commitment was slow in coming.

WORLD WAR II AND THE DEMAND FOR NURSES

In 1940 nursing leaders from the national organizations and several government agencies formed the Nursing Council for National Defense to help prepare American nursing for war. With financial assistance from the PHS, this council conducted the first exhaustive survey of professional nursing resources ever attempted in the United States and also prepared a plan to expand basic nursing education facilities to cope with the potential demands of the war. Ultimately, a weakened version of this plan was approved by Congress; it authorized some funding for basic nursing education as well as refresher and postgraduate courses to be administered under the Public Health Nursing section of the Division of States Relations of the PHS. Significantly, this marked the first time that the federal government provided funds to support basic nursing education.

The initial federal appropriation of $1.2 million for FY 1942 was small in relation to the country's needs. The money covered only tuition and subsistence for students in basic nursing programs and some advanced programs; no new programs could be initiated. By December of 1941, federal funds had accounted for a total increase in admissions of 9%, but more money was needed just to maintain this small advance. Admissions threatened to decrease, and in any case, facilities could not really accommodate any more significant increases in enrollment.

Just after Pearl Harbor, military recruitment of nurses diminished, and conscription of nurses into the armed forces was seriously considered as a means of averting nursing shortages at home and overseas. Unfortunately, RNs in general hospitals, whose services were vital to their schools of nursing and nursing services, represented the principal source of military recruits. Nursing leaders steadfastly opposed conscription and also opposed any effort to reduce the student nurse training period (suggested to accelerate the entry of young women into the profession) because they feared a massive collapse of the already meager educational standards.

U.S. CADET NURSE CORPS

By late 1942, nursing leaders had begun to accept the necessity for an accelerated program of nursing education for the duration of the war and threw their support behind Dr. George Baehr of the Office of Civilian Defense, whose plan came to be called the U.S. Cadet Nurse Corps program. The student who joined the Corps would obtain complete preparation for professional nursing in either a 24-month or a 30-month program and would receive free tuition, maintenance, uniforms, and a monthly stipend, which increased with her training; most of this would be financed by the federal government at an estimated cost of $60 to $70 million per year for some 65,000 new participants annually.

In early 1943, Congresswoman Frances Payne Bolton introduced the authorization for the Cadet Nurse Corps into Congress. After much tes-

Figure 6–4. The 1942 recruitment poster distributed by the federal government to inspire young women to seek admission to nursing education programs. (Courtesy of U.S. Public Health Service)

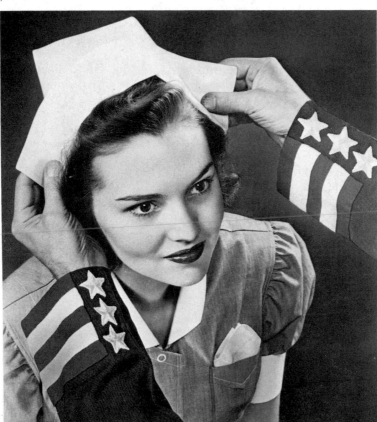

timony and several amendments, the bill was passed into law and signed by President Roosevelt on June 15, 1943, laying the groundwork for what would become the largest experiment in federally subsidized education in the history of the United States up to that time. The Cadet Nurse Corps was administered under the direction of PHS surgeon general, Thomas Parran, who created a new Division of Nurse Education (DNE) and appointed Lucile Petry, a distinguished and popular nurse educator, to head the division and direct the Cadet Nurse Corps.

In order to counteract the attractiveness of lucrative war work and the appeal of the women's auxiliary forces, the corps embarked upon a publicity program unprecedented in the history of any civilian profession in America. The recruitment campaign took the form of newspaper and magazine advertisements and stories, radio spots, posters, movies, and celebrity-studded events. While many disapproved of the tone of the publicity campaign, which emphasized the glamour, excitement, and opportunity of the new nursing program, no one could deny the dramatic success it achieved in more than meeting the recruitment goals set early in the war.

And there was also little disagreement concerning the question of the Corps' overall positive effect. The wartime acceleration and enlargement of nursing programs appeared in many cases to have improved the quality, as well the quantity, of nursing students; educational facilities benefited from additions to libraries and laboratories and from a significant number of curricular refinements. The incentive of federal money and the guidance of Division of Nurse Education consultants impelled a large number of poorer schools to improve. The collapse of nursing service in both civilian and military hospitals was averted, while data collected by the DNE contributed to the continuing reform of nursing education by generating pressures for improvement.

Some two dozen consultants from the Division of Nurse Education visited the 1125 schools participating in the corps, monitoring the quality of their programs and communicating their problems to Washington. Thus, the Cadet Nurse Corps educated the federal government in the conditions and needs of basic nurse preparation. One major problem which appeared early on was the creation of housing for the expanded student enrollments. Since the Bolton Act contained no provision for construction, housing problems were at least partially solved through the provisions of the National Defense Housing Act, which channeled over $17 million in funds from the Federal Works Administration to over 200 nursing education and dormitory facilities, the money going primarily to hospital schools. This program had far-reaching effects: it represented the first use of federal funds in nursing school construction, and the experience of reviewing and consulting on applications for physical facilities supplied the nurse consultants with a valuable background in building design, which schools would draw on later.

As a result of Cadet Nurse Corps activities, an acute nurse faculty shortage was soon identified in schools of nursing. Most of the appointments were dual in nature, with nurse faculty members performing service duties as well. The lion's share of instruction in the physical and social sciences had been done by non-nurse faculty before the war; one important devel-

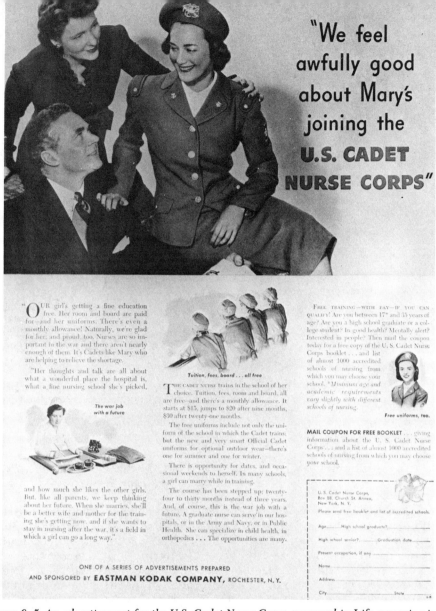

Figure 6–5. An advertisement for the U.S. Cadet Nurse Corps appeared in Life *magazine in late 1943 and elicited thousands of inquiries about this government sponsored program. (Courtesy of U.S. Public Health Service)*

opment of the war was the fact that nurse instructors began to take the place of scarce physician-lecturers in theory classes; many of these nurse-lecturers adopted new teaching methods that focused on the patient rather than on the disease. Consultants noted that the quality of a nursing school directly corresponded to the general educational background of its faculty. Although there were very few baccalaureate or graduate degrees among nurse faculty in 1945, the Bolton Act enabled several thousand faculty to undertake some postgraduate training in their field of specialization. Per-

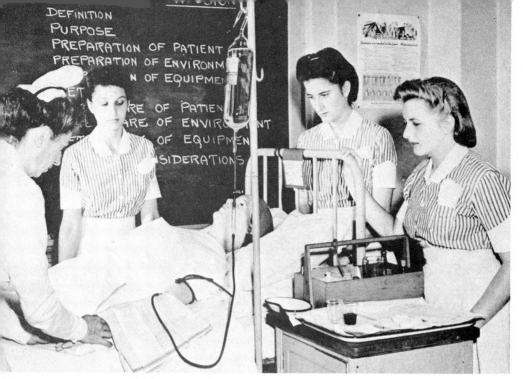

Figure 6–6. Under the leadership of the Division of Nurse Education, the quality of teaching in nurses' preparation programs was substantially upgraded. (Courtesy History of Nursing Collection, University of Michigan)

haps more important, the pressures applied by the Division of Nursing Education made schools more aware of the need for the advanced training of their faculties.

One particular concern of the Division of Nurse Education was the budgetary status of the nursing schools: most schools of nursing up until that time did not have budgets of their own. To meet federal accounting requirements, the monies made available by the Bolton Act created the need for separate nursing school budgets. One lasting effect of these special budgets was the first step in the identification of the actual costs of nursing education and its segregation from the overall hospital budget. Additionally, the Bolton Act both allocated federal money for library improvement and encouraged the schools to establish book funds as fixtures in their budget requests. Another and less tangible effect of the budgets was the fact that they allowed directors of nursing programs their first taste of relative autonomy. The experience was to be a memorable, if temporary, one.

PHS LEADERSHIP IN ADVANCING PUBLIC HEALTH NURSING

The Cadet Nurse Corps was the most dramatic example of the war's intensification of the relationship between nursing and the federal government, but other less dramatic developments also exemplify this trend. In 1941, Congress authorized the Public Health Service to engage in "Emergency Health and Sanitation Activities" related to the war effort. With this congressional appropriation, the PHS provided short courses for nurses who were later assigned to help carry out public health programs in extracantonment and defense industrial zones. PHS nurses under Pearl McIver helped to develop postgraduate training centers for public health nurses, participated in community nursing services in war-impacted areas, relieved local nurses on educational leaves, and helped to establish or improve special programs such as tuberculosis, cancer, and venereal disease control. The tuberculosis program achieved particularly notable success, as did a program that provided maternity care to the wives of servicemen and to others in underserved communities. Because of such efforts, the infant mortality rate was held to a record low during the war.

The assignment of permanent nurse consultants throughout many of the offices of the government led nursing leaders to call for better coordination of nursing activities in the PHS. This situation was brought to a head by the streamlining of the PHS at the end of 1943, whereby all service functions were separated into four divisions: the Office of the Surgeon General, the

Figure 6–7. Nurses were employed by the U.S. Public Health Service to engage in Emergency health and sanitation activities in war-impacted areas. (Courtesy of U.S. Public Health Service)

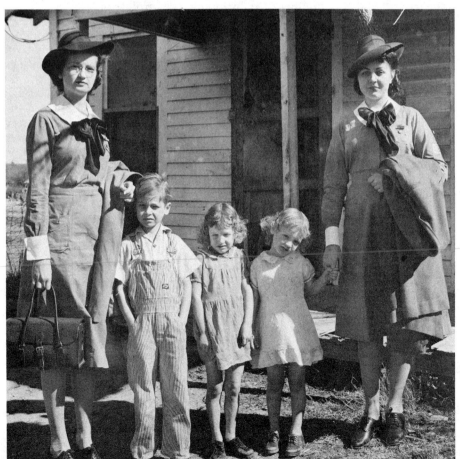

National Institute of Health, the Bureau of Medical Services, and the Bureau of State Services. Pearl McIver, director of public health nurse consultants, recommended that a division of public health nursing be created within the Bureau of State Services and that it be given general supervision over all nursing activities in that bureau, including the work of public health nurses assigned to district offices and to other agencies. Surgeon General Parran found this plan acceptable. All public health nursing would be organized under the Office of Public Health Nursing in the Bureau of State Services, whereas the Office of Nursing in the Bureau of Medical Services would supervise the activities of nurses in the hospitals and clinics of the U.S. Public Health Service. The Division of Nurse Education would continue to operate out of the Office of the Surgeon General.

The growth of the PHS during the war was reflected in both the expanding body of its personnel and the increasing value of federal appropriations: personnel increased from 9600 in 1940 to 16,000 in 1944, and the appropriation swelled even more, from $20 million to $109 million, the new Division of Nurse Education itself accounting for nearly 50% of the total annual budget.

This state of affairs engendered a climate of optimism and ambition among nursing leaders, particularly those of the National League of Nursing Education and the National Organization of Public Health Nursing; it also engendered a desire to finally consolidate the profession under a comprehensive federal agency with authority to assist the continued development of both nursing education and nursing services. But unlike nursing leaders, the federal government, especially the increasingly conservative-minded Congress, regarded its unprecedented involvement in nurse preparation as an emergency wartime measure, like rationing, acceptable only for a time and only as part of the war effort. While the Public Health Service Act of 1944 codified all legislation pertaining to the PHS and authorized the establishment of a Division of Nursing, it omitted a provision authorizing postwar programs of aid to nursing education and service. The Cadet Nurse Corps was to be phased out after the war along with its administering body, the Division of Nurse Education. Nursing leaders were in effect told not to look to the government for financial support of any master plan for nursing's future.

POSTWAR REFORMS

Several of these leaders, members of the National Nursing Council for War Service, decided to promote their own study of nursing education; they found a sponsor in the Carnegie Corporation and a director in Esther Lucille Brown of the Russell Sage Foundation. Using information on nursing schools, which had been gathered through the administration of the Cadet Nurse Corps, Dr. Brown surveyed the current state of nursing education: its problems, needs, and priorities. The final product of this effort was entitled, *Nursing for the Future;* the closing of weak schools and the development of nursing programs in universities and colleges were recommended. It was published in 1948 and met with a tremendous popular response.

With studies like the Brown Report, an acute RN shortage, and a ready supply of war-trained nurses' aides and practical nurses, the postwar period marked the dawn of widespread activity in planning for the most efficient modes of the delivery of nursing care. At the war's end, nursing faced a double crisis in the quantity and the quality of its personnel. Nursing school admissions declined drastically with the phasing out of the Cadet Corps, and hundreds of hospitals were faced with severe nursing shortages. Concomitantly, a survey conducted among physicians by the AMA indicated widespread dissatisfaction with the quality of care delivered by nurses.[4]

Nursing leaders believed that the general educational standards for nurse preparation continued to remain far too low because 97% of the nursing schools were controlled by hospitals: a diploma school's service to its hospital generally took priority over its role as an educational institution. While the baccalaureate-oriented portion of the nursing community was advancing its own plans for reform, the AMA instituted a Committee on Nursing Problems in 1948, which, upon consultation with nursing leaders, recommended that the profession be divided into professional and practical

Figure 6–8. Although massive shortages of nurses in the late 1940s prompted extensive advertising (such as this sign in Times Square, New York City), the political climate nearly forced a termination of federal assistance in resolving this problem. (Courtesy of U.S. Public Health Service)

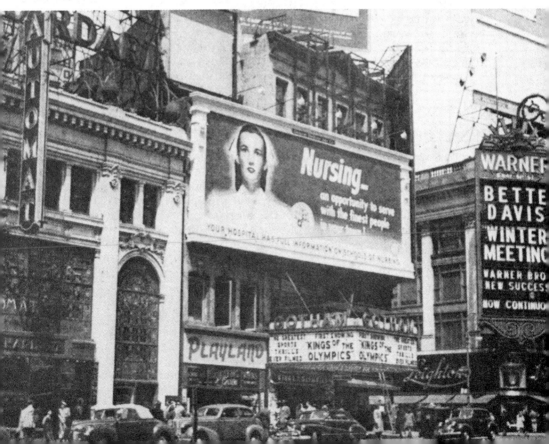

nurses with increased emphasis upon baccalaureate education for the professional nurse and upon the upgrading of practical nurse training.

The recommendations of both the Brown Report and the AMA report entailed a revision of the system whereby nurses were educated. In 1949, a comprehensive plan for a national health program was under consideration by Congress, along with legislation to financially assist the training of nurses and other health professionals. The bill reflected the request of nursing leaders for funds to improve nursing curricula and teaching. The Emergency Health Professions Training Act of 1949 included provisions for nursing scholarships as well as general support funds for schools of nursing. Although the bill passed the Senate with a unanimous vote, the newly formed National Organization of Hospital Schools of Nursing (NOHSN) claimed that the bill would enable the surgeon general to control hospital schools of nursing; marshalling opposition to the bill, it ultimately played a key role in blocking its passage in the House of Representatives. Although hospital schools would have been eligible for aid had the bill passed, NOHSN's opposition reflected recognition that hospital schools were more vulnerable to quality control mechanisms than were colleges and universities.

The postwar difficulties over a continuing federal involvement in nursing were part of the larger struggle between those who wanted to continue the New Deal's and the war's expansion of the federal role in American life and those who regarded such activities as threats to personal freedom and private initiative. Federal aid to nursing education became part of a package of health care reform whose other items included aid to medical education and federally sponsored programs of national health insurance. Such items, singly or in groups, were periodically advanced in postwar legislation and were periodically rejected by conservative Congresses. Nevertheless, their recurring appearance before each session of Congress indicated that they had acquired a permanent base of support.

ORGANIZATIONAL STRUCTURE OF NURSING IN THE PHS

The postwar period also saw a number of organizational changes in the Public Health Service. In 1946, the Division of Nursing with Lucile Petry as director, had been established within the Office of the Surgeon General, and the Division of Nurse Education was abolished. The new Division of Nursing was to act as a staff arm of the surgeon general and provide consultative, advisory, and supervisory service. It had no administrative authority, although it was granted certain broad responsibilities for evaluating the nursing personnel of the PHS. The new division consisted of three offices: the Office of Public Health Nursing (virtually autonomous in the field of public health nursing), the Office of Nurse Education and Resources (furnishing consultation concerning nurse education and supply), and the Office of Hospital Nursing (advising and evaluating in matters pertaining to nursing in the U.S. Public Health Service hospitals). Because of a lack of a viable operating budget with which to address its responsibilities, the umbrella structure of the Division of Nursing was aborted in its infancy.

During 1949, the Public Health Service was completely reorganized to better coordinate its activities. The new organization plan emphasized the

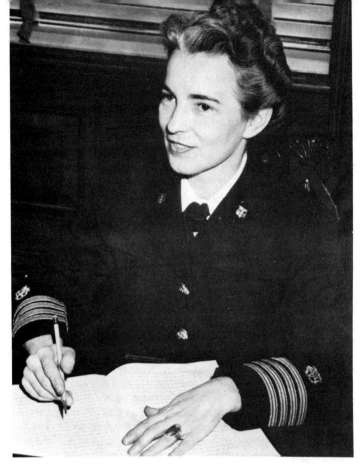

Figure 6–9. Lucile Petry administered the Division of Nurse Education during the late 1940s and then became the first chief nurse officer of the U.S. Public Health Service. (Courtesy of U.S. Public Health Service)

use of certain professional skills, and toward this end, resources divisions were established in nursing, dentistry, and engineering. Just as assistant surgeons general served as chiefs of the Bureau of Medical Services, the Bureau of State Services, and the National Institutes of Health, so the new chief nurse officer, dental officer, and sanitary engineering officer were given the rank of assistant surgeon general and served as associate bureau chiefs. In this reorganization, the Office of Public Health Nursing was given the status of a division within the Bureau of State Services, and its chief, Pearl McIver, was promoted to nurse director. This division continued to give general direction to all federal public health nursing activities, and tabulated data on public health nurses.

DIVISION OF NURSING RESOURCES ACTIVITIES IN THE 1950s

In the 1949 reorganization, staff functions were placed as close to operating programs as possible. Thus, Lucile Petry became chief nurse officer, responsible for coordinating functions for all nursing activity. The Division of Nursing in the surgeon general's office was abolished and many of its functions taken over by the new Division of Nursing Resources (DNR) of the Bureau of Medical Services, headed by Margaret Arnstein. The Division of Nursing Resources worked within the Bureau of Medical Services in promoting the effectiveness of nursing care, providing consultation services to states and institutions, and helping to conduct surveys of nursing resources. Its original structure provided for three branches, whose goals were: the improvement of nurse education, improvement of nurse utilization, and improvement of local nurse supplies; a fourth branch was set up to furnish statistical services to the other branches. The consultation and survey services were to be the DNR's mainstay over the lean years of the early 1950s as the division built up research expertise on a shoestring budget of about $90,000 annually and produced helpful publications, which guided states and hospitals in surveying the quantity and quality of nursing personnel.

Close to 335,000 professional registered nurses were employed in 1951, about half working in hospitals; in 1928, less than one-fourth had been so employed. Everyone agreed that the demand for nurses had grown, but there was much disagreement as to whether the nation needed *more* nurses above all, or *better educated* nurses, with nursing groups insisting that both needs were of equal priority. The principal controversy was the matter of collegiate education for nurses. Nursing leaders believed that schools of nursing should prepare nurses to serve in a very broad field and that such preparation could be best performed in an institution whose primary purpose was education. But the pitifully small collegiate nursing education programs could not be expanded without massive external support.

Efforts to provide federal aid to nursing education were renewed in 1951, when three separate bills were introduced in Congress providing for federal support of nursing education. One bill, modeled after the Cadet Nurse Corps plan, was part of the Korean War effort, and had as its purpose the assurance of an adequate supply of nurses for the armed forces, government hospitals, government agencies, and defense industries. Representative Bolton introduced another bill providing for scholarship aid and direct aid to schools of both professional and practical nursing. A third bill, introduced in the Senate, included most of the provisions of the Bolton Bill but also provided federal aid for the education of physicians, dentists, and other health personnel. As had happened with previous postwar efforts to obtain federal aid for nursing schools, these bills were opposed by the AMA and by representatives of a number of hospital schools, and like their predecessors, these bills went down to defeat despite the strong support of the Truman administration and most nursing organizations.

With the reality of a severe long-term shortage of professional nurses being painfully evident, more and more attention was beginning to be directed at the utilization of nursing personnel in health care institutions. About half the nursing staff of general hospitals was made up of graduate nurses and the other half of auxiliary workers. It was widely felt among the staff of the Division of Nursing Resources that the specialized knowledge of professional nurses was being improperly used, a waste which only exacerbated the nursing shortage. Surveys, job examinations, and other studies were carried out to determine the actual and appropriate levels of practice for various nursing personnel. The Division of Nursing Resources worked

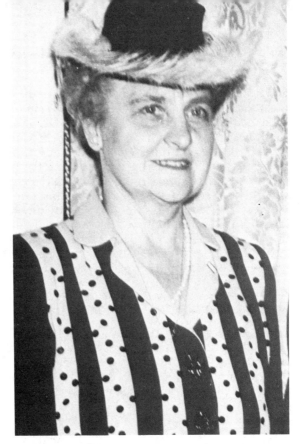

Figure 6–10. During the early 1950s, Representative Francis Payne Bolton valiantly attempted to get legislation enacted to assist nursing. (Courtesy of U.S. Public Health Service)

on a number of these projects helping state, local, and institutional authorities to attack the shortages and the inefficient use of nurses.

Once again in 1953, legislation proposing federal aid to nursing was placed before Congress. Two separate bills were introduced: Congresswoman Bolton reintroduced her 1951 bill, and several senators jointly introduced a national health bill, calling for aid to nursing schools but not for scholarships. Both bills failed, and federal aid to nursing was kept alive from 1948 to 1956 only through the program of grants for psychiatric nursing education, which had developed out of the National Mental Health Act of 1946. This act had grown from concern over the overcrowded conditions of the nation's mental institutions and the difficulty in staffing them. To promote training among mental health workers, the act authorized the PHS to make grants to nonprofit institutions for developing their training facilities and allocated training stipends to selected students in mental health fields.

In the mid-1950s the Division of Nursing Resources launched a number of impressive intramural research projects. In a cooperative study made with the Commission on Nursing of Cleveland in 1954, the division's researchers found a method of incorporating the patient's needs into their studies. In a similar but much more exhaustive study, opinions concerning nursing care were elicited from some 20,000 patients and staff members in

60 hospitals in order to determine whether satisfaction with nursing care was related to the nurse staffing. In 1957, in order to encourage hospitals to make similar studies of their own, the DNR published *Patients and Personnel Speak: A Method of Studying Patient Care in Hospitals.*[5]

The DNR continued to be the only unit in the federal government concerned with all aspects of improving the national supply of nurses. But because its support was limited, the DNR attacked only those problems that were clearly defined. As a result of this selectivity, it made considerable progress in certain areas, such as improving the use of nurse manpower and identifying the factors that lowered morale among nurses and led to high turnover rates. Through teaching and consultation the DNR also extended available nursing service, conducting institutes to help guide and direct nurses in improving their care.

FEDERAL FUNDS FOR NURSING RESEARCH AND GRADUATE EDUCATION

The second half of the decade saw the maturation of the DNR as a stimulator and producer of research. Throughout this period, the PHS in general had been receiving great increases in its extramural research appropriations. Before the war, medical research had depended chiefly upon private means of support. Then, in the 1940s, public responsibility enlarged to assume support of medical research, as it grew in so many other areas of American life. Additional institutes were created to augment the National Institutes of Health. Between 1945 and 1957 the research allocations to NIH increased from $8 million to $183 million. Finally, in 1955, nursing began to receive a relatively tiny fraction of the new research largess in the form of nursing fellowships and research grants. And in 1956, the Health Amendments Act authorized a program of traineeships for the education of nurses planning careers in teaching, administration, and supervision, as well as those preparing for public health staff positions. This represented the first significant federal appropriation for nursing education outside of the mental health program since the Cadet Corps. Despite a first year appropriation of only $2 million, the traineeship program began to answer the need for educating nurses for professional leadership. In 1957, only about half of the enrollment capacity of the graduate schools of nursing was being used, and the actual number of nurses with graduate degrees filled less than one-quarter of the estimated need. The Professional Traineeship program enabled more nurses to engage in baccalaureate, graduate, and other advanced education programs, assisting 3800 nurses to receive education beyond their basic program during the first three years of its operation alone. Short-term traineeships were largely targeted to enable nurses to participate in graduate programs.

ESTABLISHMENT OF THE NEW DIVISION OF NURSING

In 1957, Pearl McIver retired as head of public health nursing in the PHS. The public health nurses of the PHS had accomplished much in the way of local health programs, but their achievements had been overshadowed at the national level by the research and education initiatives of the PHS's younger sister, the Division of Nursing Resources, and back in 1953 their organizational entity had been reduced from a division to an office. In 1957, in an attempt to revitalize the Office of Public Health Nursing as an organization, Margaret Arnstein, who had provided outstanding leadership to the Division of Nursing Resources, was transferred to a recreated Division of Public Health Nursing, and Apollonia Adams assumed the direction of the DNR. However, the personnel change proved to be temporary. In 1960, a thoroughgoing restructuring of the Public Health Service united the Division of Nursing Resources and the Division of Public Health Nursing into the new Division of Nursing (DN). Margaret Arnstein headed the new Division of Nursing, which was placed in the new Bureau of Community Health, one of six new operating units of the Public Health Service.

In its eleven-year existence, the Division of Nursing Resources, despite very modest operating funds, had gained recognition as a national and international center for consultation on nursing education, nursing services, and nursing research. It had increased its staff from 5 to 50 and quintupled its budget between 1949 and 1960. Studies performed or encouraged by the DNR had helped to improve the use of nursing resources. For example, in one typical hospital the time spent on non-nursing activities by the nursing staff had been markedly reduced as a result of DNR recommendations, declining from 36% in 1956 to 18% in 1961. And the hospital's nursing personnel were spending more time on activities appropriate to their skill

Figure 6–11. The acute shortage of nurses in the late 1950s could literally be transformed into life or death situations. (Courtesy of History of Nursing Collection, University of Michigan)

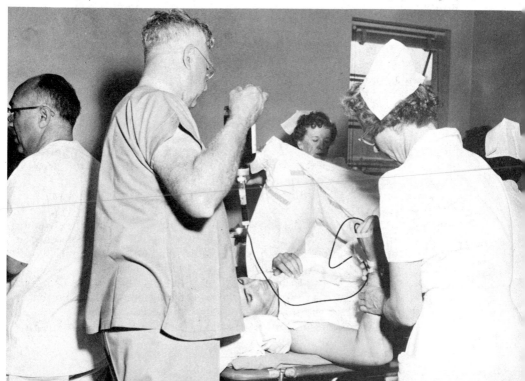

level as well as delivering more professional care. DNR consultation with the schools and the recruitment activities of nursing leaders had also produced a significant increase in the percentage of nurses enrolled in baccalaureate programs. Still, the concern over basic nursing preparation continued, and combating the ever-present threat of a shortage remained the most urgent problem in the profession. In the late 1950s there were about 240 nurses for every 100,000 people in the U.S., a proportion inadequate to the burgeoning demand for nursing care wrought by an increasingly labor-intensive health care system.

The postwar period had seen great changes in the delivery of health care. Private health insurance plans had encouraged tremendous growth in the number of Americans receiving health care each year. And although the demand for health care had skyrocketed, hospital costs per patient day had also shot up more than 250%. There had grown an increasing awareness that the aged, like other low-income groups, were particularly burdened by the rising costs of health care. The distribution of health professionals had changed as well. In 1940, hospitals had about one professional nurse for every fifteen beds and one practical nurse, or other auxiliary, for every ten beds. By 1960, one professional nurse was required for every five beds and one auxiliary for every three beds. Health care was given to a greater variety of people, and the primary focus of care had shifted from the home to the institution.

SURGEON GENERAL'S REPORT ON NURSING

As a result of increased public awareness of acute manpower shortages in health care, prospects for responsive federal health legislation began to improve, particularly after the establishment of a liberal majority in the congressional elections of 1958. The Surgeon General's Consultant Group on Medical Education published a report, *Physicians for a Growing America*, which found a worsening physician shortage in America and recommended the establishment of new medical schools, the expansion of existing schools, and the provision of financial aid to both schools and medical students. The impact of this report led leaders in the Division of Nursing to think in terms of their own consultant group, which became a reality in the summer of 1961. Chaired by Alvin Eurich, the Consultant Group on Nursing included representatives from national organizations of professional nursing, practical nursing, and nursing education, as well as physicians, medical educators, hospital administrators, and leaders from the areas of education, labor, and civil rights.[6]

The group's deliberations were to form the basis of a whole new structure of federal assistance to nursing. In its final report, *Toward Quality in Nursing*, published in 1963, the consultant group called for an estimated 680,000 professional nurses in active practice by 1970—an increase of 130,000 over the 1960 supply; they estimated that nursing schools would need to increase their number of graduates by 75% in order to meet this goal. The consultants also urged a 194% increase in the number of nurses with graduate degrees, a 100% increase in the number of baccalaureates, and a 50% increase in the number of licensed practical nurses.[7]

The group furnished a number of recommendations to enable the profession to meet these goals. To stimulate recruitment, the group recommended expanding federal aid to schools of professional and practical nursing and increasing the amount of student aid available. To improve programs, federal funds were recommended for the construction of facilities and the expansion of educational programs. Further, to increase the effective utilization of nurses, the group suggested that federal funds be used to extend consultative services and that project grants be available to strengthen programs of inservice and continuing education. Finally, the group recommended intensifying the Division of Nursing's fellowship, traineeship, and research grants programs to stimulate graduate study and research among nurses.

NURSE TRAINING ACT OF 1964

On February 7, 1963, President John F. Kennedy sent Congress a major statement on improving the nation's health. The message cited several key areas, but above all it recognized the shortage of trained health personnel as the most critical of the nation's health problems. In response to this message, Congress passed the Health Professions Educational Assistance Act, authorizing appropriations of $175 million for the construction of training facilities for physicians, dentists, nurses, and other health professionals. Although this act was directed primarily at the medical and dental professions, it authorized construction grants to nursing institutions as well. Most important, it represented the first successful major breach of the opposition to federal assistance to health education in many years, and so broke the ground for the Nurse Training Act (NTA) of 1964.

With the assistance of the Division of Nursing staff, the Johnson administration in early 1964 drafted legislation designed to meet the goals proposed by the Consultant Group on Nursing. The bill received general support, even from organizations that had opposed previous attempts to legislate federal aid to nursing.

As finally approved, the legislation *authorized* a maximum of $238 million for five programs for five years and $4.6 million for the administration of these programs, of which both amounts were subject to a variable annual appropriation:

- $90 million was authorized for construction of nursing facilities, with $55 million of this being earmarked for diploma and associate degree programs and $35 million for baccalaureate programs.
- $17 million was allocated for "teaching improvement" or special project grants available to all programs.
- $50 million was authorized for the continuation of existing traineeship programs.
- $85 million was set aside for the provision of loans—not grants—to nursing students, although those graduates who worked for five years after graduation would be forgiven half of their loan.
- $41 million was targeted specifically as formula payments to the hospital schools to "improve the quality of instruction."

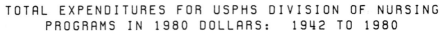

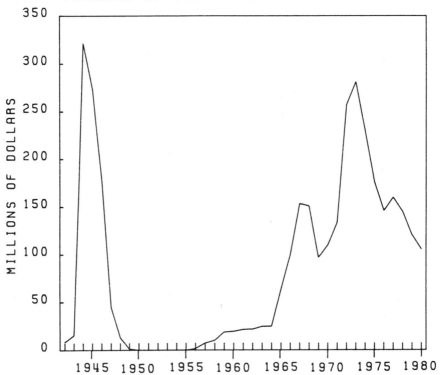

Figure 6–12. (Courtesy of History and Politics of Nursing, University of Michigan)

The act was to run until FY 1969, at which time a citizen's group would evaluate the programs and decide whether they were to continue. The National Advisory Council on Nurse Training was established to advise on policies and procedures for implementing the act and was to review applications for funds. On signing the act, President Johnson observed that the Nurse Training Act of 1964 was the most significant nursing legislation in the history of the country.

Of the 1208 nursing programs operating in 1964, 865 were eligible for some kind of grant money under the act's provisions. Only schools accredited by the National League for Nursing could receive the formula payments and construction grants while project grants, loan funds, and funds for the construction of new schools were available to schools, furnishing reasonable assurance that they would meet the NLN's standards within the grant period.

In the first years of the act, the different programs achieved varying degrees of success. The project grant program was immediately swamped with eligible applicants, whose proposals included the coordination and improvement of instruction in medical and surgical nursing, the extension of students' experience both inside and outside hospital settings, and the development of audio-visual teaching aids. The formula grants to diploma schools, on the other hand, met a less enthusiastic response. Their purpose had been to help accredited hospital programs defray a portion of the costs of enrollment increases reasonably attributable to the government. But the grants were based upon enrollment increases, and many diploma schools were already operating at full capacity. Even more frustrating to some hospitals was the exclusion of the nonaccredited schools whose need for financial support to overcome obstacles to accreditation was greatest.

The construction grants program essentially extended the construction funds already authorized under the Health Professions Act of 1963 to diploma and the fast-growing number of two-year associate degree (AD) programs. The grants were to be made for educational facilities only. Applications for student loans nearly tripled by the second year of authorization, and the number of borrowers increased from 3,645 in 1965 to 17,218 in 1967, a figure that represented 18% of the total enrollment in the participating schools. The traineeship program, operational since 1956, but newly extended, easily exhausted its first year's appropriation.

The provisions of the Nurse Training Act were seen by some as being more beneficial to collegiate programs than to diploma schools. The diploma schools had been suffering since the early 1950s: the 1100 diploma programs existing in 1949 had dwindled to 979 by 1966. Both baccalaureate and AD programs had cut into the diploma school's enrollment, the AD program exhibiting remarkable growth, which accelerated even more during the late 1960s. The conflict in the nursing community over the essentiality of the baccalaureate degree was abruptly heightened by the controversy over accreditation as the prerequisite for eligibility for federal monies. In 1965, a proposed amendment to the NTA sought to broaden the accrediting function of the NLN to regional or state approval bodies, thereby eliminating any uniform professional control over educational standards in nursing. The amendment was opposed, not only by the ANA and NLN, but also by the national hospital and dental associations, and was defeated in Congress. More successful was the amendment introduced in 1966, by Senator Jacob Javits, which provided the first scholarships for the needy nursing students. It also authorized unused construction funds earmarked for AD and hospital schools to be transferred to baccalaureate and graduate programs when AD and diploma school requests did not absorb the total monies authorized.

VIGOROUS LEADERSHIP FROM THE DIVISION OF NURSING

The passage of the first massive program of federal aid to nursing since the Cadet Nurse Corps brought a flurry of activity to the Divison of Nursing (DN). Six special consultants were borrowed by the division to interpret the act for potential applicants. Jessie Schott, who replaced Margaret Arnstein as head of the DN, announced the establishment of a new Nursing Education and Training Branch within the division to implement the legislation. The transfer of the administration of nursing research grants from the National Institutes of Health to the Division of Nursing in 1963 strengthened

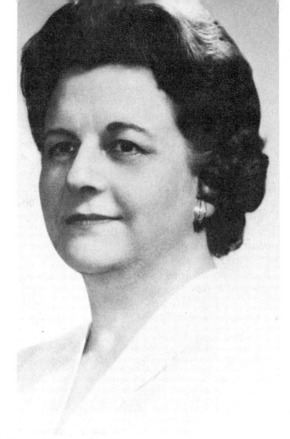

Figure 6–13. Jessie Scott administered the Division of Nursing from 1964 to 1979. (Courtesy of U.S. Public Health Service)

the ties between extramural research and other DN activities, thereby improving communication of new knowledge to the practicing nurse who applied it. This process was also facilitated by the establishment of a Division of Nursing field research center under the direction of Elinor D. Stanford, at the Public Health Service hospital in San Francisco.

The Research Grants and Fellowships Program, the smallest of the programs, had inspired a number of impressive applications from a relatively small number of schools, a concentration that was attributed to the fact that many nurses who might otherwise be motivated to do research lacked the necessary skills and supportive institutional environment. To deal with this problem, special developmental research training grants were made to schools of nursing to stimulate research capacities. By 1965, the DN had completed ten years of support for extramural research in nursing and had funded 163 studies. The record of this pioneering work was published in *Research in Nursing—1955–1965*, a compilation of abstracts of completed studies.

Just as the fortunes of nursing education improved in the expansionist atmosphere of President Johnson's Great Society, so numerous other health care items that had been voted down in the late 1940s and the 1950s were finding new favor and created new demands for health care providers.

Thus, despite the Nurse Training Act of 1964, the nursing shortage remained one of the most critical problems in health care delivery. In light of this expanded demand for nursing care and with realization that the NTA would expire in 1969, a special outside Program Review Committee evaluated the programs of the Nurse Training Act. They concluded that nursing education had made substantial progress under the impetus of the act and that the subsequent amendments had clearly improved the legislation. The committee found that by 1968, more than $100 million had been awarded through the programs of the Nurse Training Act for institutional and student assistance. Over 3300 grants had been awarded to a total of 720 schools, 490 of which were diploma programs, 55 AD, and 175 baccalaureate and graduate degree programs. Each year participation in the programs grew while faculty in the schools showed imagination in developing teaching facilities, courses, and methods.

The traineeship program had increased, by 20,000, the number of professional nurses qualifying as teachers, administrators, and supervisors since 1956. The number of nursing students studying under student loans increased to 24,500, about 23% of the total enrollment in participating schools, while the newer scholarship program had enabled some 7000 students to attend schools who would otherwise have been unable to afford higher education. However, the committee found that areas outside of nursing education remained without adequate support—particularly, planning, recruitment, and research; for this reason, the Review Committee recommended that the programs authorized by the Nurse Training Act of 1964 be expanded.

With the Nurse Training Act set to expire in 1969, congressional hearings were held on bills to extend the assistance programs. The Nixon administration proposed an omnibus bill to continue for 2 years and to strengthen all the expiring health education programs originally authorized by the various legislation of the previous 5 years. The final result of extensive hearings, the Health Manpower Act of 1968, continued most of the NTA's programs but brought a number of important changes in several of them. The new law diluted the accreditation provisions of the original NTA, defining an *accredited program* as one accredited by a recognized accrediting body or a state agency, a reflection of the new strength of the popular AD programs. A promising (but never funded) program authorized the allocation of over $250 million worth of institutional grants to all eligible schools, each school receiving an annual base of $15,000, with the rest of the money being distributed among the schools according to enrollment. Project grants were made available to institutions or agencies, which were developing new schools of nursing. The student aid provisions of the NTA were strengthened, with a much broader program of scholarship grants being authorized. Construction grants were continued, as was the traineeship program.

CONTINUED GROWTH OF FEDERAL NURSING EFFORTS

As the 1970s dawned, the health industry was the third largest industry in the U.S., employing 5% of the civilian population, or some 4,500,000 people. This represented an 80% increase over 1960, and the greatest growth had occurred in the number of nurses and allied health professionals. In 1910, for every one physician there had been two other workers, mostly nurses; in 1970, there were eleven other health workers vis-à-vis every physician.

As the pattern of health care delivery changed, the nurse's role within that pattern also evolved. Professional nurses provided less direct care to patients, and their personal satisfaction had diminished as a result of this development. Professional nurses had been directed into work in nonclinical areas, such as management, supervision, and teaching. But these alternatives were not sufficient in themselves; nurses needed to reclaim their professionalism in patient care. In the 1950s and 1960s, nursing research had been heavily concentrated on nursing education and the sociology of the nursing profession. But in the late 1960, a real effort developed to focus more specifically on patient care research, to determine precisely what the nurse does that affects patient outcomes.

In 1967, the National League for Nursing and the American Nurses' Association had jointly sponsored a study by the National Commission for the Study of Nursing Education. The final report, *An Abstract for Action* (often called the "Lysaught Report" after the commission's director, Dr. Jerome Lysaught), was published in 1970 and recommended that practice be re-established as nursing's first professional priority, that research be increased on the impact of nursing practice, and that the nurse's area of responsibility be expanded in order to increase the amount of health care available in the nation.[8] Nurses began experimenting with the role of the clinical nurse specialist, a concept that emphasized advanced nursing practice and in-depth knowledge. However, the role was not instituted as effectively as it might have been in many settings because of the unwillingness of administrators to pay for such quality oriented care. A more successful experiment resulted in the widespread popularity of Division of Nursing supported programs to prepare nurse practitioners.

In 1970 the Division of Nursing was restructured around four major areas of activity: (1) nursing manpower, (2) nursing education, (3) nursing practice and (4) nursing research. The division's intramural program represented its commitment to the long-range goals of an adequate supply of appropriately educated nurses, readily accessible throughout the country. The federal assistance administered by the division was yielding dramatic results. Between 1965 and 1971, the federal government spent more than $380 million on nursing education, this money being almost equally divided between students and institutions.

By 1972 more than 73,000 nurses had received traineeship aid for long-term, full-time study and short-term intensive courses. In the earlier years, most recipients of long-term traineeships prepared for teaching; in the early 1970s, however, an increasing number were preparing for clinical specialization in the delivery of nursing care. During the mid-1970s, doctoral programs and students in nursing began to receive more emphasis and support. Research grants were becoming the most significant factor in developing professionalism in nursing, as federal monies legitimized scientific inquiry as the basis for nursing practice. The new nurse scientist program in par-

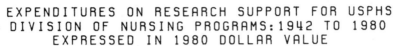

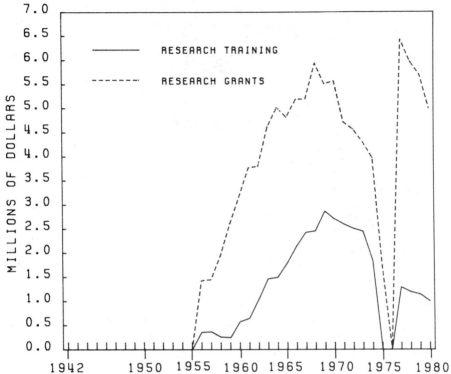

Figure 6–14. (Courtesy of History and Politics of Nursing, University of Michigan)

ticular produced several major benefits, broadening the nursing school's visions of health care, attracting more ambitious people into nursing and improving the attitude of the general intellectual community toward nursing.

Since the publication of the Consultant Group's report in 1963, the number of professional nurses with bachelor's degrees had increased by 94% and those with master's degrees, by 63%. Institutional assistance had helped to upgrade the quality of nurse preparation: $97 million having been spent for new improved facilities and $34 million for special projects to improve nursing curricula, to begin new schools, as well as to assist financially troubled schools, to establish programs for disadvantaged students, to recruit special groups into professional nursing, and to expand the role of the professional nurse. By the end of 1973 there would be more than 748,000 registered nurses in practice, a ratio of 361 nurses for every 100,000 Americans as opposed to the 1956 ratio of 259 per 100,000. But the constructive period of federal assistance was drawing to a close, and the troubles between an increasingly conservative Nixon administration and the Congress were to inflict a serious blow upon the program of federal aid to nursing.

Continuing the flow of federal dollars to nursing, the three-year Nurse Training Act of 1971 authorized the greatest expenditure in the country's history upon nursing, a total of $855 million for three fiscal years, but the bill had been the creation of a liberal Congress and was only reluctantly signed by the President, who had particularly opposed the new program of capitation grants, the first large discretionary pool of money available to schools of nursing.

FIGHT TO MAINTAIN FEDERAL FUNDS FOR NURSING

As a result of the Nixon administration's hostility toward the Nurse Training Act of 1971, schools of nursing had difficulty in securing even a modest proportion of the NTA authorizations. In both 1972 and 1973, the President's budgetary requests for nursing fell far below the amount authorized; in 1973, when Congress settled on a higher appropriation as part of the overall HEW funding bill, the President vetoed it. After Congress, unable to override, authorized a new and lower appropriation for nursing, as well as the other HEW programs, the President vetoed this bill also. When Congress voted a series of continuing resolutions, appropriating funds to tide the HEW programs over, the President impounded about one-half of the nursing money. Then the NLN filed suit in federal court and a favorable decision forced the release of some $73 million in appropriations for nursing, but this victory merely delayed the inevitable deterioration of nursing's position within the executive branch of the federal government.

The appointment of Caspar Weinberger, well-known as a budget slasher, as HEW secretary signaled a new antiexpansionist era in the federal attitude to health and welfare. In another reorganization of the Public Health Service, the last vestiges of authority were shifted from the surgeon general to the assistant secretary for health. The Division of Nursing was uprooted along with the rest of its home bureau, the Bureau of Health Manpower Education, from the prestigious National Institutes of Health and transferred to the new Health Resources Administration. In March 1973, Secretary Weinberger announced his intention of decentralizing HEW and dispersing authority from the central offices in Washington, D.C., to the ten HEW regional offices, in order to place the decision-making authority as close as possible to the performance of services.

The transfer of the Bureau of Health Manpower and the decentralization of authority diffused the program activities in the Division of Nursing. The construction grants program was decentralized in the first quarter of fiscal year 1974, while special projects and student loan and scholarship programs were decentralized in the second quarter. The initial review of grants and the awarding of grant funds was to be performed regionally, although final review of applications continued to be the legal responsibility of the National Advisory Council on Nurse Training. The move toward decentralization critically hurt the Division of Nursing. Its authorized staffing level quickly shrank from 156 positions in 1972 to 55 positions in 1975.

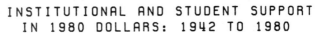

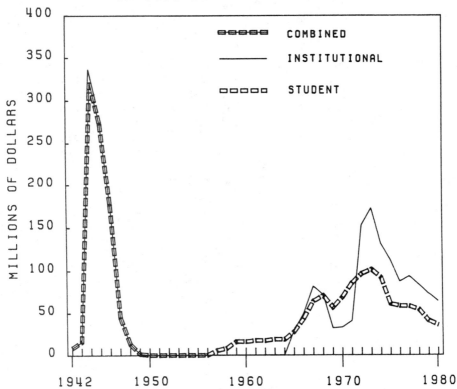

INSTITUTIONAL AND STUDENT SUPPORT
IN 1980 DOLLARS: 1942 TO 1980

Figure 6-15. (Courtesy of History and Politics of Nursing, University of Michigan)

President Nixon's 1974 budget contained more bad news for nursing: the $160 million appropriation for nursing education of 1973 was to drop to $49 million in 1974. Congressional action, prodded by the ANA and NLN among others, offset this proposed sharp reduction and the nursing programs were funded at the level of $145 million for 1974, the last year of the 1971 Nurse Training Act's authority.

PROPOSED NURSE TRAINING ACT EXTENSIONS YIELD THREE PRESIDENTIAL VETOES

On January 4, 1975, these developments reached their logical climax when President Gerald Ford vetoed the Nurse Training Act of 1974, which had made few changes in the 1971 act; he claimed that it was too expensive. No authority existed to continue provisions of the 1971 act for fiscal year 1975. Congress therefore covered this gap through the mechanism of continuing resolutions. The Ford administration in the meantime strove to end the program of nurse scholarships and to phase out the federal contribution to the student loan program, maintaining that nurses were eligible for student aid under other federal programs.

Congress's alternative, the Nurse Training Act of 1975, acknowledged the administration's blunt challenge by considerably reducing the total federal commitment to nursing, leaving a total three-year authorization of $553 million. This legislation extended the nurse training program through fiscal years 1976, 1977, and 1978. It also signified a change in emphasis as well as with a much increased emphasis on nurse practitioner programs. The measure also authorized a new advanced nurse training program to encourage the development and expansion of master's and doctoral level programs. President Ford vetoed this bill on July 26, 1975, but Congress swiftly and easily overrode the veto (the Senate on July 26, 1975 by a 67 to 15 vote [12 votes more than the two-thirds majority required to override], and the House on July 29, 1975 by a 394 to 43 vote [99 votes more than the two-thirds majority needed]). The bill then became PL 94-63.

According to the 1977 National Sample Survey of Registered Nurses, only an estimated 55,096, or 3.9% of the total registered nurse population in September 1977, had master's degrees. According to the same study, only 2304, or .2% of the registered nurse population, had doctoral degrees. Of about 1.4 million nurses, 500,000 were not practicing full-time and maldistribution compounded the problem. Nurses were still in short supply in many rural and inner-city areas, and there were not nearly enough specially educated nurses to fill teaching, administrative, and research positions.

In its report on a 1978 bill to extend the Nurse Training Act for two additional years, the Senate Human Resources Committee reported as follows that hospitals were complaining of acute nursing shortages, particularly in inner-city and rural areas, where health services of any sort were often scarce:

> This year, the President proposed major budget cuts for nurse training programs. In testimony before this committees' Subcommittee on Health and Scientific Research, officials from the administration justified this position primarily on the assertion that the current supply of nurses is adequate to meet the needs of the existing medical care system.
>
> The committee is not convinced that this is so. In a statement submitted to the Subcommittee on Health and Scientific Research, the American Hospital Association stated:
>
> 'Although some studies tended to show there no longer is a nursing shortage throughout the country, certain areas continue to suffer from chronic shortages of registered nurses. Hospitals in Texas, for example, are forced to recruit foreign nurse graduates in order to fill posted positions. Chicago hospitals presently have over 2,000 positions unfilled. The shortage of nurses to fill available positions is particularly acute in the inner cities and rural areas. The quantification of nursing shortages, furthermore, is often difficult to document where hospitals have been forced to compromise staffing patterns because of the unavailability of registered nurses in their areas.'[9]

The committee also argued that abrupt cuts in federal support would cripple nursing education and that future health policies could create additional demands for nurses. The President's negative decision was "premature and unsubstantiated," the committee said, promising a full review of national

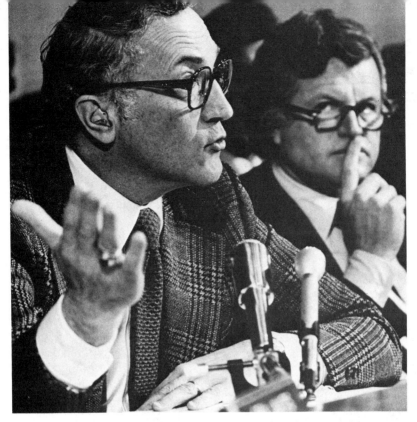

Figure 6–16. Senators Richard Schweiker and Edward Kennedy held a special hearing on January 26, 1979 in which they attacked President Carter's veto of the Nurse Training Act and his plans to nearly terminate federal assistance to nursing. (Courtesy of The Washington Post, Washington, DC)

nursing needs once several studies were finished. The Senate passed the bill on June 7, 1978, by a voice vote and the House passed the bill by a 393 to 12 vote.

On the final day of the session, Congress sent to the White House the bill extending federal support for nurse training programs for 1979 and 1980 at existing spending levels, but President Carter pocket-vetoed the measure on November 11, 1978. The veto drew an angry blast from nursing leaders who suggested that the "discriminatory" pocket-veto was motivated by sexism in the White House. "We cannot help but wonder if it [the veto] had anything to do with the fact that nursing is predominantly a woman's profession," said Barbara Nichols, president of the American Nurses' Association.[10] President Jimmy Carter, with the same viewpoint on nursing as Nixon and Ford, said he would not sign the nurse training bill because its spending levels were "excessive," particularly because two decades of federal aid to nursing schools had all but ended nursing shortages. Other forms of federal aid were available to nursing students, Carter pointed out, adding that "future federal assistance should be limited to geographic and specialty areas that need nurses most."

NURSE TRAINING AMENDMENTS OF 1979

Congress in 1979, however, was successful in enacting a much reduced one-year extension of the Nurse Training Act. The nurse training program was extended for only one year because Congress wanted to fold the program into the larger package of health manpower training programs expiring September 30, 1980. The Senate Labor and Human Resources Committee reported the bill on April 30, 1979. The committee report noted that the work of nurses in "remote, economically depressed areas" and the continuing shortages throughout the nation favored continuation of nurse training programs at least until new studies of national nursing needs and broader health manpower policies were completed. In addition, both students and administrators had told the committee that without federal aid, minority and lower-income students would be barred from nursing careers. The Senate passed the bill by voice vote on May 7, 1979. Senator Edward M. Kennedy strongly disagreed with Carter's contention that there was an adequate supply of nurses, noting that his comprehensive national health insurance plan would drastically increase the need for nurses.[11]

The House passed the nursing bill July 27, 1979, by a 344 to 6 vote, first rejecting by a 12 to 341 vote an amendment by William E. Dannemeyer (Republican, California) to slash the $103 million authorization to $14.7 million. Dannemeyer said that was the amount President Carter had requested in his budget. He said the number of nurses had risen in ten years from 300 per 100,000 population to 395 per 100,000 population. Given this improved ratio, Carter's request was "all that is needed now in the way of federal assistance," Dannemeyer asserted. Henry A. Waxman (Democrat, California), chairman of the House Commerce Subcommittee on Health, argued that there were severe nurse shortages and that Dannemeyer's amendment would "only increase an already acute problem." Carl D. Pursell (Republican, Michigan) said the Carter administration had used outdated, seven-year-old statistics to justify its proposed cuts in nursing education funds and questioned the President's rationale in gutting the longstanding program without better justification.[12]

As passed, the Nurse Training Amendments of 1979 authorized a total of $103 million in 1980 for nurse training programs. The legislation also called for a study by the Institute of Medicine (IOM) of the National Academy of Sciences to determine whether there was, in fact, a need for continued federal support for nursing. The IOM study was to make recommendations about how to encourage nurses to practice in underserved areas and how to get inactive nurses to re-enter the nursing profession. The study was also to examine the impact increased ambulatory care would have on the need for nurses in both inpatient and outpatient services. A preliminary report by the IOM was due to the Department of Health and Human Services and Congress in the summer of 1980 with the final report due early in 1981. With these provisions, Congress then sent the bill to the President, which he quietly signed September 29, 1979 (PL 96-76). The legislation, however, was enacted too late to have an effect on the regular FY 1980 appropriations act, so once again, under a stop-gap appropriations bill, Congress funded the Nurse Training Program, this time for FY 1980 at the same levels as FY 1978 and FY 1979.

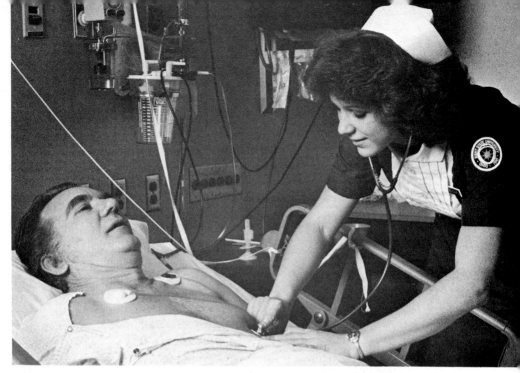

Figure 6–17. Educational programs to prepare nurses have suffered from the high degree of financial instability in federal assistance. (Courtesy of Potomac News, Woodbridge, Virginia)

From a 1980 vantage point, the educational institutions responsible for nurse preparation have been characterized by a high degree of financial instability related to continuing deficiencies and uncertainties in federal funding of nursing education. They have not been able to respond most effectively to the complicated set of demands imposed upon them. These include, in addition to a need for an increase in nurse production, an expanded program of nursing research and participation in the redesign of health service systems through federally assisted demonstrations of nursing solutions to health problems. Despite the continuance of the Nurse Training Act, no short or middle-range answers to these deficiencies are evident in the present program of federal assistance. Finally, the cost of education for nurses is increasing at a far more rapid rate than available student subsidies. This, in conjunction with a generally inflated economy, decreases the ability of prospective students to finance their own education and undoubtedly accounts, in part, for the decline in enrollments in schools of nursing in the late 1970s and early 1980s.

A challenge to all nurses is to work for the support and development of additional federal resources for nursing so that the great inequity between nursing and the other health professions, especially medicine, can be somewhat diminished. For example, while biomedical research alone accounts for well over $3 billion in federal funds annually, nursing research is currently funded at the miniscule level of $5 million per year. As documented in this chapter, the federal effort on behalf of nursing has centered predominantly on the quantitative problem of educating more nurses. This effort increasingly needs to be accompanied by expanded funds for research and development of all aspects of quality nursing care.

References

1. Quoted in Doyle A: Development of federal public health functions in the United States. Public Health Nurse 12:723–727, 1920
2. The United States Public Health Service: Its evolution and organization. Public Health Rep 36:1165–1176, 1921
3. Kalisch P, Kalisch B: Federal Influence and Impact on Nursing. Washington, DC, United States Government Printing Office (in press)
4. Brown EL: Nursing for the Future. New York, Russell Sage Foundation, 1948
5. Abdellah FG, Levine E: Patients and Personnel Speak: A Method of Studying Patient Care in Hospitals. Washington, DC, United States Government Printing Office, 1954
6. U.S. Public Health Service: Physicians for a Growing America. Report of the Surgeon General's Consultant Group on Medical Education. Washington, DC, United States Government Printing Office, 1959
7. U.S. Public Health Service: Toward Quality in Nursing: Needs and Goals. Report of the Surgeon General's Consultant Group on Nursing. Washington, DC, United States Government Printing Office, 1963
8. National Commission for the Study of Nursing and Nursing Education: An Abstract for Action. New York, McGraw-Hill, 1970
9. U.S. Congress. Senate. Committee on Human Resources: The Nurse Training Amendments Act of 1978, pp 1–2. Report to accompany S 2416. Washington, DC, United States Government Printing Office, 1978
10. Washington, DC, Washington Post, Nov 12, 1978
11. Congressional Record, pp S5421–S5424, May 7, 1979
12. Congressional Record, pp H6788–H6796, July 27, 1979

7–Key Federal Health Agencies

The federal government is divided into three major branches: legislative (the Congress), executive (the President), and judicial (the courts). A basic feature of the Constitution of the United States is the distribution of national powers among these three branches, which are all given constitutional and political independence from one another. The President's (or the executive) power, for example, does not come from Congress, nor does congressional power emanate from the judiciary. The personnel of each of the three branches are chosen by way of different procedures and hold office independently of the other branches. It is this independence of the three branches, not just the distribution of functions, which is the central feature of our system of separation of power. Great Britain also has executive, legislative, and judicial branches, but the British government is not established according to the separation-of-power principle inasmuch as the legislature chooses the executive (prime minister), and the executive depends upon the legislature both for retention of office and for authority.

In addition to separate functions and considerable political and constitutional independence, each branch has weapons with which to keep the others in check. For example, the President has a veto over Congress, and the courts interpret the laws, but it is the President and the Senate that select the judges. The designers of the Constitution constructed government in this way because they feared concentration of power in a single branch. Separation of power and checks and balances serve to prevent the situation where a single segment of the population could gain complete control of the government.

The complexity of the executive branch is reflected in Figure 7–3, which shows its formal structure and administrative agencies. The *Department of Health and Human Services* (HHS) is the cabinet-level department of the executive branch most concerned with the health of people and most involved with the nation's human health concerns. In one way or another—whether it is mailing out Social Security checks or improving the quality of American nursing or making health services more widely available—HHS touches the lives of more Americans than any other federal agency. It is literally a department of people serving people, from newborn infants to our most elderly citizens. HHS (now minus the education programs) was formerly called the Department of Health, Education and Welfare, which was created on April 11, 1953, under legislation proposed by President Dwight Eisenhower and approved by the Congress on April 1, 1953. That legislation abolished HEW's predecessor organization, the Federal Security Agency, and transferred all its functions to the new department. In addition, it transferred all responsibilities of the Federal Security Administrator to the secretary of Health, Education and Welfare.

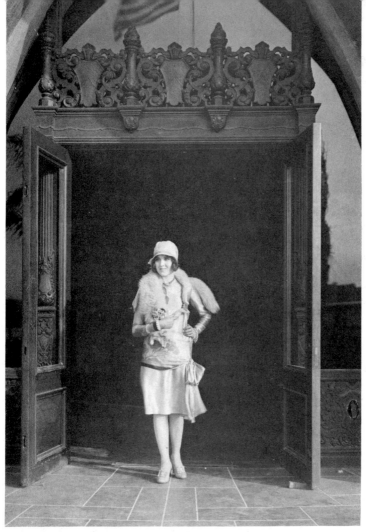

Figure 7–1. An understanding of the organization of the federal government has been essential for women since 1920, when they were first allowed to enter the political arena by the passage of the 19th amendment to the Constitution. (Courtesy of History of Nursing Collection, University of Michigan)

THE SECRETARY OF HHS AND ASSISTANT SECRETARY FOR HEALTH

The secretary of HHS advises the President on health, welfare, and income security plans, policies, and programs of the federal government. The secretary directs department staff in carrying out the approved programs and activities of the department and promotes general public understanding of the department's goals, programs, and objectives. The Office of the Assistant Secretary for Health provides leadership and direction for Public Health Service activities. Plans and strategies for accomplishing health goals are formulated for implementation in the headquarters and regional offices. Guidance is provided to the various HHS agencies on a variety of administrative, management, program-planning, and evaluative functions.

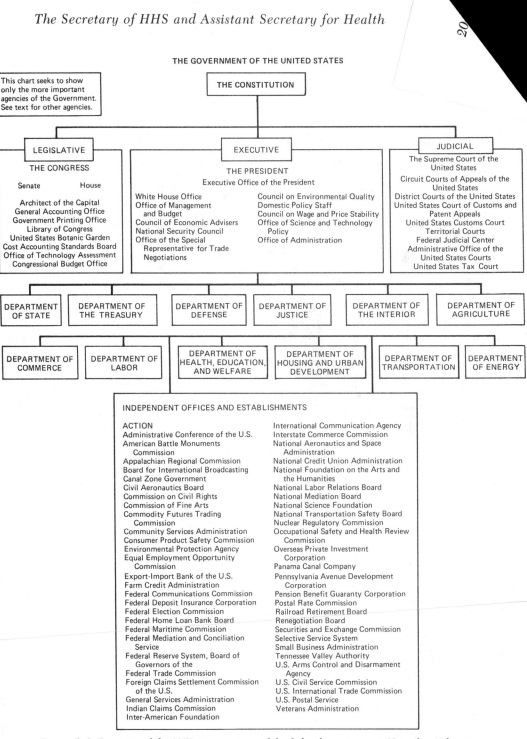

THE GOVERNMENT OF THE UNITED STATES

THE CONSTITUTION

This chart seeks to show only the more important agencies of the Government. See text for other agencies.

LEGISLATIVE

THE CONGRESS

Senate   House

Architect of the Capital
General Accounting Office
Government Printing Office
Library of Congress
United States Botanic Garden
Cost Accounting Standards Board
Office of Technology Assessment
Congressional Budget Office

EXECUTIVE

THE PRESIDENT
Executive Office of the President

White House Office
Office of Management
  and Budget
Council of Economic Advisers
National Security Council
Office of the Special
  Representative for Trade
  Negotiations

Council on Environmental Quality
Domestic Policy Staff
Council on Wage and Price Stability
Office of Science and Technology
  Policy
Office of Administration

JUDICIAL

The Supreme Court of the
  United States
Circuit Courts of Appeals of the
  United States
District Courts of the United States
United States Court of Customs and
  Patent Appeals
United States Customs Court
Territorial Courts
Federal Judicial Center
Administrative Office of the
  United States Courts
United States Tax Court

DEPARTMENT OF STATE

DEPARTMENT OF THE TREASURY

DEPARTMENT OF DEFENSE

DEPARTMENT OF JUSTICE

DEPARTMENT OF THE INTERIOR

DEPARTMENT OF AGRICULTURE

DEPARTMENT OF COMMERCE

DEPARTMENT OF LABOR

DEPARTMENT OF HEALTH, EDUCATION, AND WELFARE

DEPARTMENT OF HOUSING AND URBAN DEVELOPMENT

DEPARTMENT OF TRANSPORTATION

DEPARTMENT OF ENERGY

INDEPENDENT OFFICES AND ESTABLISHMENTS

ACTION
Administrative Conference of the U.S.
American Battle Monuments
  Commission
Appalachian Regional Commission
Board for International Broadcasting
Canal Zone Government
Civil Aeronautics Board
Commission on Civil Rights
Commission of Fine Arts
Commodity Futures Trading
  Commission
Community Services Administration
Consumer Product Safety Commission
Environmental Protection Agency
Equal Employment Opportunity
  Commission
Export-Import Bank of the U.S.
Farm Credit Administration
Federal Communications Commission
Federal Deposit Insurance Corporation
Federal Election Commission
Federal Home Loan Bank Board
Federal Maritime Commission
Federal Mediation and Conciliation
  Service
Federal Reserve System, Board of
  Governors of the
Federal Trade Commission
Foreign Claims Settlement Commission
  of the U.S.
General Services Administration
Indian Claims Commission
Inter-American Foundation

International Communication Agency
Interstate Commerce Commission
National Aeronautics and Space
  Administration
National Credit Union Administration
National Foundation on the Arts and
  the Humanities
National Labor Relations Board
National Mediation Board
National Science Foundation
National Transportation Safety Board
Nuclear Regulatory Commission
Occupational Safety and Health Review
  Commission
Overseas Private Investment
  Corporation
Panama Canal Company
Pennsylvania Avenue Development
  Corporation
Pension Benefit Guaranty Corporation
Postal Rate Commission
Railroad Retirement Board
Renegotiation Board
Securities and Exchange Commission
Selective Service System
Small Business Administration
Tennessee Valley Authority
U.S. Arms Control and Disarmament
  Agency
U.S. Civil Service Commission
U.S. International Trade Commission
U.S. Postal Service
Veterans Administration

Figure 7–2. Diagram of the 1979 organization of the federal government. Note that Education was established as a separate department in 1980. (Courtesy of U.S. General Services Administration)

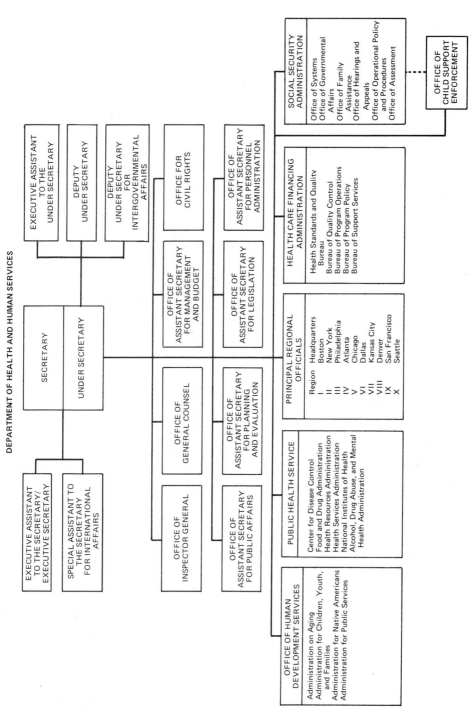

Figure 7–3. The organization of the Department of Health and Human Services, 1980. (Courtesy of U.S. General Services Administration)

OFFICE OF ASSISTANT SECRETARY FOR HEALTH

Several agencies operate directly out of the office of the Assistant Secretary for Health. The mission of the *National Center for Health Services Research* (NCHSR), funded at a level of $34 million in 1980, is to undertake and support research, demonstrations, and evaluations of problems in the organization, delivery, and financing of health care services. It also serves as the focal point for coordination of health services research within the PHS and endeavors to disseminate the findings of health services research to policy and decision makers in the public and private sectors.

The *National Center for Health Statistics* (NCHS), with a 1980 appropriation of $45 million, has responsibility for the collection, maintenance, and dissemination of statistics on the extent and nature of illness and disability of the U.S. population. It also develops indicators of the impact of illness and disability on the economy of the United States, monitors environmental, social, and other health hazards as well as health resources and the uses of health care. Finally, it collects data on births, deaths, and infant mortality.

The *National Center for Health Care Technology* (NCHCT), funded in 1980 at $3.25 million, conducts or sponsors assessments of health care technologies through a program of grants and contracts, with the use of outside experts, and the use of its own staff. These assessments include analysis of safety, of efficacy, of cost-effectiveness, and of the economic, social, and ethical impacts associated with the use of particular health care technologies.

The newly established *Office of Adolescent Health Services* with a 1980 budget of $17.5 million provides coordination, integration, and linkage to community efforts directed toward reducing the incidence of unwanted adolescent pregnancies and providing comprehensive services to the already pregnant adolescent. The extent of this problem is substantial, with nearly 1 million adolescent girls becoming pregnant each year, 600,000 going to full-term, and 90% keeping their babies. Without intervention, approximately 25% of these teenagers become pregnant again within the first year, and 44% have repeat pregnancies within two years. Children born to adolescents are more likely to be low birth weight and have a higher rate of birth defects and concomitant physical and physiologic deficiencies. The program is carried out through project grants and contracts. Technical assistance is provided to grantees and prospective grantees in the effort to encourage the development of innovative approaches to meeting the comprehensive health, educational, and social services needs of the pregnant adolescent.

The *Offices of Smoking and Health, Physical Fitness and Health Information and Health Promotion,* under the direction of the Assistant Secretary for Health, are responsible for developing and conducting a National Health Promotion Program, which is a coordinated series of activities designed to facilitate individual understanding of the importance of certain personal habits in improving health. Along with smoking, major health-risk factors that exist in the American population include high serum cholesterol, lack of adequate physical exercise, alcohol abuse, and hypertension. An analysis of the leading causes of mortality and morbidity in this country today indicates that if changes could be effected in just these three behavioral areas, substantial reduction in the incidence of heart disease, cancer, stroke, motor vehicle accidents, cirrhosis of the liver, arterial sclerosis, and diabetes would result. Funded with a $15 million appropriation in 1980, this program provides health information and education in a variety of settings: school, worksite, community, and home (including television and radio). The target emphases of the program are balanced diet, smoking reduction, hypertension control, and physical exercise. The 1979 publication, *Healthy People: The Surgeon General's Report on Health Promotion and Disease Prevention*, sets measurable health goals to be achieved by 1990 for five major age groups and identifies the most pressing needs.[1]

TODAY'S U.S. PUBLIC HEALTH SERVICE

The Public Health Service (PHS) contains the major health units of the Department of Health and Human Services. It is the federal agency charged by law to promote and ensure the highest level of health attainable for every individual and family in America. The major functions of the service are: to stimulate and assist states and communities with the development of local health resources and to further the development of education for the health professions; to assist with improvement of the delivery of health services to all Americans; to conduct and support research in health and related sciences and to disseminate scientific information; to protect the health of the nation against impure and unsafe foods, drugs, cosmetics, and other potential hazards; and to provide national leadership for the prevention and control of communicable disease and other public health functions. The PHS consists of six operating agencies, with the Assistant Secretary for Health exercising direct line authority over the top agencies.

In 1980, the total budget for the PHS was over $8 billion, of which the National Institutes of Health took about $3½ billion, the Health Services Administration approximately $2 billion, the Alcohol, Drug Abuse, and Mental Health Administration $1¼ billion, the Health Resources Administration $633 million, the Center for Disease Control $366 million, the Food and Drug Administration $328 million, and the Office of the Assistant Secretary for Health $285 million.

NATIONAL INSTITUTES OF HEALTH

The mission of the $3.5-billion National Institutes of Health (NIH) programs is to provide leadership and direction to programs designed to improve the health of the people of the United States. To accomplish this, NIH conducts and supports research about the cause, diagnosis, prevention, and cure of human diseases, the processes of human growth and development, the biologic effects of environmental contaminants, and the sciences related to health. In addition, NIH supports the training of research personnel, the construction of research facilities, and the development of other research resources, and it directs programs for the collection, dissemination, and exchange of information in medicine and health.

NIH is, as just stated, one of the six agencies constituting the U.S.

Public Health Service. NIH is under the leadership of a director who reports to the Assistant Secretary for Health of HHS and the Surgeon General of the PHS. NIH is comprised of eighteen bureaus, institutes, and divisions. There are eleven research institutes (two of which have legislated status as bureaus), one research resources division, three service divisions, a research hospital called the Clinical Center, the National Library of Medicine, and the Fogerty International Center. With the exception of the National Institute of Environmental Health Sciences, which is located at Research Triangle Park, North Carolina, NIH is located in Bethesda, Maryland. Smaller NIH research installations are located in other areas of the United States.

Among the several institutes that make up NIH, the *National Cancer Institute*, funded at $1 billion, is the largest. It conducts a National Cancer Program to expand existing scientific knowledge on cancer's cause and prevention as well as on the diagnosis, treatment, and rehabilitation of cancer patients. Research activities, carried out in the institute's laboratories

Figure 7–4. The National Center for Health Care Technology assesses the efficacy, cost-effectiveness, and ethical impacts associated with the use of particular technologies. (Courtesy of Arizona Daily Star, Tucson, Arizona)

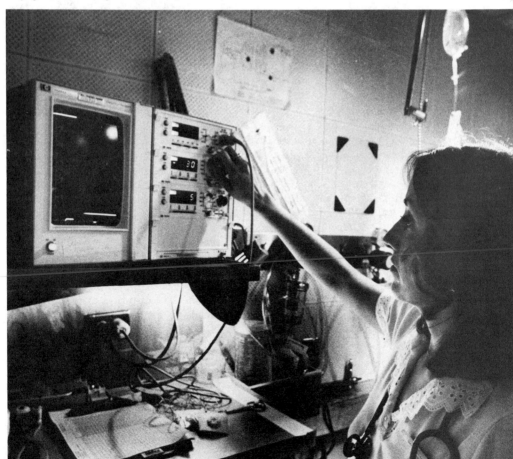

or supported through grants or contracts, include many investigative approaches to cancer through chemistry, biochemistry, biology, molecular biology, immunology, radiation physics, experimental chemotherapy, epidemiology, biometry, radiotherapy, and pharmacology. Cancer research facilities are conducted with National Cancer Institute support, and training is provided under university-based programs. The institute, through its cancer control element, applies research findings as rapidly as possible in preventing and controlling human cancer.

The *National Heart, Lung, and Blood Institute* uses its $528 million annual budget to provide leadership in a national program for diseases of the heart, blood vessels, blood, and lungs. It conducts studies and research into the clinical use of blood and all aspects of the management of blood resources, and it supports training of manpower in fundamental science and clinical disciplines for participation in basic and clinical research programs relating to heart, blood vessels, blood, and lung diseases. This institute coordinates its activities with other research institutes and with all federal agency programs related to the previous diseases, including programs in hypertension, stroke, respiratory distress, and sickle cell anemia. Also, this institute conducts educational activities, including the collection and dissemination of educational materials about these diseases, with emphasis on prevention for health professionals and the lay public.

The *National Institute of Arthritis, Metabolism and Digestive Diseases*, with its $342 million budget, conducts, fosters, and supports basic and clinical research for the causes, prevention, diagnosis, and treatment of the various arthritic, metabolic, and digestive diseases. It covers the broad areas of arthritis, bone, and skin diseases, diabetes, blood, endocrine, and metabolic diseases, digestive diseases and nutrition, and kidney and urologic diseases.

The *National Institute of Allergy and Infectious Diseases*, funded at $216 million, conducts and supports broadly based research and research training on the causes, characteristics, prevention, control, and treatment of a wide variety of diseases believed to be attributable to infectious agents (including bacteria, viruses, and parasites), to allergies, or to other deficiencies or disorders in the responses of the body's immune mechanisms. Among areas of special emphasis are asthma and allergic disease, clinical immunology (including organ transplantation), venereal diseases, hepatitis, influenza and other viral respiratory infections, disease control measures, antiviral substances, and hospital-associated infections.

Six additional institutes address human diseases. The *National Institute of Child Health and Human Development* ($210 million) conducts and supports biomedical and behavioral research on child and maternal health, on problems of human development with special attention to mental retardation, and on family structure, the dynamics of human population, and the reproductive process. The *National Institute of Dental Research* ($69 million) supports and conducts clinical and laboratory research directed toward the ultimate eradication of tooth decay and a broad array of oral-facial disorders. The *National Institute of Environmental Health Sciences* ($84 million), located in Research Triangle Park, North Carolina, conducts and supports fundamental research concerned with defining, measuring, and understanding the effects of chemical, biological and physical factors in the environment on the health and well-being of humans.

The *National Institute of Neurological and Communicative Disorders and Stroke* ($242 million) conducts and supports fundamental and applied research on human neurologic and communicative disorders such as Parkinson's disease, epilepsy, multiple sclerosis, muscular dystrophy, head and spinal cord injuries, stroke, deafness, disorders of speech, and language development problems. This institute also conducts and supports research on the development and function of the normal brain and nervous system to better understand normal processes related to disease states. The *National Eye Institute* ($133 million) conducts and supports fundamental studies on the eye and visual system, and on the causes, prevention, diagnosis, and treatment of visual disorders. The *National Institute on Aging* ($70 million) conducts and supports biomedical and behavioral research to increase the knowledge of the aging process and associated physical, psychological and social factors resulting from advanced age. Incontinence, menopause, susceptibility to diseases, and memory loss are among the areas of special concern.

Three other NIH components round out this world-wide health care resource. The *National Institute of General Medical Sciences* ($313 million) provides programs of basic biomedical science research and research training. The activities include cell biology, genetics, pharmacology, and systemic response to trauma and anesthesia. The *NIH Clinical Center* is designed to bring scientists working in the center laboratories into close proximity with clinicians caring for patients so that they may collaborate on problems of mutual concern. The research institutes select patients, referred to NIH by clinicians throughout the United States and overseas, for clinical studies of specific diseases and disorders. A certain percentage of the patients are "normal volunteers," healthy persons who provide an index of normal body functions against which to measure the abnormal. Normal volunteers come under varied sponsorships, such as colleges, civic groups, and religious organizations.

The *National Library of Medicine* (NLM) ($5 million) serves as the nation's chief health and medical information source. The NLM is authorized to provide medical library services and on-line visual graphic searches, such as Medline, Toxline, and so forth, to public and private agencies and organizations, institutions, and individuals. It is responsible for the development and management of the Biomedical Communications Network, applying advanced technology to the improvement of biomedical communications, and it operates a computer-based toxicology information system for the scientific community, industries, and other federal agencies. In addition, the library acquires and makes available for distribution audio-visual instructional material and develops prototype audio-visual communication programs for the health educational community. Through grants and contracts, the library administers programs of assistance to the nation's medical libraries, supporting a Regional Medical Library network, research in the field of health and medical library science, establishment and improvement of the basic library resources, and biomedical scientific publications of a nonprofit nature.

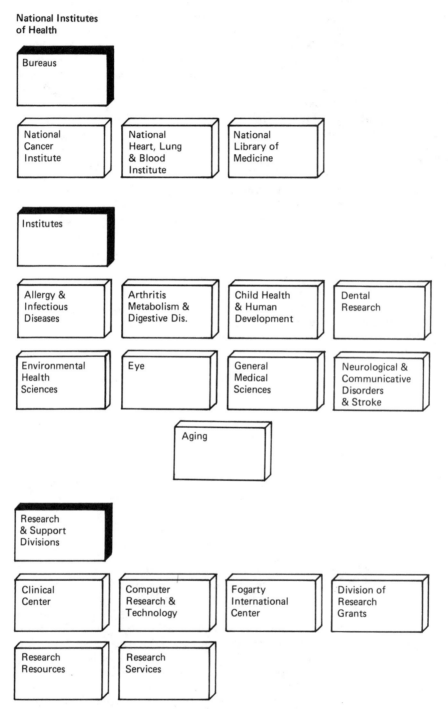

Figure 7–5. The National Institutes of Health is composed of three bureaus, nine institutes, and six divisions. (Courtesy of National Institutes of Health)

How Grants Are Awarded

With limited exceptions, NIH may not award grants for biomedical and behavioral research unless the awards are recommended by a scientific peer-review committee. The NIH peer-review system is based on two sequential levels of review known as the dual-review system. The initial review is performed by Initial Review Groups (IRGs) or study sections composed of research scientists who are experts in their fields. The members of the IRGs generally are not federal employees, but each IRG has a nonvoting executive secretary who is an NIH employee. There are about eighty permanent IRGs. In addition, ad hoc IRGs are formed as needed. The second part of the dual review is carried out by National Advisory Councils (NACs) composed of both lay persons and scientists as required by law.

Although not a part of NIH, the nursing research project closely follows the NIH rules for the grant process. Applications for grants are considered

Figure 7–6. Eye surgery is among the areas investigated by the National Eye Institute. (Courtesy of Paul Cromer, Fort Hamilton, Hughes Memorial Hospital Center, Hamilton, Ohio)

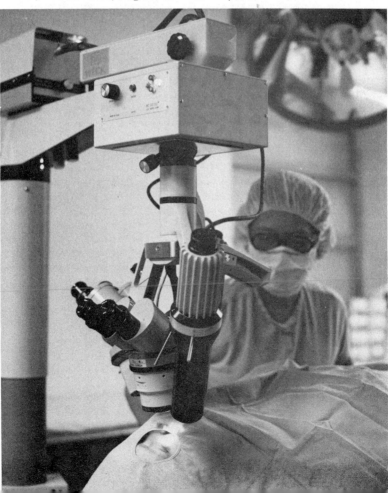

three times a year with deadline dates for submission dependent on the type of grant being sought. For instance, new research grant applications must be received by March 1 to be considered by the IRGs meeting in June, by July 1 for IRG's meeting in October and November, and by November 1 for the IRG's meeting in February and March. All applications for other than new research grants must be submitted one month earlier, that is, by February 1, June 1, and October 1. The applications are received in the Referral Branch of the Division of Research Grants, which assigns them to the appropriate executive secretary of the IRG and to the appropriate institute.

The executive secretary sends a copy of each application (except those considered to be incomplete and in need of additional data) to each member of the IRG. The IRG may have ten to twenty members. At the time the applications are sent out, they are also assigned to at least two members with the responsibility for detailed analysis and written summary. It is not unusual for an IRG member to be assigned as many as ten to fifteen applications for detailed analysis and write-up, plus general review of all of the applications, totaling perhaps 100. The IRGs meet for two or more days; most of the meetings are held in Bethesda, Maryland, but some are held elsewhere in the country. The executive secretary devotes perhaps thirty minutes to general matters, and then the IRG proceeds to consider each of the applications on the agenda. The executive secretary gives to each IRG member a worksheet listing each application and the amounts requested for the initial and subsequent years. There are columns for the IRG member to record his or her recommendations of approval, disapproval, or deferral and a column for recording a numerical priority score. The IRG members that have been assigned the task of detailed review orally present their summary of the application and their views, which are followed by general discussion. At the conclusion of the discussion, a vote is taken on whether to approve, disapprove, or defer the application, with a simple majority prevailing. If the application is disapproved, there is no further action by the IRG. If it is approved, a private priority score (with 1.0 being excellent and 5.0 marginally acceptable) is assigned by each individual reviewer with no discussion or disclosure among members about scores.

The roles of the IRGs and NACs differ in that the IRG evaluates applications solely from the standpoint of scientific and technical merit—without regard to national priorities, program goals, funding availability, or other applications or other research being performed in the same field. The NACs, in addition to reviewing specific applications, are charged with providing review and evaluation of agency programs, the identification of and resolution of problems, making recommendations concerning agency policies in the context of national health policies, and providing advice and guidance on policy making. In reviewing and making recommendations with respect to specific applications for grants, the NACs not only consider the adequacy of the scientific and technical reviews done by the IRGs, but also decide whether the proposed research is of appropriate relevance to the mission of the agency.

All of the grants, however, are dependent upon annual congressional appropriations. The role that the key members of the House and Senate Labor-HHS Appropriations Subcommittee (former Senator Warren Magnuson and others) play in the effectiveness of NIH was highlighted in a 1980 feature in the *Washington Post:*

U.S. senators are important people, accustomed to public toasts, but few could compare with the little surprise the University of Washington gave Warren G. Magnuson. During a big football weekend in 1977, the marching band spelled out Maggie on the field to honor a man who once played football for the Huskies. But a more significant tribute came that weekend. The university's Health Sciences Center, six schools housed in a 2.4-million-square-foot building, was renamed for the Democratic senator. Over a period of 30 years, a good deal of federal money had helped build the center. It was due in large part to the influence Magnuson had collected since 1937 in Congress, where he is called Mr. Health.

Dr. Jack Lein, from the school of medicine, was talking about that federal connection when he hit the punch line. Looking over at Senator Magnuson, he quipped: If you don't keep it coming, Maggie, this will become the world's largest Christian Science reading room. Even Magnuson had to laugh, but Jack Lein was putting his finger on one of the verities of life in the world of medicine and biomedical research. Without the vast infusion of federal money, medical research of the kind that developed the first artificial kidney 20 years ago at Lein's university wouldn't get very far. Magnuson is a key figure in the money-to-research transfer.

The bulk of the nation's biomedical research is paid for, channeled through and conducted by the National Institutes of Health, for which President Carter is seeking $3.6 billion in his fiscal 1981 budget. There will be much debate in

Figure 7–7. The National Institute of Child Health and Human Development awards grants for research on infant/newborn care. (Courtesy of Orlando Sentinel Star, Orlando, Florida)

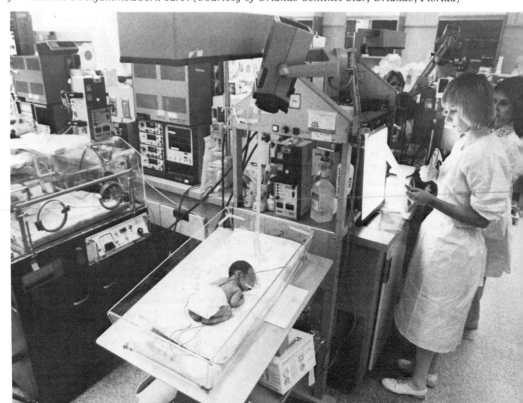

Congress over the amount and its intended uses, but it will be guided and decided in the main by Magnuson and a handful of other legislators who are the fiscal overlords of NIH. Overlord is not an excessive word. Congress controls the federal purse-strings, and it is in the appropriating committees that the string-pulling power lies. Legislators battle for vacant seats. The central forum for the debate over NIH will be the Labor–HEW subcommittees, which have begun annual hearings on the President's proposals. Decisions they make during coming months will determine in large degree what NIH does and spends in fiscal 1981.

Between them, the House and Senate subcommittees have 27 members. While representing a range of political philosophies, they tend to be generous and sympathetic toward NIH. Year after year, Congress has given NIH more than presidents have requested. This happens for many reasons. Magnuson likes to call NIH the first link in a long chain of disease prevention. Put the money in basic research and the dividends will be handsome, the argument goes. But there are other influences. New institutes and programs have come into existence at NIH because health associations lobbied Congress to push NIH into diseases they were fighting. Other times, constituents pressured for more research and more cures. Legislators or their families suffering from specific ailments provided impetus.

A light was shed on this last year by Representative Robert H. Michel (R-Ill.), the ranking Republican on the House subcommittee, who usually advocates budget cuts for NIH. Michel showed a new interest in the National Cancer Institute's (NCI) work on screening for cancer of the cervix. He told a dramatic, touching story of his wife suffering from concern over a tumor that turned out to be benign. Research and screening took on new meaning. But other legislators have become outspoken champions of certain research programs—and in a position to make a difference through their subcommittee positions. Senator Birch Bayh (D-Ind.) long has pushed for intensified cancer research, last year urging Magnuson to allow NCI's budget to reach $1 billion—which it did. Bayh's wife, Marvella, died of cancer. In 1976, he underwent surgery for removal of a spot on his lung that was diagnosed as noncancerous.[2]

ALCOHOL, DRUG ABUSE, AND MENTAL HEALTH ADMINISTRATION

The basic mission of the Alcohol, Drug Abuse, and Mental Health Administration (ADAMHA) is to prevent, control, and treat alcoholism, drug abuse and mental illness primarily through research, training, and service programs. Additionally, ADAMHA provides technical assistance to states and communities as they establish and operate alcohol, drug abuse, and mental health programs, and serves as the major federal agency in educating the public about these problems. Special emphasis has been placed on preventing problems and illnesses in these areas before they reach the point of requiring special treatment. The agency consists of three institutes with direct responsibility for the three ADAMHA health areas.

The *National Institute of Mental Health* (NIMH) ($620 million spent in 1980) provides leadership, policies, and goals for the federal effort in the promotion of mental health, the prevention and treatment of mental illness, and the rehabilitation of affected individuals. In carrying out these responsibilities, the institute conducts and supports research in the biological, psychological, sociologic, and epidemiologic aspects of mental health and illness. NIMH also supports the training of professional and paraprofessional personnel in the promotion of mental health and the prevention and treatment of mental illness. The purpose of this program is to assure an adequate, balanced, and properly distributed supply of mental health service providers and mental health researchers. This mission is accomplished through state manpower development and through the clinical training program by awarding grants and contracts for mental health services, education, research and demonstration efforts. In 1980, a total of $90 million was awarded for training, about $10 million of which went for the education of psychiatric nurses.

ADAMHA conducts a full range of drug abuse prevention activities through its *National Institute on Drug Abuse* (NIDA), which had a 1980 budget of $275 million. In carrying out these activities, NIDA supports a wide range of research programs to gain new knowledge on the causes and effects of narcotic addiction and drug abuse. This effort ranges from fundamental research on the basic chemistry of abused substances to applied research and development activities having direct impact on treatment services. It also supports training programs to assure the availability of qualified manpower for drug abuse treatment, prevention, and research programs, and it assists communities in maintaining treatment programs for drug abusers through the award of project grants. Finally NIDA demonstrates more effective methods for drug abuse treatment and prevention services and collects and disseminates scientific information on drug abuse from federal, state, and local prevention activities.

The *National Institute on Alcohol Abuse and Alcoholism* (NIAAA), established by law in 1970 and carrying a 1980 budget of $150 million, serves as a focal point for federal activities in the area of alcoholism. The basic mission of the NIAAA is to acquire a better understanding of the nature of alcoholism and its causes, while building the capacity of the states and communities to establish, sustain, and improve viable programs of alcohol prevention, treatment, and rehabilitation. The problem of alcohol abuse in this country is clearly enormous, touching millions of lives and costing more than $42 billion each year. In carrying out its mission, this institute supports research on the biological, psychological, and sociologic aspects of alcohol abuse as well as training of clinical and research personnel in alcohol-related fields. It also funds community-based programs of prevention, treatment, and rehabilitation and assists states in the development of comprehensive alcoholism programs.

HEALTH SERVICES ADMINISTRATION

The mission of the Health Services Administration (HSA) is to provide professional leadership in the delivery of health services. It is composed of three units: (1) the Bureau of Community Health Services, (2) the Bureau of Medical Services, and (3) the Indian Health Service. The *Bureau of Community Health Services* has the largest budget with over $1 billion. It was established to help communities find the best way of meeting their health needs. Its role is to serve as a national focus in improving the organization and delivery of health care by initiating activities, which provide alternatives in health care service delivery and administering programs that support health services to specific population groups, including mothers and children, and migrant workers and their families. Assuring the effective relationship of the delivery of good quality health care with health services financing resources is a high priority concern. The Bureau of Community Health Services is responsible for the management of several health care programs, including Maternal and Child Health, Community Health Centers, Migrant Health, Family Planning, and the National Health Service Corps. Primary concerns are for the development of health service delivery capacity for medically underserved areas and population groups and for the improvement and expansion of state or local systems of health care for mothers, children, and adolescents. Management emphasis is placed upon the coordination and integration of grant and other resources to meet community needs for primary health care.

The purpose of the $380-million maternal and child health services program is to provide formula and discretionary grants to states to reduce infant and maternal morbidity and mortality. Under SECTION 503 and 504 of Title V of the Social Security Act, the Maternal and Child Health Program provides formula grants ($345 million in 1980) to the states and territories to extend and improve health services for mothers and children, including crippled children. Emphasis is placed on the reduction of infant mortality and morbidity. A full range of health services addressing the needs of unserved and underserved populations is provided. Title V also authorizes under SECTION 505 special project grants to state health agencies to provide prenatal and postnatal health care to mothers and infants, necessary intensive infant health care and family planning services, with the aim of reducing the incidence of mental retardation and other handicapping conditions associated with childbearing. Special project grants to state agencies are also authorized to promote the health of children and youth of school or preschool age.

Under SECTION 511, project grants ($27 million in 1980) are available to

Figure 7–8. Senator Warren Magnuson of the state of Washington was a leading congressional advocate of federal support for biomedical research. (Courtesy of U.S. Senate)

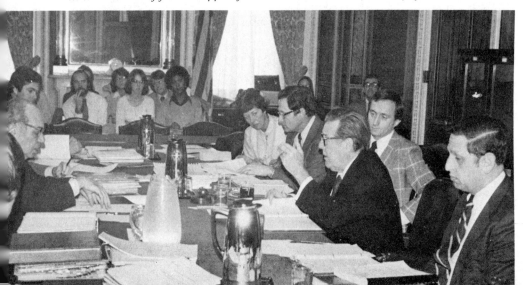

support training programs in institutions of higher learning and affiliated organizations, which provide specialized health professionals with the expertise and health services delivery for mothers, children, and handicapped children; and under SECTION 512, research grants ($5 million in 1980) are available to identify methods for improving services and service delivery systems providing care for mothers, children, and handicapped children. In 1981, it is estimated that under this program there will be 399,104 women receiving physician maternity services, 2,803,782 children receiving physician's services, 1,075,671 preschool children having assessments, and 766,000 handicapped children receiving basic and specialty assessment services.

The *Bureau of Medical Services,* with $225 million in 1980, provides comprehensive health care services to designated federal beneficiaries, provides occupational health care and safety services for federal employees, administers programs concerned with the development, improvement, expansion, and integration of emergency medical services systems and provides health care personnel and other support services to the health care program of the Federal Bureau of Prisons and the United States Coast Guard. The remaining Public Health Service hospitals and clinics serve as training centers for medical residents and other health professionals.

The *Indian Health Service,* with a $623-million budget, operates a program of comprehensive health services for eligible American Indians and natives of Alaska and provides hospital and medical care services and preventive and rehabilitative health services for Indians. It also develops innovative health services delivery systems, conducts tuberculosis and other communicable disease control activities, encourages and assists in the development of water supply and waste disposal systems, and provides training for Indian health personnel.

CENTER FOR DISEASE CONTROL

The mission of the $366-million-budgeted Center for Disease Control (CDC) is to assist state and local health authorities and other health-related organizations in stemming the spread of communicable diseases, protecting against other diseases or conditions amenable to reduction, providing protection from certain environmental hazards, improving occupational safety and health, and promoting good health. This mission is carried out through a program that includes formula grants for prevention programs, health education, and risk-reduction demonstrations. It also provides targeted disease prevention programs to states and communities, such as venereal disease control, immunization programs, floridation programs, and control of infectious diseases, environmental hazards, and chronic diseases. CDC supports state health activities with epidemic services and analysis of disease problems and trends. The center also directs and enforces quarantine activities and regulations; provides consultation and assistance in upgrading the performance of clinical laboratories; evaluates and licenses clinical laboratories engaged in interstate commerce; and administers a nationwide program of research, information, and education in the field of smoking and health. To assure safe and healthful working conditions for all working people, occupational safety and health standards are developed, and research and other activities are carried out through the center's *National Institute for Occupational Safety and Health.*

FOOD AND DRUG ADMINISTRATION

The Food and Drug Administration's (FDA) activities are directed toward protecting the health of the nation against impure and unsafe foods, drugs, and cosmetics, and other potential hazards. On a 1980 budget of $328 million, the FDA enforces a number of laws, four of which authorize most of the agency's activities:

- The *Federal Food, Drug, and Cosmetic Act,* which requires that foods be safe and wholesome, that drugs and medical devices be safe and effective, and that cosmetics be safe. All these products must be truthfully labeled.
- The *Fair Packaging and Labeling Act,* which requires that labeling enables consumers to compare the values of products they purchase.
- The *Radiation Control for Health and Safety Act,* which protects consumers from unnecessary exposure to radiation.
- The *Public Health Service Act,* one part of which establishes FDA's authority over vaccines, serums, and other biological products and is also the basis for FDA rulings on milk and shellfish sanitation, restaurant operation, and interstate travel facilities.

Figure 7–9. The Bureau of Community Health Services of the Health Services Administration funds programs in family planning. (Courtesy of U.S. Public Health Service)

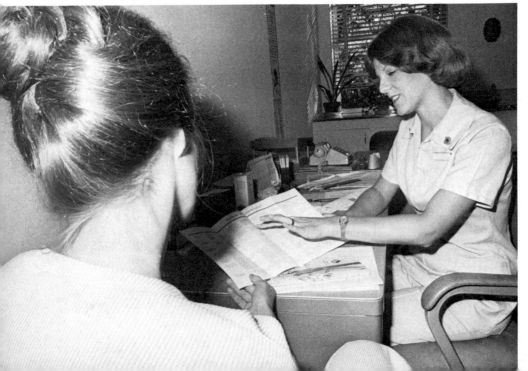

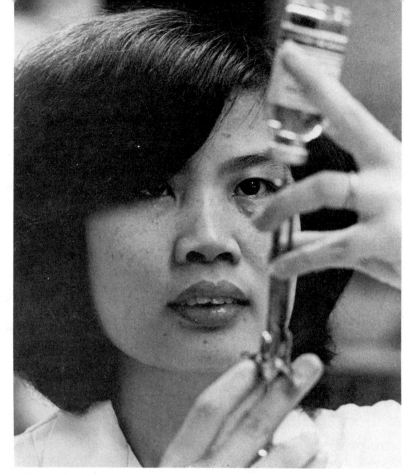

Figure 7–10. The Food and Drug Administration protects the health of the nation against unsafe drugs. (Courtesy of Philadelphia Bulletin, Philadelphia, Pennsylvania)

No new drug can be put on the market until its manufacturer provides FDA with evidence of its safety and effectiveness. FDA wants to know that a drug does what it's supposed to do and that its benefits outweigh its risks. FDA also tests and certifies every batch of insulin and most antibiotic drugs before they are released for sale. Licensing controls, which FDA maintains over biological products such as serum and vaccines, include authority over the nation's blood banks to ensure the safety of transfusions.

FDA also is concerned about drugs used by veterinarians, about cosmetics, foreign goods, and electronic devices that produce radiation. This concern is evidenced in a variety of ways. For example, FDA sets standards for consumer products—for foods that are made according to a set recipe (such as peanut butter), and for electronic equipment (such as x-ray machines, microwave ovens, and color televisions). The agency issues public warnings when hazardous products have been identified, and it can initiate removal of a product from the market when new scientific evidence reveals unacceptable or unexpected risks. FDA can go to court to seize illegal products and to prosecute the manufacturer, packer, or shipper of adulterated or mislabeled products. It can take legal action against false and misleading labeling on the products it regulates.

HEALTH RESOURCES ADMINISTRATION

The mission of the Health Resources Administration (HRA) is to provide leadership related to requirements for and distribution of health resources, including manpower training. The *Bureau of Health Planning and Resources Development*, with a $167-million 1980 budget, provides leadership and administration of a program of federal, state, and areawide health-planning and health-delivery systems development through grants, contracts, loans, and loan guarantees. The *Bureau of Health Professions Education*, with a 1980 budget of $504 million, plans, develops, and administers programs in planning, coordinating, evaluating, and supporting the development and use of the nation's health professionals. This bureau is also concerned with increasing the supply and improving the quality and distribution of the nation's health professionals. To do this, the bureau supports programs of education, training, and construction, which produce workers in the fields of nursing, medicine, osteopathy, dentistry, optometry, pharmacy, podiatry, veterinary medicine, and public health.

As of 1980, the major nursing office in the federal government, the *Division of Nursing* (DN), is located in the Health Resources Administration, Bureau of Health Professions Education. The objectives of the Division of Nursing include improving the quality of nursing education and practice, and supporting nursing research. Emphasis is placed on increasing the supply of qualified applicants to and graduates from all kinds of nursing pro-

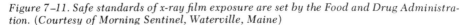

Figure 7–11. Safe standards of x-ray film exposure are set by the Food and Drug Administration. (Courtesy of Morning Sentinel, Waterville, Maine)

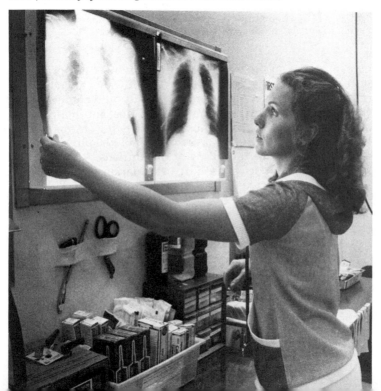

grams. The Division of Nursing also provides consultation and technical assistance to educators of associate degree, diploma, baccalaureate, and graduate programs to bring about needed changes in educational programs, to assist in the creation and development of new programs and the construction and renovation of schools of nursing. Much of the DN's work is directed by the various programs of federal assistance to schools of nursing and to students under the provisions of the Nurse Training Act.

The *Capitation Grant Program* authorizes financial support grants on a formula basis to eligible nursing educational programs in an effort to assure quality and stability of the nursing programs and to ensure an adequate supply of professional nurses. This program requires either increasing first year enrollment or conducting projects in areas such as the preparation of nurse practitioners; encouraging enrollment and retention of students from disadvantaged backgrounds; fostering clinical training and facilities geographically remote from the school location; and providing for continuing education for registered nurses. In 1980, the average amount allotted per capita student was $140 in diploma programs, $155 in associate degree programs, and $225 in baccalaureate programs. Of the total $25 million appropriation, $3 million went to the hospital schools, $8 million to associate degree programs, and $13 million to baccalaureate schools.

The *Advanced Nurse Training Program* provides institutional support through grants to collegiate schools of nursing to plan, develop and operate, expand or maintain programs for the preparation of professional nurses at the masters or doctoral level to be clinical nurse specialists, teachers, administrators, and researchers. In 1980, $12 million supported 80 projects with a student enrollment in these funded programs numbering 1600. The average award was $150,000 for each graduate program that received support.

The *Nurse Practitioner Program* provides grants and contracts to public or nonprofit private schools of nursing, medicine, and public health; public or nonprofit private hospitals, and other public or nonprofit private entities to plan, develop and operate, expand or maintain programs to educate nurse practitioners in primary health care, in such clinical areas as geriatrics, pediatrics, school nursing, and working with nursing home patients. Special traineeships are also provided for nurse practitioner students who are residents of a health manpower shortage area. These traineeships require service payback commitments in designated primary care shortage areas. In 1980, 67 nurse practitioner programs were supported with $11,500,000 in federal funds while 250 trainees received financial aid.

The *Nursing Special Project Grant Program* provides support for improving the geographic distribution of nurses, with a focus on areas with low-income populations. It also provides funds to increase nursing education opportunities for individuals from disadvantaged backgrounds, to develop innovative nursing methods emphasizing primary care and prevention to help meet the needs of high-risk groups, especially the elderly, children, and pregnant women, and to stimulate programs of continuing education for practicing nurses. In 1980, awards were made for 146 special projects at an average cost of $103,000 each with the $15,000,000 appropriated by Congress.

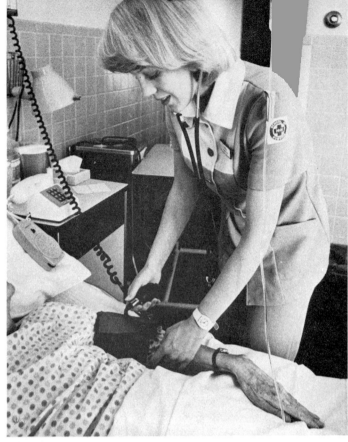

Figure 7–12. Capitation grants to schools of nursing stimulated the expansion of enrollments and fostered the development of enhanced clinical experiences. (Courtesy of Lubbock Morning Avalanche Journal, Lubbock, Texas)

From 1964 to 1976, the *Construction Grants* for schools of nursing provided essential financial assistance to build new buildings and to expand the educational capacity of existing schools. Construction grants were also awarded for new programs and to replace or rehabilitate existing facilities that were obsolete and affected enrollment and quality of education. All collegiate, associate degree, and diploma schools of nursing that were accredited or had been given reasonable assurance of being accredited upon completion were eligible for these grants. The federal share of construction costs could be as high as 75%. In addition to grants, the federal government had authority to guarantee up to 90% of the principal of a loan made to a private, nonprofit school for construction costs. The interest subsidy provision allowed the government to pay to the lending institution, on behalf of the school, amounts that would reduce the net effective interest rate paid by the school of nursing up to 3%. This authorized program has not received an appropriation since the mid-1970s; thus, no new school of nursing buildings have been assisted by the federal government since that time.

The *Nursing Student Loan Program,* funded at $13,500,000, authorizes long-term, low-interest loans of up to $2,500 per academic year or an aggregate of $10,000 to assist nursing students who are either full- or half-time and need financial assistance in undertaking the course of study leading to a diploma, associate degree, baccalaureate, or graduate degree in nursing.

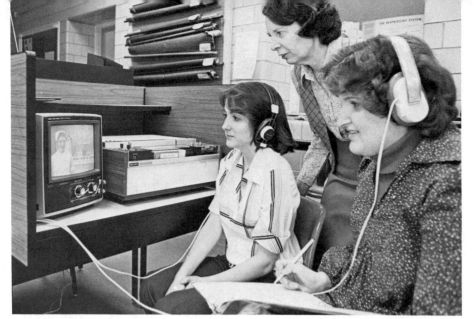

Figure 7–13. Special project grants from the Division of Nursing facilitated the development of software for learning laboratories. (Courtesy of Bridgeport Hospital, Bridgeport, Connecticut)

Funds for this program are allocated by a legislative formula to participating accredited schools of nursing located in the United States, Puerto Rico, Guam, and the Virgin Islands, who in turn administer the funds to the students. Loans are repayable over a ten-year period following completion of training. Borrowers can defer repayment of a nursing loan pending completion of study for advanced professional education in nursing and for a service in the armed forces or Peace Corps.

The nursing scholarship program provides scholarships of up to $2000 per academic year to assist qualified and motivated students who have exceptional financial need and who will undertake the course of study leading to a diploma, associate degree, baccalaureate degree, or graduate degree in nursing. Funds for this program are allocated to participating schools of nursing on the basis of a legislative formula. The schools, in turn, make scholarship awards to the students. The nursing scholarship program provided $9 million in 1980 to support students in 1339 nursing programs. As will be noted, funds are far short of the level of demand:

NURSING SCHOLARSHIP PROGRAM
Academic Year 1978–79

DEGREE PROGRAM	NUMBER OF PROGRAMS	ESTIMATED ENROLLMENT	AMOUNT REQUESTED	AMOUNT ALLOCATED	ESTIMATED RECIPIENTS
Associate	592	87,102	$19,124,558	$3,028,517	3,028
Diploma	237	37,659	6,924,263	1,280,364	1,280
Baccalaureate	391	121,650	28,739,651	4,315,683	4,316
Graduate	90	8,418	2,085,900	289,750	290
	1,310	254,739	$56,874,372	$8,914,314	8,914

The *Nursing Professional Traineeships Program* provides financial assistance to registered nurses working on graduate degrees in order to qualify for various leadership positions. Traineeships provide tuition, a stipend, and dependence allowances. In 1980, the $13 million available for this program was able to support only a small number of the 949 registered nurses who were enrolled in doctoral programs and the 13,105 in nursing master's degree programs.

The nation has very few nurse investigators qualified to carry on nursing research. In 1977, there were only 2304 nurses out of 1.4 million nurses in the entire United States with earned doctorates, the usual qualification for beginning researchers. The number of students enrolled in doctoral programs offering a major in nursing increased from 258 in 1968 to 949 in 1980. Of these, the percentage who were attending on a full-time basis varied during the period from a low of 37% to a high of 59%. Although considerable growth is in evidence, it still falls far short of demand, and this shortage of qualified nurse researchers has limited the conduct of research in nursing and the participation of nursing in the interdisciplinary research in patient care. Thus, the *National Research Service Awards* are the major source of support for individuals who have demonstrated potential and can undertake full-time predoctoral or postdoctoral study in the physical, biological, or behavioral sciences. The period of award for student support may not exceed five years in the aggregate for predoctoral training and three years in the aggregate for postdoctoral training. In 1980, $1 million supported 92 National Research Service Awards to nurses for specified research training to prepare them to conduct independent research and to collaborate in interdisciplinary research, an amount far short of the demand for these funds.

Nursing research is fundamental to the improvement of nursing practice, education, and administration through scientific investigation of the many unknowns that limit progress in these areas. Studies have shown, for example, that nursing care contributes significantly to the ability of the patient and his family to cope with problems related to achieving health, both in the hospital and in the home. More needs to be known about the scientific basis of nursing. The *Nursing Research Grants Program* provides grants to public or nonprofit public organizations and institutions to support high quality research projects in areas related to nursing practice, education, or administration. These project grants have particular emphasis on clinical interventions, psychosocial management aspects of patient care as well as primary care, development, and testing of research instrumentation, and technology transfer. In 1980, the $5 million appropriation supported 49 projects with an average cost of $102,000 per project.

HEALTH CARE FINANCING ADMINISTRATION

Although not a part of the U.S. Public Health Service, the Health Care Financing Administration (HCFA), with a 1980 appropriation of $23 billion, is responsible for a very large share of the Department of Health and Human Service's expenditures by virtue of its jurisdiction over the Medicare and Medicaid programs. For the $18-billion federal Medicare program,

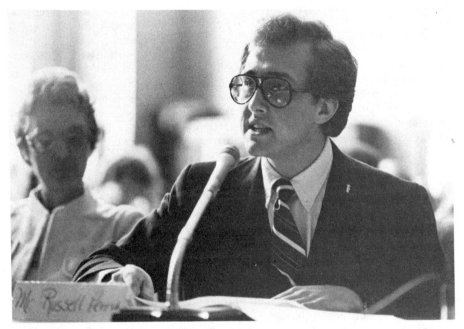

Figure 7–14. Seeking funds for scholarships and loans, Russell Perry, nursing student at Trenton State College, testifies before the Senate Health Subcommittee on the 1980 extension of the Nurse Training Act. (Courtesy of National Student Nurses' Association)

the agency is concerned with the development of policies, procedures, and guidance related to the program recipients; with the providers of services such as hospitals, nursing homes, and physicians; and with the insurance companies who handle the claims. Under the $15 billion federal share of the Medicaid program, HCFA is responsible for developing approaches to meet the needs of those who cannot afford adequate health care and for providing technical assistance to states and local organizations to improve the scope, content, and quality of health care programs for the needy. The professional standards review organization (PSRO) program is also operated by HCFA with a 1980 cost of $29 million. Finally, the agency funds a large number of research, demonstration, and evaluation projects on hospital costs ($7 million), physician reimbursement ($4 million), long-term care ($14 million), alternative forms of health-care organization ($4 million), quality of care ($3 million), and beneficiary impact ($6 million).

OFFICE OF HUMAN DEVELOPMENT

The major welfare branch of the Department of Health and Human Services is the Office of Human Development, which is responsible for the federal administration of $5 billion in programs for children, youth, the aged, the handicapped, and native Americans. In addition, it contains a number of programs aimed at improving the quality of life for the vulnerable segments of the nation's population.

For example, the *Administration for Children, Youth, and Families* supports $796 million in programs and activities designed to improve child care and youth services delivery systems and improve the quality of life for children and youths and their families. The primary emphasis is on meeting the developmental needs of preschool children from low-income families and on developing better services for vulnerable children, particularly those in need of child care, foster care, or adoption; foster children in institutions; youths who are runaways or homeless; and children who are abused or neglected. The Administration for Children, Youth, and Families funds research and demonstration programs designed to improve the quality of programs for children and to measure their impact on children and their families. One example of the health dimension of this program is the Child Abuse and Neglect program. This program is designed to help improve and increase national, state, community, and family activities for the prevention, identification, and treatment of child abuse and neglect through research, demonstration, evaluation, information dissemination, technical assistance, training, and state grants. Between 1976 and 1978, states reported an increase in the total number of child abuse cases from 416,000 to 614,000, or a jump of 48%, and they also reported that 40% of these cases had been substantiated. Reports of child sexual abuse rose approximately 100% as a proportion of the total number of reports. As part of its efforts, the administration in 1980 published and widely distributed a manual entitled *The Role of Nurses in the Prevention and Treatment of Child Abuse and Neglect* and funded the development of a curriculum specifically for use by community health nurses.

Another important agency in the Office of Human Development is the *Administration on Aging*. The elderly population in the United States is growing at a faster rate than any other age group within the population. By the year 2030, two out of every eleven Americans will be over sixty-five years of age, and 86% of these elderly persons will have some degree of functional impairment. The Older Americans Act of 1965, as amended, seeks to foster independence of the socially and economically needy elderly and to provide alternatives to institutional treatment. In order to achieve the goals, the act provides for the development of a system of community-based social and nutrition services coordinated by state agencies. Under the direction of the Administration on Aging, the program's aim is to alleviate, arrest and/or prevent functional impairments through services that:

- secure and maintain maximum independence and dignity in a homelike environment for older individuals capable of self-care with appropriate supportive services
- remove individual and social barriers to economic and personal independence for older individuals
- provide necessary services to the vulnerable elderly, among which are the elderly Indians.

OTHER FEDERAL HEALTH AGENCIES

Among the federal agencies involved in health outside of the Department of Health and Human Services is the *Occupational Safety and Health Admin-*

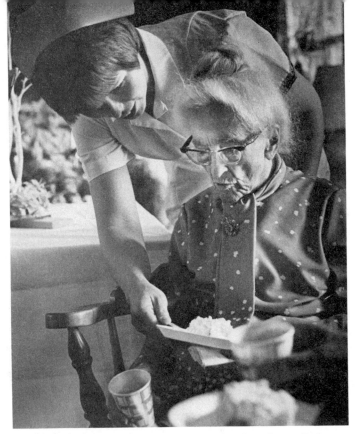

Figure 7–15. The rapidly growing elderly population is served by the Administration on Aging. (Courtesy of Muncie Press, Muncie, Indiana)

istration (OSHA). It is an agency within the Department of Labor headed by the Assistant Secretary of Labor for Occupational Safety and Health (one of the seven assistant secretaries in that department). Broadly, OSHA undertakes two kinds of tasks. First, it promulgates regulations regarding workplace conditions related to employee safety and health. These regulations state, for example, that machine parts must be guarded, floors must be kept uncluttered, stairways must have handrails, and employees may be exposed to no more than a certain concentration of harmful chemicals. Second, OSHA inspects work places to determine compliance with the regulations. These two tasks define the essential organizational division within the agency. OSHA's Washington headquarters is the locus of standards development, while OSHA's eighty-nine area offices are the loci of compliance activities.

In determining the content of regulations, OSHA must decide how far it wishes to require reductions of risks to which workers are exposed. Each reduction of risk costs money, and successive reductions cost successively larger amounts of money. The statute establishing OSHA gives the agency power to promulgate regulations requiring employers to eliminate specific conditions judged unsafe or unhealthy. These regulations have the force of law, yet they are adopted not by the legislature, but by administrative agencies consisting entirely of appointed officials. Furthermore, the statute gives the agency considerable discretion about the content of the regulations. OSHA's goal, as stated in the statute in extremely general terms, is "to assure so far as possible every working man and woman in the nation safe and healthful working conditions."

The modern *Veteran's Administration* (VA) hospital system is a post-World War II development. The system, which was originally established in 1921, was modified in the late 1940s to provide high-quality health care for the large number of veterans emerging from the Second World War with service-connected disabilities. This load has decreased with time, and the purposes of the system have changed, partly because of the changing patient load and partly because of changes in operating policy and the authorizations under which the system operates. As the number of veterans requiring hospitalization for service-connected disabilities decreased during the 1950s and 1960s, an increase occurred in the proportion of patients who were admitted for non-service-connected disabilities. It has been estimated that about 75% of the patients in VA hospitals are now hospitalized for non-service-connected disabilities. However, the VA system has become increasingly involved in the support of health care research and in the education of medical and nursing students in association with their affiliated medical and nursing schools. These activities are not simply responsive to the internal needs of the system, but also relate to needs of the nation as a whole.

PRESIDENT REAGAN'S ATTACK ON FEDERAL HEALTH AGENCIES

In its February 18, 1981, "Program for Economic Recovery," the Reagan administration proposed dismantling the array of categorical grant programs built up over the years to attack specific health problems, and replacing

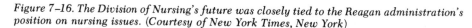

Figure 7–16. The Division of Nursing's future was closely tied to the Reagan administration's position on nursing issues. (Courtesy of New York Times, New York)

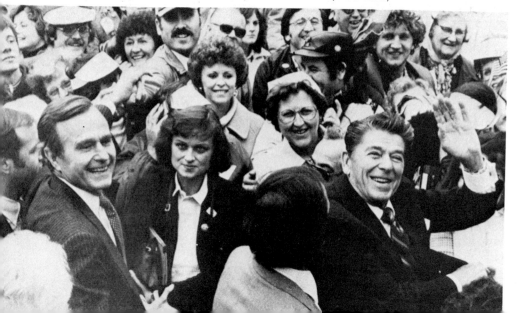

them with unrestricted block grants to states. There is a call for abolition of the nation's health planning system and professional standards review organizations (PSROs)—the two regulatory mechanisms by which the government has attempted to hold down health care costs and insure proper distribution of services. It also recommended capping the federal contribution to Medicaid, the health care program for the poor, ending subsidies to health maintenance organizations (HMOs), shutting down the eight hospitals operated by the Public Health Service, and eliminating subsidies for training physicians and other health professionals.

The Reagan administration proposed to take more than forty health and social service categorical grants programs—dealing with problems ranging from lead-base paint poisoning to venereal disease—and lump them together into block grants. Funding would be cut by 25%, but because of administrative savings by states, the administration claimed that the cut "need not result in a reduction of services." According to the administration the proposal would reduce federal spending by $2.5 billion in 1982 and by almost $4 billion a year by 1986. Block grant funds would be divided into four basic categories: preventive health services, basic health services, social services, and emergency services. In fiscal year 1982 each state would get 75% of the total grant money it would have been entitled to under the various old distribution formulas and would be free, for the most part, to spend the money as it pleased. Fighting against the change to block grants were the various health interest groups that would rather have Congress target funds for their programs than trust the states to do so.

This chapter has attempted to set out the framework of the basic federal health agencies. As noted in chapters 4, 5, and 6, there is a wide range of views and values to be accommodated in the effective administration of health care programs, and decisions should no longer be allowed to be dominated by physicians and other elite groups. If a nurse finds that the present balance of governmental power affecting the development of health service is unsatisfactory, indeed undemocratic, then she should look to the Congress to make changes in our central governmental machinery that would improve the performance of the federal health agencies. The following three chapters will present the essential three-phase process for legislating, implementing, and financing change.

References

1. Hamburg A: Healthy People: The Surgeon General's Report on Health Promotion and Disease Prevention: Background Papers. Washington, DC, United States Government Printing Office, 1979
2. Sinclair W: Sen. Magnuson is "Mr. Health" to NIH. Washington, DC, Washington Post, Feb 19, 1980

8–The Legislative Process: Authorizations

The Constitution assigns Congress *all legislative power* and grants it explicit and implied responsibilities. Congress *enacts* the laws, the President *executes* them, and the Supreme Court *interprets* them. As a representative institution, Congress and its members respond to the needs and interests of the various states and congressional districts. The nation's diversity is given full expression in Congress by legislators whose future service rests on the continued support of their constituents. The members of Congress, because they represent their constituents, survive and remain members by producing scarce resources for voters.

CHARACTERISTICS OF CONGRESS

Congress is an exceedingly complex institution, not only because there are two distinct Houses but also because the party leadership must compete with the rival leadership, which the two-party system produces. Consequently, power is widely dispersed throughout. Gathered in the nation's capital to exercise its legislative responsibilities is a Congress of 100 senators and 435 representatives elected from fifty states extending from Maine to Hawaii and from Florida to Alaska. Membership in Congress is no longer a part-time job: Congress meets in almost year-round sessions, and its concerns are massive. A House of Representatives is elected for a two-year period and constitutes a Congress. Under the Twentieth Amendment to the Constitution, adopted in 1933, a new Congress begins at noon January 3 of each odd-numbered year and ends at noon January 3 of the next odd-numbered year. Congresses are numbered consecutively, and the Congress that met in January, 1981, was the 97th in a series that began in 1789.

With elections for the House of Representatives being held every two years, each of the 435 representatives is almost constantly reflecting on his or her last election or preparing for the next one. Members of the Senate serve six-year terms, and because the terms are staggered, only about one-third of the senators are up for re-election in each biannual election. Recent academic studies reveal that the 95% re-election rate for House incumbents compares with less than 70% for senators. This fact has much to do with the reality that House challengers are less well known and visible than Senate challengers. House members have benefited from the heightened political awareness of voters during the past twenty years. As government has become more important, the representative's contact with voters has increased. There is more media attention and more need for personal contact. Whereas senators usually face prominent opponents (including many well-known House members), it is often difficult to find a local notable or politician who can rival the name recognition of the local House member. A University of Michigan survey supports this hypothesis: 93% of

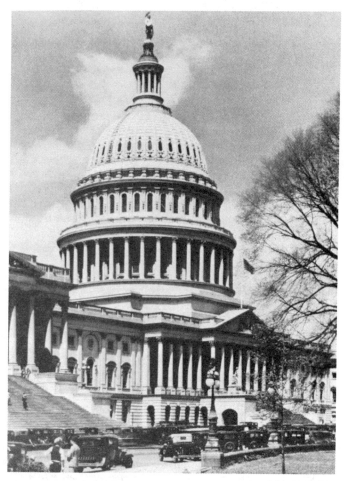

Figure 8–1. Congress and its members have responded to the health care needs and interests of the various states and congressional districts since the era of Franklin D. Roosevelt. (Courtesy of National Archives)

respondents recognized the House incumbent's name against only 44% for the challengers. By contrast, name recognition of Senate incumbents and challengers was almost equal.

Party control of Congress is of great importance to Democrats and Republicans. The Democrats have kept comfortable control of the House since 1955. Their biggest victories came in 1958, 1964, and 1974, when they gained 49, 37, and 49 seats respectively. Only in 1960, 1966, and 1980 did they lose more than 20 seats. One of the most significant elections in the cycle came in 1976, when by all odds the GOP should have regained many of the seats they lost to Democrats because of the Watergate scandal. Instead, the Republicans defeated only 2 of the 74 Democrats who were originally elected in 1974 and sought re-election in 1976. The "Watergate"

Democrats did not do quite so well either in 1978, when 8 of the 68 members who sought re-election were defeated, or in 1980, when 9 of the 57 House Democrats of the class of 1974 seeking re-election were defeated.

As a result of the 1980 election, for the first time since 1954, Republicans control the Senate. And, for the first time since 1932, different parties control the House and the Senate. The GOP held onto all 10 of its Senate seats that were at stake in the 1980 election, while the Democrats lost 12 of their 24 seats. This resulted in a 53 to 46 Republican majority in the Senate, compared with a 58 to 41 Democratic edge in the previous Congress. Independent Harry F. Byrd, Jr. of Virginia continued to sit with the Democrats. The most recent comparable Senate shift came in 1958, when Democrats picked up 15 seats, 2 of them from the newly admitted state of Alaska.

In the House, Republicans defeated 27 Democratic incumbents and scored a net gain of 33 seats, to cut the Democratic majority from 273 to 179 Republicans (with three Democratic seats vacant in 1980) to a lesser majority of 243 Democratic seats to 192 Republicans in the 1981–1982 Congress. There were even greater shifts in the House after the 1948, 1964, and 1974 elections, but one has to go all the way back to the Franklin D. Roosevelt landslide of 1932 to find comparable changes in both chambers at the same time that control of the White House moved from one party to the other.

The magnitude of the electoral turnover is perhaps best illustrated by these statistics: when the new 97th Congress convened in January, 1981, only 46 of the Senators and 236 of the House members had been in Congress longer than four years. The 1980 election brought 18 new Senators to the 97th Congress, all but 2 of them Republicans. President Ronald Reagan had 192 Republicans in the House to work with, compared to the 1980 figure of 159. Because there were at least 30 generally sympathetic Southern Democrats, it might be said that the "conservative coalition" controlled the House as it did a generation ago.

As may be noted in Table 8–1, there were 20 women legislators, including two senators and 18 House members in the 97th Congress. During the 96th Congress, only one Senator and 16 House members were women. In the Senate, joining Nancy Landon Kassebaum, Republican of Kansas, was Paula Hawkins, Republican of Florida. In the House, only one district that was represented by a woman member in 1980 was represented by a man in 1981, New York's 16th District. In that district, Representative Elizabeth Holtzman, a Democrat, ran for the Senate rather than seek re-election. Occupying Holtzman's former seat was Representative Charles Schumer. Representatives Bobbi Fiedler (Republican of California), Lynn Martin (Republican of Illinois), Marge Roukema (Republican of New Jersey), and Claudine Schneider (Republican of Rhode Island) were the four women who were newly elected to the House in 1980.

There were 16 blacks in Congress; in addition, the delegate from the District of Columbia, Walter E. Fauntroy, was a nonvoting member. No incumbent black was defeated in the 1980 election, and two blacks won seats formerly held by whites.

In most cases, House members are regarded as safe if they received at least 60% of the vote in the previous election. However, election analysts

Table 8-1.   *Women in Congress*, 1920–1981*

YEAR	NUMBER IN CONGRESS			NUMBER OF SEATS	% WOMEN
	Senate	*House*	*Both*		
1921	0	0	0	531	0
1925	0	3	3	531	.5
1931	1	7	8	531	1.5
1935	1	7	8	531	1.5
1941	1	9	10	531	1.8
1945	0	11	11	531	2.0
1951	1	10	11	531	2.0
1955	1	16	17	531	3.2
1961	2	18	20	535	3.7
1965	2	10	12	535	2.2
1971	1	11	12	535	2.2
1975	0	19	19	535	3.5
1981	2	18	20	535	3.7

* *Refers to both the House of Representatives and U.S. Senate.*

sometimes place incumbents with 60% or more in the marginal categories if their victory totals dropped from previous years, or if there are controversial local issues. The last decade has seen an inordinately large turnover in both the House and the Senate as seen in the following:

	Senate (100 members)		House (435 members)	
	Elected this Congress	Elected since 1971	Elected this Congress	Elected since 1971
1971–72 (92nd)	13	13	61	61
1973–74 (93rd)	13	25	78	128
1975–76 (94th)	11	36	98	201
1977–78 (95th)	22	53	70	249
1979–80 (96th)	20	61	79	290
1981–82 (97th)	18	79	74	364

Election returns are perhaps the most impressive indicators of constituent opinion. A member of Congress is highly conscious of the margins by which he and his predecessors have been elected. Because so many factors affect voting patterns—candidate personality, party affiliation, specific issues, and so forth—the bare figures give only crude hints of local sentiment. Breakdown of these figures by neighborhood may indicate which interest groups supported or opposed a member, and inferences can be drawn to explain the causes of that support or opposition.

As of May 16, 1981, 39% of U.S. adults said they were Republicans or leaned toward Republican party policies, compared to 40% for the Democrats and 21% for Independents. This was a 9-point gain for Republican sympathizers since June, 1980, and an 11-point loss for the Democrats. There were segments of society, however, where the shift away from Democrats had been particularly strong:

- *Males.* The Democrats had lost 14 points, with 11 going to the Republican column and 2 going to "independent."
- *Young adults* 18 to 24 years of age. Within this group, the Republicans had picked up 13 points, almost all of which had come from the independent column. This indicated that the new wave entering the electorate, which in times past might have been expected to have Democratic sympathies, now leaned toward Republican.
- *By region,* Republicans had enjoyed disproportionate gains in the Midwest farm belt (21 points), Middle Atlantic states (15 points), and Deep South (20 points). In all three areas, they had drawn from both the Democrat and independent columns.
- The shift of right-wing religious groups away from the Democrats had been, proportionately, no larger than that of other religious groups. The attraction of Republicanism and Ronald Reagan to the born-agains appeared to have been exaggerated; in fact, more (42%) identified with the Democrats than with the Republicans (32%).
- With *labor union families,* the Democrats had lost 11 points—but the percentage of those siding with the Democrats (48%) was still much larger than those with the Republicans (38%).

The one bright spot for Democrats was the black electorate, which showed a five-point gain over the previous year, with 87% siding with their traditional party in mid-1981. In the case of the Hispanic population, the shift away from the Democrats was more to the independent rather than the Republican column. The question for the future, of course, was to what degree these past-year gains solidify for the Republicans and hold on through the 1982 elections, and the degree to which they were rooted in Republican political philosophy versus the personal popularity of President Reagan.

As members come to appreciate the way in which the House and Senate operate, they recognize how little a freshman member can accomplish even if he or she works hard and is both intelligent and forceful. To become someone important one must gain seniority, for it is on the basis of years of service that much of the power of Congress is allocated. To obtain seniority, of course, one must be re-elected time and time again.

The record of the longest service in Congress, fifty-six years, is held by Carl Hayden of Arizona, who retired from the Senate in 1968 at the age of ninety-one. Hayden gave up his job as a county sheriff to become Arizona's first representative in 1912. He was sworn in on February 19, 1912, five days after Arizona became a state, and served in the House for fifteen years. In 1927, he moved to the Senate where he served seven six-year terms. When Hayden retired, he was president pro tempore of the Senate and chairman of the Senate Appropriations Committee. Runner-up to Hayden

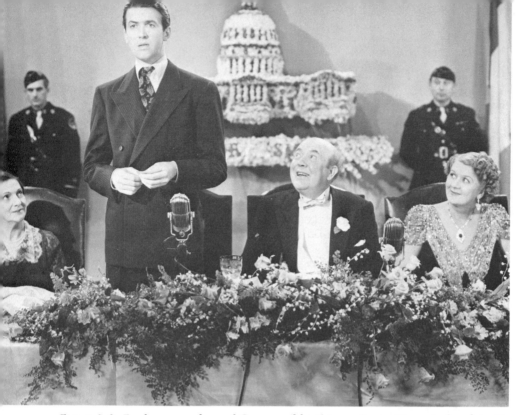

Figure 8–2. Freshmen members of Congress, like the one Jimmy Stewart played in Mr. Smith Goes to Washington, *quickly come to recognize how little a new member can accomplish* (*Courtesy of Nursing in the Mass Media Collection, University of Michigan*)

was Representative Emanuel Celler of New York, who served in the House for twenty-five consecutive terms (1923–1979). Cellar was defeated in a Democratic primary in 1972.

As can be noted below, the average age of House members has fallen from 52.9 years in 1957 to 48.4 years in 1981; the drop in the Senate was from 57.9 to 52.5 years as can be noted in Table 8–2. Not only the age, but also the occupation of a representative or senator prior to his election has an important influence on the perspective that he brings to Congress (Table 8–3). Lawyers dominate both the House and Senate with businessmen and educators enjoying good representation. Whereas physicians have been elected quite regularly, no nurse has ever served in either branch.

SENATE AND HOUSE LEADERSHIP

The leadership structures in both houses have great influence over the course a bill might take; few important bills become law without the support of the majority leadership. In the Senate, the Vice-President is the constitutional president of the Senate, and in his absence, the president pro tempore or (more commonly) a temporary presiding officer presides, but neither of these individuals has the power that is accorded the Senate majority leader. The majority leader is the most influential officer, because neither the Vice-President nor the president pro tempore has substantive powers over the chamber's proceedings. Thus, the majority leader is the

Table 8–2. *Age Structure of Congress,*
            1957–1981

YEAR	HOUSE	SENATE	CONGRESS
1957	52.9	57.9	53.8
1959	51.7	57.1	52.7
1961	52.2	57.0	53.2
1963	51.7	56.8	52.7
1965	50.5	57.7	51.9
1967	50.8	57.7	52.1
1969	52.2	56.6	53.0
1971	51.9	56.4	52.7
1973	51.1	55.3	52.0
1975	49.8	55.5	50.9
1977	49.3	54.7	50.3
1979	48.8	52.7	49.5
1981	48.4	52.5	49.2

Table 8–3. *Members' Occupations as of 1981*

	HOUSE				SENATE			
Occupation	*D*	*R*	*Total**	*Percent*	*D*	*R*	*Total**	*Percent*
Agriculture	11	17	28	5.5	2	7	9	6.9
Business or banking	58	76	134	26.2	13	15	28	21.4
Education	39	20	59	11.5	5	5	10	7.6
Engineering	2	3	5	1.0	1	1	2	1.5
Journalism	9	12	21	4.1	4	3	7	5.3
Labor leaders	4	1	5	1.0	0	0	0	0.0
Law	114	80	194	37.9	33	26	59	45.0
Law enforcement	4	1	5	1.0	0	0	0	0.0
Medicine	2	4	6	1.2	1	0	1	.8
Public service/politics	31	21	52	10.2	6	7	13	10.0
Clergymen	2	1	3	.6	0	1	1	.8
Scientists	0	0	0	0.0	0	1	1	.8

* The above totals exceed the memberships of the House and Senate respectively by at least seventy-five for the House and thirty for the Senate owing to many members having two professions.

chief strategist and floor spokesperson for the controlling (majority) party. He is elected by his party colleagues and is virtually program director for the Senate.

The Senate minority leader is also elected by the members of his party in the Senate. Everyday duties for the minority leader correspond to those of the majority leader, except that the minority leader has no authority over scheduling. The minority leader speaks for his party and acts as field general on the floor. It is the minority leader's duty to consult ranking minority members of various committees and encourage them to follow adopted party positions. If the minority party occupies the White House, its leader will probably be the President's spokesperson in the House. Each party appoints a whip and a number of assistant whips to assist the floor leader in execution of the party's legislative program. The *whip* canvasses party members on a pending issue and gives the floor leader an accurate picture of the support or opposition expected for the measure. Whips are also responsible for making sure that party members are on hand to vote. The Senate leadership of the 97th Congress (1981–1982) was as follows:

- President Pro Tempore—Strom Thurmond, Republican, South Carolina
- Majority Leader—Howard H. Baker, Jr., Republican, Tennessee
- Majority Whip—Ted Stevens, Republican, Alaska
- Minority Leader—Robert C. Byrd, Democrat, West Virginia
- Minority Whip—Alan Cranston, Democrat, California

In the House, the formal leadership consists of the Speaker, who is both the chamber's presiding officer and the majority party's overall leader; the majority and minority leaders; whips from each party; assistants to the whips; and the various committees to assist with party strategy, legislative scheduling, and the assignment of party members to committees. Speakers, who are chosen by vote of the majority party, achieve their influence largely through personal prestige, persuasion, legislative expertise, and the support of the members. The Speaker's primary powers are: presiding over the House, deciding points of order, referring bills and resolutions to the appropriate House committees, scheduling legislation for floor action, and appointing members to joint and conference committees. The Speaker may participate in debate and may vote, like any other member, although most Speakers have only voted to break a tie. Like the Senate, the House has other key leadership positions. For the 97th Congress, they were filled by the following:

- Speaker—Thomas P. O'Neill, Jr., Democrat, Massachusetts
- Majority Leader—Jim Wright, Democrat, Texas
- Majority Whip—Thomas S. Foley, Democrat, Washington
- Minority Leader—Robert H. Michel, Republican, Illinois
- Minority Whip—Trent Lott, Republican, Mississippi

The Senate is a more personal and individualistic institution than is the House. It functions to a large extent by unanimous consent, in effect adjust-

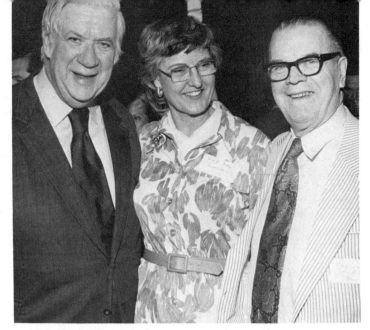

Figure 8–3. House Speaker Tip O'Neill (on the left) meets with the executive director of the Massachusetts Nurses' Association. (Courtesy of American Nurses' Association, Kansas City, Missouri)

ing or disregarding its rules as it goes along. It is not uncommon for votes to be rescheduled or delayed until an interested senator can be present. Senate party leaders are careful to consult all senators who have expressed an interest in the legislation; in the House, the leadership can consult only key members, usually committee leaders, about floor activities. Unlike the average representative, senators find it easier to exercise initiative in legislation and oversight, to have their floor amendments adopted to legislation reported from committees on which they are not members, to influence the scheduling of measures, and, in general, to participate more widely and equally in all Senate and party activities. The Senate is comparatively less concerned with the technical perfection of legislation and more involved with cultivating national constituencies, formulating questions for national debate, and gaining general public support for policy proposals. Policy-generating roles are particularly characteristic of senators with presidential ambitions, who need to capture both headlines and national constituencies.

Since senators represent a broader constituency than House members, this compels them to generalize as they attempt to be conversant on numerous national and international issues that affect their state. With their six-year term, senators are less vulnerable to immediate constituency pressures and can afford to be more cosmopolitan in their viewpoints than House members. A result of their generalist role is the necessity for greater reliance by senators on knowledgeable staff aides for advice and decision making. A House member, on the other hand, is more likely to be an expert on particular policy issues. If not, he often relies more on informed colleagues than on staff aides for advice on legislation. Consequently Senate staff aides generally have more influence over the laws and programs of the nation than do their counterparts in the House.

It is a time-consuming and often tedious task to get any group of decision makers to change the way things are, and this is true with Congress. This is not always due to the decision maker's desire to protect the status quo; it may be due simply to the innate difficulty human beings often have in accepting change of any sort. When the stakes are not large, a member with a local-interest bill usually must depend on his or her own skill and resources in gaining support from among colleagues. Success under such circumstances usually depends on how cooperative one has been when other members have been in similar positions. The more senior a member is the greater the resources he or she usually has, especially those members who are subcommittee or committee chairpersons. But the most important ingredient for success with a bill is the lack of opposition, especially from a powerful organized interest group.

THE LEGISLATIVE PROCESS

The legislative process itself is complex and technical. Formally, the process consists of a number of steps. Briefly, these can be outlined as follows:

1. Formal introduction of a bill in either the House or the Senate.
2. Referral to a standing committee and then, in most situations, referral to a subcommittee. The overwhelming number of bills go this far and no further.
3. Hearings by the subcommittee (from witnesses representing the Administration, citizens, lobbyists, and interested members of Congress).
4. *Marking up*—the term employed when a committee (or subcommittee) has come to the point where it decides legislation should go further and makes the changes it wants to make in the language of the bill.
5. Reporting the bill to the floor.
6. Debate on the bill, including consideration and acceptance or rejection of amendments.
7. Final passage of the bill and referral to the other House, where essentially the same process takes place.
8. After passage by the second House, referral to the Conference Committee, when the language of the bills is not the same.
9. Final vote of acceptance in the Conference Committee Report, in which the differences have been reconciled.
10. Referral to the President for signature or veto.
11. In the case of a veto while Congress is in session, referral back to Congress where, if both Houses vote to override the veto, the bill becomes a law.

Each step represents a whole process of struggle and pressure that in the end determines which bills become law and the form they will take.

INTRODUCING LEGISLATION

Legislative proposals may originate in a number of different ways. A member of Congress may himself develop the idea for a piece of legislation

[H.R. 1143, Introduced by Mr. STAGGERS on January 18, 1979
Cosponsored on March 8, 1979, by:
 Mr. WAXMAN, Mr. OTTINGER, Mr. WALGREN, Mr. GRAMM, Mr.
 YATES, Mr. ANDREWS (ND), Mr. LONG (MD), MR. MCDADE,
 Mr. DUNCAN (TN), Mr. WOLFF, Mr. MONTGOMERY, Mr. ANDERSON
 (CA), Mr. GINN, Mrs. HOLT, Mr. JOHNSON (CO), Mr. TRAXLER, Mr.
 AMBRO, Mr. BEARD (RI), Mr. BEDELL, Mr. D'AMOURS, Mr. JEF-
 FORDS, Mr. OBERSTAR, Mr. RICHMOND, Mr. FOWLER, Mr. LEACH,
 (IA), Mr. YOUNG (MO), Mr. WEISS, Mr. GREEN, Mr. LEACH, (LA),
 Mr. TAUKE; and
H.R. 1820, introduced by Mr. SATTERFIELD on February 1, 1979;
H.R. 2489, introduced by Mrs. HECKLER on February 28, 1979,
are identical as follows:]

96TH CONGRESS
1ST SESSION **H.R. 1143**

To amend title VIII of the Public Health Service Act to extend for two fiscal
years the program of assistance for nurse training.

IN THE HOUSE OF REPRESENTATIVES

JANUARY 18, 1979

Mr. STAGGERS introduced the following bill; which was referred to the Committee
on Interstate and Foreign Commerce

A BILL

To amend title VIII of the Public Health Service Act to extend
for two fiscal years the program of assistance for nurse
training.

1   *Be it enacted by the Senate and House of Representa-*

2   *tives of the United States of America in Congress assembled,*

3   TITLE I—NURSE TRAINING

4   SECTION 101. (a) This Act may be cited as the "Nurse

5   Training Amendments of 1979".

6   (b) Whenever in this Act (other than section 204) an

7   amendment or repeal is expressed in terms of an amendment

8   to, or repeal of, a section or other provision, the reference

Figure 8–4. Title page of a House bill. (Courtesy of U.S. House of Representatives)

and then go to the Office of Legislative Counsel in the Senate or the House for help in drafting it and putting it into legislative language. Interest groups are another fertile source of legislation. Many such organizations not only provide detailed technical knowledge in specialized fields, but also employ experts in the art of drafting bills. Constituents, either as individuals or groups, also may propose legislation. Frequently a member of Congress will introduce such a bill "by request" whether or not he supports its purposes.

Today the bulk of legislation considered by Congress originates in the executive branch. Each year the President outlines his legislative program in his State of the Union address and in budget and special messages. Executive departments, such as the Department of Health and Human Services, develop and transmit drafts of proposed legislation to Congress through the president to carry out the President's program. These bills usually are sent to the Speaker or Senate Majority Leader, referred to com-

---

96TH CONGRESS
1ST SESSION **S. 230**

To amend title VIII of the Public Health Service Act to extend through fiscal
year 1980 the program of assistance for nurse training, and for other purposes.

IN THE SENATE OF THE UNITED STATES

JANUARY 25 (legislative day, JANUARY 15), 1979

Mr. JAVITS (for himself, Mr. KENNEDY, Mr. WILLIAMS, Mr. RANDOLPH, Mr.
EAGLETON, Mr. CRANSTON, Mr. RIEGLE, Mr. SCHWEIKER, Mr. STAFFORD,
Mr. LEVIN, and Mr. DOLE) introduced the following bill; which was read
twice and referred to the Committee on Human Resources

A BILL

To amend title VIII of the Public Health Service Act to extend
through fiscal year 1980 the program of assistance for nurse
training, and for other purposes.

1   *Be it enacted by the Senate and House of Representa-*

2 *tives of the United States of America in Congress assembled,*

3   TITLE I—NURSE TRAINING

4   SEC. 101. (a) This Act may be cited as the "Nurse

5 Training Amendments of 1979".

6   (b) Whenever in this Act (other than section 204) an

7 amendment or repeal is expressed in terms of an amendment

II—E●

---

*Figure 8–5. The Senate bill extending the Nurse Training Act, which was eventually passed
by both houses of Congress and signed into law. (Courtesy of U.S. Senate)*

---

mittee, and then introduced by the chairperson of the committee or subcommittee having jurisdiction over the subject involved, or by the ranking
minority member, if the chairperson is not of the President's party. For
example, the following letter (which outlines the bill's provisions and argues for congressional support) was sent with the President's 1979 bill to
extend the Nurse Training Act at a severely reduced level:[1]

March 14, 1979

The Honorable Thomas P. O'Neill
Speaker of the House of Representatives
Washington, D.C. 20515

Dear Mr. Speaker:

Enclosed for consideration by the Congress is a draft bill "To amend and extend
provisions of law concerned with nurse training, and for other purposes."

    The draft bill supports a targeted approach to Federal assistance for nurse
training for fiscal year 1980. The Administration's health professions education

assistance proposal, to be submitted within a few months, will address the training of all health professionals, including nurses, in relation to a national health strategy for the medically underserved. Since 1956, Federal nurse training assistance programs have provided $1.5 billion in student and institutional support to stimulate growth in the supply of nurses. The Federal government's efforts have proven very successful:

- Since 1964, graduations from nursing programs have more than doubled.
- The overall supply of nurses is more than ample to meet the nation's current nursing needs.
- The outlook for an adequate overall supply of nurses over the next two decades is good, even if Federal support is substantially reduced.

The enclosed draft bill recognizes that there is no longer a need to accelerate growth in the overall supply of nurses. Rather, future Federal assistance should be targeted to assist in the training of nurse practitioners and to address certain other specific problems.

The Administration's bill would authorize appropriations of $13 million for fiscal year 1980 for the training of nurse practitioners, who are in short supply and have proven to be a cost-effective means for increasing the availability of primary care services, especially in medically underserved areas.

The draft bill would also authorize appropriations of $1,743,000 for fiscal year 1980 for nurse training special projects, including projects to improve the geographic distribution of nurses, to increase the representation of individuals with disadvantaged backgrounds in the nursing profession, to develop innovative nursing techniques emphasizing primary care and prevention, to enhance clinical skills, to provide continuing education opportunities, and to provide advanced nurse training.

In addition, the Administration's bill would expand student assistance opportunities for nursing students. The bill would eliminate the 10% limit on National Health Service Corps (NHSC) scholarship support available to health care practitioners other than physicians and dentists, would broaden the Health Education Assistance Loan (HEAL) authority to include nurses in graduate programs, and would repeal a restriction on the eligibility of nursing students for National Direct Student Loans. These proposed changes, along with the current general student assistance programs, including Basic and Supplemental Educational Opportunity Grants, would assure nursing students access to financial aid on the same basis as all other undergraduate or graduate health professions students.

We urge the Congress to give the draft bill its prompt and favorable consideration.

The Office of Management and Budget advices that enactment of the draft bill would be in accord with the President's program.

> Sincerely,
> Joseph A. Califano, Jr.
> Secretary

No matter how a legislative proposal originates, it can be introduced only by a member of Congress. In the House a member may introduce any one of several types of bills and resolutions by handing the measure to the clerk of the House or by placing it in a box called the hopper; he or she need not seek recognition for the purpose. A senator wishing to announce the introduction of a bill must first gain recognition of the presiding officer. If objection is offered by any senator, introduction of the bill is postponed until the following day. If there is no objection, the bill is read twice by title and referred to the appropriate committee. A House bill is considered read

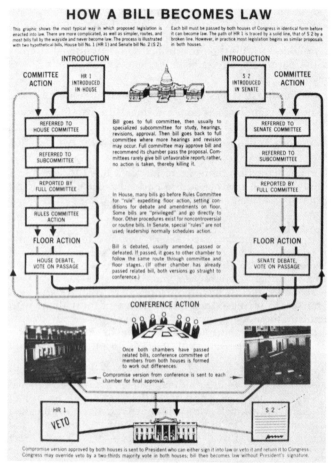

HOW A BILL BECOMES LAW

This graphic shows the most typical way in which proposed legislation is enacted into law. There are more complicated, as well as simpler, routes, and most bills fall by the wayside and never become law. The process is illustrated with two hypothetical bills, House bill No. 1 (HR 1) and Senate bill No. 2 (S 2).

Each bill must be passed by both houses of Congress in identical form before it can become law. The path of HR 1 is traced by a solid line, that of S 2 by a broken line. However, in practice most legislation begins as similar proposals in both houses.

INTRODUCTION

COMMITTEE ACTION   HR 1 INTRODUCED IN HOUSE

S 2 INTRODUCED IN SENATE   **COMMITTEE ACTION**

REFERRED TO HOUSE COMMITTEE

REFERRED TO SUBCOMMITTEE

REPORTED BY FULL COMMITTEE

RULES COMMITTEE ACTION

Bill goes to full committee, then usually to specialized subcommittee for study, hearings, revisions, approval. Then bill goes back to full committee where more hearings and revision may occur. Full committee may approve bill and recommend its chamber pass the proposal. Committees rarely give bill unfavorable report; rather, no action is taken, thereby killing it.

In House, many bills go before Rules Committee for "rule" expediting floor action, setting conditions for debate and amendments on floor. Some bills are "privileged" and go directly to floor. Other procedures exist for noncontroversial or routine bills. In Senate, special "rules" are not used; leadership normally schedules action.

REFERRED TO SENATE COMMITTEE

REFERRED TO SUBCOMMITTEE

REPORTED BY FULL COMMITTEE

FLOOR ACTION

HOUSE DEBATE, VOTE ON PASSAGE

Bill is debated, usually amended, passed or defeated. If passed, it goes to other chamber to follow the same route through committee and floor stages.. (If other chamber has already passed related bill, both versions go straight to conference.)

FLOOR ACTION

SENATE DEBATE, VOTE ON PASSAGE

CONFERENCE ACTION

Once both chambers have passed related bills, conference committee of members from both houses is formed to work out differences.

Compromise version from conference is sent to each chamber for final approval.

HR 1 VETO

S 2

Compromise version approved by both houses is sent to President who can either sign it into law or veto it and return it to Congress. Congress may override veto by a two-thirds majority vote in both houses; bill then becomes law without President's signature.

Figure 8–6. How a bill becomes law. (Courtesy of Congressional Quarterly Inc., Washington, D.C.)

for the first time when it is referred to committee. As the next step, in the House and the Senate, the bill is numbered (in order of introduction), referred to committee, labeled with the sponsor's name, and sent to the Government Printing Office so that it can be printed to facilitate subsequent study and possible action.

There is no limit to the number of bills a member may introduce. Senate bills may be jointly sponsored and carry several senators' names. The House permits multiple sponsorships of bills, with a limit of twenty-five cosponsors on any one bill. The Constitution stipulates that all bills for raising revenue shall originate in the House of Representatives and this stipulation has generally been interpreted to include appropriation bills. All other bills may originate in either chamber; major legislation usually is introduced in both houses in the form of companion bills.

Measures considered and acted upon by the House and the Senate include not only bills but also a variety of resolutions. *Bills* are prefixed with

HR when introduced in the House and with *S* when introduced in the Senate, followed by a number assigned in the order of introduction from the time that particular Congress began. Bills are used as the form for most legislation, whether general or special, public or private. When passed by both chambers in identical form and signed by the President (or passed again overriding his veto), they become public or private laws. *Joint resolutions* are designated *HJ Res* or *SJ Res*. A joint resolution requires the approval of both houses and the signature of the President, just as a bill does, and has the force of law if approved. There is no real difference between a bill and a joint resolution. The latter is generally used in dealing with limited matters, such as a single appropriation for a specific purpose. Joint resolutions are used also to propose amendments to the Constitution when ratified by three-fourths of the states.

Each bill introduced must pass the House and the Senate in identical form within the two-year term in order to become law. In fact, because Congress normally adjourns prior to the end of the term, bills usually have less than two years to become law. Bills that have not completed the required procedural journey prior to final adjournment of a Congress automatically die and must be reintroduced in the new Congress. Inaction or postponement at any stage of the process can ultimately mean the defeat of a bill. Many ideas require years or even decades of germination before they are enacted into law. Controversial proposals—reintroduced in successive congresses—may need a four-, six-, or eight-year period before enactment. Many of the 1960s policies of Presidents Kennedy and Johnson, for example, were first considered during the Congresses of the 1950s.

COMMITTEE REFERRAL

Nearly all bills are referred to committees. Although 20,000 to 30,000 pieces of legislation were introduced in each Congress over the past decade, and about 2,500 were reported from committees, only a few hundred became law. The number of bills that made it through the full process and were signed into law during the past six Congresses is as follows:

Congress	Year	Public Laws
91st	1969	190
91st	1970	505
92nd	1971	224
92nd	1972	483
93rd	1973	247
93rd	1974	402
94th	1975	205
94th	1976	283
95th	1977	223
95th	1978	410
96th	1979	187
96th	1980	426

S. 1750   June 23, 1977.

Mr. Kennedy (for himself and others)

To amend the Public Health Service Act and the Federal Food,
    Drug, and Cosmetic Act, as amended, to conduct studies con-
    cerning toxic and carcinogenic substances in foods, to conduct
    studies concerning saccharin, its impurities and toxicity and the
    health benefits, if any, resulting from the use of nonnutritive
    sweeteners including saccharin; to ban the Secretary of Health,
    Education, and Welfare from taking action with regard to
    saccharin for eighteen months, and to add additional provisions
    to section 403 of the Federal Food, Drug, and Cosmetic Act,
    as amended, concerning misbranded foods.
June 28, 1977. Reports requested from Department of Health,
    Education, and Welfare, General Accounting Office, and Of-
    fice of Management and Budget.
June 29, 1977. By unanimous consent it was requested that if
    and when the bill S. 1750 is reported by the Committee on
    Human Resources that it be subsequently referred to the Com-
    mittee on Commerce, Science, and Transportation for con-
    sideration on matters under its jurisdiction, until July 27, 1977.
June 29, 1977. Considered in open executive session by Subcom-
    mittee on Health and Scientific Research and ordered reported
    to full committee.
July 13, 1977. Considered in open executive session by full com-
    mittee and ordered reported to Senate, amended.
July 19, 1977. Reported to Senate by Mr. Kennedy (S. REPT.
    95-353).
July 22, 1977. Referred to Committee on Commerce, Science,
    and Transportation.
(July 26, 1977. Considered in open executive session by Commit-
    tee on Commerce, Science, and Transportation and ordered
    favorably reported to Senate, amended.)
(July 27, 1977. Reported to Senate by Mr. Hollings from the
    Committee on Commerce, Science, and Transportation (S.
    REPT. 95-369).)
Sept. 7, 1977. Amdt. No. 834 by Mr. Cannon (for himself,
    Messrs. Cranston, Domenici, Goldwater, Hayakawa, Stevens,
    Stone, Thurmond, Tower, Wallops, and Zorinsky).
Sept. 14, 1977. Amdt. No. 855 by Mr. Cranston.
Sept. 15, 1977. PASSED BY SENATE, 87 yeas; 7 nays.
Sept. 16, 1977. Referred to House Committee on Interstate and
    Foreign Commerce.
Oct. 17, 1977. House Committee on Interstate and Foreign Com-
    merce discharged from further consideration.
Oct. 17, 1977. PASSED BY HOUSE with an amendment in the
    nature of a substitute and a title amendment (text of H.R.
    8518, H. REPT. 95-658), as passed by House, 375 yeas; 23
    nays.
Oct. 25, 1977. Senate requested conference and appointed con-
    ferees (see Conference and Conferees).
Oct. 27, 1977. House agrees to conference and appointed con-
    ferees (see Conference and Conferees).
Nov. 2, 1977. Conferees met in executive session and agreed to
    file conference report.
Nov. 3, 1977. Conference report filed in House by Mr. Staggers
    (H. REPT. 95-810).
Nov. 3, 1977. Conference report AGREED TO BY HOUSE.
Nov. 4, 1977. Conference report AGREED TO BY SENATE.
Nov. 23, 1977. APPROVED. PUBLIC LAW 95-203.
(See H.R. 8518.)

*Figure 8–7. This history of a controversial Senate bill as recorded on the official calendar
shows its long and laborious journey to passage. (Courtesy of U.S. Senate)*

Committees are the primary graveyard for most bills that die in Congress. Stated positively, committees select from the vast number of bills
introduced, those that merit further consideration. A bill is referred to the
appropriate committee by the House parliamentarian on the Speaker's order
or by the Senate president, subject to the will of the chamber. In the Senate,
the sponsor of a bill may indicate a committee preference for referral, but
this is not binding. Generally, custom and rule govern the referral of legislation to committee; the jurisdiction of the standing committees is spelled out
in House Rule 10 and Senate Rule 25. The standing and temporary committees of the 97th Congress are given in Table 8–4. Nearly all of them, at some
time, consider legislation that is related directly or indirectly to nurses and
nursing.

The standing committees are the keystone of the legislative process,
because they have the power to review legislative proposals and report bills

Table 8–4.   *Committees and Number of Seats in the 97th Congress (1981–1982)*

HOUSE	SENATE
Agriculture (43)	Agriculture, Nutrition, and Forestry (17)
Appropriations (55)	Appropriations (29)
Armed Services (45)	Armed Services (17)
Banking, Finance, and Urban Affairs (45)	Banking, Housing, and Urban Affairs (15)
Budget (30)	Budget (22)
District of Columbia (15)	Commerce, Science, and Transportation (17)
Education and Labor (34)	Energy and Natural Resources (20)
Energy and Commerce (42)	Environment and Public Works (16)
Foreign Affairs (37)	Finance (20)
Government Operations (40)	Foreign Relations (17)
House Administration (19)	Governmental Affairs (17)
Interior and Insular Affairs (42)	Judiciary (18)
Judiciary (28)	Labor and Human Resources (16)
Merchant Marine and Fisheries (36)	Rules and Administration (12)
Post Office and Civil Service (27)	Veterans' Affairs (12)
Public Works and Transportation (46)	Select Committees*
Rules (16)	Aging (15)
Science and Technology (40)	Ethics (6)
Small Business (40)	Indian Affairs (7)
Standards of Official Conduct (12)	Intelligence (15)
Veterans' Affairs (31)	Small Business (17)
Ways and Means (35)	
Select Committees*	
Aging (52)	
Intelligence (14)	
Narcotics Abuse and Control (29)	

* Temporary committees

to the floor. Under the Legislative Reorganization Act of 1946, Senate and House committees were organized along similar but not precisely parallel lines. The committees were in general regrouped to follow the major organizational divisions of the federal government. Responsibility for overseeing the executive branch is now divided roughly as follows: the Appropriations Committee is to review requests for spending authority; the Government Operations Committee oversees administration of appropriations and the quality of administration in general; and legislative committees design and oversee policy in their respective fields. The size of the standing commit-

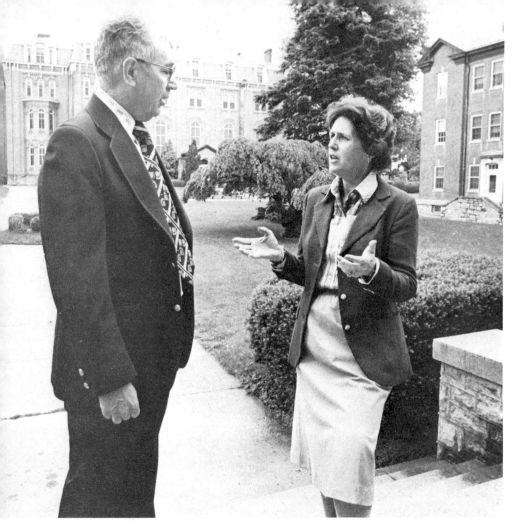

Figure 8–8. Explaining the nation's defense posture, Representative Beverly B. Byron of Maryland is one of three women on the House Armed Services Committee. (Courtesy of Representative Beverly B. Byron)

tees is fixed by the rules of their parent chamber: in the 97th Congress, House committees range in size from 12 (Standards of Official Conduct) to 55 (Appropriations), and Senate committees from 12 (both the Rules and Administration and the Veterans' Affairs Committees) to 29 (Appropriations). Traditionally party ratios on the committees have corresponded roughly to the party ratio in the full chamber, which in 1981 was 56% Democrat to 44% Republican in the House and 53% Republican to 47% Democrat in the Senate.

From the 19th century up to the early 1970s almost absolute power was vested, through the seniority system, in representatives and senators who had served longest on a particular committee and thus managed to become committee chairpersons. Their power, exercised primarily through the committee system, rarely was challenged successfully. The changes wrought in the 1970s overturned these traditional power preserves. By the beginning of the 94th Congress, in January 1975, after three sitting committee chairmen in the House had been ousted from their positions by the Democratic (majority party) caucus, the rigid seniority system was partially broken as the primary method by which members rose to power. The system still functions as a useful device for ordering the hierarchy on committees, but it no longer enables members to automatically attain committee chairpersonships by remaining on the committee longer than anyone else, to retain the chairpersonships without fear of challenge or removal, and to exercise a dominant power in the legislative process. In the House in particular, mechanisms have been established by which committee work is spread more evenly among a much larger number of subcommittee chairpersons as well as rank-and-file members, and committees now operate under written and continuing procedures that cannot be undercut by chairpersons.

Most of the legislative decisions of Congress actually are made in committee. Modern lawmaking requires an understanding of many complex subjects, and the committee system provides the means by which members can attain a high degree of specialization in different areas. A committee that has subjected a bill to expert scrutiny expects its decisions to be upheld on the floor. Traditionally, new members of Congress have had to serve an apprenticeship on minor committees before being appointed to major committees. Less desirable committees in the House include those pertaining to the Post Office and Civil Service, to Public Works and Transportation, and to Science and Technology. Much sought after assignments are the slots on the Rules Committee, Appropriations Committee, and Ways and Means Committee. Once on a congenial committee, a member of congress usually re-

Figure 8–9. Most of the legislative decisions of Congress are made in committee. Here Rosalie Abrams, RN, of the Maryland State Senate testifies before a U.S. Senate committee. (Courtesy of Ankers Capitol Photographers, Washington , DC)

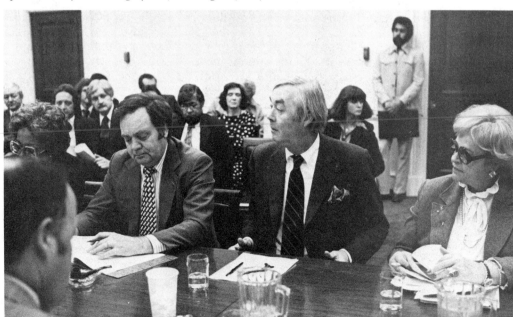

mains there, ideally working his way up by longevity to the position of chairperson or ranking minority member. He may have an opportunity to transfer from one committee to another, but he would have to start again at the bottom of the seniority ladder. Or, if a very junior member, he or she may be bumped from a much valued committee as a result of party realignments following an election.

House members have the opportunity to become highly skilled legislative technicians because they are not ordinarily permitted to serve on more than a single major committee and a single minor committee. This allows them to develop a greater degree of expertise than senators, who often serve on two or three major committees and two or more minor committees as well. As House members see it, this senatorial spread makes a member of the upper house a jack-of-all-trades and a master of none. The superior expertise of House members is especially evident in one of the most important aspects of Congress's work, the appropriations process. In the House, a member of the Appropriations Committee almost never sits on a second committee, devoting himself or herself almost exclusively to budgetary matters; he or she may eventually become a genuine expert, particularly in the subjects with which the subcommittee deals.

A committee has several options with respect to a piece of legislation: it may consider and report it favorably, with or without amendments, rewrite it entirely, reject it or report it unfavorably, or simply refuse to consider it. Failure of a committee to act on a bill usually is equivalent to killing it; the measure can be withdrawn from the group's preview only by a discharge petition signed by a majority of the House membership on House bills, or by adoption of a special resolution in the Senate. Discharge attempts rarely succeed.

Bills supported by influential members of Congress stand a good chance of receiving attention in committee. Bills taking up the largest percentage of committee time tend to be those prepared and drafted by the executive branch or by major pressure groups. They are most often introduced by committee chairpersons or other influential members of Congress and are supported by the majority party leadership. They also deal with issues in which a significant segment of the public and the membership of Congress believe that some sort of legislation is required. Bills with these characteristics do not necessarily become law, but they are the major bills before Congress each year and as such are repeatedly brought up at presidential news conferences and covered in the broadcast and print media. Such attention-getting bills account for perhaps only a hundred or so of the more than 20,000 introduced during each two-year Congress.

When a committee decides to take up a major bill, its normal procedure is as follows: While the bill may be considered by the full committee, normally the committee chairperson assigns the bill to a subcommittee for possible study and hearings. Many subcommittees themselves have become relatively autonomous policy-making bodies. It is these miniature legislatures, because of their concern with a narrow area of legislation, that have now acquired the reputation for expertise on the areas under their jurisdiction. There is a tendency to defer to their knowledge and convictions on bills to which they have devoted detailed scrutiny. This tendency is considerably reinforced by the well-understood principle of reciprocity in Congress. Members of one subcommittee expect the members of other subcommittees to respect their judgment. As a result, the full committee, which is made up of the members who also sit on other subcommittees of that particular committee exercise minimal influence on the legislation produced by its other subunits. Because members of a given committee usually sit on two or three or even more subcommittees, this simply reinforces their tendency to defer to the judgment of the subcommittees. The number of House subcommittees increased from 119 to 148 between 1971 and 1981. In the Senate, the number of subcommittees actually decreased from 121 to 90 as the result of the merger or abandonment of weaker subcommittees.

In the House, most legislation pertaining to nursing and other health issues passes through the Subcommittee on Health and the Environment of the House Committee on Energy and Commerce, chaired by Representative Henry Waxman (Democrat, California). This subcommittee has jurisdiction over the subjects of public health and quarantine, hospital construction, mental health, health professions training and research, health promotion, Medicaid and national health insurance (jointly with the Ways and Means Committee), foods and drugs, drug abuse, and environmental protection. In 1981 the membership on this subcommittee was as follows:

HENRY A. WAXMAN (CALIF.), CHAIRMAN

Democrats	Republicans
James Scheuer (N.Y.)	Edward Madigan (Ill.)*
Thomas Luken (Oh.)	Clarence (Bud) Brown (Oh.)
Doug Walgren (Pa.)	William Dannemeyer (Calif.)
Barbara Mikulski (Md.)	Robert Whittaker (Kan.)
Ron Wyden (Ore.)	Donald Ritter (Pa.)
James Florio (N.J.)	Cleve Benedict (W.Va.)
Anthony (Toby) Moffett (Conn.)	Thomas Bliley (Va.)
Richard Shelby (Ala.)	James Broyhill (N.C.), ex officio
Phil Gramm (Tex.)	
Mickey Leland (Tex.)	
John Dingell (Mich.), ex officio	

The counterpart to the above House subcommittee in the Senate is the Labor and Human Resources Committee, chaired by Senator Orrin G. Hatch (Republican, Utah). In 1981, Chairman Hatch organized the Senate Labor and Human Resources Committee, and he disbanded its health subcommittee. His action was certain to slow down the full committee that would handle both the preliminary look at health legislation (normally handled by the health subcommittee) as well as go through the full committee process of bill markup. Senator Hatch reportedly feared that ranking minor-

* Ranking minority member.

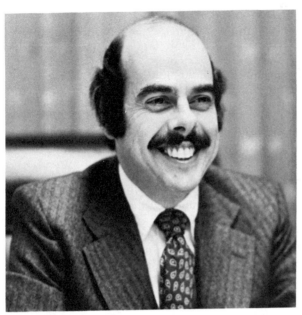

Figure 8–10. Representative Henry A. Waxman, chairman of the House Subcommittee on Health. (Courtesy of Henry A. Waxman)

ity member Senator Edward M. Kennedy would overpower the proposed health subcommittee chairman, Senator Gordon J. Humphrey (Republican, New Hampshire). The composition of this full committee in 1981 was as follows:

ORRIN G. HATCH (UTAH) CHAIRMAN

Republicans	Democrats
Robert T. Stafford (Vt.)	Edward Kennedy (Mass.)*
Lowell P. Weicker (Conn.)	Harrison A. Williams (N.J.)
Gordon J. Humphrey (N.H.)	Jennings Randolph (W.Va.)
J. Danforth Quayle (Ind.)	Claiborne Pell (R.I.)
Paula Hawkins (Fla.)	Thomas Eagleton (Mo.)
Don Nickles (Okla.)	Donald Riegle (Mich.)
John East (N.C.)	Howard Metzenbaum (Oh.)
Jeremiah Denton (Ala.)	

Bills relating to programs that provide payment (from any source) for health care or health delivery systems and all bills relating to the health care programs of the Social Security Act in the House of Representatives fall into the jurisdiction of the Subcommittee on Health of the Ways and Means

* Ranking minority member.

Committee, chaired by Representative Andrew Jacobs, Jr. (Democrat, Indiana). The 1981 membership of this body included:

ANDREW JACOBS, JR. (IND.), CHAIRMAN

Democrats	*Republicans*
Charles Rangel (N.Y.)	Willis Gradison, Jr. (Oh.)*
Harold Ford (Tenn.)	John Duncan (Tenn.)
Cecil Heftel (Hawaii)	Philip Crane (Ill.)
Ken Holland (S.C.)	

* Ranking minority member.

Figure 8–11. Senator Edward M. Kennedy, Ranking Minority Member, Labor and Human Resources Committee. (Courtesy of U.S. Senate)

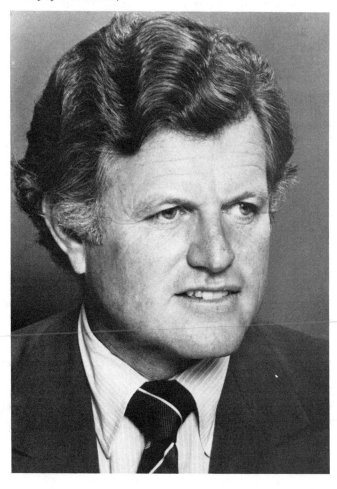

In the Senate, bills dealing with health programs under the Social Security Act and health programs financed by a specific tax or trust fund pass through the Subcommittee on Health of the Senate Finance Committee, chaired by Senator David Durenberger (Republican, Minnesota). The composition of this group in 1981 was as follows:

DAVID DURENBERGER (MINN.), CHAIRMAN

Republicans	*Democrats*
Bob Packwood (Ore.)	Russell Long (La.)*
John Heinz (Pa.)	Max Baucus (Mont.)
Robert Dole (Kan.)	Bill Bradley (N.J.)

The ranking minority member is the most influential member of the minority party on these Senate and House health subcommittees, and his or her powers include appointment of minority members to subcommittees and control of minority funds and staff. Generally, through seniority, the ranking minority member may easily become committee chairperson when there is a shift in party control of a chamber.

PUBLIC HEARINGS

During legislation, the key stages in committee consideration of a bill are hearings, the markup, voting, and the report. This process is controlled largely by subcommittee and committee chairmen who have many resources at their disposal to expedite, delay, or modify legislation. Chairmen choose tactics on the basis of their assessment of the many political and legislative factors in play and their long-range objectives for the bill. The sources of the chairperson's authority are many; a brief listing includes control of the subcommittee's legislative agenda, management of subcommittee funds, and control of the subcommittee staff. The chairman usually has long service on the subcommittee and is likely to be better informed than most other members on issues coming before the subcommittee. Chairmen can use these and other resources to delay, expedite, or modify legislation.

A chairman who opposes a bill can simply refuse to schedule hearings on it until it is too late for final congressional action on the bill. The same result can be achieved by allowing the hearing to drag on throughout the session. A chairman having strong negative feelings about a bill can also instruct the subcommittee staff to *stack* the witnesses testifying on it, that is, asking witnesses holding opposing views to submit statements only rather than appear in person. Subcommittee members who will raise dilatory questions or employ obstructive tactics can be recognized before others (who are for the bill), and, through control of subcommittee funds and the power to hire and fire most committee staffers, the chairperson can effectively block action on a bill by directing the staff to disregard it. On the other hand, a chairman who favors a bill can give it top priority by mobilizing staff

---

* Ranking minority member.

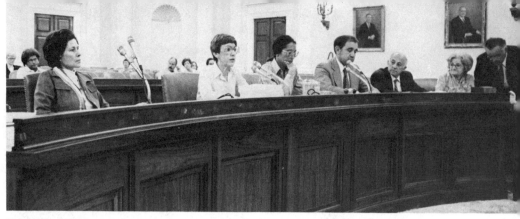

Figure 8–12. Jane Brennan, executive director of the VNA of Memphis, testifying on Medicare–Medicaid Amendments. (Courtesy of National League for Nursing)

resources, compressing the time for hearings and markups, and, in general, encouraging expeditious action by subcommittee members.

The subcommittee usually schedules public hearings on the bill, inviting testimony from interested public and private witnesses. Other witnesses may testify at their own request. For example, the Subcommittee on Health of the Senate Finance Committee invited testimony for the June 25, 1979, hearing on S 1204, A Bill to Strengthen and Improve Medical Services to Low-Income Children and Pregnant Women, with the following press release:[2]

The Honorable Herman E. Talmadge (D., Ga.), Chairman of the Subcommittee on Health of the Committee on Finance, announced today that the Subcommittee will hold a hearing on Monday afternoon, June 25, 1979, on a proposal to expand health assistance for low-income children.

The hearing will begin at 2:00 P.M., Monday, June 25, 1979, in Room 2221 Dirksen Senate Office Building.

Senator Talmadge said, 'There are a variety of Federal programs which currently provide some type of health care services to mothers and children. However, population groups targeted for assistance by these programs often overlap, resulting in confusion and duplication. Moreover, many eligible persons are left without services.

'One of the major Federal programs providing child health services is Medicaid's Early and Periodic Screening, Diagnosis and Treatment (EPSDT) program. Although this program is intended to serve all children under age 21 who are eligible for Medicaid, only about 2 million of the 11 million eligible children are being reached.'

Pending before the Committee is S 1204, the administration's Child Health Care Assessment Program (CHAP). CHAP would replace the current EPSDT program with an expanded program of medical services to a greater proportion of low-income children and pregnant women.

Requests to testify. Senator Talmadge stated that witnesses desiring to testify during this hearing must make their requests to testify to Michael Stern, Staff Director, Committee on Finance, Room 2227 Dirksen Senate Office Building, Washington, D.C. 20510 not later than Monday, June 18, 1979.

Senator Talmadge said that because a large number of requests to testify are anticipated, the Committee will not be able to schedule all those who request to testify. Those persons who are not scheduled to appear in person to present oral testimony are invited to submit written statements. He emphasized that the views

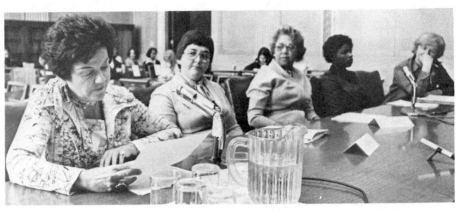

Figure 8–13. A panel group including NLN's Margaret Walsh (on left) and ANA's Constance Holloran (far right) presents testimony before the Senate on the Nurse Training Act. (Courtesy of National League for Nursing)

presented in such written statements will be as carefully considered by the Committee as if they were presented orally.

All parties who are scheduled to testify orally are urged to comply with the guidelines below:

Notification of witnesses. Parties who have submitted written requests to testify will be notified as soon as possible as to the time they are scheduled to appear. Once the witness has been advised of the time of his appearance, rescheduling will not be permitted. If a witness is unable to testify at the time he is scheduled to appear, he may file a written statement for the record of the hearing.

Consolidated testimony. The Chairman also stated that the Committee urges all witnesses who have a common position or with the same general interest to consolidate their testimony and designate a single spokesman to present their common viewpoint orally to the Committee. This procedure will enable the Committee to receive a wider expression of views on the total bill than it might otherwise obtain.

Panel groups. Groups with similar viewpoints but who cannot designate a single spokesman will be encouraged to form panels. Each panelist will be required to restrict his or her comments to no longer than a six-minute summation of the principle points of the written statements. The panelists are urged to avoid repetition whenever possible in their presentations.

Legislative Reorganization Act. The Chairman observed that the Legislative Reorganization Act of 1946, as amended, requires all witnesses appearing before the Committees of Congress to file in advance written statements of their proposed testimony, and to limit their oral presentations to brief summaries of their argument.

Senator Talmadge stated that in light of this statute and in view of the large number of witnesses who desire to appear before the Committee in the limited time available for the hearing, all witnesses must comply with the following rules:

(1) All statements must be filed with the Committee at least one day in advance of the day on which the witness is scheduled to appear. If a witness is scheduled to testify on a Monday or Tuesday, he must file his written statement with the Committee by the Friday preceding his appearance.

(2) All witnesses must include with their written statements a summary of the principal points included in the statements.

(3) The written statements must be typed on lettersize paper (not legal size) and at least 100 copies must be submitted to the Committee.

(4) Witnesses are not to read their written statements to the Committee, but are to confine their six-minute oral presentations to a summary of the points included in the statement.

(5) Not more than six minutes will be allowed for the oral summary. Witnesses who fail to comply with these rules will forfeit their privilege to testify.

Written statements. Witnesses who are not scheduled for oral presentation, and others who desire to present a statement to the Committee, are urged to prepare a written position of their views for submission and inclusion in the record of the hearings. Statements submitted for inclusion in the record should be typewritten, not more than 25 double-spaced pages in length and mailed with five (5) copies by July 9, 1979, to Michael Stern, Staff Director, Committee on Finance, Room 2227 Dirksen Senate Office Building, Washington, D.C. 20510.

Most witnesses offer lengthy prepared statements for the hearing record and then give a "boiled down" version orally. Once the testimony has been heard, each subcommittee member, usually in order of seniority, will ask the witness questions. House rules allot at least five minutes per member to question witnesses. Senate rules have no such provision. Instead, each subcommittee establishes its own rules governing internal procedures. The hearings may be brief and perfunctory, or they may go on for weeks. Because the demands on a member's time are so great, frequently only a few subcommittee members with a special interest in the subject will participate in the hearings. At the hearings on S 1204 the following witnesses testified and were questioned:[3]

- Schaeffer, Hon. Leonard D., Administrator, Health Care Financing Administration, Department of Health, Education, and Welfare, accompanied by Mary Tierney, Acting Director of Office of Child Welfare Programs
- AMA's Council on Legislation, William C. Felch, M.D., Chairman
- American Academy of Pediatrics, Birt Harvey, M.D.
- American Dental Association, William D. Allen, D.D.S., Chairman, Council on Legislation, accompanied by Hal Christiansen, Director, Washington office
- Blumenthal, Dan, M.D., W.T. Brooks Clinic, Department of Preventive Medicine and Community Health, Department of Pediatrics, Emory University School of Medicine
- Children's Defense Fund, Marian Wright Edelman, Director, accompanied by Wendy Lazarus, consultant on health issues, and Judith Weitz, program specialist in health
- Cole, Clifton A., Chief Deputy Director, Medical Care Services, Department of Health Services, State of California

NURSE TRAINING ACT AMENDMENTS OF 1979

HEARING
BEFORE THE
SUBCOMMITTEE ON
HEALTH AND THE ENVIRONMENT
OF THE
COMMITTEE ON
INTERSTATE AND FOREIGN COMMERCE
HOUSE OF REPRESENTATIVES
NINETY-SIXTH CONGRESS
FIRST SESSION
ON

H.R. 1143
(And All Identical Bills)
BILLS TO AMEND TITLE VIII OF THE PUBLIC HEALTH SERV-
ICE ACT TO EXTEND FOR 2 FISCAL YEARS THE PROGRAM
OF ASSISTANCE FOR NURSE TRAINING

H.R. 1337
A BILL TO AMEND TITLE VIII OF THE PUBLIC HEALTH SERV-
ICE ACT TO EXTEND FOR 2 FISCAL YEARS THE PROGRAM
OF ASSISTANCE FOR NURSE TRAINING

H.R. 1651
A BILL TO AMEND TITLE VIII OF THE PUBLIC HEALTH SERV-
ICE ACT TO EXTEND FOR 2 FISCAL YEARS THE PROGRAM
OF ASSISTANCE FOR NURSE TRAINING, AND FOR OTHER
PURPOSES

MARCH 22, 1979

Serial No. 96–6

Printed for the use of the
Committee on Interstate and Foreign Commerce

U.S. GOVERNMENT PRINTING OFFICE
45-406 O   WASHINGTON : 1979

Figure 8–14. Title page of the hearing record of House Health Subcommittee on the Nurse Training Act Amendments of 1979. (Courtesy of U.S. House of Representatives)

- Developmental Disabilities/Mental Health CHAP Coalition, Nancy Stone and Nancy Porter-Morrill
- Jollie, James E., Director, Recipient Management, Department of Social Services, State of South Carolina
- National Association of Community Health Centers, Inc., James T. Speight, Executive Director, East of the River Health Association

Organizations that did not send witnesses but instead submitted a letter or comments on the bill to be inserted at the end of the printed proceedings of the hearings were the following:[4]

- American College of Obstetricians and Gynecologists
- American Dental Hygienists' Association
- American Hospital Association

LEGISLATIVE HEARING ON S. 544—HEALTH PLANNING AMENDMENTS OF 1979; S. 230—NURSE TRAINING AMENDMENTS OF 1979; AND S. 590—CLINICAL LABORATORY IMPROVEMENT ACT OF 1979

HEARING

BEFORE THE

SUBCOMMITTEE ON
HEALTH AND SCIENTIFIC RESEARCH

OF THE

COMMITTEE ON
LABOR AND HUMAN RESOURCES
UNITED STATES SENATE

NINETY-SIXTH CONGRESS

FIRST SESSION

ON

S. 544

TO AMEND TITLES XV AND XVI OF THE PUBLIC HEALTH
SERVICE ACT TO REVISE AND EXTEND THE AUTHORITIES
AND REQUIREMENTS UNDER THOSE TITLES FOR HEALTH
PLANNING AND HEALTH RESOURCES DEVELOPMENT

S. 230

TO AMEND TITLE VIII OF THE PUBLIC HEALTH SERVICE ACT
TO EXTEND THROUGH FISCAL YEAR 1980 THE PROGRAM OF
ASSISTANCE FOR NURSE TRAINING, AND FOR OTHER
PURPOSES

S. 590

TO AMEND THE PUBLIC HEALTH SERVICE ACT TO REVISE
AND STRENGTHEN THE PROGRAM UNDER THAT ACT FOR THE
REGULATION OF CLINICAL LABORATORIES

MARCH 16, 1979

Printed for the use of the Committee on Labor and Human Resources

U.S. GOVERNMENT PRINTING OFFICE
45-450 O   WASHINGTON : 1979

Figure 8–15. Similar testimony on the Nurse Training Act was collected by the Senate Health Subcommittee. (Courtesy of U.S. Senate)

- American Nurses' Association
- Axelrod, David, M.D., Commissioner, New York State Department of Health
- Bates, Jacquelyn D., Chairman, Child Advocacy Program, for the Association of Junior Leagues, Inc.
- Bonk, James, Vice President, DDPA Affairs, Delta Dental Plans Association
- Brown, Cameron G., Executive Director, Wisconsin Health Care Review, Inc.
- Clough, Donald P., Executive Director, American Social Health Association
- Child Welfare League of America

- Shorey, Clyde E., Jr., Vice President for Public Affairs, the National Foundation—March of Dimes
- Wattleton, Faye, President, Planned Parenthood Federation of America

Hearings, which are published and represent an important part of the legislative history of a bill, contain the oral testimony and written material submitted to committees of Congress in public sessions held for the purpose of hearing witnesses.

MARKING UP THE BILL

After the hearings have ended, the subcommittee meets to *mark up* the bill, that is, to consider line by line and section by section the specific language of the legislation needed for recommendation to the full committee. The House in 1973 and the Senate in 1975 decided to hold most of their markup sessions in public view. In the markup session subcommittee members redraft portions of the bill, attempt to insert new provisions and delete others, bargain over final language, and, in general, determine the final subcommittee product. Frequently the subcommittee proposes amendments to the bill. If they are substantial and the legislation is complicated, the subcommittee may order introduction of a *clean bill* embodying the proposed amendments. The original bill is then put aside, and the clean bill, with a new number, is reported to the full committee. If the amendments are not extensive, the original bill may be reported with amendments.

The subcommittee may thus approve the bill unaltered, amend it, or rewrite it—or block it altogether. The subcommittee then reports its recommendations to the full committee. When the full committee receives the bill, it may repeat the subcommittee's procedures, all or in part, or it may simply ratify the action of the subcommittee. Unless a bill is highly controversial, the three health subcommittees (along with the full Labor and Human Resources Committee in the Senate, which has no subcommittee) are the last places where the substance of most legislation can be strongly affected by outside groups such as nurses. The full committees generally endorse the views of the subcommittees.

REPORTING THE BILL

If the full committee decides to send the bill to the House or Senate, it justifies its actions in a written statement called a *report*, which must accompany the bill. Reports are designated *H Rept* or *S Rept*. The chairperson has the subcommittee staff prepare a report describing the purposes and scope of the bill. Committee reports accompanying bills are almost entirely staff products. Often the reports are the only reference concerning the legislative matter being considered. Staff aides consult with the chairperson or the majority members to decide what should be emphasized or de-emphasized in the report, including minority views. Then the staff writes a report, usually conforming to a standard format. Reports usually include three basic ingredients: (1) the main body, which explains the bill and gives background and interpretation; (2) the section-by-section analysis of the

Calendar No. 103

96TH CONGRESS	SENATE	REPORT
1st Session		No. 96–101

NURSE TRAINING AMENDMENTS OF 1979

APRIL 30 (legislative day APRIL 9), 1979.—Ordered to be printed

Mr. KENNEDY. from the Committee on Labor and Human Resources,
submitted the following

REPORT

[To accompany S. 230]

The Committee on Labor and Human Resources, to which was referred the bill (S. 230) to amend title VIII of the Public Health Service Act to extend through fiscal year 1980 the program of assistance for
nurse training, and for other purposes having considered the same,
reports favorably thereon with an amendment in the nature of a substitute and recommends that the bill as amended do pass.

CONTENTS

SUMMARY—S. 230

S. 230 is a 1-year extension (through fiscal year 1980) of existing
authorities under the Nurse Training Act (Title VII of the Public
Health Service Act). The purpose of the 1-year extension is twofold: First. it will permit the completion of a study (authorized in
the bill) designed to assess the country's needs with respect to the
nursing supply. Second, it will bring the review of the nursing train-

Figure 8–16. Report from the Senate Committee on Labor and Human Resources. (Courtesy of U.S. Senate)

provisions of the bill; and (3) a written comparison of the bill with existing
law. The report usually includes the views of the executive branch agencies
consulted. Committee members opposing the bill will often submit dissenting minority views. Any committee member may file minority, supplemental, or additional views, which are printed in the back section of the
committee report. A report always favors the passage of a bill; a committee
does not report its recommendations when it disapproves of a bill. Reports
are an important element in the legislative process because they provide an
explanation of a bill's intent.

Committee prints are committee documents requested by committees
that are compiled by their research staffs, outside consultants, or the Congressional Research Service. Committee Prints are authorized by a particular committee at the time of a hearing. They are used for background information and consideration of a bill and are often of a technical or research
nature. Also, they often contain summaries of staff findings, histories of

96TH CONGRESS ⎱ HOUSE OF REPRESENTATIVES ⎰   REPORT
  1st Session ⎰   ⎱ No. 96–183

NURSE TRAINING AMENDMENTS OF 1979

MAY 15, 1979.—Committed to the Committee of the Whole House on the State
of the Union and ordered to be printed

Mr. STAGGERS, from the Committee on Interstate and Foreign
Commerce, submitted the following

REPORT

together with

MINORITY VIEWS

[To accompany H.R. 3633]

[Including cost estimate of the Congressional Budget Office]

The Committee on Interstate and Foreign Commerce, to whom was
referred the bill (H.R. 3633) to amend title VIII of the Public Health
Service Act to extend for 1 fiscal year the program of assistance for
nurse training, and for other purposes, having considered the same,
report favorably thereon with amendments and recommend that the
bill as amended do pass.

The amendments (stated in terms of the page and line numbers of
the introduced bill) are as follows:

Page 8, line 7, strike out "the Secretary shall report" and insert in
lieu thereof "the Secretary and the entity conducting the study shall
each report".

Page 8, line 10, strike out "preliminary recommendations" and insert
in lieu thereof "their respective preliminary recommendations".

Page 8, insert before the period in line 16 the following: "and shall
include in that report the report submitted to the Secretary pursuant
to subsection (b)(3)".

Page 9, line 21, insert "(a)" after "202." and after line 2 on page 10
insert the following:

(b)(1) Such section 752(b)(5)(A) is further amended by
adding after the first sentence the following: "With respect
to an individual receiving a degree from a school of veterinary
medicine, optometry, podiatry, or pharmacy, the date referred to in paragraphs (1) through (4) shall be the date upon
which the individual completes the training required for such

(1)

*Figure 8–17. Report from the House Committee on Interstate and Foreign Commerce, now
called House Energy and Commerce Committee. (Courtesy of U.S. House of Representatives)*

previous legislation and congressional efforts, and the implications of a bill
if it were to be passed. Committee prints are often proposed for complex
and controversial legislation such as proposals for national health insurance.

Bills unanimously voted out of committee stand a good chance on the
floor. A sharply divided committee vote, combined with dissenting minority
views, usually forewarns of an equally sharp dispute on the floor. Reports
are directed primarily at members of the House and Senate and seek to
persuade the membership to endorse the committee decision when it comes
up for a vote on the floor. For many members, or their staff aides, the report is
the only document they read before deciding how to vote on an issue. The
report is thus the principal formal means of communicating a committee
decision to the entire chamber. Reports are numbered, by Congress and
chamber, in the order in which they are filed with the appropriate clerks of
the House and the Senate (H Rept 97-1, S Rept 97-1, and so forth). Both the

96th Congress } 1st Session }	COMMITTEE PRINT	{ CP 96–20

Comparison of Major Features
of Health Insurance Proposals

Prepared by the Staff of the

COMMITTEE ON FINANCE
UNITED STATES SENATE

RUSSELL B. LONG, *Chairman*

Prepared with the assistance of the Congressional
Research Service

JUNE 1979

Printed for the use of the Committee on Finance

U.S. GOVERNMENT PRINTING OFFICE
47-388   WASHINGTON : 1979

Figure 8–18. Committee staff gather pertinent information on pending legislation into special documents, which are published as committee prints. (Courtesy of U.S. Senate, Committee on Finance)

reported bill and its accompanying report are then assigned to the appropriate House and Senate calendars to await scheduling for floor action.

To assist in administrative details and other aspects of committee work, each standing committee in the House and the Senate is provided with legal counsel and other highly professional staff personnel. In recent years, committee staff personnel and resources have multiplied and played an increasingly important role in committee work. Staff influence on the legislative process has been a matter of growing concern. Although it is difficult to evaluate the extent of staff influence, committee staff experts undoubtedly play an important role in the legislative process. Committee staffs formulate legislative proposals for the consideration of their bosses, help to schedule and plan committee hearings, line up witnesses for and against a particular proposal, and otherwise influence the legislative process.

Staffers set up hearings on legislation and current issues. They select witnesses, prepare questions, inform the press, brief committee members, and occasionally substitute for members or chairpersons who cannot attend hearings. In many instances, if he cannot be present, a member prepares a list of questions for aides to ask witnesses. Much original research is conducted by staff members on issues that come before a committee. This usually involves looking into existing legislation, court decisions, and current practices. Committee staff sometimes travel to areas directly affected by the pending legislation to collect additional data and secure information from citizens. Although staff members occasionally may actually write bills and amendments, they usually serve as liaisons between the Office of Legislative Counsel, committee members, government agencies, and special interest groups during the drafting of measures. The top committee aides often will accompany a bill's sponsor in the House or Senate to assist him during the floor action.

The majority of congressional committees tend to have dual staffs, one professional and one clerical. These are generally headed by a *staff director* and a *chief clerk* respectively. Although the distinction between professional and clerical staff is blurred on many committees, the duties of each can be roughly separated. The *clerical staff* is responsible for keeping the committee calendar up to date, for processing committee publications, for referring bills to the appropriate departments for comment, for preparing the bill dockets, for maintaining the files, for stenographic work, and for opening and sorting mail. The *professional staff* is primarily responsible for policy matters handled by the committee. Its members fill the need for legal, public relations, statistical, accounting, investigative, and various technical services.

Notable for the nursing profession is the fact that during the 97th Congress a nurse, Sheila Burke, holds the key responsible slot of Chief of the health professional staff on the Senate Finance Committee and brings a nursing perspective to the majority (Republican) views on Medicare, Medicaid, maternal and child health, and national health insurance issues. Ms. Burke, a graduate of the University of San Francisco School of Nursing, comments on the importance of having nurses in these positions: "It is very clear that long before legislation becomes law, there are discussions which take place among a committee staff, such as the one that I am involved with, about the direction and content of legislation. These discussions are critical in terms of the long range planning for health care delivery. That's where the influence really can begin. While the role of special interest groups is very important in influencing this process, actually having a professional colleague as a staff person, someone who you can gain access to, is critical. This role in health care policy is not as far removed from the practice of nursing as one might think. Take, for example, the need for an emphasis on wellness. Unless health care policy addresses this need, wellness care cannot be delivered. Nurses need a role in all areas including policy, not just the actual delivery of care."[6] It is hoped that at least one nurse will have a staff position on all of the major subcommittees that authorize health legislation in the near future.

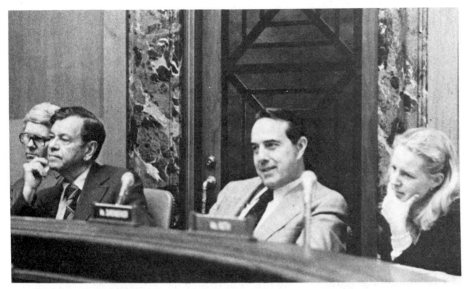

Figure 8–19. Sheila Burke, RN, chief of professional health staff of the Senate Finance Committee, seated along with Senators Robert Dole and Herman Talmadge at a committee hearing. (Courtesy of Sheila Burke)

HOUSE RULES COMMITTEE AND PARLIAMENTARY PROCEDURE

The relatively few bills that win a majority vote in committee (and generally in a subcommittee before that) usually have been subjected to grueling controversy and numerous amendments. In the House, most important legislation must then go from a standing committee to the Rules Committee, which determines if and when the bill will arrive on the floor of the entire House. It is not uncommon for several dozen bills a year to die in the Rules Committee. In the Senate, the scheduling of debate for bills reported out of committee is primarily determined by the majority leader.

The Rules Committee normally limits debate by the entire House of Representatives to one or two hours per bill, with the time divided between and controlled by the chairperson and ranking minority member who are on the committee reporting the bill. The Rules Committee occasionally prohibits amendments from being proposed from the House. In the Senate, any bill that gets out of committee may be brought to the floor by any senator, usually as scheduled by the majority leader. While it is easier to get a bill before the Senate than the House, the absence of time limits on debate make it harder to bring to a vote. If a bill's opponents resort to a *filibuster*, that is, obstructive tactics such as long speeches, it is very difficult to muster the support necessary to stop this delaying tactic as it takes a three-fifths vote by the Senate to invoke *cloture* (closing debate and causing an immediate vote), the process by which a filibuster can be ended.

The detailed parliamentary procedures used in the House and the Senate can be found in the manuals of rules for each body, which are revised biennially. They are as follows:

- U.S. Congress. House. *Constitution, Jefferson's Manual and the Rules of the House of Representatives.* Washington, D.C., United States Government Printing Office, 1979.
- U.S. Congress. House. *Deschler's Precedents of the United States House of Representatives.* Washington, D.C., United States Government Printing Office, 1979.
- U.S. Congress. Senate. Committee on Rules and Administration. *Senate Manual Containing the Standing Rules, Orders, Laws and Resolutions Affecting the Business of the United States Senate.* Washington, D.C., United States Government Printing Office, 1979.
- U.S. Congress. Senate. *Senate Procedure: Precedents and Practices.* Washington, D.C., United States Government Printing Office, 1979.

The floor action on a bill can be followed by consulting the *Congressional Record: Proceedings and Debates of the Congress,* which is a daily record of the proceedings of Congress. The 1981 subscription price for one year was $135.00 per year. It consists of four sections: (1) proceedings of the House; (2) proceedings of the Senate; (3) extensions and remarks; and (4) the "Daily Digest" of the activities of Congress. The proceedings are indexed by subject and individual. The "History of Bills and Resolutions" section is arranged by bill and resolution number. The *Congressional Record* is not a literal transcription of the floor debates. Members of Congress or their staffs have a chance to edit it before it goes into print, and again before it goes into the permanent bound volumes. The daily edition is therefore somewhat more accurate than the annual bound volumes. Normally the ability to edit makes little difference, but in hard-fought debates over a controversial bill where tempers sometimes flare, there may be considerable editing.

CONFERENCE COMMITTEE

After a bill has passed one house of Congress, it is sent to the other, where the procedure begins anew with a referral to a standing committee. If the second house passes the bill in the same form as the first, it is sent directly to the President for his signature. But if new amendments are added, the revised bill must be returned to the originating chamber for approval of the changes. Should that body refuse to approve, which happens about 10% of the time, both the Senate and the House versions of the bill are sent to a conference committee. The members of this committee are usually chosen by the presiding officers from the two standing committees that considered the bill earlier. Then a conference committee of about a dozen senators and representatives attempts to hammer out a compromise. When the compromised version goes back to the Senate and the House of Representatives for a final vote, no further amendments are permitted, and the bill is usually passed. Conference reports are generally accepted by both chambers for two important reasons—the members' disinclination to repeat the entire legisla-

United States
of America

Congressional Record

PROCEEDINGS AND DEBATES OF THE 96th CONGRESS, FIRST SESSION

Vol. 125   WASHINGTON, FRIDAY, JULY 27, 1979   No. 105

House of Representatives

NURSES TRAINING AMENDMENTS OF 1979

Mr. WAXMAN. Mr. Speaker, I move that the House resolve itself into the Committee of the Whole House on the State of the Union for the further consideration of the bill (H.R. 3633) to amend title VIII of the Public Health Service Act to extend for 1 fiscal year the program of assistance for nurse training, and for other purposes.

The SPEAKER. The question is on the motion offered by the gentleman from California (Mr. WAXMAN).

The motion was agreed to.

IN THE COMMITTEE OF THE WHOLE

Accordingly the House resolved itself into the Committee of the Whole House on the State of the Union for the further consideration of the bill, H.R. 3633, with Mr. SEIBERLING in the chair.

The Clerk read the title of the bill.

The CHAIRMAN. When the committee rose on Monday, July 23, 1979, all time for general debate on the bill had expired.

Pursuant to the rule, the Clerk will now read the bill by titles.

The Clerk read as follows:

H.R. 3633

Be it enacted by the Senate and House of Representatives of the United States of America in Congress assembled,

TITLE I—NURSE TRAINING

SEC. 101. (a) This title may be cited as the "Nurse Training Amendments of 1979".

(b) Whenever in this Act (other than sections 205 and 214) an amendment or repeal is expressed in terms of an amendment to, or repeal of, a section or other provision, the reference shall be considered to be made to a section or other provision of the Public Health Service Act.

SEC. 102. Section 801 (relating to authorizations for construction grants) (42 U.S.C. 296) is amended by striking out "and" after "1977," and by inserting after "for fiscal year 1978" the following: "and $2,000,000 for the fiscal year ending September 30, 1980".

SEC. 103. (a) Subsections (a) and (b) of section 805 (relating to loan guarantees and interest subsidies) (42 U.S.C. 296d) are each amended by striking out "1978" and inserting in lieu thereof "1980".

(b) Subsection (e) of such section is amended by inserting after "in fiscal year 1978" the following: "and in each of the next two fiscal years".

SEC. 104. Subsection (f)(1) of section 810 (relating to capitation grants) (42 U.S.C. 296e) is amended by inserting after "fiscal year 1978" the following: "and $24,000,000 for the fiscal year ending September 30, 1980".

SEC. 105. The first sentence of subsection (d) of section 820 (relating to special project grants and contracts) is amended by striking out "and" after "1977," and by inserting before the period the following: ", and $17,000,000 for the fiscal year ending September 30, 1980".

SEC. 106. Subsection (b) of section 821 (relating to advanced nurse training programs) (42 U.S.C. 296l) is amended by striking out "and" after "1977," and by inserting after "for fiscal year 1978" the following: ", and $13,500,000 for the fiscal year ending September 30, 1980".

SEC. 107. Subsection (e) of section 822 (re-

lating to nurse practitioner programs) (42 U.S.C. 296m) is amended by striking out "and" after "1977," and by inserting before the period the following: ", and $15,000,000 for the fiscal year ending September 30, 1980".

SEC. 108. Subsection (b) of section 830 (relating to traineeships) (42 U.S.C. 297) is amended by striking out "and" after "1977," and by inserting before the period ", and $15,000,000 for the fiscal year ending September 30, 1980".

SEC. 109. (a) Subsection (b)(4) of section 835 (relating to loan agreements) (42 U.S.C. 297a) is amended by striking out "1978" and inserting in lieu thereof "1980".

(b) Section 837 (relating to authorizations for student loan funds) (42 U.S.C. 297c) is amended (1) by striking out "and" after "1977," in the first sentence and (2) by inserting before the period in the first sentence ", and $13,500,000 for the fiscal year ending September 30, 1980", (3) by striking out "fiscal year 1979" and inserting in lieu thereof "the fiscal year ending September 30, 1981", and (4) by striking out "October 1, 1978" and inserting in lieu thereof "October 1, 1980".

(c)(1) Subsection (a) of section 839 (relating to distribution of assets) (42 U.S.C. 297c) is amended by striking out "September 30, 1980, and not later than September 30, 1977" and inserting in lieu thereof "September 30, 1981, and not later than December 30, 1983".

(2) Paragraph (1) of such subsection is amended by striking out "1980" and inserting in lieu thereof "1983".

(3) Subsection (b) of such section is amended by striking out "1980" each place it occurs and inserting in lieu thereof "1983".

SEC. 110. (a) Subsection (b) of section 845 (relating to scholarship grants) (42 U.S.C. 297i) is amended (1) by striking out "next two fiscal years" in the first sentence and inserting in lieu thereof "next four fiscal years", (2) by striking out "1979" and inserting in lieu thereof "1981", and (3) by striking out "1978" and inserting in lieu thereof "1980".

(b) Subsection (c)(1) of such section is amended (1) by striking out "next two fiscal years" in subparagraph (A) and inserting in lieu thereof "next four fiscal years", (2) by striking out "1978" in subparagraph (B) and inserting in lieu thereof "1980", and (3) by striking out "1979" in such subparagraph and inserting in lieu thereof "1981".

(c) The amendments made by subsections (a) and (b) do not authorize appropriations for the fiscal year ending September 30, 1979, for scholarships under section 845 of the Public Health Service Act in addition to the amount available for such scholarships under section 101(a) of Public Law 95-482.

SEC. 111. Subpart I of part B of title VIII (relating to traineeships) is amended by adding after section 830 (42 U.S.C. 297) the following new section:

"TRAINEESHIPS FOR TRAINING OF NURSE ANESTHETISTS

"SEC. 831. (a)(1) The Secretary may make grants to public or private nonprofit institutions to cover the costs of traineeships for the training, in programs which meet such requirements as the Secretary shall by regulation prescribe and which are accredited by an entity or entities designated by the Commissioner of Education, of licensed, registered nurses to be nurse anesthetists.

"(2) Payments to institutions under this subsection may be made in advance or by way of reimbursement, and at such intervals and on such conditions, as the Secretary finds necessary. Such payments may be used only for traineeships and shall be limited to such amounts as the Secretary finds necessary to cover the costs of tuition and fees,

and a stipend and allowances (including travel and subsistence expenses) for the trainees.

"(b) For the purpose of making grants under subsection (a), there are authorized to be appropriated $2,000,000 for the fiscal year ending September 30, 1980.".

SEC. 112. Section 836(b)(3) (relating to student loans) (42 U.S.C. 297b(b)(3)) is amended (1) by inserting after "(3)" the following: "In the case of a student who received such a loan before the date of enactment of the Nurse Training Amendments of 1979," and (2) by striking out "any such loan" and inserting in lieu thereof "any such loan made before such date".

SEC. 113. (a) The Secretary of Health, Education, and Welfare (hereinafter in this section referred to as the "Secretary") shall arrange, in accordance with subsection (b), for the conduct of a study to determine the need to continue a specific program of Federal financial support for nursing education, taking into account—

(1) the need for nurses under the present health care delivery system and under that system as it may be changed by the enactment of legislation for national health insurance,

(2) the cost of nursing education, and

(3) the availability of other sources of support for nursing education, including support under general programs of Federal financial support for postsecondary education, under State and other public programs, and from private sources.

(b)(1) The Secretary shall first request the National Academy of Sciences (hereinafter in this section referred to as the "Academy"), acting through the Institute of Medicine, to conduct the study, required by subsection (a), under an arrangement whereby the actual expenses incurred by the Academy directly related to the conduct of such study will be paid by the Secretary If the Academy agrees to such request, the Secretary shall enter into such an arrangement with the Academy.

(2) If the Academy declines the Secretary's request to conduct such study under such an arrangement, then the Secretary shall enter into a similar arrangement with another appropriate public or nonprofit private entity to conduct such study.

(3) Upon completion of the study, the entity conducting the study shall report the results of it to the Secretary and shall include in such report any recommendations for legislation which the entity determines are appropriate.

(4) Any arrangement entered into under paragraph (1) or (2) of this subsection for the conduct of a study shall require that such study be completed and reports thereon be submitted within such period as the Secretary may require to meet the requirements of subsection (c).

(5) The Secretary shall undertake such preliminary activities as may be necessary to enable the Secretary to enter into an arrangement for the conduct of the study at the earliest date authorized by subsection (d).

(c) Not later than six months after the date the arrangement for the conduct of the study is entered into under subsection (b), the Secretary shall report to the Committee on Human Resources of the Senate and the Committee on Interstate and Foreign Commerce of the House of Representatives preliminary recommendations respecting the need to continue a specific program of Federal financial support for nursing education and, if there is a need, the form in which the support should be provided. Not later than two years after such date, the Secretary shall report to such Committees recommendations respecting such need and form of support and the basis for such recommendations.

tive process and their deference to the expertise and prestige of the conferees.

REFERRAL TO THE PRESIDENT

When a bill has been approved in the same form by both houses, it is sent to the White House. Because their electoral bases are different, it is only reasonable to expect the president and the various members of Congress to advocate different policy positions. The President can afford to ignore certain interest groups, whereas, the congressmen may do so only with considerable threat to their political futures. The Office of Management and Budget collects the views of interested agencies and also makes its own independent recommendations to the President as to whether the bill should be signed or vetoed. Advice from White House assistants will also help the President decide. By the time an important bill reaches the President's desk, it has gone through a standing committee in each house, usually also subcommittees, the Rules Committee of the House, both the Senate and House, and often a conference committee. It may bear little resemblance to any bill the President initially requested and may indeed be a bill he never wanted at all. Should he choose to veto it, a two-thirds vote is then required in both houses of Congress before it can become law.

When the President vetoes a measure, the Constitution provides that "he shall return it with his objections to that house in which it shall have originated." Neither chamber is under any obligation to schedule an override attempt. Party leaders may realize that there is no chance to override and simply not schedule a vote. If an override attempt fails in one chamber, the process ends and the bill dies. If it succeeds, the measure is sent to the other chamber, where a successful override vote makes it law. The President has another veto weapon that cannot be overridden. This is known as the *pocket veto*, and occurs when the President refuses to sign a bill that Congress has enacted within the last ten days of the session. Because a large number of bills are passed in the hectic closing days of a session, there is no lack of opportunity to use the pocket veto. The figures (from 1945–1980) in

Table 8–5.	*Results of Presidential Vetos, 1945–1980*

PRESIDENT	REGULAR VETOES	POCKET VETOES	TOTAL VETOED	VETOES OVERRIDDEN	% OVERRIDDEN
Truman	54	29	83	11	13.3
Eisenhower	36	45	81	2	2.5
Kennedy	4	5	9	0	0.0
Johnson	6	7	13	0	0.0
Nixon	24	16	40	5	12.5
Ford	35	11	46	8	17.4
Carter	13	16	29	2	6.9

Table 8-5 indicate the difficulty of overriding a presidential veto of a public bill.

President Ford vetoed two Nurse Training Act bills in 1975, the second of which was overriden by Congress. His reasons for the veto were the same for both. The text of his January, 1975, veto is as follows:[7]

The White House
Office of the White House Press Secretary
January 3, 1975
Memorandum of Disapproval

I have withheld my approval from H.R. 17085, a bill that would amend Title VIII of the Public Health Service Act to provide support for the training of nurses.

This measure would authorize excessive appropriations levels—more than $650 million over the three fiscal years covered by the bill. Such high Federal spending for nursing education would be intolerable at a time when even high priority activities are being pressed to justify their existence.

I believe nurses have played and will continue to play an invaluable role in the delivery of health services. The Federal taxpayer can and should selectively assist nursing schools to achieve education reforms and innovations in support of that objective. The Administration's 1976 budget will include funds for this purpose. Furthermore, I intend to urge the 94th Congress to enact comprehensive health personnel training legislation that will permit support of nurse training initiatives to meet the new problems of the 1970's.

This act inappropriately proposes large amounts of student and construction support for schools of nursing. Without any additional Federal stimulation, we expect that the number of active duty registered nurses will increase by over 50 percent during this decade.

Such an increase suggests that our incentives for expansion have been successful, and that continuation of the current Federal program is likely to be of less benefit to the Nation than using these scarce resources in other ways. One result of this expansion has been scattered but persistent reports of registered nurse unemployment particularly among graduates of associate degree training programs.

Today's very different outlook is not reflected in this bill. We must concentrate Federal efforts on the shortage of certain nurse specialists, and persistent geographic maldistribution. However, this proposal would allocate less than one third of its total authorization to these problems. Moreover, it fails to come to grips with the problem of geographic maldistribution.

Support for innovative projects—involving the health professions, nursing, allied health, and public health—should be contained in a single piece of legislation to assure that decisions made in one sector relate to decisions made in another, and to advance the concept of an integrated health service delivery team. By separating out nursing from other health personnel categories, this bill would perpetuate what has in the past been a fragmented approach.

The enrolled bill would also extend various special nursing student assistance provisions of current law. Nursing students are overwhelmingly undergraduates, and as such should be—and are—entitled to the same types of student assistance available generally under the Office of Education's programs for post-secondary education. These include, in particular, guaranteed loans and basic educational opportunity grants for financially hard pressed students. Categorical nursing student assistance activities are not appropriate and should be phased out, as the Administration has proposed.

Gerald R. Ford

Less than four years later, nurses were faced with another President who vetoed a Nurse Training Act extension, this time President Jimmy Carter whose veto message read:[8]

The White House
November 10, 1978

I am withholding my approval from S 2416, a bill that would extend a series of programs authorizing special Federal support for the training of nurses.

Although I support a number of its provisions, this bill would continue several Federal nurse training programs whose objectives have been accomplished and for which there is no longer a need. Moreover, the funding authorizations are excessive and unacceptable if we are to reduce the budget deficit to help fight inflation.

For the past 22 years, the Federal government has provided substantial financial support for nursing education. From 1956 through 1977, almost $1.4 billion was awarded for student traineeships, loans, and scholarships; for construction and basic support for nursing education programs; and for projects to improve nursing education and recruitment.

With the help of this support, the number of active nurses has more than doubled since 1957 to over 1,000,000 in 1978. Ten years ago, in 1968, there were 300

S. 2416   **Jan 24, 1978.**

Mr. Javits (for himself and others)

To amend Title VIII of the Public Health Service Act to extend for 2 fiscal years the program of assistance for nurse training.

Jan. 27, 1978. Reports requested from Department of Health, Education, and Welfare, General Accounting Office, and Office of Management and Budget.
Hearing. Apr. 5, 1978. (1 VOL.)
Apr. 18, 1978. Considered in open executive session by Subcommittee on Health and Scientific Research and ordered reported to full committee.
May 4, 1978. Considered in open executive session by full committee and ordered reported to Senate with amendments.
May 15, 1978. Reported to Senate by Mr. Kennedy (S. REPT. 95-859).
June 7, 1978. PASSED BY SENATE.
Sept. 19, 1978. PASSED BY HOUSE with an amendment in the nature of a substitute (text of H.R. 12303 (H. REPT. 95-1189)).
Sept. 30, 1978. By unanimous consent ordered held at desk.
Oct. 9, 1978. Senate requested conference and appointed conferees (see Conference and Conferees).
Oct. 11, 1978. House agreed to conference and appointed conferees (see Conference and Conferees).
Oct. 11, 1978. Conferees met in executive session and agreed to file conference report.
Oct. 13, 1978. Conference report filed in House by Mr. Staggers (H. REPT. 95-1785.)
Oct. 14, 1978. Conference report AGREED TO BY SENATE.
Oct. 14, 1978. Conference report AGREED TO BY HOUSE.
Nov. 11, 1978. Vetoed by the President.
(See H.R. 12303.)

Figure 8–21. The legislative history of Senate 2416, the Nurse Training Act of 1978, which was destined to die from a veto by President Carter. (Courtesy of U.S. Senate)

active nurses per 100,000 population in the United States. By the beginning of 1977, this ratio had risen to 395 per 100,000 population.

The outlook is also good for adequate, sustained growth in the supply of nurses. There is, therefore, no reason for the government to provide special support to increase the total supply of professional nurses.

This year the Administration proposed to extend only the authorities for special projects in nursing education and for nurse practitioner training programs, in order to focus Federal nurse training support on areas of greatest national need. This proposal was based on the concept that future Federal assistance should be limited to geographic and specialty areas that need nurses most.

S 2416 would authorize more than $400 million for fiscal years 1979 and 1980, mostly for continued Federal funding of a number of unnecessary special nurse training programs, at a potential cost to the taxpayer far above my budget. At a time of urgent need for budget restraint, we cannot tolerate spending for any but truly essential purposes.

I must point out that nursing training is primarily undergraduate education, and nursing students are eligible for the assistance made available by the government to all students, based on need. I recently signed into law the Middle Income Student Assistance Act, which will significantly expand our basic grant and student loan guarantee programs. Nursing students are also eligible for National Health Service Corps scholarships.

Disapproval of this bill will not cause an abrupt termination of funding of the nurse training programs, since funds are available for fiscal year 1979 under the continuing resolution.

If the Nation is to meet its health care needs at reasonable cost, Federal nursing and other health professions programs must make the greatest contribution to adequate health care at the most reasonable cost. This bill does not meet that test.

The Administration is now conducting a major review of its support for all health professions training, including nursing. Legislative proposals in this area will be made to the 96th Congress. These proposals will recognize the key role of nurses in our society and the need for nurses to play an even greater role in the efficient delivery of health care services.

Jimmy Carter

The final step of the legislative process is presidential action, but the President's veto power influences the entire legislative process. The extraordinary majority (two-thirds) required to override a veto forces the Congress to consider the White House's position from the moment the bill is introduced until it is finally passed by both houses.

When a President signs or vetoes a piece of legislation, he usually issues a brief statement, like those above, concerning its value or deficiencies. During the time a bill is proceeding through Congress, the President may also make statements concerning the merits of the bill or criticizing or praising Congress for its handling of the bill. These statements are published in the *Weekly Compilation of Presidential Documents*.

U.S. CODE

When a bill has been enacted into law, it is first officially published as a *slip* law, a separately published law in unbound single-sheet or pamphlet form.

Weekly
Compilation
of

PRESIDENTIAL DOCUMENTS

Monday, April 7, 1980
Volume 16–Number 14
Pages 567–609

Figure 8–22. Messages that accompany the president's endorsement or veto of a piece of legislation are published in the Weekly Compilation of Presidential Documents. *(Courtesy of U.S. General Services Administration, National Archives)*

Once a bill has received presidential approval, it takes two or three days for the slip law to become available. Slip laws are gathered into a series of publications known as *United States Statutes at Large.* These are chronological listings of all the laws enacted by Congress for each session; the laws are indexed by subject and individual. The final stage comes when new laws are integrated into the *United States Code,* which contains the general and permanent laws of the United States consolidated and codified under fifty titles. The fifty titles are arranged by subject, with the first six titles dealing with general subjects and the remaining forty-four titles arranged alphabetically by broad subject area. Every six years the code is revised, and after each session of Congress a supplement is issued. Title 42 contains the laws pertaining to public health. The full range of federal laws

Public Law 88-581
88th Congress, H. R. 11241
September 4, 1964

An Act

To amend the Public Health Service Act to increase the opportunities for training
professional nursing personnel, and for other purposes.

*Be it enacted by the Senate and House of Representatives of the
United States of America in Congress assembled,* That this Act may
be cited as the "Nurse Training Act of 1964".

Nurse Train-
ing Act of 1964.

SEC. 2. The Public Health Service Act (42 U.S.C., ch. 6A) is
amended by adding at the end thereof the following new title:

58 Stat. 682.

"TITLE VIII—NURSE TRAINING

"PART A—GRANTS FOR EXPANSION AND IMPROVEMENT OF NURSE TRAINING

"AUTHORIZATION OF APPROPRIATIONS FOR CONSTRUCTION GRANTS

"SEC. 801. (a) There are authorized to be appropriated—

"(1) for grants to assist in the construction of new facilities
for collegiate schools of nursing, or replacement or rehabilitation
of existing facilities for such schools, $5,000,000 for the fiscal
year ending June 30, 1966, and $10,000,000 for each of the next
three fiscal years;

"(2) for grants to assist in the construction of new facilities
for associate degree or diploma schools of nursing, or replacement or rehabilitation of existing facilities for such schools,
$10,000,000 for the fiscal year ending June 30, 1966, and
$15,000,000 for each of the next three fiscal years.

78 STAT. 908.
78 STAT. 909.

There are also authorized to be appropriated for each of such fiscal
years ending after June 30, 1966, for grants specified in clause (1) or
(2) of the preceding sentence, the amount by which the total of
the sums authorized to be appropriated under such clause for previous
years exceeds the aggregate of the appropriations thereunder for
such years.

"(b) Sums appropriated pursuant to clause (1) or (2) of subsection
(a) for a fiscal year shall remain available for grants specified in
such clause until the close of the next fiscal year.

"APPROVAL OF APPLICATIONS FOR CONSTRUCTION GRANTS

"SEC. 802. (a) No application for a grant for a construction project
under this part may be approved unless it is submitted to the Surgeon
General prior to July 1, 1968.

"(b) A grant for a construction project under this part may be
made only if the application therefor is approved by the Surgeon
General upon his determination that—

"(1) the applicant is a public or nonprofit private school of
nursing providing an accredited program of nursing education;

"(2) the application contains or is supported by reasonable
assurances that (A) for not less than twenty years after completion of construction, the facility will be used for the purposes of
the training for which it is to be constructed, and will not be used
for sectarian instruction or as a place for religious worship,
(B) sufficient funds will be available to meet the non-Federal
share of the cost of constructing the facility, (C) sufficient funds
will be available, when construction is completed, for effective
use of the facility for the training for which it is being constructed, and (D) in the case of an application for a grant for
construction to expand the training capacity of a school of nurs-

37-539 O

Table 8–6.   *History of Authorizations for Nurse Training Fiscal Years 1965–1981*
             (in thousands)

Programs*	NURSE TRAINING ACT OF 1964 (P.L. 88-581)				
	1965	1966	1967	1968	1969
Special Project Grants & Contracts (Title VIII, Part A, Section 820)	$ 2,000	$ 3,000	$ 4,000	$ 4,000	$ 4,000
Payments to Diploma Schools (Title VIII, Part A, Section 806)	4,000	7,000	10,000	10,000	10,000
Formula Grants (Title VIII, Part A, Section 806)			N/A		
Capitation Grants (Title VIII, Part A, Section 810)			N/A		
Financial Distress Grants (Title VIII, Part A, Section 815)			N/A		
Start-up Grants (Title VIII, Part A, Section 810)			N/A		
Advanced Nurse Training (Title VIII, Part A, Section 821)			N/A		
Nurse Practitioner (Title VIII, Part A, Section 822)			N/A		
Nursing Education Opportunity Grants[c] (Title VIII, Part D, Section 861)	N/A	N/A	3,000	5,000	7,000
Scholarships[d] (Title VIII, Part B, Section 845)			N/A		
Student Loans (Title VIII, Part B, Section 837)	3,100	8,900	16,800	25,300	30,900
Traineeships[e] (Title VIII, Part B, Section 830)	8,000	9,000	10,000	11,000	12,000
Construction: *Grants* (Title VIII, Part A, Section 801)	N/A	15,000	25,000	25,000	25,000
Construction: *Interest Subsidies* (Title VIII, Part A, Section 805)			N/A		
Recruitment (Full Utiliz.) Grts & Contract (Title VIII, Part A, Section 820)	N/A	N/A		f	
Nurse Anesthetists (Title VIII, Part B, Section 831)			N/A		
Loan Repayments (Title VIII, Part B, Section 836[h])			N/A		
Loan Cancellations (Title VIII, Part B, Section 836[b] (3)) ..			h		
Fellowships (NRSA) (Title IV, Part I, Section 472)			i		
TOTAL	$17,100	$42,900	$68,800	$80,300	$88,900

(*continues on facing p.*)

Table 8–6.   (*Continued*) *History of Authorizations for Nurse Training Fiscal Years 1965–1981*) (*in thousands*)

Programs*	HEALTH MANPOWER ACT OF 1968 (P.L. 90-490)		NURSE TRAINING ACT OF 1971 (P.L. 92-158)		
	1970	1971	1972	1973	1974
Special Project Grants & Contracts (Title VIII, Part A, Section 820)	$15,000[a]	$ 15,000[a]	$ 20,000	$ 28,000	$ 35,000
Payments to Diploma Schools (Title VIII, Part A, Section 806)	N/A			N/A	
Formula Grants (Title VIII, Part A, Section 806)	20,000[a]	25,000[a]		N/A	
Capitation Grants (Title VIII, Part A, Section 810)	N/A		78,000	82,000	88,000
Financial Distress Grants (Title VIII, Part A, Section 815)	N/A		15,000	10,000	5,000
Start-up Grants (Title VIII, Part A, Section 810)	N/A		4,000	8,000	12,000
Advanced Nurse Training (Title VIII, Part A, Section 821)	N/A			N/A	
Nurse Practitioner (Title VIII, Part A, Section 822)	N/A			N/A	
Nursing Education Opportunity Grants[c] (Title VIII, Part D, Section 861)	N/A			N/A	
Scholarships[d] (Title VIII, Part B, Section 845)	(32,000)[d]	(33,000)[d]	(55,500)[d]	(58,000)[d]	(59,000)[d]
Student Loans (Title VIII, Part B, Section 837)	20,000	21,000	25,000	30,000	35,000
Traineeships[e] (Title VIII, Part B, Section 830)	15,000	19,000	20,000	22,000	24,000
Construction: *Grants* (Title VIII, Part A, Section 801)	25,000	35,000	35,000	40,000	45,000
Construction: *Interest Subsidies* (Title VIII, Part A, Section 805)	N/A		1,000	2,000	4,000
Recruitment (Full Utiliz.) Grts & Contract (Title VIII, Part A, Section 820)	f		3,500	5,000	6,500
Nurse Anesthetists (Title VIII, Part B, Section 831)	N/A			N/A	
Loan Repayments (Title VIII, Part B, Section 836[h])	N/A			g	
Loan Cancellations (Title VIII, Part B, Section 836[b] (3)) ..	h			h	
Fellowships (NRSA) (Title IV, Part I, Section 472)	i			i	
TOTAL	$95,000	$115,000	$201,500	$227,000	$254,500

(*continues on p. 276*)

Table 8-6.   *(Continued) History of Authorizations for Nurse Training Fiscal Years 1965-1981 (in thousands)*

| Programs* | NURSE TRAINING ACT OF 1975 (P.L. 94-63) | | | |
	1975	1976	1977	1978
Special Project Grants & Contracts (Title VIII, Part A, Section 820)	$ 35,000	$ 15,000[b]	$ 15,000[b]	$ 15,000[b]
Payments to Diploma Schools (Title VIII, Part A, Section 806)		N/A		
Formula Grants (Title VIII, Part A, Section 806)		N/A		
Capitation Grants (Title VIII, Part A, Section 810)	88,000	50,000	55,000	55,000
Financial Distress Grants (Title VIII, Part A, Section 815)	5,000	5,000	5,000	5,000
Start-up Grants (Title VIII, Part A, Section 810)	12,000	N/A		
Advanced Nurse Training (Title VIII, Part A, Section 821)		15,000	20,000	25,000
Nurse Practitioner (Title VIII, Part A, Section 822)		15,000	20,000	25,000
Nursing Education Opportunity Grants[c] (Title VIII, Part D, Section 861)		N/A		
Scholarships[d] (Title VIII, Part B, Section 845)	(59,000)[d]	(75,000)[d]	(78,000)[d]	(78,000)[d]
Student Loans (Title VIII, Part B, Section 837)	35,000	25,000	30,000	35,000
Traineeships[e] (Title VIII, Part B, Section 830)	24,000	15,000	20,000	25,000
Construction: *Grants* (Title VIII, Part A, Section 801)	45,000	20,000	20,000	20,000
Construction: *Interest Subsidies* (Title VIII, Part A, Section 805)	4,000	1,000	1,000	1,000
Recruitment (Full Utiliz.) Grts & Contract (Title VIII, Part A, Section 820)	6,500		b	
Nurse Anesthetists (Title VIII, Part B, Section 831)		N/A		
Loan Repayments (Title VIII, Part B, Section 836[h])		g		
Loan Cancellations (Title VIII, Part B, Section 836[b] (3)) ..		h		
Fellowships (NRSA) (Title IV, Part I, Section 472)			j	
TOTAL	$254,500	$161,000	$186,000	$206,000

(continues of facing p.)

Table 8–6.   (*Continued*) *History of Authorizations for Nurse Training Fiscal Years 1965–1981 (in thousands)*

Programs*	CONTINUING RESOLUTION (P.L. 95-482) 1979	NURSE TRAINING AMENDMENTS OF 1979 (P.L. 96-76) 1980	CONTINUING RESOLUTION (P.L. 96-536) 1981
Special Project Grants & Contracts (Title VIII, Part A, Section 820)	$ 15,000	$ 17,000	$ 17,000
Payments to Diploma Schools (Title VIII, Part A, Section 806)	N/A	N/A	N/A
Formula Grants (Title VIII, Part A, Section 806)	N/A	N/A	N/A
Capitation Grants (Title VIII, Part A, Section 810)	30,000	24,000	24,000
Financial Distress Grants (Title VIII, Part A, Section 815)	N/A	N/A	N/A
Start-up Grants (Title VIII, Part A, Section 810)	N/A	N/A	N/A
Advanced Nurse Training (Title VIII, Part A, Section 821)	12,000	13,500	13,500
Nurse Practitioner (Title VIII, Part A, Section 822)	13,000	15,000	15,000
Nursing Education Opportunity Grants[c] (Title VIII, Part D, Section 861)	N/A	N/A	N/A
Scholarships[d] (Title VIII, Part B, Section 845)	(9,000)[d]	(78,000)[d]	(78,000)[d]
Student Loans (Title VIII, Part B, Section 837)	22,500	13,500	13,500
Traineeships[e] (Title VIII, Part B, Section 830)	13,000	15,000	15,000
Construction: *Grants* (Title VIII, Part A, Section 801)		2,000	2,000
Construction: *Interest Subsidies* (Title VIII, Part A, Section 805)		1,000	1,000
Recruitment (Full Utiliz.) Grts & Contract (Title VIII, Part A, Section 820)	b	b	b
Nurse Anesthetists (Title VIII, Part B, Section 831)	N/A	2,000	2,000
Loan Repayments (Title VIII, Part B, Section 836[h])	g	g	g
Loan Cancellations (Title VIII, Part B, Section 836[b] (3)) ..	h	h	h
Fellowships (NRSA) (Title IV, Part I, Section 472)	j	j	j
TOTAL	$105,500	$103,000	$103,000

(*Table 8–6 footnotes, p. 278*)

* Note: The section numbers referenced are those sections of the law in which the programs were authorized in the most recent legislation.

a = Combined authorization of $35 million in fiscal year 1970 and $40 million in fiscal year 1971 for Project Grants and Formula Grants; first $15 million to Project Grants.

b = Authorization for Special Projects includes Recruitment and Full Utilization Grants and Contracts.

c = As added by P.L. 89-571, Allied Health Professions Personnel Training Act of 1966.

d = No specified amount authorized—amounts based on formula in the legislation. Amounts are not included in totals.

e = Authorized for "such sums as necessary" under P.L. 84-911, Health Amendments Act of 1956, for fiscal years 1957–1959 and P.L. 86-105, Health Amendments Act of 1956, Ext., for fiscal years 1960–1964.

f = Authorized originally by P.L. 89-751, Allied Health Professions Personnel Act of 1966, dated November 3, 1966, which authorized "such sums as necessary" for contracts to encourage full utilization of nursing educational talent.

g = Authorization for "such sums as necessary."

h = Mandatory authorization for "such sums as necessary."

i = Section 301 of the Public Health Service Act provided open-ended authority for Research Grants, Fellowships, Research Training Grants and Direct Operations until enactment of the National Research Act of 1974, P.L. 93-348. This Act authorized the Fellowship and Research Training Programs under section 472 (see footnote j). The Nursing Research Grant and Direct Operations Programs are still authorized under section 301. The dollar level of authorizations remains unspecified.

j = The Health Research and Health Services Amendments Act of 1976, P.L. 94-278, reauthorized Nursing Research Training and Fellowship Grants. Such grants are presently authorized under the Biomedical Research and Research Training Amendments of 1978, P.L. 95-622. National Research Service Awards are administered by the National Institutes of Health. The Nurse Fellowship Program is a small portion of the NRSA total authorization amount. Also included under this authority are Research Training Grants.

Figure 8–24. Slip laws are annually gathered into a volume known as the United States Statutes at Large. (*Courtesy of U.S. Government Printing Office*)

UNITED STATES
STATUTES AT LARGE

CONTAINING THE

LAWS AND CONCURRENT RESOLUTIONS
ENACTED DURING THE FIRST SESSION OF THE
NINETY-FIFTH CONGRESS
OF THE UNITED STATES OF AMERICA

1977

AND

REORGANIZATION PLANS,
RECOMMENDATIONS OF THE PRESIDENT
AND PROCLAMATIONS

VOLUME 91

IN ONE PART

UNITED STATES
GOVERNMENT PRINTING OFFICE
WASHINGTON : 1980

that regulate all aspects of life in the United States and that are compiled into the titles of the *United States Code* are as follows:

TITLES OF UNITED STATES CODE

1. General Provisions
2. The Congress
3. The President
4. Flag and Seal, Seat of Government, and the States
5. Government Organization and Employees
6. Surety Bonds
7. Agriculture
8. Aliens and Nationality
9. Arbitration
10. Armed Forces
11. Bankruptcy
12. Banks and Banking
13. Census
14. Coast Guard
15. Commerce and Trade
16. Conservation
17. Copyrights
18. Crimes and Criminal Procedure
19. Customs Duties
20. Education
21. Food and Drugs
22. Foreign Relations and Intercourse
23. Highways
24. Hospitals and Asylums
25. Indians
26. Internal Revenue Code
27. Intoxicating Liquors
28. Judiciary and Judicial Procedure
29. Labor
30. Mineral Lands and Mining
31. Money and Finance
32. National Guard
33. Navigation and Navigable Waters
34. Navy
35. Patents
36. Patriotic Societies and Observances
37. Pay and Allowances of the Uniformed Services
38. Veterans' Benefits
39. Postal Service
40. Public Buildings, Property, and Works
41. Public Contracts
42. The Public Health and Welfare
43. Public Lands
44. Public Printing and Documents
45. Railroads
46. Shipping
47. Telegraphs, Telephones, and Radiotelegraphs
48. Territories and Insular Possessions
49. Transportation
50. War and National Defense; and Appendix

CONGRESSIONAL SUPPORT AGENCIES

There are four congressional support agencies which assist in the legislative process and serve as the major investigative tools for the legislative branch of government. They are the Congressional Research Service (CRS) of the Library of Congress, the General Accounting Office (GAO), the Office of

UNITED STATES CODE

1976 EDITION

SUPPLEMENT III

CONTAINING THE GENERAL AND PERMANENT LAWS OF
THE UNITED STATES, ENACTED DURING THE
95TH CONGRESS AND 96TH CONGRESS, FIRST SESSION

Prepared and published under authority of Title 2, U.S. Code, Section 285b,
by the Office of the Law Revision Counsel of the House of Representatives

JANUARY 4, 1977, TO JANUARY 8, 1980

VOLUME ONE

TITLE 1—GENERAL PROVISIONS

TO

TITLE 18—CRIMES AND CRIMINAL PROCEDURE

UNITED STATES
GOVERNMENT PRINTING OFFICE
WASHINGTON : 1980

Figure 8–25. The United States Code *contains all of the laws of the United States of which* Title 42 *"The Public Health and Welfare" has major impact on the practice of nursing.* (*Courtesy of U.S. Government Printing Office*)

Technology Assessment (OTA), and the Congressional Budget Office (CBO). CRS, an autonomous part of the Library of Congress, is a ready-reference service whose strength is the speed with which it responds to countless daily requests for information from members of Congress and their staffs. "Quick and dirty" is a common description of CRS work as the vast majority of requests to CRS can be answered in a matter of hours. CRS was authorized by the 1970 Legislative Reorganization Act to assist congressional committees in analyzing federal programs under their jurisdiction.

Created in 1921, the General Accounting Office originally was intended to be the government's auditor. With its personnel stationed in nearly every government office building in Washington, the GAO still makes sure that the executive branch spends money the way Congress intended. In the past decade, the GAO's mission as a congressional support agency has expanded from auditing the executive branch's books to evaluating its programs. When the GAO issues a report containing recommendations regarding financial operations, management, or program performance to the head of any federal agency, that agency is required, under the 1970 Legislative Reorganization Act, to submit written reports to the House and Senate Appropriations Committees and government operations committees, informing them of the actions taken in response to these recommendations.

The Office of Technology Assessment's basic function is to provide congressional committees with assessments that identify a broad range of intended and unintended consequences, social as well as physical, which will accompany the uses of technology. Congress created OTA in 1972, although the new agency did not begin operating until January, 1974. It attempts to pull together scientific and engineering information and present it in the context of policy issues.

The Congressional Budget Office gives Congress an overview of the federal budget and weighs the priorities for national resource allocation. The Congressional Budget Office, the newest of Congress's four staff support agencies, was established by the 1974 Congressional Budget and Impoundment Control Act, which is discussed in more detail in the next chapter. Its basic purpose is to supply Congress with the budgetary information it needs to implement the budget process. Under the Budget Reform Act, the House and Senate Budget Committees are the CBO's chief clients. But the Office also must perform regular tasks for the appropriating and authorizing committees, and individual Members of Congress may ask the CBO to supply them with information that it has already prepared for a committee. The task that makes the CBO a part of the day-to-day operation of the new budget process is budget estimating. Specifically, the CBO is charged with the following tasks:

- Keep the Congress regularly informed of how the legislation it has enacted compares with its most recent budget resolution. (This is called the score-keeping function.)
- Help committees that process spending and tax expenditure legislation, especially the Appropriations, Ways and Means and Finance Committees, compare their legislation to the most recent budget resolution.
- Project for five years the costs of carrying out the provisions of every authorizing bill reported by a House or Senate committee.
- Issue a report soon after the beginning of each fiscal year, projecting total spending, revenue and tax expenditures for the next five years if federal budget policies remain unchanged.

Members of Congress, the direct custodians of the levers of change in health care, have traditionally been nurses' best champions in the fight over reallocation of health care resources. While each member has his or her individual approach to the job, representatives and senators generally emphasize different combinations of these goals: helping their constituents (and enhancing their prospects for re-election); acquiring power in the House or Senate; and honestly trying to help make good public policy. With regard to the latter, nurses can definitely assist by learning the process by which a bill becomes law, as thoroughly as they learn clinical nursing procedures. Indeed, the political process is the keystone to the new kind of professionalism, which recognizes that, in a very fundamental way, political decisions and governmental authorization laws and appropriations shape clinical roles and quality of patient care.

References

1. U.S. Congress. House. Subcommittee of the Committee on Appropriations: Departments of Labor, Health, Education, and Welfare, and Related Agencies Appropriations for 1980, p 161. Hearings before the Subcommittee, Part 4. Washington, DC, United States Government Printing Office, 1980
2. U.S. Congress. Senate. Committee on Finance, Subcommittee on Health: Health Assistance for Low-Income Children, p 6. Hearings before the Subcommittee. Washington, DC, United States Government Printing Office, 1979
3. Ibid, p 3
4. Ibid, p 4
5. Washington Monitor: Congressional Yellow Book Spring '80, Sec 3, pp 16–18. Washington, DC, Washington Monitor, 1980
6. Interview with Sheila Burke, Mar, 1980
7. Ford GR: Nurses' training: Memorandum of disapproval, Jan 4, 1975. In Congressional Quarterly Almanac, 93rd Congress, 2nd Session, 1974, Vol 30, p 63-A. Washington, DC, Congressional Quarterly, 1974
8. Carter J: Nurse Training Act veto, Nov 10, 1978. In Congressional Quarterly Almanac, 95th Congress, 2nd Session, 1978, Vol 34, p 68-E. Washington, DC, Congressional Quarterly, 1979

9–The Legislative Process: Appropriations

A bill that has been enacted into law is only an authorization. It signifies approval of a program that, unless open-ended, puts a ceiling on monies that can be used to finance it. By itself, the authorization provides no funds for putting the program into effect. What must come next is an *appropriations* bill, as it does little good to pass a law without money to implement it. The Congress controls the federal purse strings through appropriations bills, which allocate funds to all programs and agencies of government for their operating expenses. Congress's control over the federal purse is the most important source of its power. Although policy initiative belongs almost exclusively to the president, he can never act to translate an idea into an activity unless Congress provides the necessary funds to put it into effect.

The Constitution gives the House power to originate tax bills, but it contains no specific provision to that effect concerning regular appropriations. However, the House of Representatives has traditionally assumed the responsibility for initiating all appropriations bills and has jealously guarded this self-assumed prerogative. The practical result, as far as appropriations are concerned, is that the House Appropriations Committee is more powerful than its counterpart on the Senate side. The bulk of basic appropriations decisions are made in the House committee. The general shape of any appropriations bill is derived from House consideration of the measure. The Senate tends to review the House action and to hear appeals from agencies and outside groups seeking changes in the allotments accorded them by the House. The Senate is free to make alterations as it deems necessary, but important changes usually are limited to revisions in the financing for a relatively small number of significant or controversial federal programs.

The President's budget, submitted to Congress shortly after it assembles each January, offers the framework of the President's program for the nation in the coming year and forms the basis for congressional hearings and legislation on the year's appropriations. Together with the State of the Union address and various special messages, it forms the basis of legislative action to meet the needs of more than 230 million Americans. The budget estimates or requests that it contains are for the fiscal year, which will begin the following October 1st.

The development of the federal budget is a fascinating, almost yearlong exercise. Decisions are fashioned from a variety of political, economic, social, and sometimes emotional considerations that come into play when government policy makers divide limited dollars among a multitude of competing claims. For the Department of Health and Human Services, the Office of the Secretary devotes countless hours to budget development. Like most government agencies, HHS uses the budget process not only to chart its spending plan, but also to develop a legislative package for submission to Congress as part of the President's overall policy agenda.

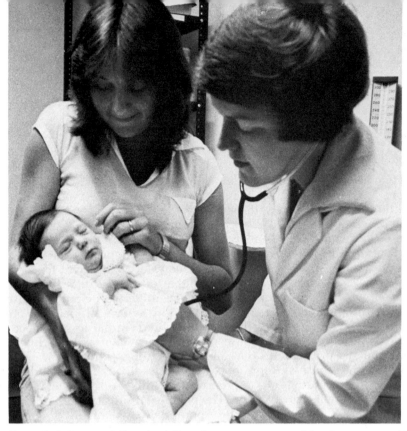

Figure 9–1. Services follow the dollars that are appropriated for their support. (Courtesy of Thomasville Times-Enterprise, Thomasville, Georgia)

BUDGET PROCESS

The budget process starts every spring at HHS, about eighteen months before it will actually go into effect, when the department establishes internal spending ceilings for each of its operating agencies. These agencies, such as the Division of Nursing, begin work on their new budgets after receiving their ceilings. In practice, the operating agencies virtually always exceed their allowances, hoping to increase their own budgets. In July, the President's Office of Management and Budget (OMB) establishes its own budget ceiling for the individual departments and agencies. Between July and the following December, the department is engaged in an internal debate over its priorities and also is involved in a similar exercise with OMB, the agency that protects the President's interests in the budget process. The central task of the OMB is to mold the spending requests of all the executive departments and agencies into an annual presidential budget. The President makes the final decisions on the major budget issues, but the OMB, with about 125 professionals working on the budget, settles dozens of issues for every one that goes to the President.

This process may be illustrated by looking at the course of the 1980 budget recommendations for the Division of Nursing. A $105 million request left the DN in the spring of 1978, and in December 1978 only a small fraction of the original left the OMB. The process of the budgetary erosion of the Division of Nursing's request is depicted in Table 9–1. The figure of $14 million was then recommended by the President in his 1980 budget request that was published and presented to Congress in January 1979.

The budget of the United States is a major instrument of national policy making. Far more than simply an economic document, it is also a political document, reflecting the level of support that the administration wants Congress to approve for the full range of federal activities. It also bears a significant relationship to the general economic condition of the nation, for a budget can be designed to stimulate the economy or to cool it off, whichever course of action seems to be the wiser one under the prevailing economic circumstances. The budget that the president submits and the actions that Congress takes in response constitute a crucial set of political decisions. These decisions are, in effect, official answers in the debate about what the federal government should do and how it should finance its activities.

During the early 1980s, many of these decisions will revolve around the controversy of spending for national defense versus spending for human resources (including health, education, and welfare programs). In constant 1979 dollars, the federal government has moved over the past quarter of a century toward more and more expenditures for human resources and appears to have reached the limits of widespread public support for the proportion of the budget going for these purposes. The statistics in Table 9–2 from the 1980 *Budget of the United States Government* indicate this trend.

Both Congress and the president, moreover, must confront a persistent and perplexing feature of budgetary politics—the contradictory attitudes of the public toward government spending. The public is typically upset about the size of the federal government and by increases in income taxes and federal spending, and it wants something to be done about these things. But the public also supports a wide range of governmental commitments— particularly with respect to health and social welfare—that inevitably require more federal intervention, increased spending, and more taxes. On the whole, however, tax revenues as a percentage of the value of all the goods and services produced in the United States in a year (GNP) have averaged about 18% to 19% as indicated in Table 9–3.

Note that in 1980 the nation's GNP was over $2.5 trillion; of course, much of its rise has been fueled by inflation. Pressure for tax cuts appears to rise significantly as the tax share of the GNP hits 20%. What this means for nursing is that the total amount of federal dollars for all human resources programs is finite, and nurses will have to fight for health care dollars that are presently going for purposes less worthwhile than quality nursing services for the public. This fight is an important task that nurses as the have-nots of the health care industry must carry out. It should not be expected that groups with less justifiable tax-supported health programs will voluntarily give up part of their share of the federal health care dollar.

CONTROLLABLE AND UNCONTROLLABLE EXPENDITURES

When President Jimmy Carter sent his fiscal year 1980 health budget recommendations to Congress January 22, 1979, as part of his overall spending proposal for the federal government for the year to start October 1, 1979, he

Table 9–1. The Course of the Fiscal Year 1980 Division of Nursing Budget in the Executive Department: How $105 million was cut to less than $15 million

	DN REQUEST	BHP ALLOWANCE	HRA ALLOWANCE	PHS ALLOWANCE	DHHS ALLOWANCE	OMB ALLOWANCE
Capitation	$30,000	$30,000	0	0	0	0
Advanced nurse training	12,000	12,000	15,300	10,000	0	0
Nurse practitioner	18,000	18,000	25,000	15,500	13,000	13,000
Special projects	20,000	20,000	7,500	7,500	7,500	1,743
Loans	0	0	0	0	0	0
Scholarships	0	0	0	0	0	0
Traineeships	15,000	15,000	13,000	8,000	0	0
Fellowships	2,000	2,000	1,500	1,000	0	0
Research grants	8,000	8,000	0	0	0	0
	$105,000	$105,000	$62,300	$42,000	$20,500	$14,743

KEY:
DN = Division of Nursing
BHP = Bureau of Health Professions
HRA = Health Resources Administration
PHS = Public Health Service
DHHS = Department of Health and Human Services
OMB = Office of Management and Budget

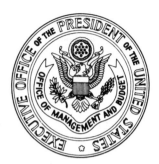

THE BUDGET OF THE UNITED STATES GOVERNMENT

FISCAL YEAR 1979

Figure 9–2. The Budget of the United States Government determines which national needs will receive priority. (Courtesy of U.S. Office of Management and Budget)

proposed an expenditure of $56.6 billion for HHS's health programs through the Public Health Service and Health Care Financing Administration. This request amounted to an $8 billion increase over comparable spending in FY 1979. It is essential to note that *controllable* health programs are those subject to annual appropriations by Congress and consist primarily of the categorical health services, training, and research programs. The *uncontrollable* programs, such as Medicare and Medicaid, provide benefits to people who become *entitled* because of age, disability, or economic status. The federal government is obligated to pay for the benefits

Table 9–2.   *Comparison of Federal Budget Expenditures for Defense with Human Resources Expenditures, 1955–1980*

Fiscal Years	Budget Total	NATIONAL DEFENSE Amount in Billions	Percent	HUMAN RESOURCES Amount in Billions	Percent
1955	185.8	108.0	58.1	39.6	21.2
1956	185.3	104.5	56.4	41.5	22.3
1957	195.3	108.0	55.3	45.0	23.1
1958	206.7	109.6	52.9	54.5	26.3
1959	225.7	112.6	49.9	59.4	26.3
1960	222.2	108.8	49.0	61.6	27.7
1961	233.6	111.2	47.7	69.5	29.8
1962	250.4	115.0	45.9	72.2	28.8
1963	257.2	115.8	45.0	75.2	29.2
1964	269.9	117.2	43.5	77.6	28.8
1965	263.7	105.5	40.1	78.7	29.9
1966	290.3	118.3	40.7	90.1	31.1
1967	331.3	143.0	43.1	106.6	32.2
1968	358.4	157.9	44.0	116.1	32.4
1969	352.1	151.4	43.0	122.6	34.8
1970	355.9	142.2	40.0	132.9	37.4
1971	364.4	130.5	35.9	154.6	42.5
1972	383.9	126.7	33.0	173.1	45.1
1973	386.3	116.7	30.2	182.3	47.2
1974	384.4	111.0	28.8	188.6	49.0
1975	424.3	111.2	26.2	219.5	51.7
1976	453.3	110.7	24.4	245.0	54.1
1977	470.4	113.9	24.2	252.0	53.6
1978	495.9	115.7	23.3	258.9	52.2
1979	493.7	117.7	23.8	259.4	52.5
1980	507.2	130.9	26.1	263.9	52.0

regardless of the cost. The only way expenditures under these programs can be controlled is through legislated changes in the authorizing legislation.

Thus, although the $191 billion that went for income security programs, such as Medicare and Medicaid, were automatically extracted from the budget because they were legislated as *entitlements,* countless other authorizations never got the appropriation needed to give them the substance that their sponsors had originally hoped they would have. As a general

Table 9–3.   *Federal Taxes as a Percent of the Gross
National Product* All Amounts in Billions*

YEAR	GNP	TAX REVENUES	TAXES AS A PERCENT OF GNP
1956	411	74	18.1
1957	433	80	18.5
1958	442	80	18.0
1959	473	79	16.7
1960	497	92	18.6
1961	508	94	18.6
1962	547	100	18.2
1963	576	107	18.5
1964	616	113	18.3
1965	657	117	17.8
1966	721	131	18.1
1967	774	150	19.3
1968	830	154	18.5
1969	904	188	20.8
1970	959	194	20.2
1971	1019	188	18.5
1972	1110	209	18.8
1973	1238	232	18.8
1974	1359	265	19.5
1975	1455	281	19.3
1976	1624	299	18.4
1977	1835	357	19.5
1978	2043	401	19.6
1979	2289	456	19.9
1980	2520	504	20.0

** GNP is essentially the annual market value of the Nation's output of
goods and services.*

proposition, it is far easier to obtain approval for programs from legislative authorizing committees and from Congress as a whole, than to convince the appropriations committees to recommend that any figure near the maximum amounts authorized be appropriated. Starving an already-authorized program is, in fact, one of the major ways in which Congress makes public policy and economizes, taking advantage of the fact that the appropriations process affords those who originally opposed the authorizing legislation another opportunity to assert their disapproval. Without bills to supply funds, no wheel of government can turn. This extremely important fact is true because of the existence of a short and simple constitutional provision: "No Money shall be drawn from the Treasury, but in Consequence of Appropriations, made by Law."

CONGRESSIONAL BUDGET TIMETABLE

Probably the most significant recent statutory change in the appropriations process was the enactment in July 1974 of the Congressional Budget and Impoundment Control Act (Public Law 93-344). Until then, Congress had reviewed the annual presidential budget in separate parts, adopting spending bills as they came to the floor from the Appropriations Committee without ever stopping to consider their overall fiscal impact. The congressional budget law requires Congress to set total spending and revenue limits each year and to stay within them when enacting appropriations bills.

The Budget Act created a congressional budget process, two budget committees, and a Congressional Budget Office. The congressional budget process requires the enactment of budget resolutions that target spending amounts for groups of related programs. By setting these targets, Congress establishes priorities among the seventeen budget *functions*. Budget accounts are generally placed in the single budget function (e.g., national defense, health) that best reflects its major end purpose addressed to an important national need, regardless of the agency administering the program. The budget resolutions go beyond the establishment of target budget priorities. They also specify appropriate levels for overall federal outlays. Unlike the resolution-setting budget function targets, the figures on overall spending are binding. Neither house is to consider any measure that would cause spending to exceed the total amount specified in the resolution.

Under the new procedures, Congress, no later than May 15, must adopt

Table 9-4.   *Congressional Budget Timetable*

DEADLINE	ACTIVITIES
November 10	Current Services budget received
January 18	President's budget received
March 15	Advice and data from all congressional committees
April 1	Congressional Budget Office reports to budget committees
April 15	Budget committees report out first budget resolution
May 15	Congressional committees report new authorizing legislation
May 15	Congress completes action on first budget resolution
Labor Day + 7	Congress completes action on all spending bills
September 15	Congress completes action on second budget resolution
September 25	Congress completes action on reconciliation bill
October 1	Fiscal year begins

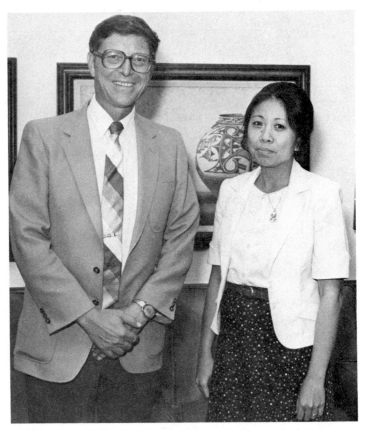

Figure 9–3. Senator Pete J. Domenici of New Mexico, Chairman of the Senate Budget Committee, with 1980 ANA Fellow and University of Michigan nursing doctoral student, Magelende R. McBride. (Courtesy of Magelende R. McBride)

a budget resolution, setting totals for receipts, outlays, and budget authority. In approving the conference report on the first fiscal 1982 budget resolution (H Con Res 115—H Rept 97–46), Congress agreed to reconciliation instructions designed to carry out President Reagan's budget-cutting plan. The instructions required 14 Senate committees and 15 House committees to revise existing programs to achieve fiscal 1982 spending cuts of approximately $36 billion. The fiscal 1982 targets, as compared to fiscal 1981 spending for the seventeen categories, are given in Table 9–5.

Congress then considers the specific revenue and appropriations bills. By September 15, action is to be completed on these measures and on a second budget resolution, which sets binding ceilings on both outlays and budget authorities and places a floor plan on receipts for the ensuing fiscal year. Any changes in revenue or spending bills already enacted or changes in the statutory limit on the debt necessitated by this second resolution must then be accomplished by September 25 so that the congressional budgetary process will be completed by October 1, when the new fiscal year begins.

Table 9–5. *The 17 Categories of the Federal Budget (Rounded Off to Nearest $Billion)*

CATEGORY	\$BILLIONS	
	1981	*1982*
National Defense		
Budget Authority	$181.0	$226.3
Outlays	162.9	188.8
International Affairs		
Budget Authority	23.6	17.4
Outlays	11.3	11.2
General Science/Space/Tech.		
Budget Authority	6.5	7.2
Outlays	6.2	7.0
Energy		
Budget Authority	7.3	4.5
Outlays	9.8	6.0
Natural Resources & Environment		
Budget Authority	10.5	8.2
Outlays	13.6	12.4
Agriculture		
Budget Authority	5.6	5.5
Outlays	2.7	4.5
Commerce & Housing Credit		
Budget Authority	6.6	7.7
Outlays	3.4	4.0
Transportation		
Budget Authority	25.0	21.2
Outlays	23.9	20.4
Community & Regional Development		
Budget Authority	8.3	7.1
Outlays	11.4	8.7
Education/Training/Employment/Social Services		
Budget Authority	30.8	26.2
Outlays	31.8	26.9
Health		
Budget Authority	72.2	83.5
Outlays	66.8	73.4
Income Security		
Budget Authority	250.4	262.7
Outlays	227.6	239.7
Veterans Benefits & Services		
Budget Authority	23.3	24.8
Outlays	22.8	24.1
Administration of Justice		
Budget Authority	4.4	4.3
Outlays	4.7	4.5
General Government		
Budget Authority	5.3	5.0
Outlays	5.0	4.9
General Purpose Fiscal Assistance		
Budget Authority	6.1	6.5
Outlays	6.8	6.4
Interest		
Budget Authority	79.5	85.7
Outlays	79.5	85.7

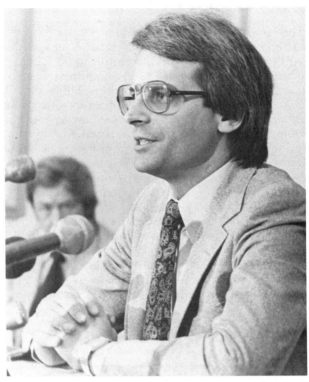

Figure 9–4. David Stockman, as director of the Office of Management and Budget, sets priorities in the President's proposed budget that is sent to Congress. (Courtesy of David Stockman, Director, Office of Management and Budget)

The totals for each budget function, such as health, are primarily targets at which Congress aims its appropriations work, but they are difficult ones to breach without compensating savings elsewhere.

The first budget resolution for fiscal year 1982 provided for total federal expenditures of $695 billion compared to income of $658 billion. The deficit for the year was, thus, to be $37 billion. Budget authority was to be limited to $771 billion. That resolution called for outlays for the health function of the budget (called the 550 function) for FY 1982 of $73 billion, while budget authority was set at $83.5 billion. The health function, however, did not include all funds for federal health activities. Included in the function were all HHS health expenditures, such as Medicare, Medicaid, the so-called controllable health programs of the Public Health Service, and several smaller programs such as mine safety, occupational safety and health, and benefits for federal employees. Excluded from this function were the health programs of the Department of Defense and the Veterans Administration, which cost nearly $12 billion in FY 1982. The amount of the resolution earmarked for HHS's controllable health programs, or those subject to annual appropriations, was to be about $10 billion in outlays and $10.6 billion in budget authority.

APPROPRIATIONS SUBCOMMITTEES

The House Committee on Appropriations has been generally recognized as extremely powerful and influential. It is a large committee (55 members during the 97th Congress, comprising 33 Democrats and 22 Republicans), which operates through 13 subcommittees, each of which exercises substantial discretion within its jurisdiction. The Senate Appropriations Committee consists of 29 members (14 Democrats and 15 Republicans). It also works through 13 subcommittees, which correspond to those in the House. Thus, when the President's budget is received, the complex and detailed work of examining and deciding on appropriations requests is conducted within these subcommittees. Both House and Senate appropriations subcommittees are set up along functional lines: Agriculture, Defense, District of Columbia, Department of Energy, Housing and Urban Development, Interior, Labor, Health and Human Services, and so on, roughly paralleling the thirteen regular appropriations bills cleared by Congress. The 1980 appropriations bills governing the spending of over $365 billion in tax funds are indicated in Table 9–6.

Generally, the members of the subcommittees become very knowledgeable and often expert in their assigned areas. The annual appropriations subcommittee hearings expose a subcommittee member to the thou-

Table 9–6.   *How Congress Directed the Expenditure of $365 Billion in 1980*

PROGRAM	AMOUNT
Agriculture, Rural Development and Related Agencies (Public Law 96-108)	$ 16,697,854,000
Defense (Public Law 96-154)	130,981,290,000
District of Columbia (Public Law 96-93)	374,200,000
Energy and Water Development (Public Law 96-69)	10,851,578,400
HUD—Independent Agencies (Public Law 96-103)	71,842,684,000
Interior (Public Law 96-126)	30,304,887,000
Labor—HHS and Ed. (Public Law 96-123)	72,552,613,000
Legislative (Public Law 96-86)	1,157,985,400
Military Construction (Public Law 96-130)	3,770,152,000
State-Justice-Commerce-Judiciary (Public Law 96-68)	8,345,591,000
Transportation (Public Law 96-131)	9,561,312,439
Treasury-Postal Service-General Government (Public Law 96-74)	8,837,278,100
Continuing Appropriations, 1980 (Public Law 96-86)	172,300,000
Further Continuing Appropriations, 1980 (Public Law 96-123)	39,800,000
Chrysler Corp. Appropriations (Public Law 96-183)	1,518,000
Total, bills for fiscal 1980	365,461,043,339

sands of purposes for which federal tax dollars are used. Because these representatives and senators are charged with the responsibility for determining the annual level of funding for each authorized program, they must constantly evaluate the worth of numerous competing interests. The 1981 membership of the House Appropriations Subcommittee on the Departments of Labor, Health and Human Services, Education and Related Agencies, chaired by Representative William H. Natcher (Democrat, Kentucky), was made up of the following twelve representatives:

WILLIAM H. NATCHER, KENTUCKY, CHAIRMAN

Democrats	Republicans
Neal Smith (Iowa)	Silvio Conte (Mass.)*
David Obey (Wis.)	George O'Brien (Ill.)
Edward Roybal (Calif.)	Carl D. Pursell (Mich.)
Louis Stokes (Ohio)	Robert Livingston (La.)
Joseph Early (Mass.)	John Porter (Ill.)
Benard Dwyer (N.J.)	

The corresponding subcommittee in the Senate, chaired by Senator Harrison Schmitt (Republican, New Mexico), was comprised of these fifteen senators:

HARRISON SCHMITT, NEW MEXICO, CHAIRMAN

Republicans	Democrats
Mark Hatfield (Oreg.)	William Proxmire (Wis.)*
Lowell Weicker (Conn.)	Robert Byrd (W.Va.)
Ted Stevens (Alaska)	Ernest Hollings (S.C.)
Mark Andrews (N.Dak.)	Thomas Eagleton (Mo.)
James Abdnor (S.Dak.)	Lawton Chiles (Fla.)
Warren Rudman (N.H.)	Quentin Burdick (N.Dak.)
Arlen Specter (Pa.)	Daniel Inouye (Hawaii)

APPROPRIATIONS FOR NURSING, 1975–1981

Each of the HHS appropriations subcommittees hold annual hearings that probe administration witnesses on the budget to fund the various health programs, including the Nurse Training Act authorities. For example, executive branch budget policy going back to the last year of the Nixon administration has attempted to slash federal support of nursing education to very limited and specific programs. It is fortunate for the development of nursing education in the nation that the Congress has defended the value and importance of continuing support of both schools of nursing and needy students. A review of the House Subcommittee on Labor-HEW or Labor-HHS appropriations hearings for fiscal years 1975 to 1980 reveals that the various

---

* Ranking minority member

Presidents and their spokespersons from HEW and HHS have held several fixed ideas regarding the adequacy of the number of nurses and quality of nursing education, ideas which have varied little from year to year. Subcommittee members' responses and reactions to the arguments put forward by administration spokespersons demonstrate that the Congress often doubts the validity of the administration's information about nurses and prefers to continue federal support of nursing education rather than jeopardize the health care delivery system. Extracts from hearings illustrate the longstanding differences between the administration's viewpoints and those held by HHS appropriations subcommittee members.

On April 30, 1975, the subcommittee heard witnesses from the administration in support of rescissions of over $54 million, which called for an elimination of capitation funds for nursing schools, of financial distress grants, and of nurse traineeships that supported graduate nursing students. In addition, cutbacks on awards for health teaching facilities construction would halt all new federal support for expanding nursing teaching facilities. In his opening remarks, Dr. Henry Simmons, acting deputy assistant secretary for health, announced the administration's policy on health manpower programs: "These reductions reflect our proposal to change the focus of health manpower programs from a primarily categorical emphasis to one which attempts to alleviate the problems of geographical and specialty distributions." Specifically the administration's conclusions with regard to nursing education were that "across-the-board federal subsidies of nurse training are not warranted," because the increased supply of registered nurses demonstrated both the attractiveness of the profession and the responsiveness of the nursing labor market.[1]

During questioning by the subcommittee members, several problems emerged with regard to the administration's conclusion about nursing education. For example, Representative Daniel Flood (Democrat, Pennsylvania) referred Dr. Kenneth Endicott, administrator of the Health Resources Administration, to the impressive and comprehensive report issued by the House Committee on Interstate and Foreign Commerce that was compiled in conjunction with the Nurse Training Act of 1975. This report stated that there was a current shortage of 50,000 nurses. When Dr. Endicott had no response to the Interstate and Foreign Commerce Committee's report, he simply changed the subject to an explanation of the current status of diploma school nurse preparation. Other committee members brought up the question of the supply of nurses. Neal Smith (Democrat, Iowa) remained unimpressed with Dr. Simmons' figures that the U.S. would have one nurse for every 100 people by 1980; the representative noted that "in my observation, in spite of the high unemployment rates we have, no nurse is looking for a job if she wants to work." Edward Patten (Democrat, New Jersey) asked, "Where do you have a surplus? I know everything I see and hear in my area shows we are in a tough bind for nurses."[2]

Administration and congressional leaders also have interpreted the evidence on the effect of capitation support for nursing schools in different ways. Dr. Endicott noted that "the Administration has always opposed capitation to nursing schools" because the greatest growth in nursing enrollments occurred before the use of capitation grants. Furthermore, the admin-

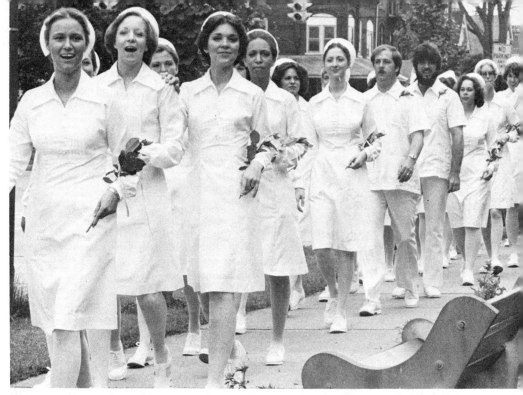

Figure 9–5. *Representative Neal Smith observed that, contrary to the administration's views, there was a strong demand for the graduates of nursing education programs. (Courtesy of Call-Chronicle, Allentown, Pennsylvania)*

istration felt that because capitation represented little more than 10% of nursing schools' incomes, the amount could be easily absorbed by increased tuitions. Mr. Patten of New Jersey, however, recounted the value of capitation grants to schools of nursing in his area, which essentially used the funds to develop and expand training in clinical specialties and in graduate programs. Silvio Conte (Republican, Massachusetts) brought up another direct result of eliminating capitation funds: the immediate increase in tuition payments that would have to be met by low- and middle-income families. Dr. Endicott claimed that the nurses could receive assistance from the same funds as any other student, through the guaranteed loan program of the Office of Education. But Mr. Conte argued that when he spoke with a representative from the Office of Education, it was stated "that Office of Education programs don't really work for professional and paraprofessional training in the health fields, including nursing." With regard to graduate education support, which was to be eliminated, Dr. Endicott admitted that a nurse would need about $15,000 a year to participate in a graduate nursing program. But he felt that graduate nurses "would do as other graduate students do; that is, borrow the money."[3]

In discussion regarding the management staff of the Health Resources Administration, Mr. Smith of Iowa asked Dr. Endicott, "How many management personnel are directly under you?" to which Dr. Endicott answered, "There would be about 100." Mr. Smith: "How many of them are nurses?" Dr. Endicott: "In my immediate staff, none." Mr. Smith proceeded to note, "It seems to me that maybe in the management of an agency or administration like yours, where you have 100 people and you are dealing with nurses' training, it seems a little bit strange to me we wouldn't have any nurses in on the management, helping to make the decisions . . . [where] decisions are going to be made as to whether or not you will support or not support nurses' training." Despite Endicott's attempt at a defense, he had to admit that nurses were not represented at his level.[4]

MORE OF THE SAME

Hearings for the fiscal year 1976 Division of Nursing budget, early in the Ford administration, covered much the same territory. For the coming fiscal year, the administration proposed a nurse training budget of $33.5 million, which cut out capitation grants and financial distress grants entirely, limited advanced nurse training grants to $1 million, eliminated all traineeship support, and substantially cut funds designated for student loans. With regard to the traineeship grants, Dr. Endicott felt that the "sufficient promise of increased earnings" would continue to attract nurses to graduate schools without the incentive of federal scholarship support.[5]

The subcommittee once more went over the issue of the supply of nurses as Dr. Endicott boldly claimed, "The most pressing problem which confronts the nation is the maldistribution of nurses, with surpluses and even unemployment [of nurses] in some areas." He argued that adjusting the pay scales of nurses would be more effective in relieving shortage problems than anything else. However, upon questioning by Bob Michel (Republican, Illinois), Dr. Endicott could not "name a specific place where a surplus exists," claiming that nursing surpluses relate to temporary general economic trends. Endicott did recognize a shortage of baccalaureate prepared nurses, perhaps reflected in the retention of some funds in the budget for loans and scholarships.[6]

In hearings for the fiscal year 1977 budget for nurse training, February 19, 1976, the administration proposed a reduced level of support similar to that advanced for FY 1976. That is, the budget for nurse training would provide modest support for loans and scholarships for undergraduates, no money for capitation or traineeships for graduate students, and an increased amount for support of nurse-practitioner training ($2 million increased to $7 million). As Neal Smith (Democrat, Iowa) noted, "Now, I noticed in the justifications the same old story with regard to nursing assistance. It's been going on for several years . . . . You are not basing a reduction like that in nursing assistance on the theory there isn't any nursing shortage, are you?" Secretary of HEW, David Mathews, spokesperson for the administration, answered, "No, as a matter of fact, we have some new initiatives in training for nurses." However, these "new initiatives" were merely more attempts to correct the geographic maldistribution of nurses by offering to forgive their guaranteed student loans. After Mathews admitted the administration's resistance to nursing support, Smith remarked, "That's an annual exercise." Secretary Mathews argued that the department had no evidence that increasing the total supply of nurses helped the maldistribution problem, but Congressman Smith countered, "Put it another way, there is no evidence that increasing the number of nurses in that area wouldn't help us there."[7]

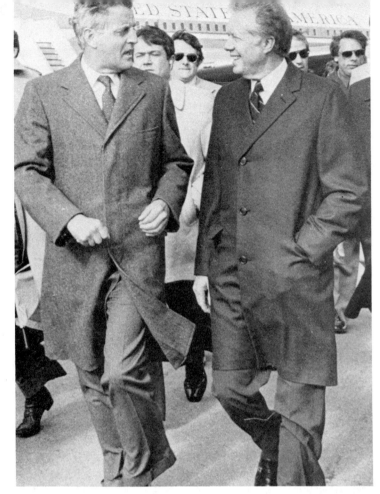

Figure 9–6. *The Carter administration consistently refused to recognize the need for federal assistance for nursing education and nursing research. (Courtesy of New York Times, New York)*

The president's budget for fiscal year 1978 again proposed no funds for capitation, financial distress grants, advanced nurse training, loans, traineeships, or loan repayments. The only support to nurses deemed necessary by President Carter was $9 million for nurse practitioner training, $6 million for special projects, and $9 million for scholarships. HEW Secretary Joseph Califano, Jr. presented the administration's viewpoint on this issue by stating that "it is basically that we feel we are able to get an adequate number of nurses without federal funds for these training programs." When Mr. Califano was asked to speak specifically to the cuts in support of nurse training, the secretary admitted that he knew very little about the matter: "I guess I would have to say in all candor, I take the judgment of the people in whom I have confidence . . . that the nurses would be there without this federal contribution." Califano submitted the following in his written rationale for the cutbacks: "There is no serious overall shortage of nurses which would justify a continuation of general federal support for nursing schools."[8]

In hearings for the fiscal year 1979 budget, February 21, 1978, Mr. Califano again admitted his lack of absolute certainty of his information

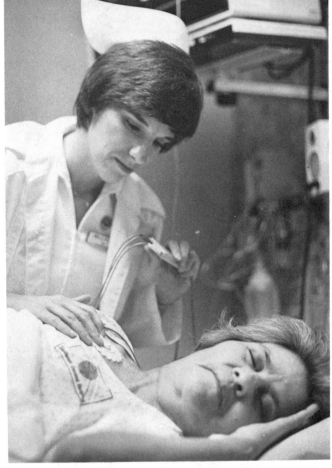

Figure 9–7. Who cares for those who care? Congressman Silvio Conte bluntly suggested that "the nurses have been done in" as far as the 1979 budget was concerned. (Courtesy San Antonio Express News, San Antonio, Texas)

about nurses. "I am, in all candor, surer of our judgment with respect to doctors and the excessive numbers of doctors in specialties than I am of our numbers with respect to nurses." However, Mr. Califano felt no difficulty in asking the Appropriations subcommittee to limit support to nurse training to a paltry $20.5 million, which would cover only nurse practitioner grants and special projects. Silvio Conte of Massachusetts suggested bluntly, "The nurses have been done in here," and reminded the secretary that the demands made by a new national health system would undoubtedly require more nurses. Mr. Califano expressed a further lack of thought when he defended his belief in a "surplus of nurses" because of a comparison with the widely publicized surplus of schoolteachers. He feared that registered nurses would soon find themselves in the position of the nation's schoolteachers—unable to find work. Joseph Early (Democrat, Massachusetts) then asked the secretary about the discrepancy between his estimate of the future demand for nurses and that prepared by the Department of Labor, which listed nursing as a "shortage profession." Mr. Califano didn't understand why the discrepancy existed, but promised to "get [together] with Secretary Marshall."[9]

CONTINUED OPPOSITION BY THE PRESIDENT

In January and February of 1980, the subcommittee again heard the testimony of administration officials, this time regarding the proposed budget for fiscal year 1981. The total budget authority of the Department of Health and Human Services proposed for 1981 stood at $223 billion, of which the subcommittee was asked to approve $56 billion. The budget request for the nursing programs was only $28 million, down from $106 million appropriated in the 1980 budget. All support for capitation grants, advanced nurse training, nursing scholarships, professional traineeships, nurse fellowships, and research grants was eliminated from the 1981 budget. In addition to the budget proposed for 1981, administration officials suggested that their new health manpower legislation, which would replace both the Health Professions Educational Assistance Act and the Nurse Training Amendments, would reflect the administration's belief that health manpower plans needed to be directed toward alleviating specific problems of geographic and specialty maldistribution rather than toward encouraging the growth in the aggregate number of health professionals.

Several members of the Appropriations Subcommittee questioned administration officials on the manner in which the nursing education programs had been routinely ignored by the administration. In general, they expressed concern that the Department of Health and Human Services was decreasing governmental encouragement of nursing education without having found any solution to the problem of a nursing shortage. Patricia Roberts Harris, Secretary of Health and Human Resources, answered Mr. Conte's question on why the President insisted upon eliminating support for nursing students despite the notorious shortage of nurses that could be documented in almost every newspaper in the country. She simply reiterated the administration's already-established argument that there were enough "trained nurses" and concluded that the problem was that too many nurses were not active in nursing jobs. It was her opinion that the nurse training funds were being used improperly to train nurses who ended up as secretaries and administrative assistants.[10]

During testimony from several officials of the Public Health Service, Congressman Pursell made frequent attempts to discover the locus of decision making on health policy, especially with respect to nursing, within the administration. At one point he suggested that, in fact, the OMB, not the Department of Health and Human Resources, was formulating health policy, and hoped that one day nurses might participate in the area of national health policy formulation. Pursell asked Dr. Henry Foley, administrator of the Health Resources Administration, that in relation to the composition of the National Council of Health Planning and Development, whether or not any nurses were included on the council. Foley replied that there were no nurses and that the authorizing statute did not indicate the need for including nurses on the council. Representative Pursell again tried to pin down the source of decisions on health policy during the testimony of Charles Miller, Deputy Assistant Secretary for Health Operations. Miller, although offering to provide the information in the future, claimed it was "virtually impossible" to draw a line around any specific number of those who contributed to the formulation of health policy, but he promised to give it a try.[11]

Throughout the hearings, congressmen returned to the subject of nursing education. Mr. Conte repeated his question, asked earlier of Secretary Harris, to Dr. Julius Richmond, Assistant Secretary for Health and the Assistant Secretary for the Surgeon General, about the reason for the administration's repeated attempts to eliminate support for nursing education. Dr. Richmond restated the premise that increasing the output of nurses would not solve the nursing shortage and pointed to the study of the Institute of Medicine as a hope for finding a better solution. Representative Conte felt that the supply should not be cut down during the study. Furthermore, Conte suggested that the Public Health Service look into providing financial support for hospital schools: "What is happening now is that 99 percent of the nurses are coming out of college and they all want to be in administration and nobody wants to change the bed pan or give a back massage. Those were the great nurses . . . . We have gotten away from it. We have to get back to that." Dr. Richmond agreed with Mr. Conte's nostalgic reflection on the merits of nurses past and pointed out that there is a great deal of confusion among nurses today, stemming in a large part from concerns about professional status.[12]

HOW THE COMMITTEES WORK

In reviewing the consideration of the nursing budget over the past few years, it is important to note that the House Appropriations Committee is composed in large part of senior members in the House elected from safe congressional districts. It is a predominantly conservative body that believes it has a duty to reduce the budget to a level that the nation can afford. This attitude is exemplified by the distinctive vocabulary used by committee members. When describing what they often do to the budgetary bills submitted by the administration, they use verbs such as cut, curb, slice, prune, whittle, squeeze, wring, chop, and slash. The tools of the trade are likewise referred to as knife, blade, meat-axe, scalpel, meat-cleaver, hatchet, shears, ringer, and fine-tooth comb.

As noted earlier, Senate Appropriations subcommittees are viewed more as appellate groups that listen to various witnesses requesting the restoration of funds cut by the House. The Senate members have additional committee assignments, sometimes serving on both the authorizing committee and the appropriations subcommittee for an agency or program. Senate subcommittees generally do not engage in the lengthy or detailed work of the House subcommittees. The Senate Appropriations subcommittees frequently restore some of the funds denied by the House, although they may make cuts in other places.

The decision-making process on Senate appropriations legislation is much less subcommittee-dominated than it is in the House; as a consequence the independent influence of the Senate Appropriations Committee is considerably less than that of the House counterpart. The full Senate itself may add or restore more when the bill reaches the floor. Many recent health appropriations bills have carried larger total amounts when they passed the

Senate than when they passed the House. The differences are resolved in conference, generally by splitting the difference between the two chambers.

Another important function performed by the appropriations process occurs in the course of the hearings. The subcommittees do not confine themselves to the examination of budgetary requests for the future operations of the agency. Instead, they often devote considerable time and effort to a review of the agency's performance in the past. In this manner, the subcommittees perform what has become increasingly the major preoccupation of Congress: *oversight,* or the supervision of policy implementation in the executive branch. This function of oversight affords subcommittees ample opportunity to have an impact on agency policy. Critical comments made by subcommittee members about the ways an agency has been performing are disregarded by HHS officials only at extreme peril. Retaliation in the form of budgetary cuts for the unresponsive witnesses' home agency in HHS provides a sanction of great effectiveness, the next time around. On occasion, specific policy directives are contained in the subcommittees' reports, which accompany the appropriations bill to the floor. The appropriations process thus serves a dual policy-making role. It establishes the level of funding for an agency and also provides an agency with specific policy guidelines.

AFTER THE MONEY HAS BEEN APPROPRIATED

Once the necessary legislation has been passed to provide an agency with an appropriation for the fiscal year, the director of OMB (acting for the president) is responsible for ensuring that the budget authority is used in an effective and orderly manner. This is usually accomplished by apportioning funds to the agency, usually on a quarterly basis or in relation to certain activities or programs. If, despite the apportionment, additional funds are urgently needed, requests for supplemental appropriations may be sent to Congress where they are considered in supplemental appropriations bills for the current fiscal years.

It is also possible for the President to recommend to Congress that budget authority provided for an agency program not be used. If this non-use is to be temporary, it is called a *deferral* and the President transmits a special message to Congress with his request and supporting information for temporarily holding up expenditure of the appropriated funds. If either the House or Senate disapproves the request, the funds must be made available for obligation. In no case can a deferral go beyond the fiscal year. If the President determines for reasons of fiscal policy or otherwise that the appropriated money for a program is not needed at all, or may essentially be wasted if used, he sends to Congress a special message requesting a *rescission* of the funds. If not approved by both houses of Congress within forty-five working days, the rescission request fails, and the funds must be made available for obligation. This procedure, adopted in 1974, substantially restricts the President's discretionary spending authority and is designed specifically to prevent impoundment, the refusal to spend appropriated funds.

These new procedures were legislated after President Nixon, unable to gain congressional approval of many of his 1973 budgetary cuts, simply refused to spend appropriated money for an enormous range of social and domestic programs. Beneficiaries of the programs went to federal courts to challenge his impoundments, and nearly every judge ruled in their favor. In an unprecedented move in the nursing circles, the National League for Nursing in 1973 filed suit against Roy Ash, director of the Office of Management and Budget, and Caspar Weinberger, Secretary of the Department of Health, Education and Welfare, to compel the release of $22 million appropriated for capitation grants to schools of nursing. The NLN complaint alleged that "the acts of the Secretary and the OMB Director are illegal. The reduction of the amounts obligated for such annual capitation grants by the Secretary and the failure to obligate all funds appropriated for the grant program violates the intent of Congress in passing the Act and in appropriating funds for its implementation."[13]

On June 29, 1973, Judge John Pratt of the U.S. District Court of the District of Columbia granted a temporary restraining order as a result of the legal action taken by the NLN. The restraining order in effect froze the nursing funds and thus prevented the monies from reverting to the U.S. Treasury Funds at the end of the fiscal year, midnight June 30, 1973. On

Figure 9–8. The release of impounded federal funds facilitated the continuation of nursing education programs throughout the nation. (Courtesy of Public Relations Department, Bridgeport Hospital, Bridgeport, Connecticut)

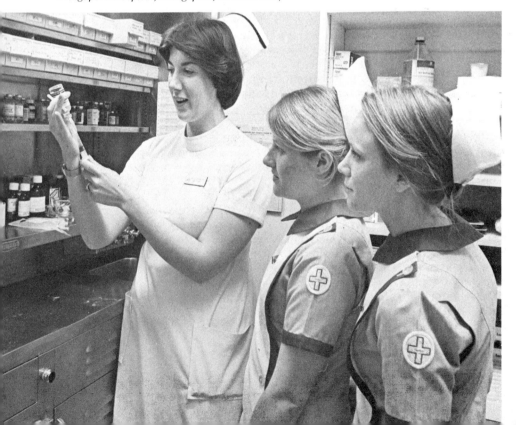

July 10, a preliminary injunction was issued by a U.S. District Judge, in favor of the NLN in its suit. Six months later a federal judge ordered the release of the $22 million of impounded federal funds to schools of nursing that were members of the National League for Nursing. Thus, the Department of Health, Education and Welfare released the impounded capitation grant funds to 948 programs of nursing in hospitals, colleges, and universities throughout the United States. After this action, an additional $52 million of additional impounded nursing program appropriations were also released. Court action, however, was a time-consuming and contentious process; Congress wanted procedures of its own to put a stop to such impoundments, and those procedures became part of the 1974 Congressional Budget and Impoundment Control Act.

President Gerald Ford tried to bend the rescission procedure to force his spending policies on Congress. For fiscal 1975, he reported rescissions and deferrals totaling $29 billion, $10 billion more than President Nixon ever had impounded at one time. He regularly proposed to rescind appropriations in the identical amounts by which Congress had exceeded his own budget requests. Ford took advantage of the impoundment control provision that allowed him to withhold funds proposed for rescission for forty-five days of continuous congressional session, while Congress was deciding whether to approve the rescission. At least twice, he waited until after he had already withheld the funds for some weeks before proposing rescissions, and in some cases this action came late enough in the fiscal year so that authority to spend the funds expired before the forty-five days of continuous congressional session. Thus, there was no way for Congress to force the President to spend money.

THE 1979 BATTLE TO KEEP NURSING FUNDS

Rescissions have proved to be a common problem for nurses. One of the more serious attempts to cancel part of an appropriation for nursing came on February 22, 1979, when the subcommittee of the Committee on Appropriations of the House of Representatives heard testimony from administration witnesses who defended President Carter's request to rescind $84 million from nurse training programs from the fiscal year 1979 budget.

Dr. Henry Foley, administrator of the Health Resources Administration, argued that because the number of active nurses had grown from 291 per 100,000 population in 1968 to 395 per 100,000 population in 1977, the continuation of current support for nurse training could not be justified.

Foley identified the greatest problems in nursing manpower as the geographic maldistribution of nurses within the country and the lack of incentives to induce nurses to work unpopular hospital shifts or to work in nursing homes; he reiterated throughout his testimony that the nation currently had enough nurses to meet health needs and that projected needs until 1990 also appeared to be met with current numbers of nurses. Furthermore, he maintained that the use of capitation funds and special scholarship funds for nurses did not contribute toward the easing of geographic maldistribution or the kinds of current vacancies in the nursing job market. The subcommittee also heard the testimony of Suzanne H. Woolsey, associate director for Human Resources, Veterans and Labor, from the Office of

Management and Budget. Ms. Woolsey re-emphasized the major policy decisions inherent in Foley's proposed rescission of health manpower funding: to restrain the growth in federal spending by retargeting resources and reducing low-priority programs such as assistance to the nursing profession. The OMB fully supported Foley's proposed nursing rescissions.

It was a great shock for nurses to learn that on February 22, 1979, the House of Representatives Labor-HEW Appropriations Subcommittee had voted to rescind $38.7 million from these funds. The committee restored funds over Carter's request, but cuts still took $10 million from capitation, $6 million from advanced nurse training, $7.5 million from special projects, $3.5 million from scholarships, $6.5 million from traineeships, $750,000 from loan repayments, $647,000 from fellowships, and $3,899,000 from research. Almost all of the remaining funds left in these categories had already been expended in the first and second quarters of the year. Thus,

Figure 9–9. If the President had his wish, a substantial proportion of the 1979 appropriations for nursing student loans and scholarships would immediately become unavailable, and the quantity and quality of patient care would suffer. (Courtesy of Fort Wayne News-Sentinel, Fort Wayne, Indiana)

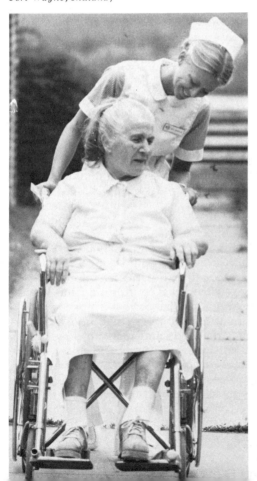

projects could be shut down as early as April 1, 1980, not even leaving two weeks for termination notices to employees.

ACTION MOVES TO THE HOUSE FLOOR

Action then moved to the full 55-member Appropriations Committee and then to the House floor. Endorsing its subcommittee decision, as usual, on Thursday, March 1, the House Appropriations Committee voted, without debate, to recommend the rescissions to the 435-member House of Representatives. On March 6, 1979, the House turned its attentions to the consideration of the Rescission Bill. Jamie Whitten (Democrat, Mississippi), Chairman of the House Committee on Appropriations, introduced the bill and urged his colleagues to accept it as recommended. After Mr. Whitten's opening remarks, Harley Staggers (Democrat, West Virginia) introduced an amendment to the bill, which restored $17 million in funds for advanced nurse training, traineeships, nursing research, and nursing fellowships.

Representative Staggers opened his argument by reminding his colleagues: "We have an obligation to our fellow citizens to assure that an adequate supply of well trained, highly competent health professionals continues to be available to all in need." Mr. Staggers explained that the Nurse Training Act of 1978 (vetoed by the president) had directed the Department of HEW to prepare a "comprehensive study of the need for continued federal financial support for nursing education and to make legislative recommendations to the Congress based on the findings." Because the study had been scrapped with the legislation, neither the administration nor Congress had the "data . . . necessary to make the informed decisions that are needed." More incredible to Mr. Staggers was the fact that the President had gone on record in support of advanced training and expanded roles for nurses, yet his rescissions cut the heart out of the advanced training programs.[14]

William Natcher (Democrat, Kentucky), chairman of the House HEW Appropriations Subcommittee, led the opposition to the Staggers amendment by calling attention to the fact that the rescission proposal was the "first test" of the House's ability to support the President's policy of controlling the federal budget. Mr. Natcher claimed, "Not a single member of this subcommittee [Labor-HEW Appropriations] is against the nursing training program," and as if to emphasize his sympathy with the nurses, he pointed out the funds that had *not* been rescinded as requested by the President. The weight of Natcher's defense of the rescissions rested upon his repeated assertion that no authorizing legislation had been passed to allow the House to appropriate money for nurse training in 1979, as the program had been funded by a continuing resolution. Natcher urged Staggers and his committee to produce a bill so that the Appropriations Committee could consider it according to formal rules. Representative Staggers answered Natcher's remarks by reminding him that there had not been time to authorize a bill yet, although the first bill that he had introduced in the 96th Congress had been the nurse training bill; furthermore, the continuing resolution had promised interim authorization until the bill could be passed formally. Congressman Natcher finally identified his main objection when he noted: "I do not believe that any bill during the calendar year of 1979 that carries any money in it and is vetoed by the President of the United States will be overridden on this floor." In other words, Mr. Natcher doubted Staggers' ability to carry through authorizing legislation for nurse training beyond the $15 million earmarked by the administration in the 1980 budget.[15]

However, several persuasive speakers rose in defense of Staggers amendment. Tim Lee Carter (Republican, Kentucky), although noting that he shared the president's concern about inflation, submitted to the House that the rescissions would have a severe impact on programs that trained health personnel throughout the country. Dr. Carter listed all the effects that losing $17 million would have on nurse training programs: the "abrupt termination of faculty" on 23 graduate nursing programs; the loss of tuition support for 2000 enrolled graduate nursing students; the termination of 60 special projects; 3500 undergraduate nursing students from low-income families would lose their scholarships; capitation support to nursing schools would be cut by 33%; and 30 nursing research projects would have to be terminated. Representative Carter felt that these cuts would have an adverse effect nationwide and knew the adverse effects which would occur in his own state, which was already "medically underserved." He concluded that without full information on the nation's nursing needs, the members should wait until the Health subcommittee reviewed nursing programs before "altering our policies with regard to nurse training."[16]

Robert Drinan (Democrat, Massachusetts) rose in support of restoring all funds to nursing programs. He felt the cutbacks were bound to have a "detrimental effect on nursing education and our health delivery system." In Massachusetts alone, 65% of nursing undergraduates depended upon federal tuition support, and some 3500 students nationwide came from low-income families. In addition to striking a blow to education opportunities for the poor, the proposed rescissions would further "limit . . . career opportunities and advancement" for women who still comprised the majority of nurses. Furthermore, Drinan reminded the House that as "we move toward a program of national health insurance, we can only expect these roles [for nurses] to be further expanded."[17]

Congressman Carl Pursell followed up these remarks by identifying an underlying problem affecting the quality of any future federal role in supporting nurse training legislation: "the proposed new Nurse Training Act is being developed by a task force in the Administration without any input at this time from the nursing profession in the United States of America—I think that is an insult to the nurses." Representative Waxman seconded Pursell's remarks and added his own concerns about the harm rendered to ongoing programs if funding was abruptly terminated. Mr. Waxman continued by repeating the adverse effects upon both the nursing profession and the health care system mentioned earlier by Representatives Carter and Drinan. Waxman also felt that many poor and rural communities depended upon nursing professionals with advanced training for their only health care, and the House risked exacerbating the health problems of these communities if they cut off funds for advanced training. He ended his remarks with this advice: "We ought to wait until the authorization committee goes forward with full hearings, before determining the fate of advanced education for nurses."[18]

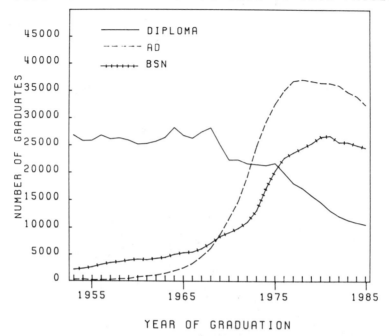

GRADUATIONS FROM BASIC RN PROGRAMS:
1953 TO 1979 ACTUAL AND 1980 TO 1985 PROJECTED

YEAR OF GRADUATION

Figure 9–10. Aware of the decline in graduations from schools of nursing, Representative Carl Pursell charged that the Carter Administration's refusal to consider nursing input into federal nursing decisions was "an insult to the nurses." (Courtesy of History and Politics of Nursing, University of Michigan)

Jamie Whitten, who introduced the proposed rescissions, rose for a full-scale defense of the cuts. He felt it necessary to explain to his colleagues that $13 million of the amount to be recovered was earmarked to "enable certain nurses to get a graduate degree or a Ph.D. degree." Since Whitten could not fathom the value of advanced degrees for nurses, he appeared to expect his fellow representatives to be likewise shocked by this news and join him in support of the rescission. When Mr. Staggers rose to defend the need for nurses with advanced training, Mr. Whitten changed the subject quickly by moving to a new rationale: "I believe we should stay with the committee recommendations because this is a kind of test about our fiscal resolve."[19]

Silvio Conte, member of the House Labor-HEW Appropriations Subcommittee, also spoke in support of the rescission, hoping to "clear the air on it." In a fulsome speech, Mr. Conte related, ". . . it grieves and it hurts me" to go along with the rescission. After all, he pointed out, his own wife was a registered nurse, and "I think I know something about nurses." But his sense of fiscal responsibility impelled him to "urge the Members to accept" the proposed rescissions. Despite the objections to the Staggers amendment, the full House of Representatives embarked on the unusual move of overturning its Appropriations committee's recommendation on a vote of 262 to 139 and restored $17 million of the nursing funds (leaving $21 million to be rescinded). It was now the Senate's turn to consider the rescission bill.[20]

THE SENATE CONSIDERS THE RESCISSION BILL

The Senate Appropriations Committee, chaired by Senator Warren Magnuson, submitted its recommendations on HR 2439 for full Senate consideration on March 14, 1979. The committee proposed to cut only $16 million from nurse training funds, an improvement of $5 million over the House figures. The first amendment to the committee's proposal was submitted by

Figure 9–11. The women members of the House of Representatives in the 96th Congress consistently supported funding for the Nurse Training Act. (Courtesy Dale Wittner, Camera 5, New York)

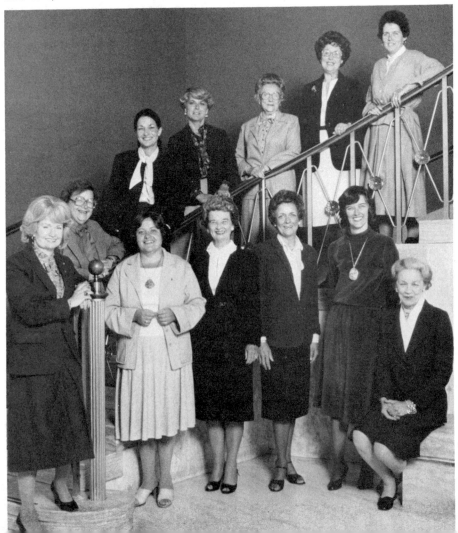

J. Bennett Johnston, Jr. (Democrat, Louisiana), who asked that his colleagues support the President's entire $84 million rescission request.
Senator Edward Kennedy spoke against the Johnston amendment, referring
his "good friend and colleague" from Louisiana to a number of Louisiana
newspaper articles documenting the nursing shortage in various parts of
Johnston's home state.[21]

Robert Morgan (Democrat, North Carolina) also supported Kennedy
and offered the most pro-nursing stand heard in the afternoon's debate. In
addition to his opinion that President Carter would be better off to concentrate his efforts on the proposed 1980 Nurse Training Act instead of reneg-
ing on current commitments, Morgan asked a very pertinent question: Who
could say that 395 nurses per 100,000 of the population was an adequate

*Figure 9–12. Can more than a thousand newspaper editors be wrong? Senator Morgan was
skeptical of the Carter administration's "evidence of a nurse surplus" (Courtesy of Carolyn
Hohnke, Nursing in the Mass Media Research Project, University of Michigan)*

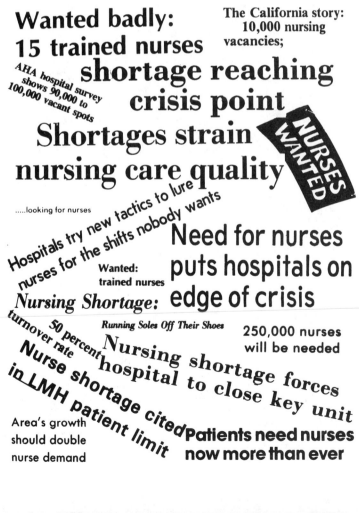

number? The Senator from North Carolina asked to see some guidelines or standards by which to judge what was an adequate number of registered nurses. In very clear reference to the 1978 and early 1979 survey of newspaper articles documenting the nation's nurse shortage, which had been gathered by the Nursing in the Mass Media Research Project of the University of Michigan School of Nursing, Senator Morgan argued that the question of nursing supply definitely remained to be resolved.

The Johnston amendment failed by a vote of 83 to 14, and the full Senate went along with its Appropriations Committee's recommendation of a $16 million cut in the 1979 funds for nursing. The bill then went to a conference committee where it was agreed that the lesser cuts of the Senate for the nursing programs be endorsed. Both the full House and the full Senate agreed on this course of action on March 27, 1979, and the 1979 nursing appropriation survived as the focal point of a very serious attempt to destroy federal assistance for nursing education and nursing research.

The recent appropriations battles between the executive branch and the Congress over the continuance or near termination of federal funds for nursing education have brought more nurses into contact with their representatives and senators than ever before. As some of the nurses who have been involved in the lobbying activities have come to realize, in the American system, congressmen's relationships to their constituencies are paramount. Even though both Republican and Democratic presidents have backed the efforts to cut nurses out of the federal budget despite all rational evidence to the contrary, same-party representatives and senators have voted on the basis of constituency interests. Up to the present time, these interests have been often expressed quite independently of what one might call the *nurse vote*. The next chapter discusses activities that can make the term *nurse vote* as potent a political force as the *teacher's vote* and the *physicians' vote*.

References

1. U.S. Congress. House. Committee on Appropriations: Departments of Labor and Health, Education and Welfare Appropriations: Rescissions for FY 1975. Hearings before the Committee. Washington, DC, United States Government Printing Office, 1975
2. Ibid
3. Ibid
4. Ibid
5. U.S. Congress. House. Committee on Appropriations: Departments of Labor and Health, Education and Welfare Appropriations for 1976. Hearings before the Committee. Washington, DC, United States Government Printing Office, 1975
6. Ibid
7. U.S. Congress. House. Committee on Appropriations: Departments of Labor and Health, Education and Welfare Appropriations for 1977. Hearings before the Committee. Washington, DC, United States Government Printing Office, 1976
8. U.S. Congress. House. Committee on Appropriations: Departments of Labor and Health, Education and Welfare Appropriations: 1978. Hearings before the Committee. Washington, DC, United States Government Printing Office, 1977
9. U.S. Congress. House. Committee on Appropriations: Departments of Labor and Health, Education and Welfare Appropriations for 1979. Hearings before the Committee. Washington, DC, United States Government Printing Office, 1978

10. U.S. Congress. House. Committee on Appropriations: Departments of Labor and Health, Education and Welfare Appropriations for 1981. Hearings before the Committee. Washington, DC, United States Government Printing Office, 1980
11. Ibid
12. Ibid
13. Division of Nursing Documents Unpublished, DN Office Files: Interview with Ray Blackburn. Bethesda, Md, Jan 22, 1975
14. Congressional Record, pp H1071–H1072, Mar 6, 1979
15. Ibid, p H1073
16. Ibid, pp H1074–H1075
17. Ibid, p H1075–H1076
18. Ibid, p H1076
19. Ibid, p H1079
20. Ibid, pp H1080–H1083
21. Congressional Record, Mar 14, 1979

10–Political Participation

Who is active in politics and who is not? Why do people become politically active, and to what degree do nurses participate in politics? The answers to this set of questions are of vital concern to a growing number of nurses who realize the necessity of *expanded political participation,* which refers to activities of citizens aimed at influencing the selection of governmental leaders and the actions that they take once in office. The goal of political participation is to make a continuing impact on decisions made by the government, not just to participate during elections. The nurse who becomes involved in a variety of political acts can effectively expand her influence far beyond a single vote.

Nurses, like all other individuals in a democracy, may run for public office; take part in marches, demonstrations, and sit-ins; make financial contributions to political candidates or causes; attend political meetings, speeches, and rallies; and write letters to public officials or newspapers. They may also join organizations that support particular candidates and take stands on certain public issues, wear political buttons or place bumper stickers on their cars, attempt to influence friends while discussing candidates or issues, vote in elections, or merely follow an issue or campaign in the mass media. Participation in the political system is the core of democracy. It makes possible the formulation of societal goals on the basis of widespread citizen involvement. Besides allowing for the expression of the wants and needs of nurses, political activities foster a feeling of satisfaction, of belonging, and of responsibility. As a result of participation, a personal investment in and consequent positive regard for our government despite its imperfections, typically occurs.

LEVELS OF PARTICIPATION

Milbrath classified citizens into four distinct groups according to level of political participation: (1) the apathetics, (2) the spectator activities, (3) the transitional activities, and (4) the gladiatorial activities (Fig. 10–2).[1] Starting at the bottom of the hierarchy, the apathetics, or inactives, engage in virtually no political activity, whereas the gladiators participate in the highest forms of politics such as working actively to get someone elected or running for office themselves.

These kinds of political participation require different amounts of effort and yield different amounts of return. Some participation makes only minimal demands on the citizen in terms of time, preparation, personal commitment, and risk. Other forms are much more expensive and are therefore engaged in by far fewer people. In general, the return that follows from any individual's investment in participation is directly related to the quantity and quality of involvement. For example, exposing oneself to political stim-

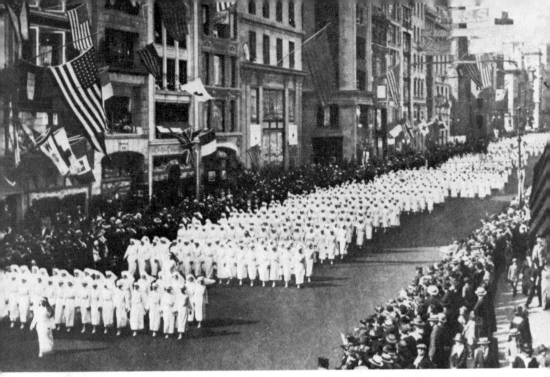

Figure 10–1. *While nurses have been the leaders among all groups of women in defending our democracy, they have been remiss in most forms of political participation. Nurses rally for the defense of the nation in World War I. (Courtesy of History of Nursing Collection, University of Michigan)*

uli or being subservient to the law are kinds of participation that are almost passive and yield little if any return in terms of the individual's personal resources. Voting requires slightly more investment and yields more of a return. Joining a group, becoming active in a group, and leading a group all increase both the investment and the potential for control of additional

Figure 10–2. *A hierarchy of political involvement. (Milbrath LW: Political Participation, p 18. Chicago, Rand McNally, 1965)*

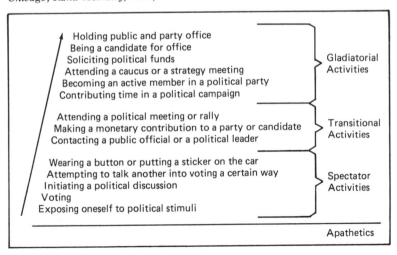

Holding public and party office
Being a candidate for office
Soliciting political funds
Attending a caucus or a strategy meeting
Becoming an active member in a political party
Contributing time in a political campaign

Gladiatorial Activities

Attending a political meeting or rally
Making a monetary contribution to a party or candidate
Contacting a public official or a political leader

Transitional Activities

Wearing a button or putting a sticker on the car
Attempting to talk another into voting a certain way
Initiating a political discussion
Voting
Exposing oneself to political stimuli

Spectator Activities

Apathetics

resources. Finally, election to public office makes intense personal demands, but also has the highest probability of maximizing that person's influence on public events. In other words,

Political acts differ in what they *can get the citizen:* Some kinds of activities supply little more than the gratification from taking part, whereas, other political acts can lead to more specific and concrete payoffs. Political acts differ in what they can *get the citizen into:* some activity is likely to bring him into open conflict with others, some is not. And political acts differ in what *it takes to get into them:* some activity calls for initiative, time, resources, skill, some does not.[2]

In looking at another study of political participation, Verba and Nie found, in a survey of 2549 persons in 200 locales, that *political acts* fall into four categories: (1) voting; (2) campaigning; (3) communal acts (aimed at influencing broader social issues in the community or society); and (4) personalized contacts (aimed at personal issues or those that affect his or her family). They identified six kinds of *political actors,* each practicing a different mixture of political acts:

1. *The Inactives.* This group, which made up 22% of the total, were found to have no involvement in politics.
2. *The Voting Specialists.* Another one-fifth of the population (21%) fell into the category of voting regularly but not trying to influence government in any other way.
3. *The Parochial Participants.* Only 4% of the population fell into this category. These persons made personalized contacts but did not engage in campaign work or communal acts and held average records of voting.
4. *The Communalists.* This group, which made up 20% of the total, was characterized by a high degree of communal activity and a low degree of campaign involvement. In other words, these persons were interested in dealing with community problems but not with conflict-oriented campaigns.
5. *The Campaigners.* The direct opposite of the communalists, these persons, who constituted 15% of the population, engaged heavily in political campaigns but virtually no communal activities.
6. *The Complete Activists.* These individuals were found to engage in all of the kinds of activities and in large quantity. Approximately 1 in 10 Americans was classified with-in this segment (11%).

The inactives and the voting specialists showed psychological detachment from politics, low levels of political skill and competence, decreased desire to be involved in conflict, and a low level of civic-mindedness. The complete activists, on the other hand, showed a high degree of political efficacy and skill and psychological involvement in politics, as well as a large amount of political information. They also showed a high level of civic-mindedness and ability to cope with conflicts.[3]

APATHETICS OR INACTIVES

The apathetics show virtually no involvement in politics. They do not vote, and they are largely unaware of and indifferent to the political life of their community and the nation. To call them apathetic, however, distorts the meaning of participation in their personal lives. They engage in a variety of activities that either support the political system or place demands on it. They work, obey laws, pay taxes, use public services, collect benefits from government programs, raise families, send their children to school, serve in the armed forces, and support the national economy through purchases.

Nonparticipants tend to be heavily concentrated among the less wealthy people and those who do not belong to organizations. Most middle-class professional people (lawyers, physicians, business people, college professors, etc.) can rearrange their work schedules in order to take a few hours off to engage in such political activities as testifying before a legislative committee or government agency, to vote or to carry out some other political activity in the middle of the day. This is impossible for the hourly wage-earning person whose pay will be docked for time missed from work. The professional or business person also tends to have access to such resources as an office telephone, a secretary, copying machines, and other office assets that ease the task of preparing position papers, contacting people, and arranging meetings. The hourly wage earner has none of these resources. Finally, if a babysitter has to be hired to watch children while the parent

Figure 10–3. Political apathetics have been found to fear conflict with authority figures. (Courtesy of Nursing in the Mass Media Collection, University of Michigan)

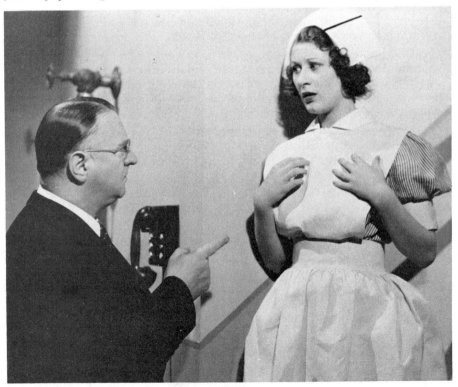

attends a political event, the babysitter costs will be much more significant to the lower-income family than to the more affluent family. Another factor reducing political participation among working-class people is the lack of organizations to mobilize them. Labor unions are the exception in that they make strenuous effort to mobilize their members to participate.

Most nurses, unlike many other professionals and more similar to the hourly wage earner, find it difficult to leave their jobs in the middle of the day owing to the pressing demands for continuous nursing care. They also lack job-related resources to facilitate political activity and are generally either unorganized or when organized are less cohesive as a group to be effective in political matters. Nurses' salaries are typically low and thus extra money for political purposes is indeed hard to generate.

Most nurses are prepared in the course of their professional education for what might be described as "direct service roles." The emphasis that schools of nursing place upon conformity and acceptance of the established health care system may have unplanned consequences. Characteristics such as docility and conformity have been traditionally prized in schools of nursing, but they are unlikely to lead to a healthy questioning of, or an open-minded consideration of, the political process surrounding health care or the attendant labor and economic issues. These factors, plus others which are discussed later in this and other chapters, lead nurses, we believe, to be overrepresented in this inactive category.

SPECTATOR ACTIVITIES

One basic spectator activity is being *exposed to political stimuli* such as viewing television, listening to the radio, reading newspapers, newsletters, or other materials. Collecting information in this way is fundamental to all other political acts. The mass media literally flood citizens with political information and immerse them in politically significant data. Nurses are exposed to this information either by accident or because they seek it out. As with everyone, nurses like some media better than others, but every nurse has the opportunity to be exposed at some level to this information. Yet some nurses are remarkably able to avoid the political stimuli that surrounds them. Most, however, respond to the stimuli by increasing their political participation. For example, those nurses from families that have experienced a high degree of political involvement are more likely to be active.

In addition to general political information, nurses need in-depth data about the relationship between nursing, health care financing, and political decisions. Just as political stimuli raise the political participation of people in general, nurses who are exposed extensively to information about nursing and health care politics are more likely to become involved in the political process. Newspapers, television, radio, and news magazines tend to include only the broadest information about the details of legislative matters. Consequently other methods of exposure must be used.

Professional organizations (ANA, NLN, AACN, ACNM, and so forth) regularly send out position statements, newsletters, directives, and other communications to their membership or to selected parts of the membership

EVANS-NOVAK POLITICAL REPORT

WHAT'S HAPPENING . . . WHO'S AHEAD . . . IN POLITICS TODAY

Mental Health Reports

American Academy of Pediatrics

Government Activities Report

WASHINGTON ACTIONS ON HEALTH
THE HEALTH PROFESSIONAL'S WEEKLY
GUIDE TO SIGNIFICANT DEVELOPMENTS
AND DOCUMENTS IN NATIONAL HEALTH

"The Blue Sheet."
Founded 1957 – $230.00 a year

National Health Insurance
report

WASHINGTON
HEALTH RECORD.

THE BARON REPORT
November 21, 1980
LR XXI-LR18

LR LEGISLATIVE ROUNDUP

A Report on National Medical Legislation

VOL. 17 NO. 3
JANUARY 23, 1981

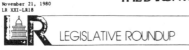

hospital week.
©1981 by the American Hospital Association

Figure 10–4. A weekly reading of the various Washington health care newsletters provides vital information on which to base political action. (Courtesy of History and Politics of Nursing, University of Michigan)

(such as legislative committees). In addition to these important sources, newsletters on health care politics, published on a daily, weekly, or monthly basis, are very useful. The number of these publications has increased markedly in recent years and includes such titles as: *Washington Report on Health and Medicine, Health Manpower Report,* and *National Health Insurance Report.* Each hospital, school of nursing, and health care agency should subscribe to these publications and make them available to their nurse employees because they tend to be quite expensive (owing to the heavy expense of researching the day-to-day events on Capitol Hill) and not easily affordable on a personal subscription basis for individual nurses.

Another publication from which nurses can gain political information is the *Congressional Record,* which is published each day Congress is in session and reports proceedings of both the House and Senate verbatim as well as how each senator and representative voted on issues acted on that day. This official publication, which can be subscribed to or reviewed in libraries, is quite long and too detailed for most persons to use on a regular basis. The *Congressional Quarterly Weekly Reports* and the *National Journal*, on the other hand, provide more focused weekly reports on significant activities in Congress. Listings of how senators and representatives voted on major issues are also usually published the following day in the *Washington Post*, which is subscribed to by many academic and public libraries. Committee hearings are also published and available at governmental depository libraries, for purchase at the U.S. Government Printing Office or from congressmen/women or senators, particularly if the issue is under the jurisdiction of a committee they serve on. Unfortunately similar data for state and local legislative activities are not generally available.

The second most frequent mode of spectator political participation is *voting*, which has been called a "blunt but powerful instrument of control over government."[4] Voting in the United States was originally confined to a small minority of citizens, that is, white males with property. Gradually the white-males-only restriction and the property requirement disappeared, and three extensions of the U.S. Constitution extended the vote to black males (1870), to women (1920), and to persons 18 to 21 (1970). Although the Civil War gave blacks the vote, some years later, numerous states, particularly in the South, created barriers to disfranchise most blacks. Even as late as the early 1960s, Southern blacks were often blocked from exercising their voting rights, and as a result, the *black vote* began only in the mid-1960s to exert a significant impact on American politics. While the women's suffrage victory increased the proportion of eligible voters most dramatically by doubling the number, many women still chose not to vote. The addition of the younger age group of voters has more potential than it has real impact on American politics because this group's participation tends to be lower than expected.[5]

Voting takes little time or initiative as contrasted to other political acts. The first step involves registering at a city hall or some designated place in the community. (In some states, it can even be done by mail.) Being registered is a fundamental step to having any influence in government. At the time persons register as voters, they have an opportunity to become members of one of the political parties. This allows participation in the activities of that party, including eligibility to vote in primaries, when candidates are selected. It also provides opportunities to become involved in the political process. Once registered, a person is able to vote in any election. Registration is typically permanent, but a few states require repeated registration every few years. Actual voting is done at the precinct or district poll. The voter's name is checked on the voting list to ensure that he or she is qualified and registered; it also prevents people from voting in the wrong place or from voting more than once. The voter then steps into the voting machine, pulls a lever to close the curtain which guarantees privacy and makes his or her decisions. Voting for candidates all of the same political party is known as a *straight ticket*. Selecting individuals from more than one party is a *split ticket*. A person can elect not to vote for a position, or can vote a *write-in* by putting the name of a person not listed on the ballot.

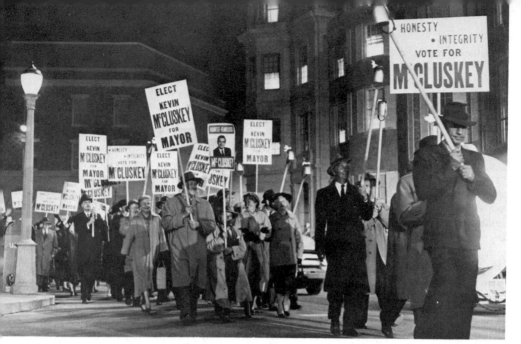

Figure 10–5. Carrying a sign for a favorite candidate is one form of revealing one's partisanship. (Courtesy of Nursing in the Mass Media Collection, University of Michigan)

Higher on the pyramid, actions *revealing one's partisanship* through political discussions, displaying bumper stickers, and wearing campaign buttons are the next most frequent activities engaged in by a large percentage of the population. Political discussions vary greatly in quantity and quality. Campaigns naturally increase political talk, and these interchanges continue to escalate as the campaign progresses. Persons with more time available, more contacts in communities, and more memberships in organizations engage in a greater amount of political discussion than other persons. If an issue is salient to a person, it is also the subject of a greater amount of his political talk. There are some individuals who seem to be constantly involved in initiating and engaging in these interchanges, and there are others who avoid them. Generally people simply comment about political issues, whereas a lesser number seek to persuade others to see political events their way. Revealing one's partisanship by displaying bumper stickers or the like is sometimes popular for persons who do not want to be involved in the more aggressive process of trying to influence others through political persuasion. In addition, influential people are sought out for their opinions and are thus known as *opinion leaders*. Within professions, such as nursing, opinion leaders are usually persons who are more knowledgeable about political issues and processes and are involved in political events.

TRANSITIONAL TYPES

Those in the next level of political participation, the transitional types, actually *contact politicians or public officials*. Only a small proportion of the population engage in this activity. Individual contacts are confined to a one-to-one interaction, whereas cooperative citizen activity involves an organized group of persons joining together to influence governmental outcomes, such as an interest or pressure group (which will be discussed in Chapter 12).

These contacts can take the form of letter writing, telegrams, mailgrams, telephone calls, or direct contact, and the agenda for such meetings can range the gamut from personal problems to broad national issues. Legislators can be asked to cosponsor bills; to request that hearings be held on issues; to urge committees to report bills that are out; to speak to other legislators, especially committee chairpersons, about bills or other matters (sometimes in the form of "Dear Colleague" letters); or to vote for or against legislation. Nurses having direct contact with elected officials can influence the problems raised by legislators.

Legislators keep track of telephone calls, mail, telegrams, and personal visits, recording the percentage for and against particular issues. They may even quote especially strong or well-phrased arguments in their own statements at public gatherings or at legislative committee sessions. Because relatively few people participate in personal communications with officials, those who do can have unusual impact. The impact of communications are (1) leading a legislator to take a position on an issue (*i.e.*, please vote *yes* on third-party reimbursement for nurse practitioners providing care for Medicaid patients coming before the full House early next week); (2) requesting a legislator to reverse a position already taken (*i.e.*, please reconsider your previous negative stance and vote *yes* on the Nurse Training Act extension);

Figure 10–6. Developing a relationship with one's representative and senator is a key step in influencing the political process. (Courtesy of American Nurses' Association, Kansas City, Missouri)

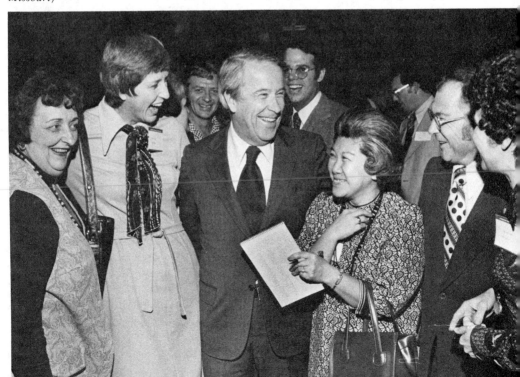

or (3) encouraging a legislator to renew his or her efforts on behalf of a previous position he or she has taken (*i.e.*, please reintroduce your legislative proposal for a national health insurance plan in the new congressional session).

Even a single communication can stand out when it shows thoughtful consideration. Much depends, however, on a policy maker's own inclinations. It is doubtful that even the best written letter or the most persuasive in-person argument will sway an official who is committed to an opposing viewpoint. Yet a well-written or well-articulated message may strengthen the resolve of an official who is predisposed in that direction. And a flood of messages may cause even contrary-minded recipients to reconsider their positions, if only to make sure they have good answers to questions raised. These opposition communications tend at least to cause the legislator to soften opinions and efforts on an issue or to be less obvious about them. They also might make a policy maker think twice when it comes up again, because most issues are rarely completely resolved. If, on the other hand, legislators support a position, communications strengthen them against the opposition and encourage them to be more active on the issue. Communications which raise issues that legislators have not yet taken a stand on can not only encourage them to take a position in favor of the contact's viewpoint but even sometimes to take an active role such as introducing a bill.

Legislators are most influenced by the people who vote for or against them. Thus communications from their own constituents will receive the greatest attention and have the potential for the most significant impact. Letters to representatives and senators from other states or districts typically receive only scant notice and are referred to the legislators of the person making the contact. There are exceptions, however. Some legislators have adopted certain issues upon which they focus their attention and become specialists and thus welcome the ideas and input from persons all over the country. Historically, Congresswoman Francis Payne Bolton, for example, was known for her special interest in nursing. Today, Senator Daniel Inouye of Hawaii has devoted a great deal of energy to pursuing third-party reimbursement for nurse practitioners and nurse-midwives, and Senator Edward Kennedy of Massachusetts has played a central role relative to most health matters, the most notable of which has been his work on national health insurance proposals. Another instance in which legislators are more responsive to contacts from persons outside their districts, but still within their state, occurs when they may be preparing to run for a statewide office, such as governor or U.S. senator. In general, the best way for a concerned individual to influence key legislators on committees dealing with nursing issues, when none of the committee members represents him or her, is to contact nurses, nurses' families, and other persons who *are* constituents of these key legislators and have them communicate the messages.

Senators and representatives and their staffs spend the largest share of their time on constituents' letters, which are usually their only contact with the majority of their constituents. The overall volume of correspondence rises and falls with public interest on legislative issues and is often suddenly expanded by pressure-group campaigns. Mail dealing with the problems of individual constituents tends to remain rather constant. Variation in the volume of mail from one office to another depends on both the characteristics of the state or district and the policies of the members. Mail ranges from 150 pieces a week for representatives from rural districts to 12,000 pieces a week for senators from the most populated states. Opinion letters on legislation or issues make up about one-third of the total. The timing of communications is vitally important. Those that occur too early tend to be forgotten, and those that come too late to influence the action of officials who have already decided their positions have no impact and show a lack of political awareness.

Although complaints about the volume of mail are commonplace, many members of Congress actively stimulate correspondence by such devices as mass mailings in which they solicit constituent opinions. Those who write are usually put on mailing lists to receive newsletters, polls, and other literature. Each newsletter can generate hundreds of letters. Mail provides a key link to voters; if a constituent makes a request and receives a prompt response that is favorable, the voter will probably not only vote for that legislator come election day but will also encourage friends to do so. The

Figure 10-7. Mail provides an essential link to voters, and widespread support for a position on an issue makes it difficult for a legislator to vote against his or her constituents' views. Jimmy Stewart as Senator Jefferson Smith in the film Mr. Smith Goes to Washington *expresses anguish over hundreds of telegrams and letters inspired by his political opponents. (Courtesy of Nursing in the Mass Media Collection, University of Michigan)*

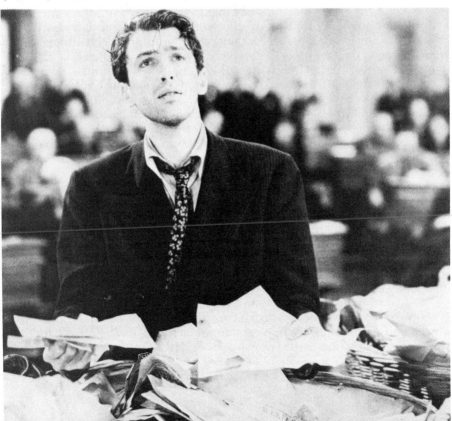

letter may even be shown to family and friends, and this positive word-of-mouth publicity for a legislator yields a popular image.

The way legislators handle their mail varies considerably and depends largely on volume. A few congressmen and congresswomen read and personally answer every piece of mail, but this is the rare exception. At the other end of the continuum, the busiest senators from larger states can personally answer only a few letters from people they know well. In order to handle the mail, legislators normally assign several of their staff to the task of reading and answering every piece of opinion mail from their own constituents as well as responding to selected persons outside their district or state. In some cases, the staffer drafts a response that is reviewed, revised as needed, and signed by the legislator himself or herself. In other instances, only letters with new policy positions are reviewed in this way, and the staffperson handles all other correspondence, signing the letters for the legislator with an automatic pen (known as "Mr. Siggie" by insiders).

Automatic typewriters and computers are also used in legislators' offices to facilitate the process of replying to correspondence. Once a policy statement is developed on an issue that is generating a large volume of mail, the staff person develops a *roboletter*, which after being edited and accepted by the legislator, is placed on a magnetic tape cassette or on punched paper tape (as in any other office). Usually there are two versions: one for those with whom the legislator agrees and one for those with whom he or she disagrees. These letters can be produced quickly and accurately. The computer uses paragraphs set up in advance, and the staffer constructs letters by combining the relevant ones together in answering the mail.

Although these methods of dealing with letters appear to be fairly mechanical, the legislator does receive and value input from constituents. Different methods are employed depending on the preferences of the legislator. Weekly or daily tallies by subject may be developed with brief summaries of the mail. Lawmakers also receive reports just before they are in a position to vote or take another action on an issue. Legislators are usually given a portion of their mail each day to allow them to read firsthand what their constituents are concerned about. The best, most thoughtfully written letters are almost always included in this group. Constituents' letters and their replies are filed by subject and also in many cases under the writer's name so that it is available for future reference.

Constituent letters produce the greatest impact if they: (1) are from individual citizens, as opposed to organized group efforts; (2) are well-written and thoughtful; (3) are limited to one page unless more is absolutely necessary; and (4) mention any prior action taken by the legislator on the issue. Letter-writing campaigns in which letters repeat the same word-for-word message or, even less desirable, use photocopied or mimeographed form letters or postcards, which are simply signed by different people, have a fraction of the impact of individually written letters. It is known as *ineffective mail*. Two-hundred letters with identical wording, particularly if from a very localized area within the district or state, make the legislator think that only a handful of people are behind the campaign. If, on the other hand, the letters are all different but expressing essentially the same point of view, serious attention would be given to them. Senator S. I. Hayakawa of California discusses the contrast between the two approaches:

> Early in 1977, I received sacks of printed postcards from union members opposing a bill before the Senate. The cards obviously were prepared by union officials and handed to members to sign and mail. Most of those cards with their canned message told me very little about what individual union members believed. However, some cards did carry a real message—those on which the signer had crossed out the printed message and written, 'I disagree.'
>
> Contrast this with the reaction to the Food and Drug Administration threat to ban the use of saccharine. I received hundreds of letters and cards. Each was a personal effort.
>
> Mothers wrote about their children with diabetes, whose few pleasures in life included an occasional sugar-free soft drink. Boys and girls wrote about younger brothers and sisters, or playmates. People wrote about their own problems with overweight, diabetes, or whatever.
>
> Each letter was a gripping personal story that I could not ignore, so I became the first Senator to call for a moratorium on the ban until further scientific research could be conducted. . . .
>
> If I were involved in a campaign to influence Senators, I would be careful of my tactics. First, I would do away with canned [preprinted] letters and cards. I would encourage people to write persuasive, personal letters, filled with facts and individual experiences. When it is necessary to prove that very large numbers of people have the same opinion, I would consider petitions as an effective device—but with enough signatures to prove that a significant percentage of the population is concerned.
>
> Yes, Senators pay attention to their mail. And they welcome it. But we are more impressed by personal correspondence than by mass-produced, engineered campaigns.[6]

Follow-up letters to legislators, or those written after receiving an answer to an original inquiry, are extremely rare and consequently have greater impact. Lawmakers typically feel that constituents are satisfied with their stated positions if they hear nothing back. Because pressure groups cannot generally produce mass follow-up responses, people who do communicate in this way are viewed as deeply committed to the issue at hand. These letters also receive more attention because they cannot be answered with a roboletter. The follow-up letter generally attempts to get the legislator to convert a negative or noncommittal or neutral position to one in favor of the writer's stance, or it contains an expression of gratitude for agreeing with an issue or for carrying out favorable actions. Those follow-up letters that point to actual votes or comments made in hearings or on the floor of Congress are particularly potent, because they communicate a close monitoring on the part of the writer and, thus, deep commitment to the issue and the legislator's relation to it.

Nurses and other citizens may also write to the President of the United States and key officials in the executive branch of government, such as the Secretary of Health and Human Services. Typically these letters are funneled downward to the agency in charge of the relevant program. Many of the letters about nursing issues end up at the Division of Nursing, which is delegated responsibility for drafting a response supportive of the Presi-

United States Senate

WASHINGTON, D.C. 20510

January 4, 1979

Professor Ruth Carey
School of Nursing
1335 Catherine Street
Ann Arbor, Michigan 48109

Dear Professor Carey:

Thank you for writing to me concerning S. 2416, the Nurse
Training Amendments Act of 1978. I was pleased to join Senator
Javits as a co-sponsor of this important legislation, and am
quite concerned about the pocket veto of this bill.

This bill extends each of the provisions of the Nurse
Training Act for two years, with one exception; the authority for
financial distress grants has been deleted and the $5-million
authorized for that purpose transferred as additional funding for
special projects. The bill as sent to the White House also
provided a grant program for the training of nurse anesthetists
and a study on federal support for nursing education.

Nursing is an integral and major part of our health care
system. Nurses have a major responsibility for most primary care
and often have the most direct patient contact. The role of the
nurse has increased greatly in recent years. A nurse is no
longer just an assistant to a doctor, but an integral part of the
team caring for a patient.

I was disappointed with the Presidential veto of this bill.
I believe that the nursing education program is vital and will
work in the 96th Congress to assure the passage of a bill that
will have the strong support of the nursing community.

Sincerely,

Edward M. Kennedy, Chairman
Subcommittee on Health and
Scientific Research

Figure 10–8. Senator Kennedy's supportive response to a nurse's plea for help in fighting the President's veto of the Nurse Training Act. (Courtesy of University of Michigan, School of Nursing)

dent's official stance on the issue. Although nurses who work in the executive branch may disagree with the President's position or that of the secretary of HHS, they are obligated to endorse the executive department's position. Thus Division of Nursing personnel must *officially* agree with President Reagan's assertion that funds for nursing education should be cut to the bare bones even though their personal views may be quite different.

Telegrams, mailgrams, and telephone calls are also used by constituents, particularly when time is of the essence. Mailgrams reach a legislator the morning after they are sent and are fairly reasonable in cost ($4.10 for 100 words). Telegrams are more expensive but communicate even more quickly and are useful in extremely urgent situations. Telephone calls, mailgrams, and telegrams are often less effective than well-written letters with details about the issue at hand but do have the advantage of speed when a vote is near. They are most effective when they reemphasize a position expressed in writing earlier.

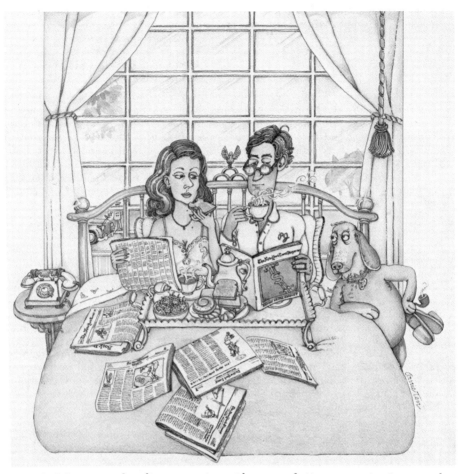

Figure 10–9. Letters to the editor transmit a wide range of views on nursing issues to the general public. (Courtesy of New York Times, New York)

Another form of transitional political activity is *writing letters to the editors of newspapers*, expressing reactions to published views. This form of influence allows readers in a community to see different viewpoints and gain additional new information about an issue. Some of the reading public will in turn contact their legislators with opinions. For example, a July 18, 1980, *Wall Street Journal* article on the nationwide nurse shortage (entitled "Nurse Shortage: Causes and Cures") elicited numerous responses from across the country. In turn, more than 600,000 readers were exposed to letters sent to the editor, as the following ones:[7]

The American Nurses' Association is proposing that in order to attain the title 'professional nurse,' a nurse must by 1985 attain at least a baccalaureate degree. What happens at that time to the thousands of nurses who for years have been rendering quality nursing care? What is the status of these nurses; nurses who graduated from hospitals' diploma schools of nursing, the places where the basics of bedside nursing evolved? In reality and as your article says the shortage is most acute in bedside nursing, not in nursing administration, research, or education.

> A. M. Lombardi, Jr.
> Executive Director
> Monongahela Valley Hospital
> Monongahela, Pa.

In your recent article concerning the nursing shortage you emphasized the fact that 'the hospital industry, the federal government and the nursing profession are taking steps to fill the vacancies' (flexible hours, recruitment gimmicks, etc.). Unfortunately, these ploys only scratch the surface of the main issue: that the nursing profession is seriously underpaid in relation to its educational requirements, training and responsibilities. Until this main issue is addressed, there will continue to be a severe nursing shortage and an increase in union organizing campaigns. Let's abandon our Florence Nightingale stereotype and compensate nurses as the professionals they are.

> Philip R. Brodeur
> Greenfield, Mass.

A probable cause of the nurse shortage is the natural result of the free market economy. The marketplace prices nurses—expressed in such mundane terms as salary, benefits, working conditions and job satisfaction—at a value less than other job opportunities. Young persons realize this and in selecting educational programs are quite rationally choosing other careers. Sixty percent of hospital expenses are payroll related; therefore, correcting this situation by improving compensation (and attitudes) will be expensive, whereas not solving the problem may require other awkward social adjustments.

A paradox exists when politicians simultaneously favor ERA and organized labor (primarily male dominated), while supporting the so-called hospital cost-containment bills. These proposals will obviously suppress the compensation of nonphysician, nonadministrative health care professionals and employees and in effect be detrimental to many working women.

> Charles Duffy
> Assistant Administrator-Finance
> Marion General Hospital
> Marion, Ind.

The critical shortage of nurses came about because the Labor Department in 1977 removed the blanket labor certification for nurses. This had allowed thousands of foreign qualified nurses to enter the U.S. annually. Perhaps the time has come for nurses to be restored to 'Schedule A' so that they can again enter the U.S. and remedy the existing shortage.

> David Scheinfeld
> New York

Although you'd never know it from your article on the subject, men are nurses, too.

'Fewer young women are entering nursing . . .' Really, now.

> Bill Alpert
> Seattle

Many fewer citizens move up to the participatory role of direct contact with political decision makers. First, there are limits on the time and energy a policy maker can devote to such contacts, and secondly, citizens do not take the initiative. Those nurses, for example, who do engage policymakers in direct conversation are atypical of the population at large and thus become quite an important source of influence. In-person contacts tend to have a great deal more impact than letters and telephone calls.

Personal contacts are made either at the legislator's home base or in Washington (or the respective state capitol). Home contacts are usually fairly rushed and take a long time to set up, because the legislator is almost always heavily engaged in various meetings and other activities. Some persons use the legislator's town hall meetings or other public events to speak with their representative. Visits to Washington, D.C., when Congress is in session are most effective when: (1) an appointment is set up ahead of time; (2) the nurse has prepared a short well-written statement of exactly what legislative action is desired and why (with name and address for future reference); (3) this statement is accompanied with research reports, pertinent news clippings, or other documentation such as anecdotal case reports in the absence of *hard* evidence; (4) points are made concisely, intelligently, seriously and are not overstated; (5) the direct impact on the legislator's constituents is highlighted; (6) the person dresses and acts in a professional, businesslike manner and demonstrates confidence; (7) the stay is kept short; (8) the conversation is kept focused on the issue (sometimes legislators like to change the subject) and a commitment is secured from the legislator; and (9) the staffperson with jurisdiction over health and nursing issues is also seen. In some cases, only the staffperson is available for personal appointments, but his key role in the legislative process makes these contacts quite significant. The various nursing associations with Washington offices typically assist nurses in making personal contacts with their representatives and senators.

Nurses who make a point to visit personally with their two state senators and their representative whenever they visit Washington become known to these policy makers. Even though particular legislation may not be imminent, general discussion of important areas of concern tend to be remembered later, particularly if followed up at the time that legislation is imminent. Attending congressional committee hearings or mark-up sessions tends to be both educational and informative. The schedule of these sessions is listed in the *Washington Post* each morning and in the daily and weekly editions of the *Congressional Monitor*. Most sessions are open to the public (unless it specifically states that they are closed). Because the rooms are small, early arrival (thirty to forty-five minutes) is often necessary to assure a place. Observation of the House and Senate in session is also valuable (passes are available from representatives and senators). Typically the galleries are crowded, particularly during the tourist season, and visitors are rotated out after a short stay. A special gallery area exists where persons can stay longer for the entire debate and the vote on issues of particular relevance.

Testifying before congressional and state legislative committees and other groups is another important form of making contact with politicians and public officials. Public hearings are held to gather information about legislation under consideration and to decide provisions of bills. They also tell legislators how much support and opposition exists for the bill. Hearings are also used to educate persons opposed to the bill by countering opponents' arguments, and to highlight an issue even if legislation has little chance of passage by the House or Senate. They are the *official* opportunity for citizens to participate in the legislative process.

As noted in Chapter 8, congressional hearings are generally held in Washington but are also occasionally set up in other locations throughout the country. Those in Washington are primarily for the purpose of gaining testimony from members of Congress, the executive branch, interest groups and organizations and experts, whereas *field hearings* are aimed at gaining the grassroots input of individual citizens and local organizations. The hearing offers the opportunity to advance an argument and offer evidence. Because they are published, hearings tend to influence lawmakers who are not in attendance or not on the particular committee or subcommittee that hears the testimony.

Some committees invite witnesses to testify whereas others announce hearings and extend an invitation for interested persons to testify. The latter tend to occur in field settings. If the list of witnesses is long, a strict time limit may be imposed. Some persons submit letters or statements for the record if they cannot testify, or they ask a sympathetic legislator to submit the statement for them. Hearings typically begin with the testimony of members of Congress. Next, they move to representatives from federal agencies, then to local elective and appointive officials, to organizations including interest groups, and finally to individuals.

Persons who testify on behalf of an organization or institution are more influential than those who talk only for themselves. Washington-based hearings typically confine all testimony to those persons representing organizations. Persons who do testify for themselves have more of an impact when they also submit statements or letters from various other people or petitions signed by others. Those who testify before various committees have also found it helpful to submit their statement and other materials to their own legislators, after making the presentation.

The content of testimony is best when it includes a solid database for the arguments presented as well as anecdotal case materials that tend to elicit the legislators' interest by making the issue a matter of deep human concern. The beginning of the statement contains the name, position, and special qualifications of the testifier presenting his or her view at the hearing and of the organization being represented, and a clear statement of position on the matter under consideration. For example, at a recent Senate Finance Committee hearing on Medicare and Medicaid reform, an ANA witness introduced herself as follows:

> Mr. Chairman, I am Dolora Cotter, the Director of the Denver Visiting Nurses' Service. I am pleased to have the opportunity to appear today on behalf of the American Nurses' Association. Before I address the problems of home health I would like first to focus on its successes. There are in this country millions of older persons who have used home health care benefits under Medicare since 1966. Only their stories of receiving the nursing, physical therapy, home health aid or other services and what it meant in terms of sustained independence and quality of life would give us the human glimpse of this issue today.[8]

The body of the statement should contain factual and logical arguments along with compelling evidence. The most important points should go first,

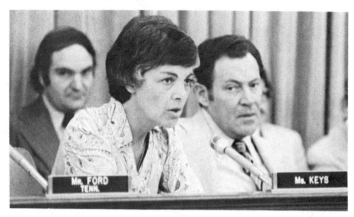

Figure 10–10. Martha Keys of the House Ways and Means Committee was strongly supportive of nursing legislation. (Courtesy of National League for Nursing, Washington, DC)

and the ending should convey an expression of thanks to the legislators for the opportunity to testify. The use of dramatic human situations by Ms. Cotter in her testimony on the need for expanded home health care by nurses before the Committee on Finance was most effective:

> In their absence, I cite the example of an 82-year-old man who died last year. He had a stroke in 1966 at 70 years of age, the year the Medicare program started. He returned home with total paralysis of the right arm, a brace on his right leg and the need to learn new skills in feeding himself, dressing and walking. He had a nurse and a physical therapist for several months the first year, then went four years without service. He had prostate surgery, lost strength with the hospitalization, required a visiting nurse for a month after he went home to help him regain his ability to walk, restore normal management for his bowels, and provide teaching to his wife to cope with his somewhat lower level of functioning. In 1973 both he and his wife had severe flu. Family members from across the country mobilized to return to help their parents for three or four weeks. An occupational therapist and nurse were needed for a month to reteach skills of independence.[9]

The written statement, which becomes part of the record, is often longer than the oral one. Sometimes visual aids (charts, graphs, slides, photographs, and so forth) are used to gain more attention. Speaking without reference to the text, concentrating on the key points, and keeping the text brief is more effective than reading verbatim from a long text. It is surprising to the uninitiated that legislators sometimes do not appear to be in full attention during the session as they may be engaging in conversations or writing during the testimony. The fact that the witnesses' statements are entered into the hearing record and may receive press coverage, however, is key to the influence of the hearing process despite the seeming lack of attention on the part of legislators themselves. Consequently, it is useful for witnesses to submit copies of their statements to the press, who typically are in attendance at hearings, and to editors of newspapers for the editorial page.

After the formal testimony, the committee members ask questions of witnesses, starting with the chairperson and the ranking minority member and then in order of seniority. Questioning is done in different ways. Those committee members in favor of an issue may use questioning of witnesses to try to persuade other members to adopt their own views. They also facilitate the performance of witnesses who represent their own inclinations on an issue. An example of this process in action occurred during the testimony of Ellen Peach before the House Subcommittee on Health relative to the extension of Medicare and Medicaid reimbursement for nurse practitioners and physician extenders in rural health clinics:

Ms. [Martha] Keys. 'Yes; I am very interested in your testimony about not requiring direct supervision but merely consultation.

Could you in any way detail a little bit more how this would work?'

Ms. [Ellen] Peach. 'I will use Idaho again because that is the State with which I am familiar. In Idaho, as I said, it is a collaborative relationship with the physician for referral and consultative purposes. Direct supervision to me infers . . . that the physician must assume legal responsibility for the nurse practitioner's practice. I am responsible for my own practice and responsible to my patient clients, accountable to them for the care that I give them.

I think that this is what we are talking about.'

Ms. Keys. 'Then, there is no physician who has the responsibility in terms of liability for your deliberative care?'

Ms. Peach. 'I have my own license under the State law and I carry my own medical malpractice insurance. We have not had a test case yet in Idaho.'

Ms. Keys. 'That is one of the areas in which there seems to be some concern. As you are saying, it works very well for you.'

Ms. Peach. 'Yes.'

Ms. Keys. 'I have one other question about the idea that we have always had of maintaining quality by physician control. I think it has been a false idea but I wonder if you could address yourself to that?'

Ms. Peach. 'Maintaining quality assurance?'

Ms. [Anne] Zimmerman. 'Maintaining the quality of care.'

Ms. Peach. 'Okay.'

'One of the ways that we have attempted to do it in Idaho—and also we are trying to set something up with a couple of our neighboring western States that have similar problems with distance and medical referral facilities—is to have a traveling team that would go around for relief purposes and information peer review and chart audit. We hope these teams will be funded through a grant. That way the nurse practitioners in some of these neighboring western States who have tried to provide these kinds of services to the patient—because that is who benefits from it—can be kept up to date and their care can be maintained.

So this is how we are trying to maintain the quality of care.'

Ms. Keys. 'Do you think that it is important that nurses be included on PSRO's?'

Ms. Peach. 'Absolutely.'

Ms. Zimmerman. 'Could I comment about that? There is legislation, as you know, that has been introduced and we feel very strongly that nurses should be a part of that PSRO legislation.'

Ms. Keys. 'I agree.'

'Thank you.'[10]

If the legislator opposes the view of the witness who is testifying, he or she may try to discredit the statement and the person who made it. The most successful reaction by a witness to hostile questioning is a calm and factual response but one that firmly conveys the message the witness wishes to express. This principle was used effectively by Margaret Arnstein of the Division of Nursing at a January 20, 1950, hearing before the HEW Appropriations Subcommittee:

> *Mr. [John] Fogarty.* 'Why do you need these eight additional positions?'
>
> *Miss Arnstein.* 'Mr. Chairman, we are not half meeting the job that we think we should be doing. We plan to use four of those new nurses in our Nursing Resources Branch, which is making these State surveys, and which must follow up on the State surveys if we are to get the benefit of our initial investment; and, also, from these State surveys have come problems that we ourselves were not aware of, which we need to solve in order to get the best use of our nurses. We plan to use three in our Nursing Education Branch, one to give consultation of the kind I have been describing, in addition to what is now being given, and two for loan purposes to universities and schools of nursing, to demonstrate the kind of education needed in nursing today.'[11]

Representative Erland H. Hedrick of West Virginia, a physician and former superintendent of Pinecrest Tuberculosis Sanitarium at Beckley, West Virginia, then had some sharp questions for Miss Arnstein:

> *Mr. Hedrick.* 'It seems ridiculous to me that Washington has to look after the nurses in the various States. I see no reason why the States would not be better and perfectly qualified to take care of the nursing situations. I would like you to answer that.'
>
> *Miss Arnstein.* 'They do. We have been operating with a staff of seven nurses for the entire country. For example, we send a nurse for one month to a state to give their group some guidance, some expert knowledge, and we bring to them the knowledge we can collect from our experiences in other States. The States do not all want our help, but more of them want it than we have staff to give it to them. We have frequently replied to requests for assistance by referring to the nurse leaders in their state.'[12]

Another transitional activity is *making campaign contributions.* Giving funds for political purposes often means giving up other material goods that the money could be used to purchase. The amount of sacrifice inherent in a contribution is not reflected in the amount of a gift but is related to the income of the giver. Thus, a nurse who gives $20 may be as intense a supporter as a physician, lawyer, or businessperson who donates $200. Legal restrictions limit contributions to $1000 to any single candidate during one election, although the nomination or primary process and run-off elections are treated as separate elections. The combined total of donations one person can make is $25,000 for federal election campaigns held during the same year. This does not include up to $500 worth of food, beverage, and space donated to a candidate or up to $500 in unreimbursed travel expenses. Multicandidate political action committees (which are discussed in the next chapter) may contribute up to $5,000 per candidate per election. Federal funds are available for presidential elections on a matching basis up to 2¢ per person of voting age during the primaries. After the national party convention is held, major party nominees are entitled to about $30 million with no matching requirement. Each major party convention also gets $2 million from the government. Campaigns are costing more and more as each election passes, and sufficient funding is becoming an absolute prerequisite for having a chance at getting elected. Speaker of the House Tip O'Neill said, "Winning campaigns have four components—money, the candidate, issues, and organization. Of course, if you don't have money, you can forget the other three."[13]

Approximately one-tenth of the population contributes money during presidential election years, but only about 20% of the population is asked to contribute and, of these, about half comply. Gallup polls show that many persons not asked would contribute at least a small amount, if they were solicited. Thus a fairly large reservoir of potential small contributors exists. As would be expected, higher-income individuals as well as professional, managerial, and business persons are more likely to donate funds, as are the party-identifiers. Republicans, who are more likely to be conservative and employed as white collar workers in business and corporations, are more likely to make contributions than Democrats, who tend to be more liberal and predominantly from the working class. Middle-aged individuals give more than younger or older persons. Funds are raised from a variety of sources: personal contributions, individual contributions, party organization contributions, group contributions, and fund-raising events. Studies show that for congressional and local elections, the candidate, his family and friends, and active partisans are the largest contributors.

Nurses who have run for elective offices have had to raise funds ranging from several hundred dollars to hundreds of thousands of dollars. Rhode Island legislator Maureen Maigret, a 1964 graduate of the Memorial Hospital School of Nursing in Pawtucket, Rhode Island, who also works as an RN in a community hospital, said her campaign cost only $700: "I raised the money the first time by holding a raffle. Each ticket cost one dollar and we raised several hundred dollars."[14] By contrast, Sandra Smoley, the nurse (University of Iowa, 1959) who has come closest to winning a seat in the House of Representatives of the U.S. Congress and who has served as an elective member of the county commission in Sacramento, California, since 1972, spent $340,000 on her 1978 bid for this federal-level office. As a Republican candidate in a Democratic district, she was able to gain 47% of the vote, an impressive showing. While this campaign was financed through contributions from individuals, political action committees, and party sources, she notes that, "The first time I ran for the Board of Supervisors, my husband's or our family money was instrumental. It accounted for $6500 of the $9000 the campaign cost. The first time out it is very difficult to raise money. People want to contribute to a winner. After that initiatl victory, I have been able to raise sufficient funds."[15] A similar story is told by a Mississippi nurse, Jan Acker (Warner Brown School of Nursing), who served as a county commissioner: "My husband, a wealthy man, financed much of $7,000–$8,000 it cost for the first time I ran for the office. Then we were divorced, and I only was able to spend $3000 the next time."[16] She lost the second election, and lack of sufficient money was probably at least somewhat responsible.

Another transitional activity is *attending political meetings*. For those people who come sporadically and just observe, this action would simply constitute a spectator activity; but for those who attend regularly and commit considerable support organizing and participating in the meetings, it is close to a gladiatorial level of participation. This is especially true when individuals are involved at the level of planning strategy or attending a caucus.

GLADIATORIAL ACTIVITIES

Gladiatorial activities, the highest level of involvement, include working for political campaigns, becoming active in political parties, and running for and holding elective offices. The role of professional politicians can be thought of as the most involved of all political roles because politicians turn over their life to political pursuits. Successful politicians know that every election campaign, regardless of the extent of commitment made, is based on the organization and use of scarce resources. An effective campaign organization is indispensible to nearly all political races. For partisan contests in states where there are strong parties, the organization may be ready-made and eager to support the party nominee. But in nonpartisan races, in states with weak parties, or in tense primary fights for the party nomination, a new organization may have to be developed from scratch. In either case, it is here that a nurse or any other citizen can become importantly involved in the political process.

There are several levels of *political campaign work,* ranging from the full-time organizational leaders to part-time volunteers. In campaigns of any size, a *campaign manager* is hired to provide expert leadership; and in more extensive organizations, a media director, a legal adviser, a research director, a finance director, a coordinator of volunteers, field organization personnel, and special group coordinators are all in evidence. These additional roles may be held by paid or unpaid personnel. Typically in larger efforts, paid professional people are employed, while smaller campaigns use unpaid amateurs in these positions. One study of House of Representatives' campaigns showed that of eight or nine full-time people only about five were paid.[17] Volunteers thus play key roles in the elective process even though only a small portion of the population engages in volunteer work. Candidates who win generally have about three times the number of volunteers as those who lose.

Volunteers typically carry out a wide range of activities: photocopying, stuffing envelopes, typing letters, making telephone calls, ringing doorbells, handing out leaflets on a street corner, holding meet-the-candidate get-togethers, arranging TV parties to hear a national candidate speak, taking people to the polls, preparing registration lists, and other similar activities. They are also involved in raising money for candidates by holding fund-raisers or by soliciting funds from other sources.

Most people who become involved in campaign work are recruited through various means (by mail, at candidate appearances, by telephone requests, etc.). Other persons contact the legislator's office themselves and volunteer their services. Legislators prefer to have a key group of conscientious volunteers whom they can count on because volunteers are known to be unreliable (not showing up on time, not doing what they promise, tiring of campaign work, not liking their assignment, and so on). Sometimes more valuable staff time is spent in organizing, training, and following up on volunteers than is gained from volunteer efforts, particularly if they quit in discouragement upon finding out that it is not all glamour. People who make the greatest contributions and are thus most appreciated by candidates are those who demonstrate steady performance and who have developed a reputation for being serious about their efforts.

In recent years, nurses have begun to work actively for both nurse and non-nurse candidates and have been making themselves known as a group that can be quite helpful in the campaign process. Although many nurses in elective offices have not had campaign assistance or support from nurses (one nurse recalls writing to the state nursing organization asking for an endorsement and receiving no answer), others indicate that nurses have played a key role. Marilyn Goldwater, who graduated from the Mt. Sinai Hospital School of Nursing in New York City and is a member of the Maryland State Legislature, explained, "The first time I ran for office, nurses weren't involved. But after I was elected, I started to work on legislation which affected nursing practice, such as the third party reimbursement for nurse mid-wives, and reached out to nurses. When I ran again, they were very helpful."[18]

Figure 10–11. Nurses were the backbone of Jean Moorhead's winning campaign for a seat in the California legislature. (Courtesy of Jean Moorhead, Berkeley, CA)

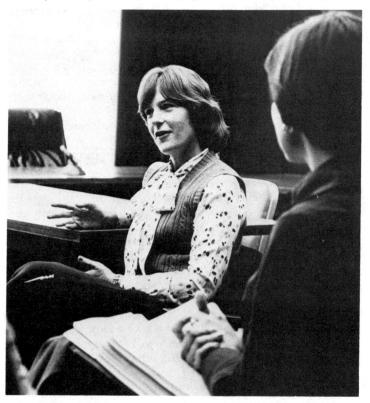

One of the most extensive involvements of nurses in a campaign was that of Jean Moorhead, who successfully ran for the California state assembly. Ms. Moorhead, the first nurse assemblywoman in the history of the California state legislature, has a BSN from Stanford University and a MS in community health nursing from San Jose State University. She served as a lobbyist for the California Nurses' Association prior to running for office in 1978. She describes the pivotal role of nurses in her campaign as follows:

> When I sat down with my campaign staff the first time they said, 'OK what is your base.' I didn't even know what they meant. They asked me if I had been involved in the schools in the community or whatever. I kept saying 'no.' They finally asked 'What have you been doing all your life?' I said: 'I've been in nursing.' They asked 'How many nurses are there in California?' I said there were 180,000 nurses and they said 'Great. If we could raise $1 from every nurse, we could finance the campaign.' Well I doubted we could get a dollar from every nurse but I paid to send a letter to every nurse who belonged to the California Nurses' Association requesting money. That brought in enough to fund me going up and down the state giving talks on nursing's need to be involved in the political process. After 2 or 3 hours, these nurse groups were so fired up, they donated to my campaign. Then we sent more letters, asking those who gave before to give a little more. My average gift was $15, which was higher than typical. By the time of the primary, we had $18,000 and that was entirely from nurses. Between February and June, 1978, we raised that much.
>
> With this much money already raised, other groups like the Realtors PAC, started paying attention. They said 'If this nurse can raise that much money, she must have something going for her,' so they contributed large amounts.
>
> I can say that I couldn't have won without the support of nurses. 150 nurses came from around the state before the election and walked the precinct, door to door. They were the backbone of my campaign.[19]

The highest form of political participation, that of actually *running for and holding an elective office,* mandates certain talents and assets. These often include intelligence, wide acquaintances, fluency, determination, charisma, an outgoing extroverted personality, a high-energy level, a pleasing physical appearance, and money, just to name a few. All of these attributes are not required for success but tend to be helpful. Although large numbers of nurses have not yet run for many elective offices, those few who have attempted the task find that success is truly within reach. For example, an impressive performance is documented by the successful political campaign of nurse–lawyer Jeanine Gisvold for a seat on the Marin, California Hospital District board as reported in the San Rafael, California *Journal* of November 14, 1978:

> Can a small group of politically naive nurses, operating on a shoestring, conduct a successful political campaign in Marin? Early last spring when a group of nurses asked her to run for the Marin Hospital District board, Jeanine Gisvold didn't think so. Last Wednesday, celebrating her election to the board—first in a field of nine contenders—Mrs. Gisvold, 33, was laughing as she recalled the first step in the campaign: she and her committee read a book on campaigning.
>
> The nurses wanted Mrs. Gisvold, assistant director of nursing at the hospital from 1972 through 1974, to run because they felt they lacked an advocate at the hospital. 'I was waiting for the results of the bar exam, so I turned them down,' said Mrs. Gisvold, who has since begun law practice with the San Rafael firm of Shaw,

Kuhn and Thomas. But the nurses were able to convince her there was a need and she was the best one to handle problems at the hospital.

She worked while she was in graduate school at the Haight Ashbury Clinic, and following receipt of the master's degree in psychiatric nursing and nursing administration, came to Marin General to direct the new Community Mental Health Center Crisis Intervention Center. In various capacities—chief administrative nurse, coordinator of the day care program and psychiatric clinical nurse specialist—she stayed at the mental health center until it was taken over by the county. Then she moved into the assistant director of nursing position, where her duties included coordination and operational management of the nursing department, including patient care, preparation of budgets, counseling, staff development, policy and decision making and scheduling.

'I am a career person,' Mrs. Gisvold, a divorcee, said. 'I could never be a housewife. I took a look at my career, and I knew 10 years down the road I didn't want to be where I was then. I had always wanted to go to law school.' She enrolled at Hastings College of the Law and continued through law school to work at the hospital as a nursing supervisor. 'I love nursing, and I will always be involved in it in some way. My practice is exclusively personal injury, so the nursing experience fits right in.'

She has taught continuing education courses for nurses at College of Marin and U.C. Medical Center and will continue to do so, especially in the areas of the legal aspects of nursing.

Figure 10–12. Jeanine Gisvold, a former hospital Assistant Director of Nursing, waged a successful campaign for an elective seat on the Marin General Hospital Board, San Rafael, California. (Courtesy of Jeanine Gisvold)

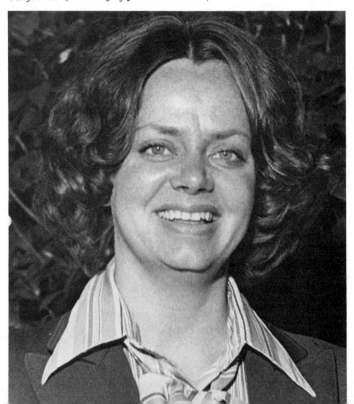

Campaigning, Mrs. Gisvold often cited the need on the board for a woman since 'there are some things about feminine health care that men do not understand.' She has 'always been an advocate for women' and feels strongly that women 'should be able to do whatever they want.' During the campaign—walking precincts, talking to constituents, attending meetings—she learned even more about women's concerns as they relate to the hospital. She will check into a claim by members of the National Organization for Women that abused and raped women receive such poor treatment at Marin General that NOW members are referring women to Ross General Hospital, she said.

It was community contact, walking at least a part of every precinct and 'millions of dollars' worth of time—walking, planning, organizing, talking—from campaign workers that won the election, she said. 'We couldn't afford to do a countrywide mailing because it costs more than $6,000.' said Mrs. Gisvold, who two weeks before the election had received a total of $6,264.41 in contributions. 'We couldn't afford large newspaper ads. Women candidates, we discovered, just don't have large sums of money, so we had garage sales. Our major fund raiser was a Monte Carlo night. That probably was the highlight of the campaign. We had a good time and raised some money.' The party put $2,358.96 into the campaign coffers. 'The most exciting part of the campaign was involvement with people. I have been in Marin for 10 years and come in contact with large numbers of people, many of them people I have done things for, things I certainly did not expect returns for. But every favor or gesture seemed to return during the campaign. It was a real boon and not anything I ever expected,' she said. As a board member, as when she was a nursing supervisor, she said, she will not tolerate inadequate patient care.[20]

The importance of having nurses in political elective offices can be highlighted by a number of examples. Marilyn Goldwater, working with Senator Rosalie Abrams, another nurse in the Maryland State Legislature, was successful in gaining passage of two bills that allow nurse practitioners and nurse-midwives direct access to third-party payers. Although they wanted all health insurers in Maryland to be required "to include in their policies benefits for expenses arising from the care, treatment, or services rendered by a nurse practitioner or nurse-midwife," in the end it was amended so that the benefit was not automatic. Ms. Goldwater explains: "The policyholder, in order to receive coverage [for these services] may have to pay a small additional premium."[21] Insurers aren't actually charging patients. This is a significant step in nursing legislation and would certainly not have occurred if Delegate Goldwater had not taken a personal interest and made a real effort to see it through the legislative process.

Another example is provided by Maureen Maigret, who in the six years she has served in the Rhode Island House has sponsored an impressive list of legislation leading to the creation of a state radiation control agency, an open records law, sexual assault or rape statutes, a department for families and children, a displaced homemaker center, and temporary disability payments for pregnancy-related diseases (previously not allowed).[22] Among her many legislative feats, Assemblywoman Jean Moorhead has, in the short three years she has been a California assemblywoman, introduced legislation that allows nurses to buy into a medical or health corporation and become a full-fledged partner in the corporation while deferring payments until later. She also sponsored legislation that would allow the state to monitor the practice sites of nurses through the relicensure process.[23]

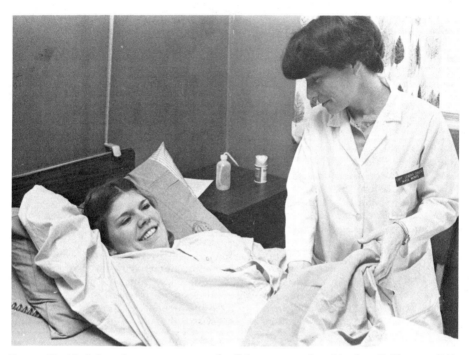

Figure 10 –13. Political participation paid off for nurses when Marilyn Goldwater, R.N., pushed bills through the Maryland State Legislature to mandate reimbursement of nurse– midwives and nurse practitioners under Blue Shield and other private insurance plans. (Courtesy of St. Petersburg Times, St. Petersburg, Florida)

Mary Cotton, a nurse in the New Hampshire legislature, tells about the time she assisted the nurses of a state hospital institution, whose salaries were abysmally low, by telling them "to come to the State House in uniform." She helped to orchestrate this lobbying effort, which resulted in the achievement of better pay and benefits.[24] South Dakota legislator Patricia Kenner, a 1951 graduate of St. Johns-McNamara Hospital School of Nursing, Rapid City, North Dakota, was instrumental in getting a progressive revised nurse practice act passed into law. On another issue she recalled, "We got a bill approved to fund nurse practitioner educational programs but the appropriations committee failed to give it any money. It was what you call a hollow victory."[25] And Jan Acker ran her whole initial campaign on correcting the drainage problems in the Mississippi Delta, where she was affectionately known as the "ditch witch."[26]

Another gladiatorial activity is participating as a delegate to conventions and caucuses of political parties. The National Education Association, for example, made good use of this mechanism by getting 302 schoolteachers selected as delegates and 162 as alternate delegates to the 1980 Democratic Convention in New York City, where they were all Carter supporters and where they hoped to win a tremendous amount of future goodwill from the candidate.

It is essential for nurses to know that political parties are organized in pyramid fashion with the base being most important in facilitating maximum party success. The *precinct*, a neighborhood where hundreds of voters are organized, is the basic unit in the political structure and the first theater of operation for party workers. These approximately 175,000 units are headed by *precinct captains*, or *precinct leaders* (other titles are also used). They may be chosen at caucuses, at direct primary elections, or in the general elections; or they may be appointed by higher party officials. This precinct executive is the direct link between voters in the precinct and the professional political group. This is the party organization person who, through block workers and other aides, knows a great deal about the individual voters in the precinct and has substantial direct influence on them. The *county committee*, the tier just above the precinct (in larger cities, just above the district, which is composed of several precincts), is a unit of major significance in the party machinery. It consists of precinct executives or alternates chosen by them. The *state committee* or state central committee forms the tier above the county committee. The state committee person is an important party figure. The authority and composition of state committees are usually spelled out in state law. Committees range in size from a handful of people to hundreds of members. Methods of selection differ widely from state to state. The chief function of state committees is to conduct campaigns through their officers and agents and to help in governing the party. The *national committee* is the top layer of party organization. It has representatives, at least one man and one woman, from each state and is of prime importance in the choosing of a President. Its chair is a top-ranking professional politician. Its powers and duties are dictated by the national convention. The titular heads of the parties are the President and the defeated nominee of the other party.

The importance of becoming involved in the party organization is emphasized by nurse Maureen Maigret, who has now risen to the position of deputy leader in the Rhode Island House:

> I entered politics with a lot of naivete. I just assumed if I was energetic and a nice person, people would vote for me. I didn't realize the importance of the grass-roots political party at the local and state level. Nurses need to get on the local precinct and ward committees and become more aware of the party structure. These are the groups that endorse candidates. Being endorsed by the party makes it much easier to win elections. Even if they don't want to run themselves, nurses can help other nurses and women gain party endorsement by serving on these committees.[27]

Methods used to choose delegates vary from state to state and between the two major parties. All systems are based on two general methods: (1) the convention or caucus and (2) the primary. Many states use a combination of conventions and primaries, selecting some delegates one way and some another. In most systems, people who want to be delegates may commit themselves to a specific Presidential candidate, or they may run uncommitted. Under the convention/caucus method of selection, delegates are chosen by party conventions. The process begins when party members meet in grass-roots local caucuses (usually at precinct level) to select delegates to

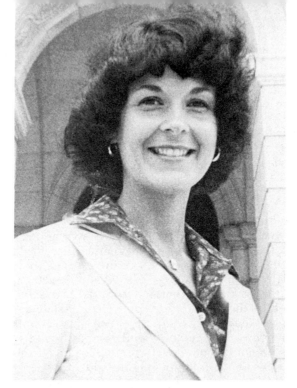

Figure 10–14. "It is important to get involved in the party organizaton," says Maureen Maigret, R.N., the Deputy Leader in the Rhode Island House. (Courtesy of Maureen Maigret)

the next level (usually the county). The county conventions then choose delegates to go to the congressional district and state conventions. In most cases, these state delegates may meet in their own congressional district to select some of the national delegates before going on to meet with the whole state convention to select the rest. Party members express their preference through an election, rather than by attending a meeting or caucus. In 1978, the Democrats ruled that state delegations must be equally divided between men and women. This creates an opportunity for nurses to emulate the National Education Association by making sure that they place a large number of nurses as delegates in this party's national political conventions. Republicans are also facilitating more and more women into their party leadership ranks, and nurses should make the effort to achieve prominent representation.

In addition to elective office, another avenue to more adequate nurse representation in political leadership is through the appointment to the numerous boards, commissions, and offices which set policy at all levels of government. While a few nurses presently hold such appointments, they are a very small number in contrast to persons from other fields. Although the process of determining which persons will be considered for *appointive offices* varies widely, those individuals who are selected often come from among those who worked diligently on political campaigns. Elected officials, or persons representing their party, are often in a position either to make these appointments or to recommend persons for various appointments. Competency is important, of course, because no one wishes to spon-

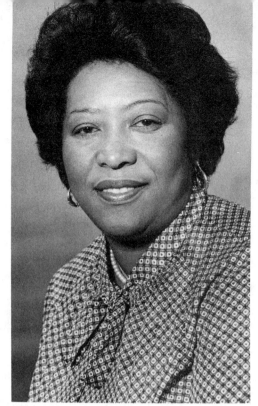

Figure 10–15. One of the key political appointments for mental health policy was filled by a nurse when Rhetaugh Dumas was named Deputy Director of the National Institute of Mental Health in 1979. (Courtesy of Rhetaugh Dumas)

sor someone who might become an embarrassment or who is obviously unqualified for the position. Appointive opportunities are more likely to occur when the individual seeking appointment represents a constituency of her or his own, such as medicine, nursing, or education. A balance of geographic, ethnic, and sex representation is also typically sought out. The appointing official sees this as important because a constituency can assist in securing support for policies or re-election if he or she is in an elective office. This fact has made it valuable for organizations and groups to develop a talent bank of persons they can suggest for a variety of appointive offices and to keep a calendar of appointments, which lists all important appointive positions, terms of office, and other information. Close monitoring of the upcoming vacancies and mounting campaigns for particular persons to fill these openings has proven quite effective. Individuals who seek appointive offices have found it facilitative to send their vitae to appointing officials along with documentation of their competency for the particular office in question.

Another kind of appointment is that of *legislative assistant* to a congressman, congresswoman, or senator or as a staff member of a congressional committee. These positions are of key importance in terms of policy, because, as we have previously noted, members of Congress must because of necessity delegate responsibility to their assistants. Therefore, despite the fact that legislative assistants cannot independently develop policy, they are

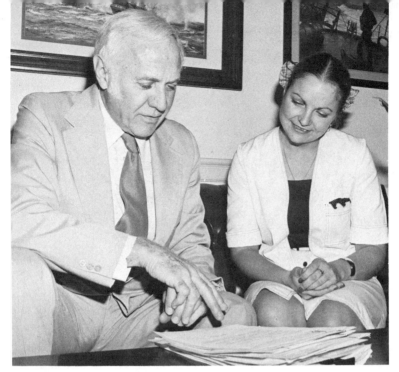

Figure 10–16. Debra Hardy, R.N., is a legislative assistant in the Office of Illinois Congressman, George O'Brien. (Courtesy of Debra Hardy)

in a key position to contribute to and influence the process. Serving as a legislative assistant has also been found to be a pathway to elective office in that many members of Congress have had such political experience prior to seeking elective office. Legislative assistants come from numerous occupations and professions ranging from law to business. Nurses have been extremely underrepresented in this group. The fingers on two hands would more than indicate the number of nurses who have ever occupied these key positions. Physicians, on the other hand, have often served in such roles.

One nurse holding a legislative assistant position is Mary Jo Dennis, who works for Representative Doug Walgren, a Democrat from Pittsburgh, Pennsylvania, and a member of the Subcommittee on Health and Environment of the Committee on Energy and Commerce. She has a master's degree in medical-surgical nursing from Catholic University and says she first became interested in politics while working with the Maryland State Nurses' Association during a student experience as a lobbyist. "It was just luck," she said, "that I was hired on in Doug's [Walgren] office after I graduated." Of the experience, she notes,

> It's fabulous. I've been here 2½ years and I've learned so much. I am able to give Doug insight into how health legislation will translate into practice. So many people on the Hill have no idea what specific health and nursing legislation will mean once it is enacted or if programs are removed. For example, I would have never gone to graduate school without a traineeship—never. I remember thinking, 'I would like to write and thank someone but I didn't know who to write to then.[28]

About nurses, she is disturbed by "their powerlessness. I could write a book about that. The schisms in nursing are very bad politically. Groups are divided as to what a nurse is and who should receive funding. It is difficult for legislators to deal with those differences."[29]

Most major political appointments are typically not permanent, and thus those professions and businesses that facilitate their own kind, helping them back into good positions once the political appointment is over, reduce the career risk for the individual's period of government service. Of course, individuals who have held such positions have often found it was facilitative of their career development despite the fact that it was short-term and may perhaps have even resulted in a dismissal for political reasons.

Another important kind of political involvement comes in the form of directed experiences working with legislators, legislative committees or other governmental agencies on a temporary basis (that is, anywhere from several weeks to one year or even longer). Such experiences are often called *legislative fellowships* or internships and allow selected sponsored persons to spend time away from their regular educational or career responsibilities and to be placed in Washington to learn firsthand about governmental and political matters. The NLN Policy Fellowship Program (formerly funded by the Robert Wood Johnson Foundation) and the ANA minority nurse fellowship program (funded by NIMH, USPHS) have provided excellent opportunities for certain nurses to have these learning experiences during several weeks in the summer. A number of nurses have also been selected for participation in the Robert Wood Johnson funded Health Policy Fellowships Program for academic health science faculty (physicians, nurses, dentists, and so on). These fellowships pay for one year of placement in an appropriate position in a federal government office. The nurses who have been a part of these various programs have served in the offices of congressmen and senators (such as those of Carl Pursell, Douglas Walgren, Andrew Maguire, Henry Waxman, Silvio Conte, John Heinz, Alan Cranston, and Daniel Inouye), on congressional committees (such as the Senate Finance Committee, the House Select Committee on Aging, the House Subcommittee on Health and the Environment, and the House Subcommittee on Oversight and on Investigations), and in executive branch offices (such as the HMO Office of the Health Care Financing Administration, the Congressional Research Service, the Office of Evaluation and Legislation in HRA, the Medical Services Administration, the Congressional Budget Office, and the Food and Drug Administration).[30]

DEGREE OF PARTICIPATION

Compared with many other countries, the United States shows a fairly high degree of political participation among its citizens. Despite this fact, political participation is not widespread. Voting in elections, for example, particularly those that do not involve voting for a president, is done by only a portion of the citizens eligible to vote, and even fewer persons engage in other kinds of political activities. Exposure to political stimuli and voting in presidential elections are the only political activities engaged in by the majority of Americans, yet the democratic process requires an involved and informed citizenry.

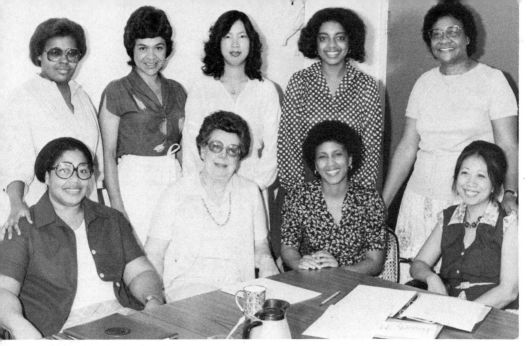

Figure 10–17. The 1980 ANA policy fellows served in a variety of federal and congressional offices. (Courtesy of American Nurses' Association, Kansas City, Missouri)

A large number of studies have been conducted in recent years, including a longitudinal study being carried out at the Survey Research Center at the University of Michigan. These findings show, for example, that only one person in three attempts to influence the voting decisions of another person. Under 10% attend political rallies or meetings during an election, and 8% donate money. No more than 5% of the citizens belong to political parties or partisan organizations. Less than 28% of the citizenry have ever attempted in any way to influence the outcome of a governmental decision in their local community, and fewer than 16% have made similar influence attempts at the national level. Because people tend to exaggerate their activities, these figures probably indicate more public participation in political activity than actually exists.

One has to consider also that it is usually the same persons who attend meetings, donate money, belong to partisan organizations, and are otherwise active in elections. Robert Lane comments, "If a person electioneers, he is almost certain to attend party meetings. If a person attends meetings, he is almost certain to be among those who contact public officers and other political leaders. If a person contacts public officers and leaders, he is almost certain to be a member of some politically oriented (though not strictly political) association. If a person is a member of such an association, he is almost certain to be a voter . . . there is a 'latent structure' pattern in most populations such that those who perform certain less frequent political acts are almost certain to perform *all* the more frequent acts."[31]

The results of another study of political participation are contained in Table 10–1. What this shows is that more than 25% do not even vote in presidential elections and less than half in local elections. Only about one-third of the citizenry is ever involved in any political activity other than

Table 10-1. *Percentage of Citizens Engaging in Twelve Different Acts of Political Participation*

TYPE OF POLITICAL PARTICIPATION	PERCENTAGE
1. Report regularly voting in Presidential elections.	72
2. Report always voting in local elections.	47
3. Active in at least one organization involved in community problems.	32
4. Have worked with others in trying to solve some community problems.	30
5. Have attempted to persuade others to vote as they did.	28
6. Have ever actively worked for a party or candidates during an election.	26
7. Have ever contacted a local government official about some issue or problem	20
8. Have attended at least one political meeting or rally in last three years.	19
9. Have ever contacted a state or national government official about some issue or problem.	18
10. Have ever formed a group or organization to attempt to solve some local community problem.	14
11. Have ever given money to a party or candidate during an election campaign.	13
12. Presently a member of a political club or organization	8
Number of Cases: weighted 3,095 unweighted 2,549	

Source: Verba S, Nie NH: Participation in America, p. 31. New York, Harper & Row, 1972

voting. Political activity involving a minor investment of time is engaged in by about 18% to 23%, about one-sixth of the population. Most of the activities that involve greater investments of time and energy have been engaged in by less than 15% of the voting-age population. For example, only 18% of the populace have ever contacted a national government official, such as their congressman, about a problem or issue, and only 13% have given money to a campaign.[32]

Still another study on the incidence of various political activities was conducted as part of a 1973 Harris Poll. For the purposes of this survey, people were considered active if they said they had participated in an activity even once in their entire lifetime. The activities engaged in by the greatest number of people surveyed, as shown in Table 10-2, are petition signing and political discussion. About two-thirds of the American adults questioned claimed to have signed a petition. About one-half said they had defended the actions of a public official in a private conversation, and almost the same number maintained they had attended a speech or rally for a

Table 10–2.   *Political Actions People Have Taken in Their Lifetime*

POLITICAL ACTION	PERCENTAGE OF ALL RESPONDENTS WHO HAD TAKEN THIS ACTION AT LEAST ONCE	PERCENTAGE OF WHITE RESPONDENTS WHO HAD TAKEN THIS ACTION	PERCENTAGE OF BLACK RESPONDENTS WHO HAD TAKEN THIS ACTION
Signed a petition	69	73	39
Actively defended the action of an elected official in private discussion	56	60	29
Attended a speech or rally for a political candidate	50	53	33
Written a letter to congressional representative	33	36	12
Contributed financially to a political campaign	33	36	15
Written a letter to a U.S. senator	25	28	4
Visited or talked in person with a congressional representative	22	24	6
Written a letter to a local government official	19	21	6
Campaigned or worked actively for a candidate for Congress	14	14	9
Visited a state legislator in the state capitol	14	15	8
Campaigned or worked actively for a candidate for president	14	15	7
Visited or talked in person with a U.S. senator	13	15	5
Campaigned or worked actively for a candidate for the U.S. Senate	11	12	6

Source: Compiled from Harris Poll reported in U.S. Senate Committee on Government Operations: Confidence and Concern, *p. 256, 1973.*

political candidate. For the other activities included in the survey, no more than one-third (usually considerably less) even claimed to have participated even once.[33]

This survey also points to the differences in participation between blacks and whites. For each of these activities, participation is greatest for white, well-educated citizens with high incomes. Although the level of activity among whites is low, that among blacks is much lower. Only 12% of those blacks surveyed had written to their congressional representative as compared to 36% of whites; only 4% of blacks had written to a senator, compared to 28% of whites.[34] These findings, together with the other study findings, have shown a rather consistent picture of who participates in political activities in the United States. It shows primarily that there is a low level of participation among the populace and that the participation which does exist is concentrated in the hands of a small proportion of people. In other words, participation is minimal, marginal, and maldistributed among the populace.

WHO IS ACTIVE AND WHY?

There are a number of different perspectives on why some people do and others do not participate in political activities. Some believe that a restrictive electoral process and cumbersome administrative procedures discourage people or bar them from participation. Others suggest that the structure is designed to encourage participation, referring for instance to the representation rules in the party structure. In fact, particularly in the Democratic Party, the rules are so cumbersome as to be understandable only to a small and relatively elite minority of the party, who consequently control the electoral process. Beyond these structural reasons Milbrath has given us a cogent explanation of why certain people participate in politics and others do not. He gives four overall factors: (1) political stimuli, (2) personal factors, (3) political setting, and (4) social position.[35] The greater the political stimuli, the more participation that occurs. For example, persons who are personally contacted about becoming involved in political matters have a greater likelihood of becoming involved. Some individuals are more prone to pick up the stimuli than others.

Personal factors, or attitudes, beliefs, and personality traits, also help determine who is active in politics. In terms of attitudes, psychological involvement in politics enhances participation as does intense identification with or preference for a political party, a candidate, or certain issues. People with a sense of political efficacy, that is, a feeling that they can get things done through the political process, are more likely to become involved in it. It has also been shown that individuals who are more effective in other aspects of life and have a high sense of duty or civic-mindedness also have a greater propensity to take part in the political process. Civic responsibility is heightened when one feels one's actions have an impact on the political process; it is worthwhile to participate because one's own political role is significant and effective. Few decisions by government affect citizens generally and uniformly. Most governmental decisions have meaningful and immediate consequences only for a relatively small part of the population at any one time. Only those citizens who expect the decisions to have important and immediate consequences for themselves try to influence the outcome. As the character and consequences of decisions change, some of the actors change; there is an ebb and flow in the number who participate. There is much looseness in the relationship between leaders and followers.

The amount and accuracy of political knowledge and the degree to which an individual has a *consistent political philosophy* are other determinants of political involvement. A higher degree of political knowledge yields enhanced interest in politics. A Gallup Organization survey uncovered a shocking and alarming lack of political information among high school juniors and seniors. Results of the survey, which was administered to 1000 17- and 18-year-olds across the country in 1978 under a grant from the

Scherman Foundation of New York, revealed that only 25% realized that at conventions the choice of presidential nominees is made. One-third didn't know which party has a majority in Congress. Ninety-seven percent knew that they were eligible to vote at 18, but only 42% had heard of absentee ballots and knew how they could get their vote counted if they were away from their home district on election day. Only 38% realized a voter can split his party choice between the President and the other offices. A scant 4% could name the three men who served as President immediately before Gerald Ford.[36] Another study compared scores of the assessments of political knowledge and attitudes of 13- to 17-year-olds and found that the most recent scores indicate a general decline in adolescents' knowledge of constitutional rights, the political process, and international affairs from adolescents at the start of the decade.[37]

The personality characteristics of sociability and ego-strength have been found to be associated with a higher level of political participation, whereas anomic alienation, cynicism, dominance, and manipulativeness are associated with lower involvement. Low self-esteem, or poor ego-strength, may place ego-satisfaction through voting very low on the citizen's list of payoffs.

Figure 10–18. Somewhat apprehensive but with considerable fortitude, nurses in the 1980s have begun climbing the ladder of politicl participation. (Courtesy of Buffalo Evening News, Buffalo, New York)

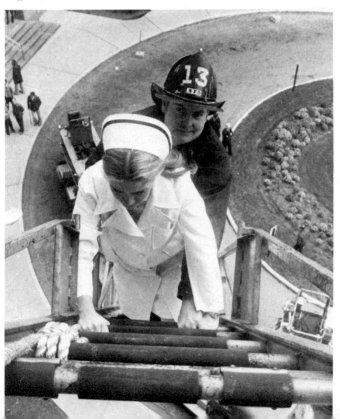

The political setting influences participation through rules of the game (*i.e.*, eligibility rules, such as who can vote and the difficulty or ease of registering to vote); the party system (*i.e.*, the degree of competition between parties increases political involvement); and special characteristics of given political events or campaigns (*i.e.*, the presence of personal contacts, closeness of the race, relative importance of elections, clear differences between candidates, and flow of propaganda).

And finally, social position impacts on political involvement; persons who occupy central roles in society are more likely to participate than those with a peripheral or distant role. Political detachment and voting irregularity are found among persons and groups who are isolated from the larger society in a disproportionately large degree. The larger the number of group memberships that a person has, the more likely that he or she will cast a ballot. In other words, the nonparticipant has few social roles in general and probably no political roles in particular that are esteemed enough to put to use. In terms of reference groups, the nonparticipating person has in mind few, if any, reference groups whose expectations include voting; the decision not to become involved may actually become a positive, rational act.

Demographic variables of education, socioeconomic status, ethnicity, age, and sex were found to vary considerably among political participants. According to recent U.S. Census Bureau statistics of voting behavior, voters are:

- Better educated: Some 80% of college graduates voted in 1976; whereas, only 37% of those who didn't finish grade school voted.
- White-collar workers: 72%; only 50% of blue-collar workers voted.
- Married people: 63%, as against about 50% of the unmarried people.
- Suburbanites, more than city or rural dwellers.
- Homeowners, more than renters.
- Midwesterners, more than those in other major regions.
- Older: median age of voters 45 years old; 35 for nonvoters.

Other studies of broader participation in political matters have shown that political actives are more likely to have higher education, higher income and higher occupational status. The active voters are also more likely to be male, older, Republican, urban dwellers, homeowners, Protestants, and Caucasians. These latter characteristics vary in degree and significance in different localities and under different political conditions. Conversely, political inactives are characterized by lower educational levels, lower income, and lower occupation and socioeconomic levels. Women, minorities, and young persons are overrepresented in the inactive group.

Age, ethnicity, and sex are discussed elsewhere in the text, but education and socioeconomic status need further explanation here. One study of young adults who were graduated from high school four and one-half years previously asked whether they had participated in various activities over the past two years. According to their responses, young adult college graduates were far more likely to register and vote in governmental elections and belong to political organizations than their counterparts with less education. Sixteen percent of young college graduates indicated that they belonged to a political club or organization, three times the participation rate of young-adult high school graduates with no college experience. Fewer than 60% of the young adults who had not gone beyond high school had registered to vote. College graduates were also more often involved in work-related organizations and in organized community and service-oriented volunteer work. Only in church-related activities were rates comparable for young adults of different educational levels.

A larger number of studies have correlated high income and high socioeconomic status with participation in political affairs. Studies of occupation and political involvement, although more difficult to study, have also indicated that occupations of higher status are more likely to have political actives as members. A job that offers time, flexibility, and development of skills that might be helpful in political action makes an important difference; professional persons are more likely to become involved than those with more restricting jobs.

Despite the relative scarcity of personal political activity among the population as a whole, such activity can be prominent and effective in shaping policy. Although the widespread lack of participation certainly cannot be considered a positive factor, the gap between the democratic ideal and the reality of political involvement creates an inordinately large opportunity for nurses to have a timely impact on the political system.

References

 1. Milbrath W: Political Participation, pp 17–19. Chicago, Rand-McNally, 1975
 2. Verba S, Nie H: Participation in America, p 45. New York, Harper & Row, 1972
 3. Ibid, pp 77–81
 4. Nie N, Verba S: Political participation. In Greenstein FI, Polsby NW (eds): Handbook of Political Science: Nongovernmental Politics, Vol 4, p 9. Reading, Mass, Addison-Wesley, 1975
 5. Flanigan WH, Zingale HH: Political Behavior of the American Electorate. Boston, Allyn & Bacon, 1979
 6. Hayakawa SI: Do senators read their mail? Public Relations J 35:32–33, 1979
 7. Nurse shortage: Causes and cures. New York City, Wall Street Journal, Aug 4, 1980
 8. U.S. Congress. Senate, Committee on Finance, Subcommittee on Health: Medicare and Medicaid Home Health Benefits, p 179. Hearings before the Subcommittee. Washington, DC, United States Government Printing Office, 1979
 9. Ibid
10. U.S. Congress. House. Committee on Interstate and Foreign Commerce, Subcommittee on Health and the Environment: Reimbursement of Rural Clinics Under Medicare and Medicaid, pp 65–66. Hearings before the Subcommittee. Washington, DC, United States Government Printing Office, 1977
11. U.S. Congress. House of Representatives. Committee on Appropriations: Department of Labor and Federal Security Appropriation Bill for 1951, pp 602–603. Hearings before the Committee. Washington, DC, United States Government Printing Office, 1950
12. Ibid, pp 603–604
13. Rockefeller SP, Testimony before the U.S. Congress. Senate. Committee on Labor and Human Resources: The Coming Decade: American Women and Human Resources Politics and Programs, 1979, p 141. Hearings before the Committee, Part 1. Washington, DC, United States Government Printing Office, 1979
14. Interview with Maureen Maigret, R.N., Aug 21, 1980
15. Interview with Sandra Smoley, R.N., Aug 15, 1980

16. Interview with Jan Acker, R.N., Aug 22, 1980
17. Agranoff R: The Management of Election Campaigns, pp 181–211. Boston, Holbrook Press, 1976
18. Interview with Marilyn Goldwater, R.N., Aug 12, 1980
19. Interview with Jean Moorhead, R.N., Aug 22, 1980
20. Nurse–lawyer runs campaign on a shoestring. San Rafael, Calif, San Rafael Journal, Nov 14, 1978
21. Goldwater M: The politics of health care. Mich Nurse 53:12–14, 1980
22. Maigret, op cit
23. Moorhead, op cit
24. Interview with Mary Cotton, R. N., Aug. 12, 1980
25. Interview with Patricia Kenner, R.N., Aug 22, 1980
26. Acker, op cit
27. Maigret, op cit
28. Interview with Mary Jo Dennis, R.N., Aug 13, 1980
29. Ibid
30. National League for Nursing: Summer Study Fellowships in Public Policy: Summers 1977–79. Unpublished document, 1979
31. Lane RA: Political Life: Why People Get Involved in Politics, pp 93–94. New York, Free Press, 1959
32. Verba and Nie, op cit
33. U.S. Senate Committee on Government Operations. Confidence and Concern, p 256, 1973 (Compiled from a Harris Poll)
34. Ibid
35. Milbrath, op cit
36. National Center for Education Statistics: The Condition of Education. Statistical Report. Washington, DC, United States Government Printing Office, 1979
37. Ibid

11–Women and Politics

Because 98% of nurses are female, understanding the role of women in politics has great significance for understanding the role of nurses in politics. How do women and men differ in political participation, in political efficacy, in policy beliefs and political socialization, and what are the causes of these differences? The answers to these and other questions offer insights into the political nature of women. Since much of the history of noninvolvement of women in politics in general parallels the noninvolvement of nurses in particular, these answers will also shed considerable light on the political status, past and present, of nurses.

Women have traditionally been thought of as nonpolitical beings. Politics has been considered "men's business," and "women's place" has been in the home. Sharon Percy Rockefeller noted in January 1979 before the Senate Committee on Labor and Human Resources that "women aren't the better half—they are the other half. But, in government, they are the *missing* half. . . . Shall we continue to ignore half our population, half our brains and half our talent in the running of our public affairs?"[1]

The battle for women's suffrage, finally won in 1920, was a significant occurrence not only because it gave women the right to vote, but also because it involved an extensive mobilization of women into lobbying efforts and the development of a nationwide organization. Yet numerous women chose not to vote, even after they were given the right to do so. The cultural and role restraints were still in place and would be for years to come. Many were afraid to vote because of the consequences of their husbands' disapproval, or they believed that they were fully represented by their husbands and thus felt no need to become involved in political matters. The strength of these social norms is highlighted by the fact that in 1838, long before women received the vote, Kentucky allowed widows with school-age children to vote in local districts. About twenty-five years later, Kansas also extended this privilege of voting in school elections to women; then many more states followed suit. The implicit notion here was that women did not need to vote because they could ask their husbands to vote for them and thus express their views about school matters. It was only in the case of his death, and only in matters of child-oriented local issues, that it seemed proper for a woman to have the right to vote.[2]

Despite the great significance of the 19th Amendment, women's suffrage had little actual impact on equalizing the distribution of men and women in positions of political power. It did little to elevate women out of the second-class citizen role they held or to convert women's concerns to public issues or to move women into public life. Only within recent years has the tendency to view women as nonpolitical beings began to dissipate somewhat.

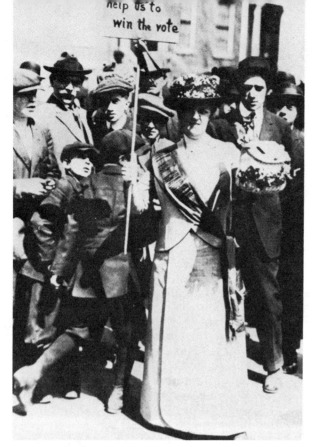

Figure 11–1. Women activists, who waged a long campaign to win the right to vote, achieved a victory in 1920. (Courtesy of History of Nursing Collection, University of Michigan)

POLITICAL PARTICIPATION OF WOMEN

Substantial differences in political participation between men and women have been reported in study after study. In examining the participation hierarchy, the apathetics have an overrepresentation of women, and the gladiatorial activities of running for and holding elective office are carried out by very few females.[3] Verba and Nie found that there were more women than men among inactives, voting specialists, and parochial participants, and more males than females among the communalists, campaigners, and complete activists.[4]

SPECTATOR ACTIVITIES

The legal right to vote has been extended to women in one country after another over the past eighty-five years. In 1893, only one country (New Zealand) enfranchised women on an equal level with men. Australia followed in 1902, and over the next twenty years another dozen countries, including the United States, extended the vote to women. Today only eight countries, all but one of which are Muslim nations, deny women the vote.[5]

Giving women the right to vote has not meant that they have automatically exercised it. Only 10% of Egyptian women vote, for example, even though they have been enfranchised since 1956. In 1924, Merriam and Gosnell explained that the traditional attitude that voting was "not something women do" continued to linger and was most evident in the southern United States.[6] Women around the world generally lag behind men in exercising their voting rights, but this gap narrows where women have had the vote for a longer period of time. Only 47% of Swedish women, as compared to 67% of men, voted when first enfranchised. By 1970, however, Swedish women voted only 1% less than men.[7]

It wasn't until the New Deal era in the 1930s that U.S. women began to vote in larger numbers. The Roosevelt administration elicited the interest of women, probably because of the emphasis on domestic problems.[8] It was also Roosevelt who appointed the first woman to a cabinet position. As can be seen in Table 11-1, the voting gap between men and women was reported to be 13% in 1948. By 1960, Campbell, Converse, Miller, and Stokes showed an 11% voting gap between women and men. They further noted that among females in the 21- to 54-year-old group, those without children voted at the same level as men. Women with children voted somewhat less.[9] Gradually, however, the differences in voting between men and women have diminished. By the 1970s, the gap between men and women had closed considerably; men voted 6% more (76%) than women (70%) in the 1972 Presidential election.[10] In 1980, men and women voted in equal numbers. Education continued to be an important factor in that there were greater differences between the voting of men and women who did not finish high school. In other words, "education affects the level of political participation more among women than among men."[11]

In other spectator activities, men and women were found in 1972 to be equal in terms of wearing political buttons or displaying bumper stickers (each 14%). This had changed considerably since 1956 when 13% of females as compared to 19% of males engaged in this activity. In trying to influence other persons on political matters, 26% of women as compared to 35% of men were reported to engage in this activity in 1972. The spread was even greater in 1956 when 36% of males and 22% of females were involved in political influence.[12]

Table 11-1.   *Sex Differences in Voting for President*

SEX	PERCENTAGE								
	1948	1952	1956	1960	1964	1968	1972	1976	1980
Men.	69	72	80	80	73	76	76	60	59
Women	56	62	69	69	70	73	70	59	59
Difference between the sexes									
(Men–Women)	13	10	11	11	3	3	6	1	0

Source: *Lansing M: The American woman: Voter and activist. In Jaquette J (ed): Women in Politics, p 8. New York, John Wiley & Sons, 1974 (1976 and 1980 data added from personal communication, U.S. Census Bureau, March, 1981)*

TRANSITIONAL ACTIVITIES

Men have been found to participate more in the transitional activities of contacting a public official (29% men, 25% females) and contributing money to a party or candidate (12% male versus 9% female). Men also showed a higher level of attendance at political meetings than women (9% versus 7%) in 1964 (data for 1972 not available).[13]

GLADIATORIAL ACTIVITIES

Gladiatorial activities showed an interesting dichotomy; women actually reported working to get someone else elected (6%) more than men (4%) in 1972. In both 1956 and 1964, men and women reported participating equally in this activity.[14] Yet in terms of actually being a candidate for office, women were abysmally absent. Lee found, in her study on why so few women hold public office, that women actually devote considerably more time to political work at the local level than men do. For example, 9.2% of men as contrasted with 16.2% of women reported spending over forty hours a week.[15] Yet despite this large time commitment, the powerful political roles have nearly always been filled by men. Figure 11-2 shows that although the number of women who serve as delegates to national conventions has grown, only the 1980 Democratic party approached the 50% proportion of women that is representative of the U.S. population.

Both elective and appointive offices range from highly visibly positions, such as those in the U.S. Congress, to obscure offices, such as local boards and commissions. Women have been found to be underrepresented in the full range of public offices. Of the total of 9699 members ever to serve in the House of Representatives, only 90 have been women; and similarly, of the 1734 senators, only 14 have been women. Starting with Representative

Table 11-2.   *Hours Per Month Devoted to Political Activities by Sex*

	SEX	
RESPONSE	WOMEN	MEN
Over 40 hours	16.2%	9.2%
30 to 40 hours	12.2	5.9
20 to 30 hours	10.8	11.8
10 to 19 hours	24.3	18.4
9 or less hours	36.5	54.6
	100 %	100 %
	(N = 148)	(N = 152)

Cramer's V = .207
Source: Lee MM: Why few women hold public office: Democracy and sexual roles. Polit Sci Q 91:302, Summer, 1976

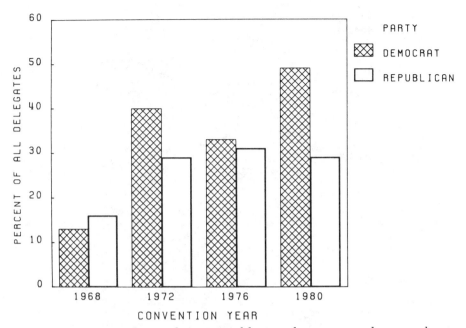

Figure 11–2. *Proportion of national convention delegates who were women by year and party.* (*Courtesy of History and Politics of Nursing, University of Michigan*)

Jeannette Rankin (Republican, Montana), elected in 1916, a total of 104 women have been elected or appointed to Congress. The total includes one woman—Margaret Chase Smith (Republican, Maine)—who served in both chambers. Even the total of 104 is misleading: Two women were never sworn in because Congress was not in session between their appointment or election and the expiration of their terms; another sat in the Senate for just one day; several were appointed or elected to fill unexpired terms and served in Congress for less than a year. Only four women have been elected to full Senate terms. By the end of 1975, 40% of the women members had entered Congress by following their husbands who had been in office. Thirty-eight were married to members who served before them; 36 of these (4 senators and 32 representatives) were appointed or elected to fill the unexpired terms of their late husbands.

Twenty women hold seats in the 97th Congress (1981–1982). Of the 435 members of the House of Representatives in 1981, only 18 seats are held by women, about the same number as twenty years ago. Only 2 women serve in the Senate. The 95th Congress (1977–1978) and the 87th (1961–1962) also had 20 women members, or about 3.7%, the highest number to date. In 1979, Nancy Landon Kassebaum of Kansas became the first woman to enter the Senate outside the route of being appointed to fill the unexpired term of a man and the first woman elected to what had been an all-male Senate since the 1972 retirement of Margaret Chase Smith. (In 1978, Muriel Humphrey and Maryon Allen were both appointed to serve out their deceased

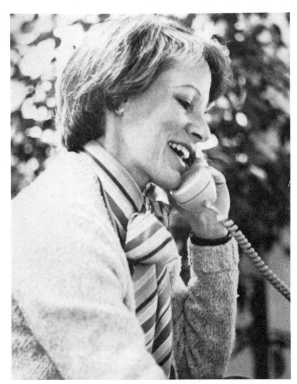

Figure 11–3. Nancy Landon Kassebaum (Republican, Kansas) pioneered a direct electoral route to the U.S. Senate in 1978. (Courtesy of Senator Landon Kassebaum)

husbands' unexpired Senate terms. Mrs. Humphrey did not run for re-election; Mrs. Allen was defeated in her bid for re-election.) Rockefeller aptly points out that "there are three times as many whooping cranes—a rare, endangered species—as there are congresswomen." She quotes David Broder as saying that the "most accessible route to Congress is still through the pain of widowhood."[16] Nancy Kassebaum's election marked a new era for women in high political office and offered hope for women achieving such positions. At 46, she lacked political experience beyond a school board term and a stint in Kansas Senator James Pearson's Washington office. Her father, however, was Alf Landon, the Republican nominee for President in 1936 and former governor of Kansas. He obviously provided a strong political role model for her. She also has substantial wealth, which is a very helpful asset in running a senatorial race, as campaign expenses are high for this select office.

In 1980 Paula Hawkins (Republican, Florida) joined Ms. Kassebaum to become the second woman senator. She was the first woman in the Senate's history to be elected to that body whose career was not based on her relationship to a male relative. Beginning as a political volunteer and community activist, Ms. Hawkins made her first try at public office in 1970, running

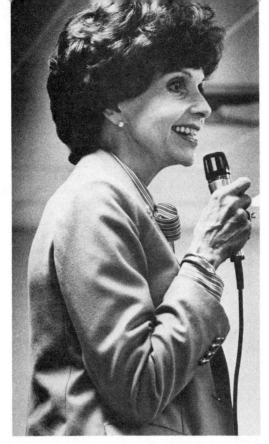

Figure 11–4. Paula Hawkins (Republican, Florida) was the first woman to win election to the U.S. Senate whose political career was unrelated to a male relative. (Courtesy of The Miami Herald, Miami, Florida)

for the Florida House. She was defeated soundly in the Republican primary by a candidate backed by a rival wing. Two years later, she was persuaded by state party leaders to run for the Public Service Commission. Dubbed the "Maitland housewife" by the press, she narrowly won the election to become the third Republican in a century to hold a statewide office in Florida. During the seven years she held that office, Ms. Hawkins established herself as a gutsy consumer champion who fought both rising utility rates and the opposition of other commission members on several issues. The recognition she achieved with her splashy investigations and frequent news conferences provided an excellent basis for her senatorial race in 1980.

Ms. Hawkins' achievement has been a hollow victory for feminists, however, in that she strongly opposes two issues many consider fundamental to women's rights: the proposed equal rights amendment and free choice for women to have abortions. "I am outraged," said Sarah Shirley Hagan, professor of psychology at Miami–Dade Community College, "that the first female elected to such a position of power, authority, and influence in Florida would be opposed to issues that would encourage and support the intellectual and emotional liberation of our own sex." "The E.R.A. is oversold, vaguely worded and ambiguous," Ms. Hawkins says. "There has been a lot too much written about it, and a lot too much said about it." When asked to explain her opposition to the proposed federal equal rights amendment, she has a stock answer: "Women already have the upper hand."

Francis Payne Bolton, a Cleveland, Ohio, area congresswoman who exerted considerable influence on behalf of nursing through passage of the Bolton Act, which created the U.S. Cadet Nurse Corps in 1943, and through numerous other activities, is a classic example of how women entered Congress through the "pain of widowhood." Ms. Bolton was active and interested for many years in nursing education and public health nursing. She funded, for example, a large portion of the Grading Committee Study of Schools of Nursing in the early 1930s and endowed the Western Reserve University School of Nursing in the 1920s (later named the Francis Payne Bolton School of Nursing, Case Western Reserve University). It was not until 1940 that she entered politics, however, when she was elected to fill the unexpired term of her deceased husband at a special election in February of that year. She didn't stop there, however, but instead sought re-election for a seat in the 77th Congress and won and continued to win in the next twelve elections serving twenty-eight years until 1968 when she was eighty-three years of age. In 1972, we (BJ Kalisch and PA Kalisch) interviewed Ms. Bolton and she told us that "the Ohio Republican party leader-

Figure 11–5. Representative Lindy Boggs (on left), one of only eighteen female House members, entered Congress through the route of widowhood. She is pictured with Marie Primm of the Louisiana Nurses' Association. (Courtesy of American Nurses' Association, Kansas City, Missouri)

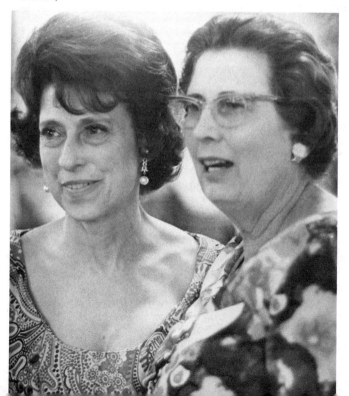

ship expected me to quietly serve out my husband's unexpired term as a memorial to his political career and then stand aside for a new male Republican nominee. I surprised them."[17]

Women governors have also been a rare occurrence. Ella Grasso of Connecticut and Dixy Lee Ray of Washington, the only women ever elected to this office in their own right, ended their administrations in 1980. No woman currently holds this important position. Three other women have served as governors, but they accomplished this feat by succeeding their husbands in office. In 1978, a record was set with the election of four women lieutenant governors, which increased the number of women holding this post to six (a figure which is still maintained in 1981).

Despite the fact that there has been a growth of women in state and local elective posts, the underrepresentation of women at these levels was, until recently, just as dramatic as in the most prestigious offices. An upsurge in political participation of women in state legislatures began to take place in the early 1970s, when the number of women elected reversed the decline of the previous decade. As a result of the November 1972 elections, out of a total of 7561 state legislators, 441 women served in the 1973 sessions. This figure represented a 28% increase over the previous two-year period. The number of women who campaigned for these offices also rose from 842 in 1972 to 1126 in 1974 and then to 1348 in 1978, an increase of 63% in six years. By 1975–1976, there were 611 females in the state houses, or about double the number who served in 1969. Immediately after the November 1976 elections, the figure rose to 685, slightly more than 9% of all state legislators. By January 1981, the total had reached 801, well over twice as many as in 1971. Table 11–3 shows the number of female legislators for the twelve-year period from 1967 to 1981 and the percent of change for each two-year period. Women hold 3% of county commissioner offices and 8% of major and township council positions. Because election to state and local office is considered a springboard to national office, the steadily growing

Table 11–3. *Number of Women Serving in State Legislatures and Percent of Change for Each 2-Year Period*

YEAR	PERCENT CHANGE	NUMBER OF WOMEN LEGISLATORS
1967		323
1969	− 5.57	305
1971	+ 12.79	344
1973	+ 28.20	441
1975	+ 38.55	611
1977	+ 12.60	688
1979	+ 2.03	702
1981	+ 14.10	801

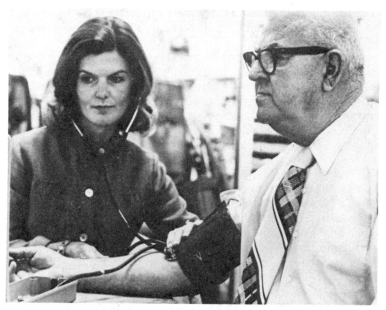

Figure 11–6. Jan Acker, a graduate of Warner Brown School of Nursing, was elected to the Washington County, Mississippi, County Commission in 1976. She became one of the handful (3%) of women county commissioners nationwide. (Courtesy of Jan Acker)

number of women achieving such positions improves the prospects of more women moving into the national political arena in the 1980s.[18]

In appointive offices, there were 468 women holding high-level posts in the federal government early in 1980. Some 18% of former President Carter's appointees to high-level federal jobs were women, including three cabinet members: Patricia Roberts Harris, then the Secretary of Health and Human Services, served earlier in the Carter administration as Secretary of Housing and Urban Development; Shirley M. Hufstedler, a former federal circuit court judge, was named Secretary of the newly established Department of Education; and Juanita M. Kreps served earlier as Secretary of Commerce. Before 1977, only three other women had ever served in the federal cabinet. Jimmy Carter also brought a large number of women into subcabinet positions. President Ronald Reagan has appointed one woman to his cabinet, Jeane Kirkpatrick, a political scientist, as Ambassador to the United Nations. Another key Reagan appointment for both women and nurses has been that of former University of Michigan School of Nursing dean Carolyne K. Davis as Administrator of the Health Care Financing Administration.

At the state government level, executive positions at the cabinet level or higher held by women were 84 in 1975 and 97 in 1977, or 11% of the estimated 904 positions. In early 1979, 110 women were serving as state appellate court judges, and 11 were on the federal bench. By late 1979, 20 women (including 4 blacks) had been included among those nominated to

Table 11–4.   *Percentage of Men and Women Holding Elective Offices in the United States in 1979*

	MEN %	WOMEN %
U.S. Population	48.7	51.3
U.S. Senate	99	1
U.S. House	96	4
U.S. Supreme Court	100	0
Federal Judges	99	1
Governors	96	4
State Representatives	90	10
State Senators	95	5
Statewide Elective/Appointive Offices	89	11
County Governing Boards	97	3
Mayors and Councilors	92	8
School Board Members	75	25

Source: Figures compiled by the National Women's Education Fund and the Center for the American Woman in Politics, Rutgers University

fill the 152 new federal judgeships authorized by the 1978 Omnibus Judgeship Act—117 new district court judgeships and 35 additional circuit court of appeals seats. As of January, 1980, 33 of the 632 federal judiciary were women. No woman has ever served on the U.S. Supreme Court.[19]

Women have increased their numerical strength in public office on every level except Congress. The greatest increases have been at the local level. Yet despite the incremental gains in female office-holding of the past few years, approximately 90% of all elective offices in the United States are still held by men. As is noted in Table 11–4, there are more women than men in the electorate, but the percentage of women officeholders continues to be extremely low. For every woman elected to a public office, there are nine men. Only at the school-board level do women reach 25% of the office-holders, which harkens back to the days when women were allowed to vote only in school elections. This is considered a proper sphere for women inasmuch as it is closely tied to concern for children.

POLICY PRIORITIES

Most experts in the field believe that a greater representation of women in all levels of political participation would have a significant effect on policy outputs. Women as a whole have different policy stands and different policy priorities than men as a group. Some of these differences center on women's issues such as the Equal Rights Amendment (ERA), but women also tend to view other matters differently as well.

In 1959, Lane emphasized a greater "moralism," which women bring

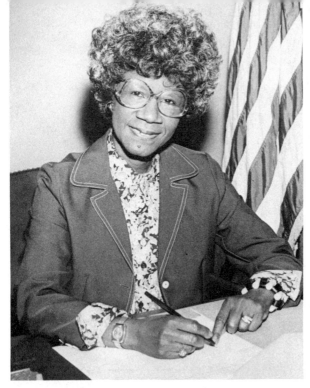

Figure 11–7. The first stage in becoming a political woman involves developing a sex-role ideology. Shirley Chisholm of New York has held a seat in the House of Representatives since 1968. (Courtesy of Shirley Chisholm)

to politics. Correlating the female vote with a "reform" (good government, anticorruption-centered), he tacitly admitted that this interpretation might be stereotypic, yet he nonetheless asserted the cyclic character of reform-dominated elections as proof. For Lane, virtually all aspects of women's political behavior are colored by traditional sex-role requirements:

> Politics is . . . an area of power, and a woman enters politics only at the risk of tarnishing, to some extent, her femininity. Although voting and talking politics are only at the threshold of this power-saturated life, the woman who seems too active in these areas, seems, to some people, to have moved from the properly dependent role of her sex and to seek the masterful and dominant role of men.[20]

In more recent years such sex-role differences continue to emerge. Women have been found to be more against war and capital punishment and against marijuana, pornography, and similar kinds of indulgences. They are more interested in health and welfare issues and less interested in tax problems, diplomatic, and military affairs than men.[21,22,23]

The fact that the Equal Rights Amendment, which was first introduced in Congress in 1923, has not yet received ratification, is perhaps one consequence of women's underrepresentation in politics. This constitutional amendment declares that "equality of rights under the law shall not be denied or abridged by the United States or by any state on account of sex." Hershey found that women were much more likely than men to be interested in the ERA issue, although she found no differences in their ex-

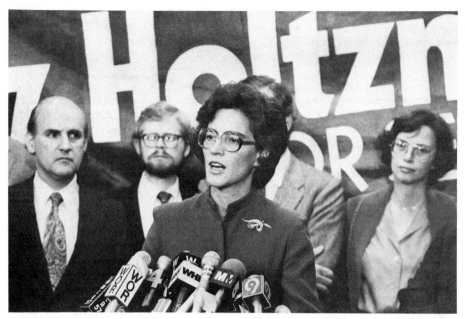

Figure 11–8. Elizabeth Holtzman of Brooklyn, who narrowly lost the 1980 U.S. Senate race in New York, was very active in pushing women's issues during her eight years in the House of Representatives. (Courtesy of John Sotomayer, The New York Times, New York)

pressed support for it. Men were more confused over what it would actually mean.[24] By the end of 1977, 35 of the 38 states required for ratification had approved the proposed 27th Amendment to the Constitution. The Congressional resolution that proposed the amendment set March 22, 1979, as the date by which the required three-fourths of the state legislators should ratify. In 1978, the United States House and Senate voted a 39-month extension of the original deadline to June 30, 1982.

WHY WOMEN HAVE LOWER PARTICIPATION

Most scholarly attempts to explain the inordinately low levels of participation of women in politics can be subsumed under three categories of reasons: (1) political socialization; (2) personality factors; and (3) situational factors.

FEMALE POLITICAL SOCIALIZATION

One prominent explanation for the lower level of political participation and the lesser degree of political efficacy of women as contrasted with men centers on the political socialization experiences of children, adolescents, and adults. The distribution of roles in society may be made on the basis of either *ascribed* or *achieved* characteristics. Sex differentiation is a system whereby roles are distributed on the basis of the ascribed sex. Unlike *distributive systems*, which are based upon achievement, *ascriptive systems* do not depend on motivation of individuals; roles are preselected on the basis of an inborn characteristic from which there is no escape. Such is the case with sex. Male dominance in politics has been assisted by this fact and by stereotypes justifying the differentiation of roles on the basis of gender, in the family, at work, at leisure, as well as in politics.

Sex-role learning begins very early in life. As we all know, infants are treated differently according to sex from the very beginning. Parents tend to reward those behaviors that are considered correct for the sex of the child, even before a child is aware of his or her own sex. Girls are talked to and cuddled more; they are jostled less than boys. Initially, boys are handled more often and more roughly than girls, but the amount of handling diminishes with age. In addition to being played with more roughly, boys are discouraged from clinging. As children grow older, these differences are accentuated. By the time a child enters kindergarten, not only are sex role stereotypes well-developed, but also the male role has traditionally been given higher value.

Because a female child has traditionally had little encouragement for independence, more parental protectiveness, and less cognitive and social pressure for establishing a separate identity, she has engaged in less independent exploration in her environment. As a result she has not as often developed skills to cope with her environment nor confidence in her ability to do so. Parents tend to encourage obedience and conformity in their daughters to a much greater degree than in their sons, and consequently girls are influenced much more easily than boys and have a much greater need for approval of others than boys do. Males are also socialized to be more interested in the outside world in anticipation of entering the more public-oriented work role, whereas girls are socialized to be concerned to a greater extent with private issues. Historically, the male has been the public-being, and the female has been the private-being, whose place is in the home and local community. All of the socialized behaviors result in a lesser interest in and knowledge of politics on the part of females in our society. To put the matter succinctly, the politically relevant norms children acquire during their formative years become lastingly important ones in structuring attitudes and behaviors in adult life.

Early research on political socialization found female nonparticipation in politics to be a predictable event, which can be accounted for by sex-role learning. It has been shown to remain durable and consistent throughout the life cycle. In a 1959 study of political socialization, Hyman found that boys were more interested in political matters than girls.[25] Hess and Torney uncovered the fact that girls showed more confidence and trust in the political change, and chose public figures for admiration more than females did. greater amount of political knowledge, were more comfortable with political change, and chose public figures for admiration more than females did. Both girls and boys indicated a preference for the father as a source of political information and opinions. Greenstein summarized the psychocultural basis of female nonparticipation as follows:

> Politics . . . is more resonant with the 'natural' enthusiasm of boys. Other psychological bases will also be found. For example, the need to conform to cultural definitions of masculinity often is bulwarked by powerful feelings . . .

women who find it especially threatening not be 'feminine' and who see politics as a male function, will be drawn into the political arena only at the cause of great psychic discomfort.[27]

The differences in political socialization of boys and girls is further highlighted by Jaros:

Are women socialized to . . . non-participatory orientations as children? If they are, girls ought to differ from boys on such dimensions at very early ages. By most measures they do, with girls decidedly less political. Girls are less oriented to various kinds of political actions and decidedly less informed. Moreover the sexual differences are seen as early as the fourth grade. Despite increased efforts to involve women in the political world, there is a cultural tradition of feminine nonparticipation transmitted in childhood.[28]

Later studies by Merelman, by Easton and Dennis, and by Orum and his associates have shown that sex differences are not as great as those reported in earlier studies. Although a sufficient amount of research has not been completed to answer this question definitively, these findings could mean that sex-role training is changing and that young girls are experiencing less inculcation into traditional sex-linked behavior. But the recent origins of these changes still dictates that the vast majority of the female population was brought up under the old standards and beliefs.[29]

Through a study of female political elites, Kelly and Boutilier identified

Figure 11–9. Highly politically oriented, Marge Roukema, a physician's wife, was victorious in a hard fought 1980 campaign for New Jersey's Seventh District seat in the U.S. House of Representatives. (Courtesy of The Record, Hackensack, New Jersey)

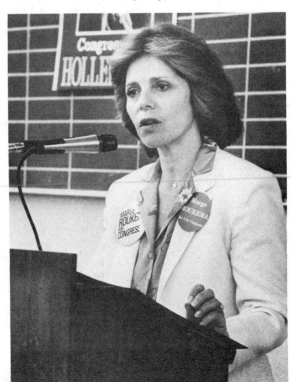

four stages of socialization that a female must pass through sequentially if she is to become politically oriented: (1) development of an activist sex-role ideology; (2) attainment and maintenance of personal control over her life space; (3) development of political salience; and (4) continued rewards and success for political participation. The first two stages, in particular, should occur during childhood, but if this does not happen, a certain degree of adult resocialization is possible.[30]

In the case of a political woman, the first stage involves the *development of an activist sex-role ideology* instead of the traditional, passive one. From Keniston's study of achievement-oriented young career women and graduate students who opted for other than traditional life-styles, some insights for the acquisition of sex-role ideology can be derived. His work identifies critical conditions for the development of women's achievement-motivation and makes it possible to identify a developmental model to assess family influences on socialization. First, there is "the availability to them, within their immediate family or close to it, [of] some individual in whom a degree of individuation and autonomy was apparent." He thus postulates two distinct conditions surrounding the availability of such persons. Among the young women he studied, Keniston found the first condition, "identification with the highly intelligent, able professional mother who has successfully combined in her own person, marriage, career, and motherhood," to be a rare occurrence.[31]

Figure 11–10. The influence of a father on the political development of a daughter was emphasized by Mary Cotton, a nurse who won election to the New Hampshire legislature in 1974. (Courtesy of Mary Cotton)

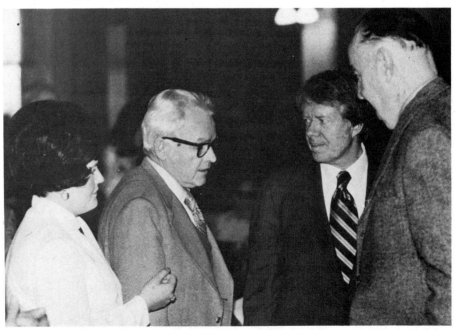

More prevalent was the second condition of "conscious identification with the father described as dynamic, energetic, creative and vigorous." Mary Cotton, a nurse (Mercy Central School of Nursing, 1964) who has run successfully several times for a seat in the New Hampshire State Legislature and who works as a staff nurse when the legislature is not in session, emphasized the importance of her father as a role model for political behavior. She noted, "My father had the idea that women could accomplish anything in life. At dinnertime, we would discuss political affairs routinely. The emphasis was always on how we could work within the system to change things."[32] This hypothesis bears more than passing similarity to the theme that has prevailed in the pragmatically oriented women's movement: it is concerned about women's role stereotypes and dependent image, as portrayed in the mass media, and it demands that young children be exposed to more varied feminine role models—particularly those of working women or of mothers who combine childrearing with employment.

The fact that sons, but not daughters, tend to have their political participation and efficacy increased by a more educated mother, reveals the tremendous impact of the prevailing sex-role ideology. Even when a mother has a higher level of education, it does not necessarily mean that she has a less traditional sex-role ideology; it can, however, provide the mother with an increased ability to educate her children to be more competent within whatever sex-role or behavior framework she does espouse. This means that a well-educated women with a traditional sex-role ideology is likely to transmit a sense of political and public competence to her male offspring. The females will learn the traditional, private, and nonpolitical competencies associated with the family life space they are expected to occupy.

Keniston also hypothesizes that another critical condition for the development of achievement-motivation in women is the existence of a family climate that promotes "open expression of personal and interpersonal conflict." This, he argues, is of fundamental importance because psychological conflict is a common dimension in the experience of achieving women. Their aspirations run contrary to the still conventional sex-role expectations and to the social environment, which continues to be largely nonsupportive. But the family's openness to conflict presents to daughters a personally useful paradigm of conflict and conflict-resolution. Later on, this paradigm is psychologically efficacious in negotiating the role-related conflicts women face in choosing less traditional roles of life-styles, as is stated in the following:

From an early age, these women seem to have learned in their families that conflicts could generally be resolved if they were directly aired. Thus quarrels between the parents were relatively open and frequent, but to the daughters they have rarely seemed very threatening. Personal conflict came to be seen simply as a routine part of people living together. This capacity to experience conflict—interpersonal or intrapsychic—openly but without being overwhelmed by it was an enduring characteristic of most of these women.[33]

Keniston's conclusion, that the family's promotion of conflict-expression and conflict-resolution is an important condition of the development of achievement-motivation in women, echoes certain analyses of politicization and role conflict. Several studies have found that politicized women show evidence of greater ability to deal with role conflicts and possess greater role freedom—that is to say, the ability to avoid the constraints imposed by traditional norms and definitions of female roles. In agreeing that policized women are freer, these studies have also hypothesized that such freedom explains their ability to combine several roles and to undertake political ones with some success, if not without strain. For the purpose of examining the social processes by which women become "different" enough from other women to confront structural barriers opposed to their political entry, Keniston's developmental model raises both role model and family climate conditions of interest.

The case for the relationship between achievement-orientation and the presence of family role models is congruent with a substantial body of findings by political scientists about the emergence of activists from politically engaged families. One of the more interesting findings from a cross study of national legislative elites is that those who were socialized to politics during childhood—37% in all cases—invariably came from intensely involved political families. Women state legislators had politically active fathers in 50% of the cases and active mothers in 40% of the cases. For example, this was the case with a former nurse legislator from North Dakota, Patricia Kenner, who said, "I grew up thinking my father was the only Democrat in South Dakota. He ran for office when it was impossible to elect a Democrat in the state."[34] Among female party delegates to national conventions studied for their political ambitions, slightly more of the ambitious ones came from politically active families. Where only one parent was active, it was the mother who more frequently affected ambition. The research

Figure 11–11. Patricia Kenner, who was elected to the South Dakota State House in 1974, attributed her own gladiatorial political activities to the activism of her parents. (Courtesy of Patricia Kenner)

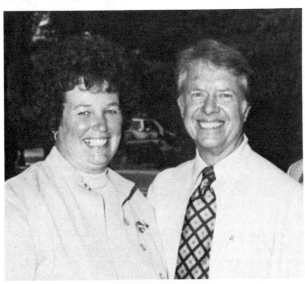

of Keniston and others confirmed the importance of role models as the key variable underlying the emergence of achieving political women.

The second stage of political development involves gaining *personal control over one's life space* and "gaining needed competencies and abilities to maintain control as the life-space expands." It is "at the interface between the individual's life-space and politics that the key to understanding political efficacy lies. . . ; the immediately relevant life-space differs for men and women and for subgroups of males and females."[35] Women have lacked control over many aspects of their lives in that they have traditionally not been able to determine for themselves such things as when they will have children, how they can use their time, and what they can do with their lives. Child care, for example, is not always predictable. Even though modern innovations (such as birth control, timesaving household appliances, pre-prepared food) and a more open society in terms of opportunities for women have actually given women more control over their lives than was formerly true, women still tend not to think of themselves as being in control and thus do not take control of their own lives. They feel they are not capable of doing so. This belief spreads to include feelings about control over other areas of life such as politics, and is underlined in the findings of a large national survey of adolescents, in which the future orientations of males and females were studied in terms of their fantasies (*i.e.*, their hopes and dreams of the future) as well as their realistic plans. They found that males' reality conceptions corresponded closer to their fantasies. Females, on the other hand, displayed much less congruence between their reality and fantasy conceptions.

The third stage of becoming political involves *developing an awareness of the salience of politics.* In order for a woman to develop politically, she must feel that politics is important to her and that it is rewarding to be involved in it. Political salience develops from political discussions with parents, peers, and teachers, from strong love for a parent involved in politics, and from political events of special significance. In other words,

> As politics becomes included in a woman's day-to-day existence, it is possible that she will begin to expand her definition of her life-space to include political activity. The greater her intellectual and emotional involvement in political activity, the more likely she is to develop a greater need for personal control over that aspect of her life-space and to develop further the beliefs and the abilities required to exercise that control.[36]

The final stage in the development of a political woman is *receiving rewards for political participation and having sufficiently successful experiences* so that she is encouraged to continue. Positive political activity or participation leads to political efficacy, which in turn leads to more participation and then to an even greater degree of efficacy. The traditional lack of political efficacy seen among women was highlighted in a study by Soule and McGrath. Employing four commonly used items to measure political efficacy, they found that females have less efficacy than males. More women felt that they have no say in government, that public officials don't care what they think, that voting is the only way to influence government, and that politics is so complicated they can't understand it.[37]

The need for the positive reinforcement stage of development is readily seen in the experiences of many nurses who have eventually sought elective office. Marilyn Goldwater, a Maryland state legislator and nurse explains that she got involved in politics after "extensive community service activities. I became well known and people came to me asking me to run."[38] Similarly Marion Spencer, a Vermont nurse (Muhlenberg Hospital School of Nursing) who has served in the state house since 1974, explains, "It was a natural progression. At first I worked for the PTA and in women's groups. Then I became a School Director, and Chairman of the District and finally I ran for the House."[39]

PERSONALITY FACTORS

Another explanation for the fact that women are less involved in politics, particularly certain aspects of political life, is that they differ from men in certain personality traits necessary for political success. Kruschke, for example, studied political women and found that they scored higher than apolitical women on sociability, optimism, willingness to risk, liberalism, and a sense of political efficacy.[39] Similarly, Werner and Bachtold found that women politicians serving in state legislatures were generally more intelligent, more assertive, more venturesome, more imaginative and unconventional, and had more liberal attitudes than women in general. They were similar to male political leaders in intelligence, boldness, and venturesomeness. Male politicians were more enthusiastic, self-assured, and self-controlled than female politicians, whereas female leaders were found to be more assertive, imaginative, and experimental.[41]

Figure 11–12. A strong social service orientation directed Marilyn Goldwater, R.N., to successfully seek elective office in the Maryland State Legislature in 1974. (Courtesy of Marilyn Goldwater)

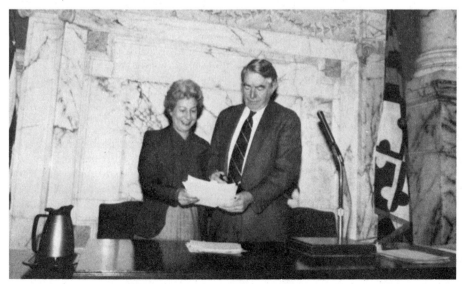

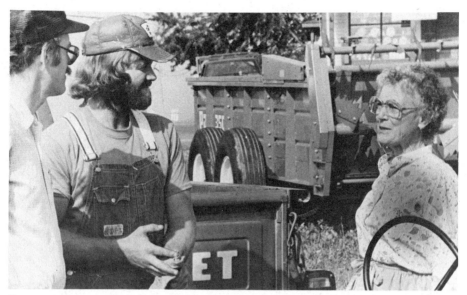

Figure 11–13. A steady progression from offices in civic organizations and the school board led Marion Spencer, R.N., to her seat in the Vermont State House in 1974. (Courtesy of Thomas M. Johnson, Vegennes, Vermont)

In comparing female political party leaders with other women, Constantini and Craik found the leaders to be more forceful, effective, ambitious, and socially ascendant individuals; they also had lower scores on abasement, succorance, and deference. In comparing these women with male leaders, they showed a fairly similar personality trait pattern. Both groups were found to be outgoing, socially skilled, capable, and persistent; but female party leaders worried more, tried harder, and felt more uncertain about themselves. Men were seen as more easygoing. These findings led to the conclusion that political women tend to be more similar to political men than to other women and that a relationship exists between certain personality attributes and success in politics. Although not empirically based, it appears that fewer women have these attributes.[42]

SITUATIONAL FACTORS

The disparity between the political behavior of men and women has also been explained in terms of certain situational factors such as level of education, unequal employment opportunities, marriage, children, sex discrimination, and traditional attitudes. As we have seen, the socialization process creates differences in the political attitudes, knowledge, and participation of males and females, but these differences linger and in some cases seem actually to become more entrenched as children move into adolescence and adulthood.

Numerous studies have shown that political participation is associated with socioeconomic level. One aspect of socioeconomic level is education, and less education has been shown to be associated with less participation. Because fewer women have college education than men, this factor can be considered to be one possible situational explanation for women's lower participation rates. Among Caucasians, 34% of men versus 22% of women had completed college in 1976. Within professions, nursing overall ranks low in educational achievement of its members. The contrast with elementary and secondary school teachers in 1977 can be noted in Figure 11-10. Even though teacher education is also largely dominated by women (70.6% versus 98% for nurses), their overall education level is higher, and thus one would predict a higher degree of participation in politics among teachers.

Another factor highly associated with the socioeconomic level is the nature of women's employment or lack of employment. In a market economy such as the United States, where the activity of an individual is rewarded in accordance with its exchange value on the market, status is largely determined by occupational participation. When the division of labor is one in which men take responsibility for participation in the economy and women engage in activities that have no exchange value (i.e., housewife), the social status of women is largely dependent on that of the man they marry. Even among women who work, family responsibilities are usually considered to be of primary importance, and involvement in work has been sometimes limited to certain periods of the life cycle and almost always confined to staff and supportive positions. Only 5% of working women, for example, held managerial or administrative positions in 1975.

Figure 11–14. Comparison of educational pyramids (professional education only) of the nation's registered nurses and active elementary and secondary school teachers in 1977. (Courtesy of History and Politics of Nursing, University of Michigan)

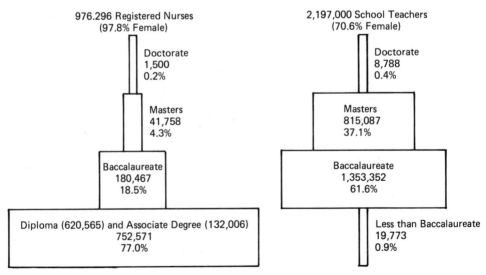

Table 11–5.   *Growth of the Working Women Population 1950–1978*

YEAR	WOMEN AGED 20+ WHO ARE EMPLOYED (IN MILLIONS)	% OF TOTAL WOMEN WHO ARE EMPLOYED	% OF WORKING ADULTS WHO ARE WOMEN
1950	17.3	33.9	29.4
1955	19.6	35.7	31.4
1960	21.9	37.7	33.3
1965	24.7	39.3	34.5
1970	29.7	43.3	37.7
1975	33.6	46.3	39.6
1980	41.0	51.2	42.4

Source: *United States Department of Labor, Bureau of Labor Statistics,* Perspectives on Working Women: A Databook. *Washington, Government Printing Office, 1980*

Income levels of women are lower than males, even for the same kind of work in many cases. Yet as Table 11-5 shows, 51% of all women were employed in 1980, and the figure is growing each year. Thus over half of all women do work, and at least half of these women are married.[43]

Women have traditionally tended to leave primary responsibility for the satisfaction of material goods to their husbands and have viewed their own educational and occupational aspirations as sources of intrinsic fulfillment, bearing little relationship to their material expectations. Women's work has thus been seen as supplementary and of less importance than men's work, which represents a full-time commitment and provides the major source of family support.

The persistence of traditional female roles in families can be seen in Figure 11–15. Seventy-eight of those polled in this survey either fully or partially agreed that a wife should put her husband and children ahead of her own career. Similarly 69% agreed that children suffer if women work, and around half felt that the wife is still the person responsible for housecleaning even if she works and that marriages benefit from the stay-at-home wife. Similarly, Figure 11–16 shows that the idea of moving to a new locale for a woman's job is relatively uncommon. There exists, then, an ambiguity about the female role and inherent conflict between a strong commitment to a career and realization of the traditional female role in marriage and parenthood. It is not surprising that females have been oriented toward achieving success in the areas that our culture has deemed most important for women. Because a woman's self-esteem has, until recently, been tied to fulfillment of the traditional female role, occupational concerns have been less important. Males, on the other hand, have been more concerned with their occupational roles because they have been central to the male role and not seen as conflicting with, but rather as contributing to, the family's well-being and future. For men, occupational accomplishments have represented

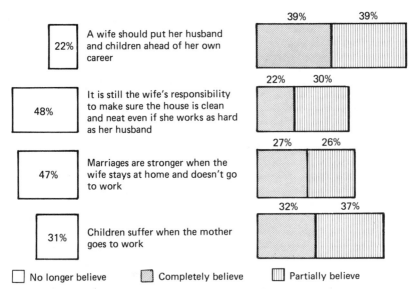

Figure 11–15. Mixed reactions to traditional female roles in family. (Courtesy of Public Opinion, Vol. 2, Jan/Feb 1979, p 36)

the major achievements rewarded by contemporary society. When occupations were grouped on the basis of the commitment they would require, only 10% of the females as compared to 47% of the males wanted jobs involving strong career commitment.

Because politics often mandates heavy commitment, it has been found not to mesh easily with traditional marriage and family life. Conflicting demands occur, and women are faced with the serious dilemma of feeling that either home or career may suffer. Women legislators, for example, have

Figure 11–16. Husband's job still governs choice of residence. (Courtesy of History and Politics of Nursing, University of Michigan)

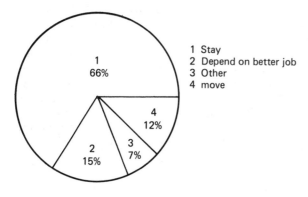

testified eloquently about the demands on them to maintain the responsibilities of both roles simultaneously: to be super-prepared for their legislative duties and to have dinner promptly on the table. Sandra Smoley, the California nurse who ran for the U.S. House of Representatives in 1978, underlined this problem: "My first husband, a physician, could not accept the fact that I came home tired and sometimes later than him. The dinner wasn't always on the table. He kept saying 'You don't have to work.'" Eventually they divorced. She remarried and her second husband's attitude "is just the opposite. He very much wants me to succeed in politics. He would have moved to Washington with me, commuting back and forth as needed to maintain his firm, if I had won the election."[44]

The attitude of husbands toward their wives' political involvement has been found to be of key importance. In 1955, Maurice Duverger described the political behavior of women as follows: "Women . . . have the mentality of minors in many fields, and, particularly in politics, they will accept paternalism on the part of men. The man—her husband, fiancé, lover, or myth—is the mediator between them and the political world."[45] Kirkpatrick reported that most female legislators would not have run for office without their husbands' approval.[46] Similarly, Stoper found that husbandly support

Figure 11–17. The strong support of her husband has been instrumental in the highly successful political career of Representative Patricia Schroeder of Colorado. (Courtesy of Representative Patricia Schroeder)

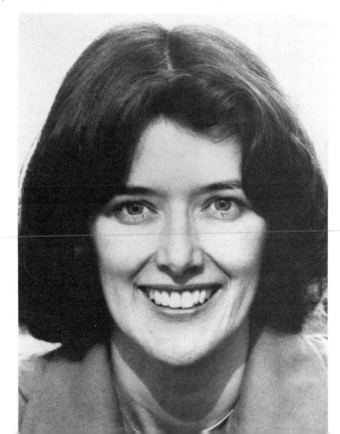

was significantly more frequently reported by women state legislators than was wifely support by male legislators. By inference, husbands' support is a critical condition for women successfully holding state office.[47]

From the available evidence it would seem that the supportive husband may be facilitative to the extent of taking an active role in his wife's political career or by assuming some of her domestic responsibilities, which, in fact, few husbands with wives involved in state or local politics do. Rather the typical husband does not impede or discourage the woman's political aspirations. When women move into congressional roles, however, more husbands become involved in household work and in more active supportive roles. More of a partnership is in evidence whereby each person is willing to sacrifice somewhat so that both individuals can have a career. Husbands have traditionally been threatened by a wife's superior or equal achievement, and this fact is still deeply rooted in our culture. Husbands who feel pleased and happy with their wife's achievements rather than threatened are essential. This is the case with Patricia Schroeder, U.S. congresswoman from Colorado. Her husband narrowly lost a bid for the Colorado state legislature in 1970. Both are lawyers, and she had campaigned for him in his attempt to win office. In 1972, he offered her name to run for the House and in turn campaigned for her. When she won the congressional seat, he relocated his law practice to Washington.[48] This is also the case with state legislator Mary Cotton, R.N., who emphasized the importance of her "extremely supportive husband. He has no ego problems. He often has dinner ready for me since I often don't get home until 7 or 8 p.m. at night. At parties, I tend to get more attention because of my position but it doesn't bother him. I couldn't do it without Jack, especially when the game gets especially rough such as the time I was attacked in the newspapers on a personal level."[49]

Related to the issue of spouse support for political efforts is the fact that societal norms make husbands' campaigning for wives more difficult than is true of the opposite case. For the male, a wife and family are assets. They can represent him at political events and thus multiply the politician's effect. For women, a husband and children in public view often leads voters to conclude that she should be at home fulfilling the traditional role. For example, Sandra Smoley, the nurse who ran for the U.S. Congress, noted, "I was continuously asked, 'what will happen to your children?' I felt compelled to carry around and show photographs of my children so that they could see they were older!"[50] Widows do better than single women because voters assume that they have already fulfilled their wifely role. This point was brought home when Congresswoman Martha Keys (Kansas), married a representative from another state and found that her marriage was a significant issue in her re-election bid. The question brought up by her opponents centered on how she could be married to a congressman from Indiana and still represent Kansas. She was defeated. Her husband, by contrast, never had their marriage raised as an issue in his re-election campaign.[51]

The problem of marital roles is compounded by the presence of young children, which decidedly inhibits younger women from political activity. The typical resolution of this *role conflict* is to wait until children have

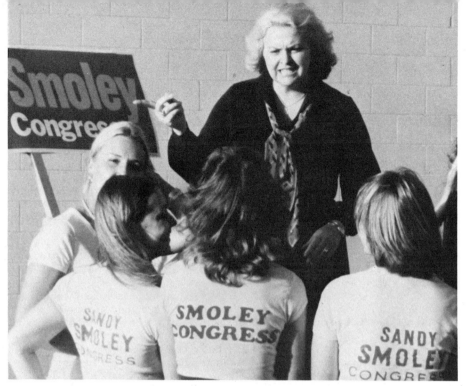

Figure 11–18. Questions about a woman's "family responsibilities to any young children" automatically crop up in a female's political campaign as they did in California nurse Sandra Smoley's race for a U.S. House seat in 1978. (Courtesy of Sandra Smoley)

grown. Lee, for example, found that having child-care responsibilities did not affect the amount of time women devoted to political activities or whether a woman served as a party district leader or not. Running for an elective office decreased, however, for women with young children, thus throwing those that did participate into the older age brackets. The typical female political activist is a middle-aged or older woman.[52] Flora and Lynn found that "becoming a mother had a definite influence on . . . political socialization. . . . The urgencies of motherhood, when one suddenly finds oneself totally responsible for a young life, have repercussions for the issues a woman is interested in." They did find that political involvement was enhanced by anticipatory socialization, husband helpfulness, and interaction networks.[53]

A number of women who have served in Congress have had no children. Martha Griffith and her husband, for example, chose not to have children in order that she could have a full-time career. Other married congresswomen without children have included Senator Margaret Chase Smith and Representatives Leonor Sullivan, Helen Meyner, Virginia Smith, and Shirley Chisholm. Ella Grasso, the first woman elected to a governorship without following in the footsteps of her husband, did have children, and the impact is described as follows:

> Ella Grasso began her political career in 1952 when she first ran for the Connecticut state legislature. Already married and the mother of a three-year-old girl and a one-year-old boy, Grasso was blessed with an extended family which

allowed her to participate in politics without feeling as if she had abandoned her husband and children. She acknowledges that without this support system she would never have committed herself to such extensive political activity. 'My husband was always very helpful. And we shared many of the tasks I might have had to assume alone. I was very lucky because I had parents who lived right across the street and I had uncles and aunts all around. My children were living in a familiar neighborhood . . . where their mother had been born. So it was almost like a little enclave, and I had no qualms.'

Although Thomas Grasso was not particularly interested or active in politics himself and did not necessarily encourage his wife to begin her political career, he was instrumental in this development insofar as he did not object and did not oppose her political activity. Her career is predicated on the acceptability of her ambitions to other members of her family. Better able to combine her private life as wife and mother with her public life at the state level, she did not seek to run for Congress until 1970, eighteen years after her entrance into politics. One might expect such a delay had she lacked the party support, or if she had been an independent spirit, an outsider who did not get along because she would not go along, but this is hardly the case. As legislator and secretary of state Ella Grasso paid her dues in backroom party chores: she canvassed, wrote Democratic planks and speeches, [and] served as floor leader in the legislature. Epitomizing the party loyalist, Grasso could well have anticipated a congressional seat earlier than she achieved it. It was the family consideration which led her not to enter Congress until she was nearly fifty years old; she would never consider going off to Washington while her children were still young and at home. The fact that her children had grown up and her husband had retired may have facilitated her taking on the congressional post, but it also meant that her power potential in the Congress was severely limited. The years of internship necessary to acquire political power were no longer accessible to her.

Grasso frankly stressed the priority of her family in her career: 'I measured all these events in my life by what my family was doing at the time.'[54]

The fact that not having motherhood responsibilities can contribute to success as a politician is just the opposite of congressmen who either benefit from having children or do not benefit politically from being childless. Lee sums it up as follows: ". . . the percentage of women holding public office is unlikely to increase by a substantial amount in the future unless radical changes occur in current sexual role assignments."[55]

Women, of course, can resolve the conflict and successfully combine political office and motherhood. This is vividly portrayed in the case of Jean Moorhead, the nurse in the California assembly. She has five children, the youngest being four and the oldest fourteen years of age. When asked how she manages, she explains, "It's difficult sometimes particularly when I have night commitments. But I didn't have to leave home to serve in office since Sacramento is the state capital. It would be extremely difficult otherwise. My husband is supportive."[56]

Sex discrimination has also been identified as a situational factor that holds women back from full participation in politics. Women cannot achieve politics and perform successfully solely through their own motivations and characteristics. Quite apart from their actual abilities, aspirations, and attitudes to achieve elective office for example, they are dependent upon approval from electorates, from political party leaders, and from office holders with the power to select others for appointed offices. Once in office,

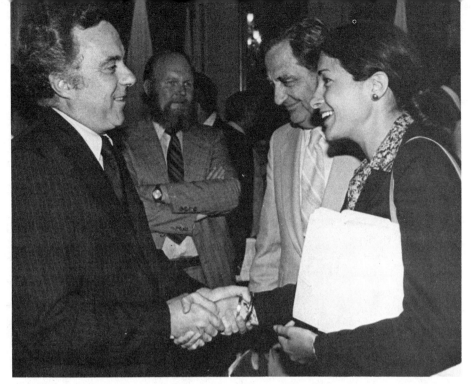

Figure 11–19. Although sex discrimination remains a major barrier for women candidates, there are a few bright success stories. Representative Olympia J. Snowe of Maine won a close race for a U.S. House seat in 1978. (Courtesy of Olympia J. Snowe)

women face additional barriers if sizeable proportions of constituents and colleagues automatically regard their competence and qualifications as suspect because of their gender. In the minds of women office holders, discrimination—especially discrimination from colleagues and party leaders—looms far larger as a difficulty of office holding than conflict with family responsibilities or deficiences of background and education. In one survey, women were asked to respond to the following question: "What special difficulties, if any, have you experienced as a result of being a woman holding public office?" Men were asked, "What do you think are the special difficulties, if any, for a woman holding office?" The responses can be seen in Table 11–6.

Women complained that they are not taken seriously; stereotyped in their characteristics; regarded as sex objects; excluded from the "old boys" network; not consulted on pending issues; discriminated against in committee assignments; asked to do clerical work and domestic chores; asked to assume an unfair share of the workload; subjected to opposition to their programs and ideas because a woman has initiated them; expected to prove their competence whereas that of men is taken for granted; and sometimes avoided or ridiculed by male constituents. Many commented simply that they confronted the "old story" of male chauvinism. More than eight in ten comments in the female comparison sample referred to such forms of discrimination.

Men were less likely than women to name sex discrimination as a problem experienced by women serving in office. Larger proportions of the dif-

Table 11–6.   Perceptions of Female Office Holders' Difficulties by Sex
of Office Holder

TYPE OF DIFFICULTY NAMED	PERCENTAGE WOMEN	PERCENTAGE MEN
Chauvinism, stereotyping	45	26
Exclusion from male networks	7	1
Discrimination in assignments	3	—
Opposition to programs, ideas	3	1
Having to prove competence	14	4
Constituent prejudice	9	17
Discomfort of minority status	6	3
Financial support	1	—
Family pressures	3	11
Personality difficulty	2	17
Deficiency in qualifications	4	17
Other	3	3
Total difficulties named = 100 pct	(574)	(288)
Total naming 1 or more	(372)	(215)
Percentage naming 1 or more	60%	68%

Source: Johnson M, Carrol S: Statistical report: Profile of women holding office, 1977.
In Center for the American Woman and Politics: Women in Public Office,
p 43A. Metuchen, NJ, Scarecrow Press, 1978

ficulties named by men focused on conflicts between office holding and the
family life of women, or on perceived inadequacies of personality and qualifications among female officials. Forty-five percent of the responses given
by men, but only 9% of those made by women were in these areas. In addition, nearly twice the proportion of men's responses (17%) as of women's
(9%) referred to the prejudice of constituents. Thus, although men in office
tend to perceive women's difficulties as related to personal qualities and
characteristics of women in office or to public antipathy to women office
holders, women officials perceive their difficulties largely in terms of the
behavior of their colleagues or of political men.

These findings are reinforced by a Louis Harris poll in which 23% of
those women responding felt that "men hold women back in politics" and
50% felt that "women are mostly given the detailed dirty work chores in
politics, while men hold the real power." Similarly, Lee found that women
believed that both men and women felt that women should participate in
politics in ways other than running for office.[57] Sharon Rockefeller further
collaborates the existence of such discrimination:

We don't have to ask why there are so few women holding public office—we
know why. And the overriding reason is not the public attitude toward women

. . . two problems . . . overshadow all others: (1) money and (2) the reluctance of the political establishment to let women into the fraternity.[58]

In terms of money, Rockefeller characterizes women as being in a Catch-22: "Women are not taken seriously as candidates until they can raise money. And they cannot raise money until they are taken seriously." Women themselves tend not to be able to contribute because they lack control over the family finances or because they don't have the money. As to entering the political establishment, Rockefeller notes that women are "on the periphery of this club. They stuff envelopes, they answer telephones . . . they serve the same functions as the clerical staffs in the thousands of business offices in this country. A few of them are fortunate enough to hold offices within the club, as long as they are not those offices which control the campaign funds or make the binding policy decisions. . . . Women . . . have spent their talents and their energies getting men elected."[59]

In looking at attitudes of women toward other women in politics, polls taken from 1931 to 1978 show that women originally showed more support for a woman president than did men in the 1930s and 1940s, but men were more willing to vote for a woman in 1963 and 1976. By 1978, it had evened out.[60] Significantly, women as a group have been less favorable toward women candidates than blacks are toward black candidates. Consequently, women have lacked the cohesive voting pattern (so often found among blacks, for example) that can warn political leaders that a social grouping has become a force to be reckoned with, requiring inclusion of its members on party slates and attention to its special concerns. The importance of this

Figure 11–20. Opinion Roundup: Men keep pace with women in support for female president. (Courtesy of Public Opinion, Vol. 2, Jan/Feb 1979, p 36)

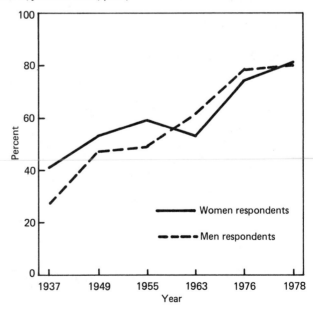

fact in the political world is suggested by the inability of women to translate vote power into public policy status. Until quite recently, it was assumed that women or nurses would not vote as a block because they would divide along family lines, voting as submissive wives and daughters.

The relationship between 98% of the nurses in the United States and men may productively be approached through the study of power distribution, measured in terms of control of valued resources. Ideologic differentiation accounts for variables in male and female political participation. Where ideologic differentiation is present, there is disagreement between the sexes as to the relative value of particular resources. Female nurses, for example, consider some male-controlled power resources relatively unimportant (*i.e.*, office holding) and value highly their own resources (*i.e.*, motherhood), while men hold the opposite valuation. During the 1970s and early 1980s males and females have been increasingly perceived as fundamentally the same, and therefore both should have equal access to important (*i.e.*, traditionally male) resources. Differential access to political power through office holding and active involvement in policy making are injustices that should be redressed, so that power is no longer distributed on the basis of sex roles. One of the means by which this goal may be attacked is through the effective use of interest groups at the national level, a subject that is addressed in the following chapter.

References

1. Rockefeller SP, Testimony before the U.S. Congress. Senate. Committee on Labor and Human Resources: The Coming Decade: American Women and Human Resources Politics and Programs, 1979, p 138. Hearings before the Committee, Part 1. Washington, DC, United States Government Printing Office, 1979
2. Stucker J: Women as voters: Their maturation as political persons in American society. In Githens M, Prestage JL (eds): The Political Behavior of the American Woman, pp 264–283. New York, David McKay, 1977
3. Milbrath L: Political Participation, pp 135–136. Chicago, Rand-McNally, 1965
4. Verba S, Nie NH: Participation in America, pp 97–100. New York, Harper & Row, 1972
5. Newland K: The Sisterhood of Man, pp 97–123. New York, WW Norton, 1979
6. Merriam C, Gosnell HF: Nonvoting, pp 109–116. Chicago, University of Chicago Press, 1924
7. Newland, op cit
8. Chafe W: The American Woman: Her Changing Social, Economic and Political Roles, 1920–1970. New York, Oxford University Press, 1972
9. Campbell A, Converse E, Miller E, Stokes E: The American Voter. New York, John Wiley & Sons, 1960
10. Lansing M: The American woman: Voter and activist. In Jacquette JS (ed): Women in Politics, p 8. New York, John Wiley & Sons, 1974
11. Soule JW, McGrath WE: A comparative study of male–female political attitudes at citizen and elite levels. In Githens M, Prestage JL (eds): A Portrait of Marginality, p 181. New York, David McKay, 1977
12. Ibid, p 181
13. Ibid
14. Ibid
15. Manning Lee M: Why few women hold public office: Democracy and sexual roles. Polit Sci Q 91:302, 1976
16. Rockefeller, op cit, p 139
17. Interview with Francis Payne Bolton, Cleveland, Oh, July 30, 1972
18. Karnig AK, Walter BO: Election of women to city councils. Soc Sci Q 56:605–613, 1976;

Sigelman L: The curious case of women in state and local government. Soc Sci Q 56:591–604, 1976

19. Diamond I: Sex Roles in the State House. New Haven, Yale University Press, 1977
20. Lane RE: Political Life: Why People Get Involved in Politics, p 213. Glencoe, Ill, Free Press, 1959
21. Hamilton RF: A research note on the mass support for "tough" military initiatives. Am Sociol Rev 33:439–445, 1968; Verba S et al: Public opinion and the war in Vietnam. Am Polit Sci Rev 61:317–333, 1976; Converse PE, Schuman H: "Silent majorities" and the Vietnam War. Sci Am 222:17–25, 1970
22. Erikson RS, Luttbeg NR: American Public Opinion: Its Origins, Content and Impact, pp 206–207. New York, John Wiley & Sons, 1973; Gruberg M: Women in American Politics. Wisconsin, Academic Press, 1968
23. Lee, op cit
24. Hershey MR: The politics of androgyny: Sex roles and attitudes toward women in politics. Am Politics Q 5:261–287, 1977
25. Hyman H: Political Socialization. Glencoe, Ill, Free Press, 1959
26. Hess RD, Torney JV: Development of Political Attitudes in Children. Chicago, Aldine, 1967
27. Greenstein F: Children and Politics, p 127. New Haven, Yale University Press, 1965
28. Jaros D: Socialization to Politics, pp 44–45. New York, Praeger, 1973
29. Merelman RM: Political Socialization and Educational Climates. New York, Holt, Rinehart & Winston, 1971; Merelman RM: The family and political socialization: Toward a theory of exchange. J Politics 42:461–486, 1980; Easton D, Dennis J: Children in the Political System. New York, McGraw-Hill, 1969; Orum AM: Sex, socialization and politics. Am Sociol Rev 39:197–209, 1974
30. Kelly RM, Boutilier M: The Making of Political Women. Chicago, Nelson-Hall, 1978
31. Keniston K: Themes and Conflicts of "Liberated" Young Women, pp 11–15. Karen Horney Memorial Lecture, New York City, Mar 24, 1971
32. Interview with Mary Cotton, R.N., Aug 12, 1980
33. Keniston, op cit, p 12
34. Interview with Patricia Kenner, Aug 22, 1980
35. Kelly and Boutilier, op cit, pp 51–52, 312
36. Ibid, p 59
37. Soule and McGrath, op cit, p 183
38. Interview with Marilyn Goldwater, R.N., Aug 12, 1980
39. Interview with Marion Spencer, Aug 14, 1980
40. Kruschke ER: Level of optimism as related to female political behavior. Soc Sci 41:67–75, 1966
41. Werner EE, Bachtold LM: Personality characteristics of women in American politics. In Jaquette JS (ed): Women in Politics, pp 75–84. New York, John Wiley & Sons, 1974
42. Constantine E, Craik K: Women as politicians: The social background, personality, and political careers of female party leaders. J Soc Issues 28, No. 2:217–236, 1972
43. U.S. Department of Labor: Handbook on Women Workers, p 91. Washington, DC, United States Government Printing Office, 1975
44. Interview with Sandra Smoley, R.N., Aug 15, 1980
45. Duverger M: The Political Role of Women, p 129. Paris, United Nations Educational, Scientific and Cultural Organizations, 1955
46. Kirkpatrick, op cit
47. Stoper E: Wife and politician: Role strain among women in public office. In Githens M, Prestage JL: A Portrait of Marginality, pp 320–337. New York, David McKay, 1977
48. Thompson JH: Career Patterns and Role Perceptions of U.S. Congresswomen Since 1916. Unpublished Ph.D. dissertation, Johns Hopkins University, 1978
49. Cotton, op cit
50. Smoley, op cit
51. Thompson, op cit
52. Lee, op cit
53. Flora CB, Lynn NB: Women and political socialization: Considerations of the impact of motherhood. In Jacquette JS (ed): Women in Politics, pp 37–53. New York, John Wiley & Sons, 1974

54. Kelly and Boutilier, op cit, pp 120–121
55. Lee, op cit, p 297
56. Interview with Jean Moorhead, Aug 22, 1980
57. Lee, op cit
58. Rockefeller, op cit, p 142
59. Ibid, pp 143–144
60. Opinion roundup. Public Opinion January–February:36, 1979

12–Interest Groups and Lobbying

An interest group is an association of people concerned with protecting and promoting shared values through the use of the political process. The function that describes the role of such groups in politics is interest-articulation. Interest groups distribute information about the group's interests, encourage support for this interest among members, organize the resources of such members to achieve these goals, and use the power of the organization to influence public decisions that could affect their ability to achieve their specific interests. Interest groups represent the policy preferences of their constituents. Interest groups are everywhere in American economic, social, and political life, representing a bewildering diversity of occupational, ethnic, and ideologic interests. *The Encyclopedia of Associations* lists more than 13,000 associations or groups. Not all of these, of course, have some interests in government, but almost all of the trade, business, agricultural, and labor organizations plus many of the educational, professional, cultural, civic, and religious groups do.

ORGANIZATION OF INTEREST GROUPS

Joining and participating in formal groups and organizations is more common among better educated people, who often hold better jobs and have higher incomes. Organizational activity is thus similar to being informed about politics, voting, and working in campaigns in that poor people are less likely to do any of these things. Self-confidence, bureaucratic skill, and verbal ability are scarcer among less-educated people, who are at a competitive disadvantage in the interest-group struggle, as they are generally. Many people join an organization for reasons other than the accomplishment of political goals. Most members of labor unions have no choice: they must join in order to work. Lawyers generally must belong to a state or local bar association to practice law, and many physicians must join local affiliates of the American Medical Association to practice in certain hospitals. Many scholars, lawyers, and physicians join their professional organizations to receive the journals published by these groups; farmers may join organizations to benefit from special insurance policies or social activities; and businessmen join trade associations to make contacts, learn new business techniques, or keep up on new products. Nurses (or nursing students) also join interest groups such as the following:

- American Nurses' Association (Membership: 181,000)
- American Association of Critical Care Nurses (Membership: 40,000)
- National Student Nurses' Association (Membership: 35,000)
- Association of Operating Room Nurses (Membership: 29,834)

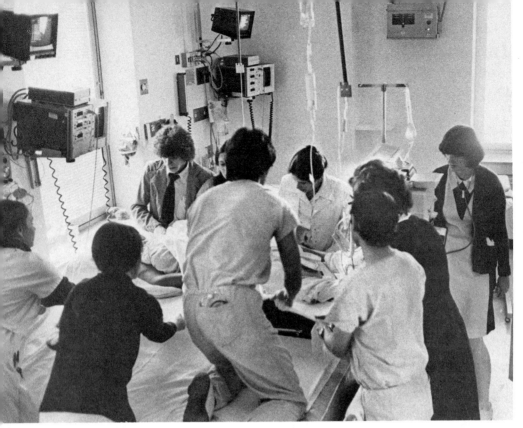

Figure 12–1. *The American Association of Critical Care Nurses, with 40,000 members, is the second largest professional nursing interest group. (Courtesy of Arizona Daily Star, Tucson, Arizona)*

- The Nurses' Association of the American College of OB/GYN (Membership: 20,000)
- National League for Nursing (Membership: 19,000)
- American Association of Nurse Anesthetists (Membership: 19,000)
- National Male Nurse Association (Membership: 14,000)
- Emergency Department Nurses' Association (Membership: 12,000)
- American Association of Occupational Health Nurses (Membership: 10,650)
- National Association of Physicians' Nurses (Membership: 4,000)
- Association of Rehabilitation Nurses (Membership: 1700)
- American College of Nurse-Midwives (Membership: 1650)
- American Association of Neurosurgical Nurses (Membership: 932)
- American Association of Colleges of Nursing (Membership: 244)

The growing importance of lobbying by nurse interest groups is related to the more general phenomenon of expanding interest-group advocacy. Medical interest groups have also increased their reliance on Washington lobbying. Extensive lobbying by interest groups is, of course, nothing new.

What has happened, though, is that government has ventured into more and more areas of American life. The regulatory spiral of more agencies and more regulations has created a demand for more interest-group lobbying. The United States is moving toward an interest-group society, one in which organized lobbies function as primary mediating structures.

Interest groups of all types have acquired a greater sophistication in their operations. Washington lobbies have become more adept at activating rank and file constituents. Assuming that it is the ordinary people back home, not the Washington lobbyists, who move policy makers, professional staffs use computerized retrieval systems to pinpoint the right citizens to be contacted. Farmers, truckers, and numerous other interest groups have taken to the streets and attempted to gain news coverage of their problems with Washington. Nothing better illustrates the new sophistication in lobbying than the ability of interest groups to rapidly inform their members of important developments in Washington. The Washington-based newsletter has become an integral part of most lobbies' ongoing operations. It is often said in Washington that "knowledge is power." If this is true, interest groups have learned how to become more powerful. Their newsletters provide a detailed, *inside* perspective on developments in various policy fields. The rank and file, regardless of where they live, are kept abreast of those issues that concern them most.

There are two components to the leadership of the major interest groups. First, there is the professional staff. These are the people who are the employees of the organization and those who work in the Washington office, or in other headquarters and branch offices, on a day-to-day basis. Second, almost all of the groups have a board of directors. These boards have legal responsibility for their organization, but their real influence within the groups varies widely. Members of the professional staffs are sometimes also members of the governing boards. In deciding which issues to lobby on, in allocating group resources, formulating strategies and tactics, and generally developing policy positions, the professional staffs tend to be the primary locus of influence.

Many interest groups, in other words, behave much the same way as social organizations generally. The mass membership is often reduced mainly to ratifying the choices already made by the leadership, which consists of a small minority of members with the time, money, and inclination to take on the responsibilities involved. When the rank and file of such an organization is encouraged to speak its mind, it is usually only an endorsement of what the leadership has already decided. The larger the organization and the more complex the problems with which it deals, the greater the likelihood that effective leadership is concentrated in a few hands. Sometimes the effective leadership is not exercised by the elected officers at all, but rather by permanent members of the organization's staff. Especially if there is a high rate of turnover in the elected leadership, officers will be compelled to lean heavily on the permanent and full-time staff. This tendency may be so highly developed that the organization's course is really set not by the elected president and fellow officers, but rather by an executive director and other staff members, such as research specialists, lawyers, and public relations experts, all equally unaccountable to the membership.

ECONOMICALLY MOTIVATED INTEREST GROUPS

Economically motivated groups have a direct economic interest in government policy. Government policies will either cost or save their members' money; business and labor are the most obvious examples. Business corporations have to be concerned with the government's taxing and spending policies. They seek to minimize their taxes and to channel government spending into areas from which they will benefit. Most of the largest corporations in the United States maintain lobbyists or contact with Washington law firms that specialize in representing businesses in government. Lobbyists and business representatives help to sell their company's services or products to governmental agencies; they handle their company's relations with administrative and regulatory agencies; and they attempt to influence legislation in which their company has an interest. Among those corporations with active Washington lobbying efforts are:

- American Express Co, New York, New York: "Legislation regarding travel, miscellaneous financial services or otherwise of interest to the business of American Express."
- Burger King Corp, Miami, Florida: "Tax, nutritional labeling, Federal Trade Commission and minimum wage legislation. . . ."
- Chrysler Corp, Detroit, Michigan: "All legislative activity relating to the motor vehicle industry."
- Merck & Co, Inc, Rahway, New Jersey: "Proposals to revise or reform existing food and drug laws, health care programs, OSHA [Occupational Safety and Health Administration], TSCA [Toxic Substances Control Act], air and water control acts and . . . taxation and foreign economic policy [proposals]."
- Merrill Lynch & Co, Inc, New York, New York: "Any and all legislation affecting the financial services industry."
- Montgomery Ward & Co, Inc, Chicago, Illinois: "Retail industry, including relations with federal agencies, manufacturers, suppliers, employees and customers."
- The Prudential Insurance Company of America, Newark, New Jersey: "Federal legislation affecting Title 26 of the U.S.C. [U.S. Code]."
- The Upjohn Co, Kalamazoo, Michigan: "Pharmaceutical, agricultural, chemical and/or health care services; S 2075, Drug Regulation Reform Act, S 23, Plant Variety Protection Act."

In addition to the lobbying carried on by individual businesses, most industries and trades have organized themselves into associations such as the Pharmaceutical Manufacturers Association, the American Trucking Association, the Association of American Railroads, the National Association of Real Estate Boards, the Savings and Loan League, and the American Petroleum Institute. Many of these associations originated in cooperative efforts by businessmen to eliminate competitive practices among themselves, such as price-cutting, and to establish standards of quality of goods. For example, the National Association of Manufacturers, representing over 13,000

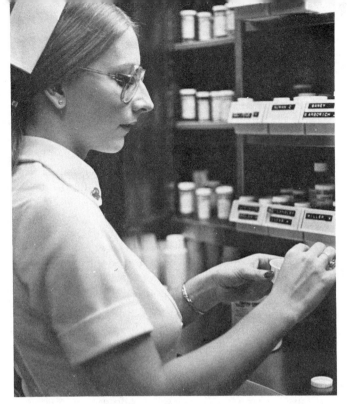

Figure 12–2. Most of the major pharmaceutical companies have active Washington lobbyists. (Courtesy of Tucson Citizen, Tucson, Arizona)

businesses, promotes conservative views about the role of government in society; it opposes most legislation and most government attempts to regulate business activity, and it fights for lower tax levels and for restricting the activities of organized labor. Among the hundreds of other trade associations with Washington representation are:

- American Petroleum Institute: "Legislation affecting the petroleum industry."
- American Society for Medical Technology: "Legislation with potential effect on medical laboratory services and personnel, health legislation, civil service legislation."
- American Textile Manufacturers Institute: "All legislation affecting the welfare of the textile industry—such as domestic and foreign trade policy, tax policy, labor policy, government controls, raw cotton and wool policy, consumer, environmental control, energy policy and lobbying legislation."
- Chamber of Commerce of the United States: "Matters of interest to the business community as to which the Chamber may wish to make recommendations or comments."
- Federation of American Hospitals: "FAH is a national trade association of investor-owned hospitals. The primary thrust of its activities is in the area of monitoring, analyzing enacted and proposed health legislation and regulations."

- National Association of Home Builders of the United States: "All legislation affecting that industry and its members."
- National Association of Truck Stop Operators: "All federal legislation affecting the operation of truck stops."
- National Restaurant Association: "Any legislation affecting the restaurant and food service industries . . . small business, labor laws, wages and hours, taxation, consumer protection, food marketing, and economic stabilization."
- National Retail Merchants Association: "Laws relating to advertising, antitrust, conditions and terms of employment, consumer affairs, credit, corporate and individual taxes, crime prevention, energy conservation, environmental protection, foreign trade, health care, housing, land use, national economic recovery, pensions, postal rates and services, regulatory reform, small business, telecommunications and transportation."[2]

Business interests have three advantages in dealing with the government. First, individual firms are already organized, so it is not necessary to form a group when a political issue arises. This is also true of trade associations. Formed for nonpolitical purposes, they have leaders, including attorneys and public relations staff, available for political purposes. Second, in dealing with government, business groups are on "home ground": they deal with familiar topics—their own economic specialties. This is not the same thing as being knowledgeable about politics, but it does give business an advantage not always shared by other groups. Further, public officials tend to find the views of individuals who are directly affected by a policy particularly important. When business groups move to general ideologic advocacy, they are far less persuasive than when they confine themselves to issues bearing directly on their businesses. Third, business organizations, whether they are individual firms or trade associations, are able to spend money liberally to attain their political ends.

LABOR UNIONS

Labor unions are also economically motivated. Labor unions, that is, organizations formed by wage earners to maintain or improve their terms and conditions of work by bargaining with employees, have existed in the United States, at least at the local level, since the 1790s. Until the 1930s, however, only a small proportion of workers belonged to unions; in 1933 union membership totaled 2.3 million members. Since then there has been a substantial expansion of union membership, although growth was most rapid in the 1930s and 1940s.

Geographically, union membership as a percentage of nonagricultural employment is highest in the Middle Atlantic, East North Central and Pacific Coast regions, whereas workers in the Mountain, South, Southwest, and West North Central regions are comparatively poorly organized. On a state basis, high rates of union membership (30% to 40%) are found in such states as West Virginia, New York, California, Michigan, Illinois, Ohio, and Pennsylvania. Low rates of union membership (less than 15%) exist in such states as North Carolina, South Carolina, South Dakota, Texas, Mississippi, and New Mexico. This situation results in part because industries with high rates of union membership tend to be concentrated in some states and regions. But other factors are also operative. In the South, for example, strong resistance by business interests in an unfavorable political climate contribute to low rates of unionization. Great disparity also exists in the membership size of various unions.

Union organizing activity was especially vigorous in the hospital sector of the health care industry during the 1970s. By 1976, over 23% of American Hospital Association member hospitals surveyed had at least one collective bargaining agreement with a labor organization. By contrast, a similar AHA survey conducted in 1970 found that only 16% of those surveyed had any collective bargaining relations. The same comparison revealed that by 1976 more than half of all larger hospitals—those with more than 550 beds—had labor agreements, and it found that urbanized institutions were far more likely to be unionized than rural and suburban institutions.

Labor unions employ two general methods in promoting and protecting their interests: collective bargaining (including strikes, picketing, and boycotts) and political activity. Political action by unions has been and is necessary because unions exist in a socioeconomic environment that has generally been critical of them, and sometimes hostile toward them, and has often produced unfavorable governmental attitudes and actions. Although "work" enjoys generally high regard in this country, the same is not true for organized labor. Thus, at the least, labor has had to defend itself in the political arena against labor injunctions, right-to-work laws, and other legislative restrictions, and executive interventions on behalf of management during strikes. To this extent, labor's political activity has appeared as a necessary condition for its survival and the opportunity to bargain collectively. But, and especially in recent decades, the political objectives of labor have been more than merely defensive or negative. Unions now rely on political action, in addition to collective bargaining, to promote the economic interests of their members.

Employees of both voluntary and investor-owned hospitals have a federally protected right to engage in union organizational activity without interference or reprisal by their employers. The National Labor Relations Act (NLRA), the federal law that confers this right upon employees, was first passed in 1935 as the Wagner Act. In 1947 the Taft–Hartley Act amended the Wagner Act to exclude from its coverage employees of not-for-profit hospitals, but the act's coverage was extended to not-for-profit hospital employees in 1974 by the Health Care Amendments. As defined by the NLRA, supervisors are not employees. Supervisors have no right to engage in union organizational activity and, if they do, in most circumstances they can be discharged.

Today, 22.5 million workers—nearly 1 of every 4 in the work force—belong to unions. Although the proportion of union members has been slowly falling, from 26% of civilian workers in 1968 down to about 24% at latest count, unions have a major impact on Washington political decisions. Their major purpose is to improve the working conditions and economic status of their members. The unions were first organized for economic objectives: better wages, hours, benefits, and working conditions. They soon

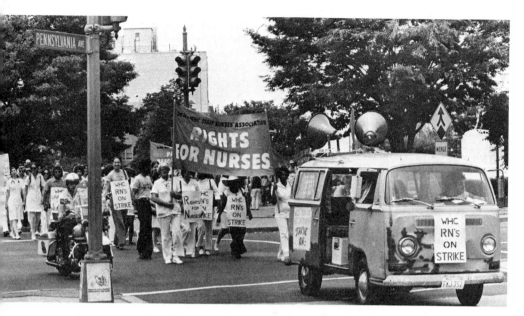

Figure 12–3. In 1974, Congress passed legislation granting nurses the right to organize and engage in collective bargaining under the provisions of the National Labor Relations Act. (Courtesy of The Washington Post, Washington, DC)

found they could make little progress if government took a hostile attitude toward the basic weapons of the working man: the rights to organize, to bargain collectively, and to strike. Thus labor turned to political activity in order to protect these organizational tools. Examples of unions with lobbyists in the nation's capital are the following:

- American Federation of State, County and Municipal Employees: "All bills affecting the welfare of the country generally and specifically bills affecting the state, county and municipal workers."
- Department of Professional Employees, AFL-CIO: "Legislation affecting labor organizations and their members, particularly those in the scientific, cultural and other professional fields."
- International Brotherhood of Electrical Workers: "Legislation dealing with electrical workers in particular and labor in general, such as: pay legislation, federal retirement, railroad retirement, social security, unemployment insurance, group health, hospitalization and surgical insurance, medical care for the aged, consumer legislation, and other liberal benefits for the working man."
- Retail Clerks International Union, AFL-CIO: "Social legislation and all matters relating to the interests of labor organizations."
- United Automobile, Aerospace and Agricultural Implement Workers of America: "Support all legislation favorable to the nation's peace and security, add to the economic and social well-being of the UAW members, their families and the nation. . . ."

- United Mine Workers of America: "Promote legislation that in UMWA opinion benefits workers in the coal mining industry and conversely to oppose legislation believed to be detrimental to coal miners."
- United Steelworkers of America: "Support all legislation favorable to the national peace, security, democracy, prosperity and general welfare. Oppose all legislation detrimental to those objectives."
- National Education Association: "Educational functions in support of legislation establishing a Department of Education."[3]

THE NATIONAL EDUCATION ASSOCIATION—A CASE STUDY OF AN ECONOMICALLY MOTIVATED GROUP

The National Education Association (NEA) has evolved over the past decade into a full-fledged labor union. In fact, it is the nation's second largest union, ranking just behind the Teamsters. It is made up of teachers, principals, and school administrators. The NEA had long been the major organization representing school teachers. Until recently, it avoided political involvement, but in 1972, the NEA formally decided to abandon this policy and move into politics. Its aim was to give teachers the decision-making authority, the public esteem, and the economic remuneration it felt teachers must have. Once the NEA decided to get into politics, its tremendous resources immediately made it a major force on the political scene. In 1980, it represented 1.8 million of the nation's 2.2 million public school teachers. Unlike most unions, where the bulk of members are concentrated in cities and in such regions as the Northeast and far West, NEA membership is broadly dispersed. There are between 400 and 6000 teachers in every congressional district, giving the organization a tremendous grass-roots lobbying potential. Teachers are more familiar with issues and more likely to vote than many other union members with less education, according to most voting studies. NEA has a president (who serves a 1-year term), a board of directors, a ten-member executive committee, and an annual budget of about $60 million.

Dues and political contributions of $186 a year support 600 Washington employees headquartered in a six-story building near the White House, one of the largest work forces of any Washington-based association. NEA's Washington operation includes a political action committee (NEA-PAC) and a large and active government relations office, with 18 registered lobbyists. As powerful as its Washington presence is, the association's real strength lies elsewhere. A force of 1436 full-time field organizers and 50 state affiliates in 1980 had combined budgets exceeding $250 million a year— financed from members' dues. Once a week the NEA sends out a lengthy Telex message from Washington to these outlying offices, keeping them abreast of Washington developments to sensitize teachers to what is going on in Congress, to stimulate grass-roots pressure. To each of the 435 congressional districts, teams of teachers have been detailed to create widespread support for NEA's legislative goals.

In 1976, the NEA endorsed its first presidential candidate, Jimmy Carter, and elected more than 325 delegates to the Democratic and Republican national conventions. In the 1978 congressional election, the group's cam-

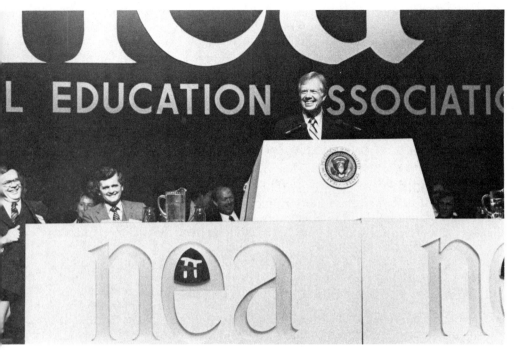

Figure 12–4. The National Education Association provided both an endorsement and strong financial support for President Jimmy Carter in 1976 and 1980. (Courtesy of National Education Association)

paign finance arm contributed $331,000 to help NEA-backed candidates win 211 House and Senate races. Two years later, the NEA emerged as one of the most powerful special interests in the 1980 campaign. Nearly all of its 302 Democratic convention delegates and 162 alternates were solidly for Jimmy Carter—accounting for one-seventh of his delegates. Eleven NEA members were on the 155-member committee that drafted the 1980 Democratic party platform. When the NEA helps a candidate, it contributes more than funds. Volunteers work on all kinds of tasks ranging from addressing envelopes to ringing doorbells.

NEA's support was crucial in numerous 1980 primaries and caucuses. The NEA set up offices and phone banks for Carter around the country. Twenty-six full-time NEA workers helped Carter defeat Senator Edward Kennedy in the Iowa caucuses, the first campaign test. Carter's first telephone call in his effort to organize the Maine Democratic caucuses went to an Auburn kindergarten teacher named Rosalie Spaulding, who apparently packed the caucuses with NEA members. And in Florida, the first stop for Carter field operatives, was the Florida Teachers' Association headquarters in Tallahassee.

The NEA's chief political objectives are collective bargaining rights for teachers and sharply increased federal aid to public schools, despite the sharply declining enrollments of the 1980's. From 1959 to 1979 federal aid to education skyrocketed from $408.5 million to $12 billion annually—more than 8% of education outlays nationwide. Despite the falling enrollments, federal education spending increased 36% in the Carter years of 1977 to 1979, and with the President's help, the NEA in 1978 defeated legislation that would have given tuition tax credits for students attending private schools. For years the NEA strongly believed that still more federal dollars would flow to schools if education became the sole concern of a cabinet-level department. Thus, the following year, the NEA got from President Carter what it had sought from every president since Calvin Coolidge, a separate Department of Education. NEA's announced goal for the 1980s is to at least double the level of federal support of education to the level of $25 billion a year and cut the student to teacher ratio in classrooms.

PROFESSIONALLY MOTIVATED INTEREST GROUPS

A second category of interest groups is the professionally motivated group. Various professional groups may exhibit many differences, but some meaningful criteria exist whereby professionals can be distinguished from non-professionals. Myron Lieberman says that a professional performs some unique and essential service; emphasizes intellectual rather than physical techniques in the performance of that service; goes through a long period of training in order to become a practitioner of that service; has a broad range of autonomy over how the service is performed; accepts responsibility for judgments made and acts performed within the scope of that autonomy; *emphasizes a service rendered rather than the economic gain* as the basis for organization with similar practitioners; forms comprehensive self-governing organizations with other practitioners; and establishes a clear and workable code of ethics for the group. Among the professional groups with Washington representation are the following:

- American Nurses' Association: "Works for the improvement of health standards and the availability of health care services for all people; fosters high standards of nursing; stimulates and promotes the professional development of nurses; and advances their economic and general welfare. The purposes are unrestricted by consideraions of nationality, race, creed, lifestyle, color, sex or age."
- American Association of Nurse Anesthetists: ". . . Legislative proposals affecting nurse anesthetists."
- American Hospital Association: "Active in various functions of the health care field, the AHA is a national association whose members consist of approximately 6,500 hospitals and other institutions and 29,000 individuals."
- American Medical Association: "A national scientific organization of physicians dedicated to promoting the science and art of medicine and the betterment of the public health."
- American Psychiatric Association: "All health legislation affecting psychiatry."

- Association of American Medical Colleges: "Works to advance medical education and the nation's health. Its activities include data collection and studies, evaluating the quality of educational programs, providing consultation and technical assistance on medical education issues, and communication among members and policymakers."
- Association of State and Territorial Health Officials: "All legislation affecting state health agencies."
- Private Doctors of America: "A professional medical association representing privately practicing doctors nationwide on all issues affecting the private practice of medicine."[4]

THE AMERICAN MEDICAL ASSOCIATION'S WASHINGTON OFFICE

Many of these professional groups are getting very close to the line where their economically oriented political activities are overshadowing their scientific and professional concerns: The American Medical Association is a good example. Originally organized to regulate entrance into the medical profession and to maintain high professional standards, the AMA has become more and more political over the years. Fearing that government-sponsored health insurance would tend to restrict physicians' fees, and claiming that service to the public would suffer as a result, the AMA has consistently resisted government attempts to include health care among Social Security benefits, and it has opposed most forms of national health insurance. The AMA never tires of insisting that it is a professional organization, intent only on maintaining and elevating the standards of the medical profession. In the long fight it waged against Medicare, it purported to base its opposition on exclusively professional grounds: a health care plan financed by the government would impair the physician–patient relationship and would undermine the very practice of medicine. It was not difficult, however, to perceive that physicians were at least as much interested in quite a different subject: protecting their advantageous economic position in society.

Organized in 1847, the AMA is a federation of 55 state and territorial medical societies and nearly 3000 local and county chapters. In five states—Arizona, Hawaii, Illinois, Oklahoma, and Wisconsin—a physician who joins on any level is automatically a member of all three (state, local, and county). In 1980, the AMA had just over 170,000 dues-paying members. Students and certain dues-exempt members, including retirees, boosted the total enrollment to over 220,000. Its headquarters, with a staff of 950, is in Chicago. Although 70% of its $61 million annual budget is devoted to scientific activities, the association maintains a large office in Washington, D.C. to protect its members' interests.

In 1980, there were five lobbyists who were articulating organized medicine's views before Congress. Three other lobbyists were assigned to the federal agencies, principally the Department of Health and Human Services. The AMA's Washington office, which has nine other professionals and eight supporting staff, occupies a floor in a modern office building at 1776 K Street. The lobbyists fan out through the city during the day, covering hearings, meeting people, attending news conferences, and so forth.

They send their "stories" back to the AMA headquarters in Chicago by telephone, teletype, telefax, and mail. The AMA's chief lobbyist is John Zapp, who previously served as deputy assistant HEW secretary in charge of legislation.

NURSING INTEREST GROUPS

The American Nurses' Association provides the most extensive Washington lobbying effort of the nursing interest groups. The purposes of the ANA include the fostering of high standards of nursing practice, the promotion of professional and educational advancement of nurses, and the development of economic and general welfare of its members. The organization is made up of a number of elected commissions, councils, and divisions, which address these areas of concern (*e.g.*, the Commission of Nursing Practice, the Commission on Nursing Research, and so forth). The main offices of the ANA are located in Kansas City, Missouri, with Myrdle Aydelotte serving as executive director of the organization. The Government Relations Office is located at 1030 15th Street, N.W., in Washington, D.C. From 1951 to 1973, Julia Thompson served as the first ANA lobbyist. She was followed by Constance Holleran, who headed the office from 1973 to 1981. A Washington staff of eight professionals, of whom two are registered lobbyists, orchestrate

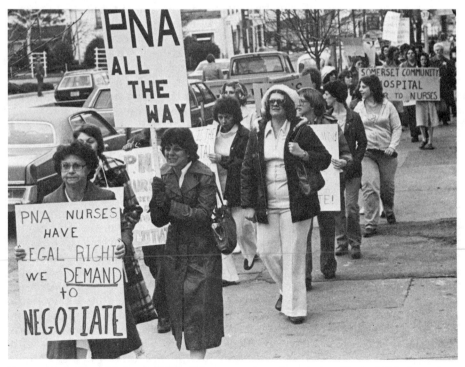

Figure 12–5. The ANA has addressed the economic and general welfare of RNs through its state affiliates. (Courtesy of Somerset American, Somerset, Pennsylvania)

the major lobbying efforts of the ANA. State nursing organizations also hire lobbyists or legislative specialists to work on state nursing issues and to assist with the federal efforts as needed.

The American Federation of Teachers (AFT) is a labor union with nursing membership. This union, originally formed to represent teachers, has begun to organize other groups including nurses. Working at 11 Dupont Circle, Washington, D.C., Karen O'Rourke is the major nurse representative, and she carries out lobbying activities on nursing issues.

In addition to these interest groups who actually have registered lobbyists and can legally be termed lobbyists, other nursing organizations have also established representation in Washington. One of these groups is the National League for Nursing, whose aim is to upgrade nursing services and education. It is particularly concerned with working for the improvement of the standards of educational programs and with the augmentation of both the quantity and quality of nurse professionals. NLN has both nurse and non-nurse members as well as individual and agency members. It is organized into councils, assemblies, and forums (*e.g.*, the Council of Baccalaureate and Higher Degree Programs, the Assembly of Constituent Leagues, and the National Forum for Administrators of Nursing Services, and so on), and it is concerned with accreditation, consultation, conferences, and research and produces various publications. The NLN, whose executive director is Margaret Walsh, is located in New York City. The government relations efforts of this organization are carried out by Pamela Maraldo, director of Public Affairs, who frequently travels to Washington. The NLN also hires a Washington-based representative to assist with its lobbying efforts and to keep in touch with the day-to-day Washington events.

The purpose of the National Student Nurses' Association, the only organization for nursing students, include upgrading nursing education, promoting community involvement of nurses, and influencing legislation impacting on health care. Among its many political activities, the organization arranges for nursing students to testify before Congress, and it publishes and disseminates legislative alerts to members. Mary Ann Tufts serves as executive director and Eileen McGee as director of program and legislative activities.

The offices of the American Association of Colleges of Nursing, whose executive director is Marion Murphy, are located in Washington, D.C. (11 Dupont Circle, Suite 430). The membership of this group is confined to deans and directors of schools of nursing, and their governmental efforts primarily concern nursing education matters. The American College of Nurse–Midwives, the professional organization for nurse-midwives in the United States, dedicated to the improvement of services for mothers and babies in cooperation with other allied groups, is also Washington based (Suite 801, 1012 14th Street, N.W.). The administration director is Faith Lebowitz, and the person in charge of governmental affairs is Sally Tom. The American Public Health Association also has a government relations department (1015 15th Street, N.W., Washington, D.C.) which deals with those issues related to public health nursing. Several other nursing organizations also retain Washington representatives: The American Association of

Nurse Anesthetists, the Emergency Department Nurses' Association, and the American Association of Operating Room Nurses. The 1980s will probably see more nursing groups become involved in governmental affairs for the purpose of furthering their particular interests at the federal level.

PUBLIC INTEREST GROUPS

A third category of interest groups is the public interest group. These groups claim to speak for *the public*. In fact, these organizations do not always express the popular view, but they also do not appeal to economic self-interest in recruiting supporters and in soliciting financial aid. Instead, they rely on idealism and ideologic commitment. Among the major public interest groups that have effective offices in Washington are the following:

- Action for Children's Television: "Appropriations for the Federal Trade Commission (FTC) and possible congressional ban on the FTC rulemaking on advertising on children's television . . ., reauthorization of the FTC and Federal Communications Commission (FCC), efforts to improve children's television programming. . . ."
- American Conservative Union: "Reform of the motor carrier industry; reform or repeal of the Occupational Safety and Health Administration; legislative issues generating sufficient public interest to warrant involvement by conservatives and expression of a conservative point of view."
- Common Cause: "Open government, campaign financing, consumer protection, freedom of information, ERA, energy policy, environmental protection, defense spending, tax reform, waste in government, voting rights, presidential nomination and confirmation process, administration of justice and reform of the criminal code, merit selection of federal judges and U.S. attorneys, intellience policy, public participation in federal agency proceedings, civil service reform, regulatory reform, reapportionment, the congressional budget process and congressional reform."
- Congress Watch: "All energy and environment-related issues and legislative matters."
- Consumer Federation of America: "Clinical Laboratory Improvement Act, National Health Insurance, natural gas, oil deregulation, conservation legislation . . . any legislation that would be to the benefit of the consumer."
- Public Citizen Inc: "Amendments to the Price-Anderson Act, food, drug and cosmetic legislation, including legislation on nitrites, legislation on saccharin and food additive policy."
- Sierra Club: "Energy, air pollution, water pollution, solid and hazardous waste, toxic substances control, occupational safety and health, and regulatory reform legislation."
- The Wilderness Society: "Boundary Waters Wilderness Act, HR 12250; Alaska National Lands Conservation Act, HR 39; Department of Natural Resources Reorganization; national forest wilderness, National Parks Concessions Policy Act."[5]

· Moral Majority: "A fundamentalist religious political action movement. Opposes legalized abortion, recognition of gay rights, toleration of pornography, and the banning of voluntary prayer in public schools. Opposes 'liberal' social programs as forms of governmental interference in family life and favors hard-line foreign and military policies."

Without question, the mass media's increasing attention to environmental, consumer, and government reform issues helped develop the constituencies that enabled the public interest group movement to flourish in the 1970s. In addition, translating citizen concern into national groups could not have been accomplished without one key ingredient—direct mail solicitation. The 1970s witnessed an explosion in the technologies of mail solici-

Figure 12–6. Public interest groups are an effective outlet for feelings of alienation that in the past have frequently resulted in civil disorders. (Courtesy of History and Politics of Nursing, University of Michigan)

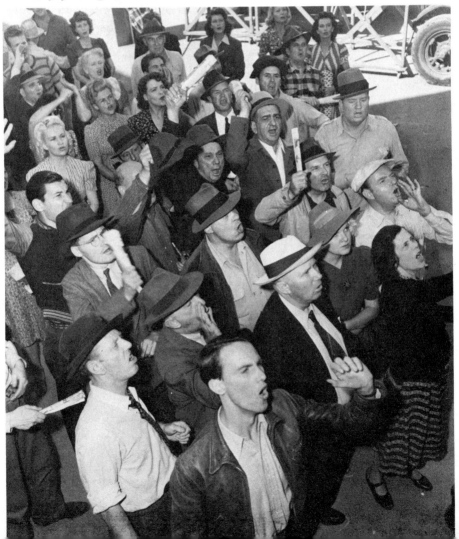

tation and in the sophistication of its practitioners. Public interest groups have found that mail as a form of fund-raising and membership solicitation is effective because it makes a specific appeal to a particular group of people. Appeals made through the mass media—radio, television, newspapers—do not. Direct mail is also flexible in that it allows the user to single out the persons who are to receive the appeal and to address the appeal to as many or as few people as desired. It also allows a group to tell a lengthy story that would be too costly to tell through another medium. Unlike other fund raising forms, particularly those made through the mass media, a good direct mail appeal provides not only the urge to take action, but the means to take action (response forms to complete easily, self-addressed envelopes, and so on).

Public interest groups often focus their efforts on modifying the goals and structures of institutions, such as large corporations, which they believe have grown powerful enough to avoid normal social and political constraints. Not only corporations, but also government agencies, legislative bodies, labor unions, health care institutions, and religious organizations tend to institutionalize past needs and perceptions and are reluctant to perceive new needs and to respond to new conditions. Some measure of institutional lag is inevitable and necessary to avoid disruptive and rapid oscillations in societies. However, in conditions of rapid technological and social change, new complexities, and interdependencies that are characteristic of the United States today, this institutional lag often becomes clearly counterproductive.

COMMON CAUSE'S CRUSADE

Common Cause, the best known of all the public interest groups, depends entirely on direct-mail membership drives and fund-raising campaigns. Founded in 1970, it had 325,000 members within four years, inspired in part by public outrage at the ethical shortcomings of the Nixon administration. As Watergate began fading into history, Common Cause's 1980 membership shrank to about 215,000; however, it is still the most influential organization of its kind and a continuing force in Washington. Unlike other public interest groups, which are composed mostly of politically inexperienced young lawyers and scientists, Common Cause's staff are seasoned veterans of the Washington scene. It has eighty full-time staff in its Washington office, supplemented by a core of over 200 experienced volunteers, and chapters in almost every state.

Owing to the effectiveness of such public interest groups as Common Cause, Congress in 1971 passed a law forcing disclosure of campaign contributions. In the middle of the decade, legislation was enacted limiting the size of political contributions by individuals and political action committees in providing for public financing of presidential campaigns. Congress was persuaded to open almost all of its committee hearings to the public, and large dents were made in the seniority system for choosing committee chairpersons. A sunshine law was passed, opening up executive branch deliberations to greater public scrutiny. Litigation by environmental groups has forced strict enforcement of the 1968 National Environmental Policy Act, which established a procedure to ensure that agencies weigh the environmental consequences of their actions. The Environmental Protection Agency, established in 1970, was greatly strengthened with passage of new laws governing air and water pollution, drinking water, solid waste, toxic substance, pesticides, and ocean dumping.

In the late 1970s, the tide in Congress began turning against the public interest groups, in part because business had greatly increased both its political contributions and its lobbying presence in Washington. The defeat in Congress of the proposed consumer protection agency in 1978 was the signal that business had amassed enough strength to block the public interest groups. Defeat of the Consumer Protection Bill was principally due to the massive coalescing of business interests and "selling" the message "to the folks back home" that the proposed bill was not in the "public interest." The combination of grass-roots strategic forces with direct and indirect interindustry forces made the difference. In 1978 the House rejected the Consumer Agency by a vote of 227 to 189. It was a larger margin than the most outspoken opponents had anticipated.

THE RISE OF POLITICAL ACTION COMMITTEES

Giving money has always been the most common form of campaign activism, but as far back as the early part of this century, it was declared illegal for incorporated groups (such as ANA) to make political campaign contributions. With recent amendments to this law, campaign giving is regulated even further by laws that set up requirements for accurate and timely reporting of contributions and spending; by limits on the amount of contributions; by public financing for presidential candidates; and by the Federal Election Commission (1325 K Street, N.W., Washington, D.C. 20463), which administers the law. A major benefit of these laws is the creation of an open, legal way for corporations, unions, and professional and other groups to contribute to candidates for elective office. The law mandates that funds collected be kept as a separate fund and that no organizational money be used for contributions to candidates, although organization monies can be used to establish and to administer such an endeavor. These separate organizations have become known as Political Action Committees (PACs) and are now the main way labor, business, professional organizations, and other interest groups contribute to campaigns. These committees are known as political action arms and are often physically located in the same office as the interest group itself, but the funding activities are kept strictly separate. Lobbying and political action are two separate activities—the first being designed to influence the decisions of persons in office and the second aimed at getting persons into office who will view legislation in the way the group wishes them to view it. Obviously, even though separate, they are highly related endeavors.

In 1974, ANA budgeted $50,000 to set up the ANA political action arm known as N-CAP (Nurses' Coalition for Action in Politics) to solicit funds for political purposes and to carry out political education of nurses. It also has worked with interested states and localities to develop their own political action committee because powerful state PACs are felt to be important. For example, medicine not only has a strong national PAC, known as American Medical Political Action Committee (AMPAC), but also has a powerful committee in each state (*i.e.*, California Medical PAC, Texas Medical PAC, and so forth). No one may give more than $5000 to a PAC, and no PAC may give more than $5000 to a candidate per election. Primaries and run-off elections are considered separate elections, so that a candidate may actually receive up to $15,000. Groups, like medicine, who are highly organized at the state level, can exert much greater influence, because the national as well as the state PAC can contribute maximum amounts to candidates. (Individual contributions can be layered on top of these gifts as well).

A look at campaign fund sources shows that major contributors fall into several categories: business and professional groups, organized labor, and other etiological organizations. According to a Common Cause study, the largest interest group contributors in the 1976 congressional races were AMPAC ($1,780,879); dairy interests ($1,362,159); and oil, natural gas, and coal firms ($809,508).

Table 12–1. *Leading Political Action Committee Contributors to 1980 Campaigns (as of June 30, 1980)*

NAME	CONTRIBUTIONS	CASH ON HAND
American Medical Political Action Committee	$542,538	$ 856,108
Automobile and Truck Dealers Election Action Committee	473,674	448,725
AFL-CIO COPE Political Contributions Committee	396,506	44,725
UAW Voluntary Community Action Program	363,135	1,302,174
Realtors Political Action Committee	348,213	1,019,725
Committee for Thorough Agricultural Political Education	228,562	1,399,993
Machinists Non-Partisan Political League	228,349	494,091
United Steelworkers of America Political Action Fund	211,610	248,202
Carpenters' Legislative Improvement Committee	198,750	117,932
Railway Clerks Political League	191,980	2,476
Attorneys Congressional Campaign Trust	189,653	159,475
National Association of Life Underwriters Political Action Committee	184,058	301,906
Communications Workers of America-COPE Political Contributions Committee	159,954	237,856
Transportation Political Education League	159,150	409,806
American Dental Political Action Committee	151,900	377,691

Source: *Federal Election Commission*

PACs generally concentrate their attention on the members of Congress who are most concerned with their particular problems. In 1978, AMPAC was ahead of all PACs in contributions to congressional candidates, with $1.64 million. The following year, campaign contributions for the American Medical Association's "political committees" played a major role in defeating the Carter administration's hospital cost-containment bill, according to a study by Common Cause. The House on November 15, 1979, voted 234 to 166 to substitute for the administration's measure a bill setting up purely voluntary limits on hospital costs. The administration's bill would have triggered a mandatory federal ceiling if the voluntary limit were exceeded. House members who voted to kill the measure received almost four times as much in campaign contributions for the AMA's political committees as did the bill's supporters. According to Common Cause:

- Two hundred and two of the 234 House members who voted for the substitute bill received AMA political committee contributions averaging $8157 per member and totaling $1.6 million.
- Of the 50 leading House recipients of AMA political committee contributions who voted on the amendment, 48 voted in favor of the AMA position. They received an average of $17,300.
- Forty-four of the 166 members who opposed the amendment received no AMA political committee contributions. The remaining 122 members opposing the amendment received substantially smaller AMA political committee contributions than those who voted in favor—an average of $2287, compared to the $8157 average for those who voted for the amendment.
- Thirty-seven of the 48 freshmen members who voted for the amendment received AMA political committee contributions during the 1978 campaigns, averaging $9454 per member. A majority of the freshmen who opposed the amendment—13 of 25—received no AMA political committee contributions. The remaining 12 members voting against the amendment received 1978 contributions averaging $4717.
- The AMA political committees contributed $3.9 million to House and Senate candidates during the last two congressional elections. Some 320 members (or two-thirds) of the present House received AMA political committee contributions during their 1978 campaigns, averaging $4176 per member. Four years earlier, fewer than half that number—154 members of the House—received AMA political committee contributions, averaging $3196.

As noted previously, getting elected to Congress has grown to be a very expensive endeavor. Sums spent on 1978 election campaigns averaged well over $200,000 for those seeking seats in the House of Representatives. Most candidates either had to be wealthy or look for contributions, which would come from those seeking legislative favors. In 1976, Senator William Proxmire's re-election cost $697. Two years later, Senator Jessie Helms of North Carolina set a record by spending over $6 million to retain his seat. His opponent, who had less than $500,000 for his campaign, called Helms "the Six Million Dollar Man." Some House winners spent under $100, but many others spent over half-a-million dollars in 1978 and 1980. In 1978, Texas oil-drilling contractor William P. Clements, Jr., also spent about $6 million in his successful bid to be the first Republican governor of Texas since the Reconstruction. Clements' opponent, Texas Attorney General John Hill, spent $2 million on his campaign, including about $600,000 in advertising. In a tight Senate race, Texas Republican John Tower spent $3,600,000 in his successful effort to retain his seat.

Many organizations, including business and medical groups, give money to both Democrats and Republicans. In 1975, 78 members of the House received 40% or more of their total contributions from PACs during the 1974 elections. In 1979, the number of House members receiving similar amounts in the 1978 election rose to 136, whereas PACs accounted for 56% of the funds spent by House committee chairpersons up for re-election in that campaign. Despite the explosive growth in many ways, PACs are still in the incubation stage. During the period from 1974 to 1978, contributions from the National Automobile Dealers Association's PAC grew 6000%, from $14,000 to almost $1 million. Over the same period, contributions from the National Association of Realtors increased from $261,000 to $1.1 million, with their PAC director being quoted as saying that this potential was just starting.

Some interest groups spread their campaign contributions among candidates with whom they are philosophically or ideologically attuned. Others single out candidates whose voting records show precisely where they have supported or failed to support positions of the donor organization. A case in point is the Air Line Pilots Association, a member of the AFL-CIO, which represents most of the nation's commercial airline pilots. In 1979, the association's PAC raised more than $200,000 among its members, many of them putting up $200 to $250, although the average contribution was in the neighborhood of $50. Five pilots serve on a steering committee that determines how their contributions are distributed. According to records on file at the Federal Election Commission, the pilots directed most of their campaign gifts to members of Congress in amounts ranging from $50 to $5,000. But a single check for $10,000 was used to help pay for a Democratic congressional fund-raising dinner.

N-CAP received $93,392 and distributed $100,410 to candidates for the two-year period of 1977 and 1978. The comparison of candidates who received the highest contribution from N-CAP as compared to AMPAC can be noted in Table 12–2. The contrast with selected other professional groups can be noted in Table 12–3.

CAMPAIGN COSTS AND PACs IN THE 1980 ELECTIONS

The costs of a 1980 election campaign was nearly double the $540 million spent in the presidential election year of 1976. Inflation was a major factor. Analysts noted that the general cost of living had shot up 46% since the 1976 presidential election, and prices of some campaign necessities rose even more sharply than that. Another major increase in expenses was the cost of television time: thirty minutes on national network could easily cost $250,000. TV was used more heavily in the 1980 campaign than ever before.

Table 12–2. *Largest N-CAP and AMPAC Contributions to Winners of House Races in 1978 Elections (Maximum Contribution of $5,000 allowed for each election, including primary, run off and general elections)*

N-CAP Representative	Amount	AMPAC Representative	Amount
Pat Schroeder (CO)	$2,000	Paul Seward Trible, Jr. (VA)	$15,000
Olympia J. Snowe (ME)	1,500	Dan Marriott (UT)	14,000
Margaret Heckler (MA)	1,100	Arlan Strangeland (MN)	13,500
Elizabeth Holtzman (NY)	1,100	Richard C. Shelby (AL)	12,000
Timothy E. Wirth (CO)	1,100	John T. Myers (IN)	11,000
John Brademas (IN)	1,000	James Abdnor (SD)	10,000
Geraldine A. Ferraro (NY)	1,000	Beryl F. Anthony, Jr. (AR)	10,000
Michael E. Lowry (WA)	1,000	Bill Boner (TN)	10,000
Gladys Noon Spellman (MD)	1,000	Carroll Ashmore Campbell, Jr. (SC)	10,000
Thomas L. Ashley (OH)	500	E. Thomas Coleman (MO)	10,000
Les Aspin (WI)	500	William E. Dannemeyer (CA)	10,000
Les Aucoin (OR)	500	H. Joel Deckard (IN)	10,000
Lindy (Mrs. Hale) Boggs (LA)	500	Robert K. Dornan (CA)	10,000
Robert M. Carr (MI)	500	Thomas B. Evans, Jr. (DE)	10,000
Shirley Chisholm (NY)	500	William Philip Gramm (TX)	10,000
William L. Clay (MO)	500	Sedowick William Green (NY)	10,000
Anthony Lee Coelho (CA)	500	Larry Jones Hopkins (KY)	10,000
Cardiss Collins (IL)	500	James P. Johnson (CO)	10,000
James C. Corman (CA)	500	Marvin Leath (TX)	10,000
William R. Cotter (CT)	500	Robert L. Livingston (LA)	10,000
Lawrence Coughlin (PA)	500	Ron Paul (TX)	10,000
Norman D. Dicks (WA)	500	John Edward Porter (IL)	10,000
Thomas J. Downey (NY)	500	John J. Rhodes (AZ)	10,000
John J. Duncan (TN)	500	Eldon Rudd (AZ)	10,000
Joseph D. Early (MA)	500	Olympia J. Snowe (ME)	10,000
Robert Eckhardt (TX)	500	Steve Symms (ID)	10,000
Robert W. Edgar (PA)	500	Joe Wyatt, Jr. (TX)	10,000
Don Edwards (CA)	500	Don Young (AK)	10,000
David Walter Evans (IN)	500	Ronald Charles Marlenee (MT)	9,900
Joseph L. Fisher (VA)	500	Harold S. Sawyer (MI)	9,500
James J. Florio (NJ)	500	Floyd D. Spence (SC)	9,500
Thomas S. Foley (WA)	500	George M. O'Brien (IL)	9,250
Harold E. Ford (TN)	500	James G. Martin (NC)	8,229
William David Ford (MI)	500	Douglas K. Bereuter (NE)	8,000
Martin Frost (TX)	500	Anthony Lee Coelho (CA)	8,000

(continues on facing p.)

Table 12–2. (Continued) Largest N-CAP and AMPAC Contributions to Winners of House Races in 1978 Elections (Maximum Contribution of $5,000 allowed for each election, including primary, run off and general elections)

N-CAP Representative	Amount	AMPAC Representative	Amount
Robert N. Giaimo (CT)	500	Donald H. Clausen (CA)	7,635
Benjamin A. Gilman (NY)	500	Harold Volkmer (MO)	7,600
John Paul Hammerschmidt (AR)	500	Tim Lee Carter (KY)	7,500
Kent Hance (TX)	500	Richard Bruce Cheney (WY)	7,500
James M. Hanley (NY)	500	Thomas J. Corcoran (IL)	7,500
Herbert E. Harris II (VA)	500	Arlen Erdahl (MN)	7,500
Augustus F. Hawkins (CA)	500	Thomas J. Tauke (IA)	7,500
Hon. Robert W. Kastenmeier (WI)	500	Harold C. Hollenbeck (NJ)	7,100
Dale E. Kildee (MI)	500	Marc Lincoln Marks (PA)	7,000
George Thomas Leland (TX)	500	Carl D. Pursell (MI)	7,000
Andrew Maguire (NJ)	500	Thomas Jerald Huckaby (LA)	6,900
Edward J. Markey (MA)	500	Martin A. Russo (IL)	6,600
Paul N. McCloskey (CA)	500	Ed Jones (TN)	6,500
Mike McCormack (WA)	500	Vic Fazio (CA)	6,000
Gunn K. McKay (UT)	500	John J. Duncan (TN)	5,829
Daniel A. Mica (FL)	500	Austin J. Murphy (PA)	5,600
Barbara Ann Mikulski (MD)	500	John M. Ashbrook (OH)	5,100
Stephen L. Neal (NC)	500	Lamar Gudger (NC)	5,100
Richard Nolan (MN)	500	James Quillen (TN)	5,100
David Obey (WI)	500	Bob Stump (AZ)	5,100
Richard L. Ottinger (NY)	500	Mendel J. Davis (SC)	5,050
Leon E. Panetta (CA)	500	Donald Allen Bailey (PA)	5,000
Edward J. Patten (NJ)	500	Robert Bauman (MD)	5,000
Claude D. Pepper (FL)	500	Robin Beard (TN)	5,000
Richardson Preyer (NC)	500	John H. Buchanan (AL)	5,000
Dan Rostenkowski (IL)	500	William Carney (NY)	5,000
Martin A. Russo (IL)	500	William F. Clinger, Jr. (PA)	5,000
James David Santini (NV)	500	James A. Courter (NJ)	5,000
James H. Scheuer (NY)	500	Daniel B. Crane (IL)	5,000
James Shannon (MA)	500	Robert W. Davis (MI)	5,000
Philip R. Sharp (IN)	500	Samuel L. Devine (OH)	5,000
Paul Simon (IL)	500	Charles Dougherty (PA)	5,000
Neal Smith (IA)	500	Jack Edwards (AL)	5,000
Stephen J. Solarz (NY)	500	Charles E. Grassley (IA)	5,000
Allan Byron Swift (WA)	500	Wayne Richard Grisham (CA)	5,000

(continues on p. 414)

Table 12-2. *(Continued) Largest N-CAP and AMPAC Contributions to Winners of House Races in 1978 Elections (Maximum Contribution of $5,000 allowed for each election, including primary, run off and general elections)*

N-CAP		AMPAC	
Representative	Amount	Representative	Amount
Frank Thompson, Jr. (NJ)	500	Sam B. Hall, Jr. (TX)	5,000
Albert Conrad Ullman (OR)	500	Kent Hance (TX)	5,000
Lionel Van Deerlin, MC (CA)	500	George Hansen (ID)	5,000
Douglas Walgren (PA)	500	Carroll Hubbard, Jr., (KY)	5,000
Henry A. Waxman (CA)	500	James Jeffries (KS)	5,000
Pat Williams (MI)	500	Richard Kelly (FL)	5,000
Howard Wolpe (MI)	500	Thomas N. Kindness (OH)	5,000
Matthew F. McHugh (NY)	400	Ray Kogovsek (CO)	5,000
Kenneth L. Holland (SC)	200	Kenneth Bentley Kramer (CO)	5,000
Joseph P. Addabbo (NY)	100	Gary A. Lee (NY)	5,000
John Anderson (IL)	100	Jerry Lewis (CA)	5,000
James T. Broyhil (NC)	100	Tom Leoffler (TX)	5,000
Robert F. Drinan (MA)	100	Daniel E. Lungren (CA)	5,000
W. G. Hefner (NC)	100	Robert T. Matsui (CA)	5,000
James Jeffords (VT)	100	Mary Rose Oakar (OH)	5,000
Raymond F. Lederer (PA)	100	Danforth J. Quayle (IN)	5,000
Louis Stokes (OH)	100	Dan Rostenkowski (IL)	5,000
Cecil Landau Heftel (HI)	20	Toby Roth (WI)	5,000
		F. James Sensenbrenner (WI)	5,000
		Gene Snyder (KY)	5,000
		Gerald B.H. Solomon (NY)	5,000
		Charles Stenholm (TX)	5,000
		William M. Thomas (CA)	5,000
		Robert "Bob" Whittaker (KS)	5,000

N-CAP and AMPAC Contributions to Winners of Senatorial Races in 1978 Elections

N-CAP		AMPAC	
Senator	Amount	Senator	Amount
Carl Levin (MI)	$2,500	John Goodwin Tower (TX)	$15,000
Charles Percy (IL)	2,000	William L. Armstrong (CO)	10,000
Larry Pressler (SD)	1,500	Howard H. Baker (TN)	10,000
Jennings Randolph (WV)	1,050	Rudolph E. Boschwitz (MN)	10,000
Max Baucus (MT)	1,000	William S. Cohen (ME)	10,000
William Thad Cochran (MS)	1,000	Pete V. Domenici (NM)	10,000

(continues on facing p.)

Table 12–2. (*Continued*) *Largest N-CAP and AMPAC Contributions to Winners of House Races in 1978 Elections* (*Maximum Contribution of $5,000 allowed for each election, including primary, run off and general elections*)

N-CAP		AMPAC	
Representative	*Amount*	*Senator*	*Amount*
Pete V. Domenici (NM)	1,000	David Durenberger (MN)	10,000
Ted Stevens (AK)	1,000	Howell Thomas Heflin (AL)	10,000
Howard H. Baker (TN)	600	Jesse Helms (NC)	10,000
		Gordon J. Humphrey (NH)	10,000
		Charles Percy (IL)	10,000
		Larry Pressler (SD)	10,000
		David Hampton Pryor (AR)	10,000
		Alan Kooi Simpson (WY)	10,000
		James Strom Thurmond (SC)	9,900
		Max Baucus (MT)	8,600
		Walter D. Huddleston (KY)	8,250
		William Thad Cochran (MS)	5,000
		James J. Exon (NE)	5,000
		Roger Jepsen (IA)	5,000
		James A. McClure (ID)	5,000
		Sam A. Nunn, Jr. (GA)	5,000
		Ted Stevens (AK)	5,000
		Donald Wilbur Stewart (AL)	5,000
		John William Warner (VA)	5,000
		Dennis Deconcini (AZ)	3,000
		Bob Packwood (OR)	3,000
		Joseph R. Biden, Jr. (DE)	2,500
		Nancy Landon Kassebaum (KS)	2,000
		Mark Odom Hatfield (OR)	1,500
		J. Bennett Johnston, Jr. (LA)	1,100
		Edmund S. Muskie (ME)	600
		Jennings Randolph (WV)	50

More than 50% of presidential campaign budgets went for media advertising, mostly on network TV. Jimmy Carter spent about $4 million for television in the final week of the campaign, and Ronald Reagan's forces doubled that amount. Experts estimated that all presidential hopefuls combined spent about $120 million seeking nomination, including public funding.

The 1980 election revealed the tremendous growth in the campaign impact of Political Action Committees. Common Cause documented some

Table 12–3.   *Selected Political Action Committees (PACs) Contributions to Political Candidates in 1977 and 1978*

NAME OF PAC	RECEIPTS	DOLLARS DISBURSED MINUS TRANSFERS TO AFFILIATED COMMITTEES	NUMBER OF PROFESSIONALS IN 1977	DOLLARS PER MEMBER OF PROFESSION
American Medical PAC	$1,657,885	$1,845,164*	362,700	$5.09
American Dental PAC	544,741	573,543	279,800	2.02
National Education PAC (National Education Association)	754,421	407,312 ⎱ 1,221,994	2,197,000	.50
Voice of Teachers for Education, Committee on Political Education (American Federation of Teachers)	796,881	814,632 ⎰		
American Nurses' PAC (N-CAP)	93,392	100,410	976,296	.09

* This does not include the funds distributed by each state medical association PAC. For example, the California Medical PAC disbursed $674,808 and the Texas Medical PAC disbursed $757,074.

$8.9 million in PAC contributions to Senate races in the first nine months of 1980, with some candidates receiving nearly half of their total contributions from PACs alone. The Democratic Study Group estimated total PAC disbursements to congresspeople of nearly $60 million in 1979–1980, compared with $39 million in 1977–1978, and only $12.5 million in 1973–1974. But the most significant changes occurred in the development of the so-called "independent" and anti-candidate PACs which were not bound by the normal $5000 per candidate per election limit. According to *Public Citizen*, these PACs spent more than $6 million to benefit the Reagan campaign, while only $18,500 was spent to benefit the Carter campaign.

The huge increases in PAC contributions were largely a result of the growth of corporate-based PACs. Only 89 corporate PACs had existed in 1974, compared to 1,127 in 1980. Over the same period, labor-related PACs increased in number from 201 to 276. Public Citizen's *Congress Watch* argued that the defeat of many of the most liberal congresspeople was a result, in part, of these PAC expenditures. They cited, as an example, the narrow defeat of Representative Bob Eckhardt of Texas who was outspent by a 3 to 1 margin by his opponent, Jack Fields. Public Citizen's analysis showed that 58% of Fields' contributions had come from oil company PACs, or executives of oil in oil-related corporations.

The 1980 election was a massive payoff for numerous conservative PACs, since many Republican challengers could not have won without these funds. For example, in the 1980 election, conservative Dallas, Texas, business PACs pumped more than $1.5 million into election campaigns throughout the country, stretching their political influence far beyond the city limits. This figure was almost twice as large as the amount of money spent in 1978. The number of Dallas businesses with Political Action Committees soared to 59, ranking Dallas second only to New York City. The Federal Election Commission reported that Texas had the most corporate PACs of any state with 151. A survey of FEC records filed by the 59 Dallas business PACs revealed the biggest spenders were the conglomerate LTV Corporation, Vought Corporation, Enserch Corporation, Texas Power and Light Company, and the Steak and Ale Restaurant chain. Each gave candidates more than $100,000 in 1980.

In Iowa, Republican challenger Charles Grassley received help from thirty Dallas corporations in his bid to defeat Senator John Culver. Diamond Shamrock Corporation with $2500 and Steak and Ale with $3500 were among Grassley's larger campaign contributors, as were Texas Oil and Gas Company with $3000, and Hunt Energy Corporation. For the Dallas Hunt Brothers, Bunker and Herbert, their corporate PAC money was a modest supplement to significant personal contributions to conservative candidates' campaigns. More than ten Hunt family members made multiple contributions of $1000 and more to Idaho Republican Steve Symms, who unseated Senator Frank Church, and to conservative Representative Larry McDonald of Georgia, a physician. In the final month of the campaign, the Hunt Energy Corporation PAC put $36,000 into the campaigns of other conservative candidates, including James Buckley in the Connecticut Senate race and Dan Quayle in his winning race against Indiana's Senator Birch Bayh.

In 1980, the new American Hospital Association PAC (HAPAC) and the Federation of American Hospitals PAC (FEDPAC) generally contributed money to incumbents holding key health committee positions. Unlike the heavyweight PACs of the American Medical Association, which contributed to unknowns if their sympathies were deemed proper, hospital PACs largely supported incumbents. Even candidates who had endorsed the Carter administration hospital cost-containment bill, for example, were occasionally supported by hospital PACs. Hospital groups noted that this was because many factors were considered in their choices beside votes on health care industry issues. Accessibility, open-mindedness, expertise in health care issues, and interest in local hospitals by the various candidates had a major bearing on the allocation of contributions. As of mid-August 1980, HAPAC had collected $92,600 and FEDPAC had close to $95,000. The hospital PACs tended to support prominent members of health-related committees such as Senator Bob Dole (Republican, Kansas), Senator Russell Long (Democrat, Louisiana), and Senator Bob Packwood (Republican, Oregon), who had received $2000, $3000, and $4000 respectively from FEDPAC, and $2750, $500, and $1250 from HAPAC. All were members of the Senate Finance Committee.

The great bulk of campaign contributions and other such assistance constitutes investment in the future goodwill of the recipient. When an interest group feels it necessary to call on a member of Congress for support, there is usually no need of a reminder of what the group has done in the past and of what it is in a position to do in the future. There is a tacit understanding about such things. The group has made contributions in the past and can be counted on again; all it wants is cooperation to the extent that it can be given. In most relationships between an interest group and a member of Congress, there is never any real question about cooperation because, to begin with, there is probably a mutuality of interests.

Critics increasingly claim that PACs can interfere with a politician's job of representing voters. "PAC money . . . obligates candidates to contributors and reduces their ties to constituents," observed Fred Wertheimer, Executive Vice President of the public interest group, Common Cause. "PACs go to first place in line and leave constituents on the sidelines." In early 1981 calls for tighter regulation of campaign funding were being drowned out by insistant demands to increase contribution limits for individuals and organizations. Republican Representative Bill Frenzel of Minnesota voiced the sentiments of many members of Congress in saying: "Election laws should be changed to encourage more giving, not less." Instead of tighter limits on political donations, observers predicted that lawmakers might increase the $1000 ceiling on individual contributions for federal races to $3000 or even $5000. Critics of that $1000 limit noted that since the ceiling had been adopted in 1974, inflation had reduced the real value to $600.

LOBBYING BY INTEREST GROUPS

Interest groups monitor governmental activity that might affect them, initiate governmental action to promote their interests, and block action that would work to their detriment. Each of these areas of activity requires access above all else, that is, access to information on what the government is doing or is about to do, and access to key decisionmakers. For a group to pursue its goals and promote its interests in the political arena, it must have access to decision makers. Regardless of the type of group, access to political decision makers is the key to group activity, and the nature of that access— the number of points of access, the ability to reach the "right" people, the type of reception from the decision makers—is directly related to the resources of the group and its ability to use them. With several hundred executive agencies and congressional panels continually formulating regulations, provisions, and laws that affect individuals and groups, the job of simply keeping up with political activity relevant to a group's interests is a massive one, even for a group with relatively narrow interests.

Lobbying is a tactic of trying to influence a decision of a legislature or some other government body. The right to lobby is constitutionally guaranteed, as it represents a form of petition for the redress of grievances. Lobbying is done directly by interest groups, by individuals, and by professional lobbyists who make a career of representing the interests of various groups before the legislature. A *lobbyist* is someone who spends much or all of his or her time representing the interests of a particular group. Some lobbyists are part-time or temporary Washington representatives for their employers or clients. Others represent several interests simultaneously or in succes-

Figure 12–7. Lobbying is the tactic used in an attempt to influence decisions of representatives and senators: Dr. Philip Kalisch and Russell Perry at work in the Senate. (Courtesy of School of Nursing and National Student Nurses' Association, University of Michigan)

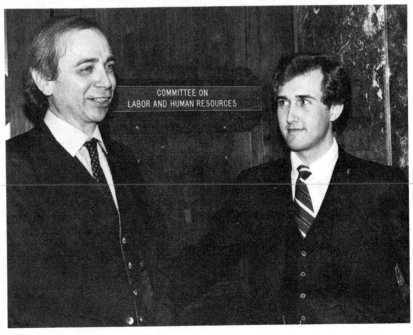

sion. Lobbyists of this sort tend to be lawyers and public relations specialists. Most of them have worked on Capitol Hill or in the executive branch, and some are former members of Congress. Many important national interest groups retain Washington law firms and also employ expensive lobbyists who serve as long-term advocates for the organizational cause. The most influential lobbyists in this category are significant figures on the Washington scene, on a first-name basis with hundreds of politicians and reporters. A good lobbyist is one who has spent years cultivating friendships in Washington and knows everybody on the congressional committees, congressional staffs, administrative agencies, and news staffs that handle affairs affecting her or his group.

In recent years, lobbying has become big business, with many organizations spending tens and, in some cases, hundreds of thousands of dollars on it. Expenditures for lobbying are estimated to be well over $1 billion a year. At the federal level, the first and only general statute governing the activities of lobbyists is the Federal Regulation of Lobbying Act of 1946. The act requires only those individuals and organizations whose *principal purpose* is to lobby, irrespective of the actual dollar amount spent, to register with the clerk of the House and the secretary of the Senate. The requirements of the act are aimed at disclosure rather than prohibition, of lobbying activities. However, owing to a number of gaping loopholes, especially ones caused by the principal purpose provision, hundreds of thousands of dollars for lobbying activities go unreported annually. The 1946 act also does not cover lobbying directed at the executive branch, and it has no enforcement mechanism.

Undoubtedly, the most significant nonsubstantive issue in recent years affecting nursing lobby groups was the Conable bill—an amendment to the Tax Reform Act of 1976 allowing nonprofit, tax-exempt organizations incorporated under SECTION 501 (c)(n3) of the IRS Code to engage in significant lobbying activities without fear of losing their tax-exempt status. Among other provisions, the new guidelines focus on legislative lobbying at the federal, state, and local levels, excluding administrative agency lobbying from the definition of covered activities. The new law also defines and sets limits on certain kinds of grass-roots (indirect) lobbying.

Lobbying by nurses is an appropriate and essential response to the serious imbalance created in the health care system, where other special interests are exerting powerful influences on federal legislative decision making by speaking with disproportionately loud voices. Lobbying involves a variety of political actions, often far removed in time and place from actual policy deliberations. These actions may be aimed at mobilizing public opinion, or they may be intended to gain access and bear leverage with decision makers. The effectiveness of the efforts of lobbying are directly related to some combination of the following factors: the amount of money spent on influence-seeking activity; the sophistication of the lobbying strategies and techniques; and the number, location, socioeconomic status, and degree of activism of the paid and volunteer representatives and members. These factors allow lobbyists to obtain privileges and superior access to decision makers and to influence the content of public-policy decisions.

The skill with which a lobbyist monitors, analyzes, and participates in the political system is a major factor in determining his or her influence on the public-policy process. Immense resources alone do not guarantee that a group will have a significant influence on policy. But a group's ability to use its unique mix of resources to influence political allies, neutral figures, and opponents is of great importance. Lobbyists often score their greatest victories when the groups they represent want to disrupt or delay legislation. A group defending the status quo derives benefits from the sheer cumbersomeness of the legislation process in Congress, and its task is relatively easy because there are so many junctures at which a negative decision can doom a bill. Congressional procedures, in fact, may appear so formidable to lobbyists that it would seem they were devised solely to prevent enactment of any particular group's favored legislation. Although proponents of a bill must win every match, the opposition often requires only a single victory.

To petition Congress, agencies, or the White House, a group must know what it wants and how to achieve it legislatively or administratively. It must translate its desires into legislative or legal language, develop supporting materials, and find a way to have its initiative routed onto a path where it will have a chance of legislative adoption or administrative approval. Membership cohesion and a sense by political actors that group lobbying is representative of group-membership opinion are also important. Without at least a modicum of unanimity, a group finds itself unable to take a position and base legislative action on it. The ability of a group to command facts, figures, and technical information in support of its position is another key organizational resource. Substantive information, to be used by legislators or bureaucrats to support their positions or to persuade individuals to change their views, is at a premium in the political process.

An inability to produce meaningful cost-benefit data has handicapped the development of nursing programs. Although a great deal of lip service has been given to the importance of expanded nursing activities, the lack of concrete evidence on cost effectiveness of nursing services has hindered their funding. The American Nurses' Association and the National League for Nursing place a high priority on expanded nursing services; unfortunately, the federal health budget does not translate that priority into dollars. Also, none of the national health insurance proposals under consideration make any real provision for funding community expanded nursing services. For example, it has been estimated that one-third to one-half of the total national health bill could be avoided if all preventive health actions that would reduce the need for medical care were instituted. Improvements in curative medical care offer nothing similar to that potential for savings. But estimates and impressions are not enough. Until reliable cost-benefit data on the advantages of greater attention to preventive health measures and the nurse's role can be provided, public-policy decisions are likely to continue in favor of nonpreventive medical care programs.

Sophisticated lobbyists are aware that costs and benefits of pending legislation may be widely distributed or narrowly concentrated. Income and social security taxes are *widely* distributed, whereas, subsidies to a particular industry or regulations imposing costs on an industry that cannot be fully passed through to consumers are *narrowly* concentrated. When

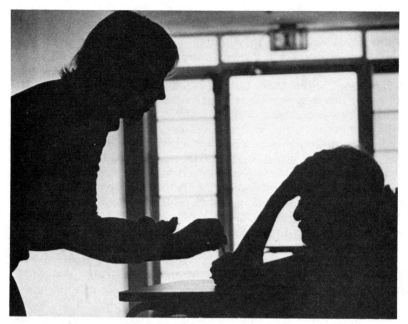

Figure 12–8. The lack of available cost-benefit data has hindered nursing's case for increased funding. (Courtesy of Urbana Citizen, Urbana, Ohio)

both costs and benefits are widely distributed, lobbyists find *majoritarian politics*. All or most of society expects to gain; all or most of society expects to pay. Interest groups have little incentive to form around such issues because no small, definable segment of society (an industry, an occupation, or a locality) can expect to capture a disproportionate share of the benefits or to avoid a disproportionate share of the burdens.

When both costs and benefits are *narrowly* concentrated, conditions are right for *interest-group politics*. A subsidy or regulation often benefits a relatively small group at the expense of another comparably small group. Each side has a strong incentive to organize and exercise political influence. The public does not believe it will be much affected one way or another, so it may sympathize more with one side than with the other; its voice is likely to be heard in only weaker general terms. When the benefits of a prospective policy are *concentrated*, but the costs widely distributed, *client politics* is likely to result. Some small, easily organized group will benefit and will thus have a powerful incentive to organize and lobby. The costs of the benefit are distributed at a low per capita rate over a large number of people, and hence they have little incentive to organize an opposition—if, indeed, they even hear of the policy.

Finally, a policy may be proposed that will confer general (though perhaps small) benefits at a cost to be borne chiefly by a small segment of society. When this is attempted, lobbyists are witnessing *entrepreneurial politics*. Antipollution and auto safety bills were proposed to make air cleaner or cars safer for everyone at an expense that was imposed, at least initially, on particular segments of industry. Entrepreneurial politics depends heavily on the attitudes of third parties. The reaction of the regulated industry is predictably hostile. The reaction of the public that is to benefit may be difficult to discern or evident only in general terms ("do something about this problem").

Although the term lobbyist often carries a negative connotation, lobbyists serve a very important ombudsman function as a communication link between constituents and public officials in the legislative and executive branches of state, local, and federal government. Their activities can be classified into two broad categories: outside lobbying and inside lobbying.

OUTSIDE LOBBYING

Outside lobbying refers to indirect, grass-roots lobbying activities intended to influence government officials. Telephone, telegram, and letterwriting campaigns, as well as press conferences, letters to the editor, and other media activities, typify grass-roots-type lobbying. Grass-roots activity is generally aimed at educating or mobilizing, at the level of the local community, the members of lobbying organizations or the general public to influence a policy decision on an issue by their elected or appointed representatives.

Grass-roots lobbying of Congress—pressure from the 50 states and the 435 constituencies, from corporate headquarters to professional communities—is extremely potent politically in the 1980s. Members of Congress are often highly adept at resisting the blandishments of the Washington lobbyists who make up the day-to-day voice of the many groups affected by the federal government. Yet the legislators' representative role compels them to weigh carefully the voices of individual constituents who contact them regarding legislation. Constituent power on issues from "the folks back home" is the language of Washington. The constituent power serves as the base for political action.

The American Hospital Association has made excellent use of hospital trustees, who by the very nature of their connection with the health care industry, are well-positioned to have a particularly strong voice with their legislators. Hospital boards are dominated by business executives, members of the legal and accounting professions, and spokespersons for medicine and hospitals. Representatives of nurses, the consumer, and the general community are very seriously underrepresented. Obviously, hospital boards are not representative of, nor do they reflect the composition of, the community in general. Despite the lack of input from the broad range of social, economic, and health care interests, the people who sit at the hospital boardroom table are uniquely equipped to take the hospital's message to political leaders. They have the special vantage point that results from their activities inside and outside the hospital, and they have special skills that make them effective spokespersons. The leadership skills that distinguish the trustees' professional, business, and personal lives carry over to their health care roles, often making them influential advocates of hospitals' interests. Their leadership abilities make them articulate and effective spokespersons for the hospitals they govern.

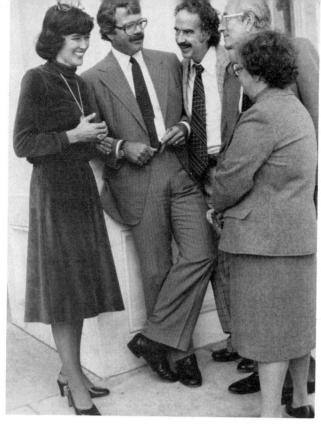

Figure 12–9. When the people back home contact them, members of Congress listen: Representatives Patricia Schroeder (Colorado) and Barbara Mikulski (Maryland) talk to constituents. (Courtesy of New York Times, New York)

Trustees who know legislators and have access to them can create opportunities to give them the hospital's perspective on pending legislation that affects health care. One of the most effective ways hospitals are making the connection between legislators and trustees and other important people in the health care sector is through the Partnership for Action program of the American Hospital Association. This is a network of contacts between health care institutions and lawmakers that is activated when a matter critical to health care is being considered.

Partnership participants, often selected because of close (first-name) relationships with their members of Congress, are encouraged to cultivate contacts with them. Aside from the more formal aspects of keeping abreast of their positions on various issues and knowing their voting records, participants are urged to invite their legislators to their hospitals, to visit them in their district or mobile offices, to take part in their public activities, or to show an interest in or contribute to their campaigns.

INSIDE LOBBYING

Inside lobbying, in contrast, is aimed at influencing decision makers in a more direct manner. It involves such activities as submission of testimony, drafting of regulations and amendments, face-to-face visits with policy makers and their staffs, vote counting and development of lobbying target lists. The most intense activities of professional lobbyists involve inside lobbying related to the formal deliberations on an issue. The bulk of legislative deliberations, for example, occurs in committee and subcommittee, where it has been estimated that as much as 90% of the work of legislative bodies takes place. It is at this level that lobbyists have their greatest impact, but it is also where the general public is least informed of the actions of lobbyists as well as of their elected representatives. It is much easier for lobbyists to try to influence the one, two, or sometimes three dozen members of a committee, than it is to try to promote their interests on the floor of the Senate or House of Representatives with its 100 members and 435 members respectively. Lobbying at the committee level becomes even more intense when focused on the marginal or swing votes—those members who are undecided on a bill or amendment at a given point in time. The ability of lobbyists to "count heads" to determine lobbying targets, to coordinate inside and outside lobbying efforts, and to use and manage organizational resources receives its biggest test during the committee process.

LOBBYING THE CONGRESS

Lobbying strategies frequently differ when it comes to handling the House of Representatives and the Senate. Representatives, because of their number, have fewer committee assignments, smaller personal staffs, and in general fewer time commitments than senators. Lobbying strategies for the House thus tend to focus on contacts with the members, whereas strategies for the Senate put more emphasis on relationships with staffs. If one wants to get something from the entire House membership, it is important to have key members in a large number of congressional districts. The interest group that is widely dispersed—and nurses *have* this advantage—is in a position to appeal directly to a large share of the House membership through their constituencies. No matter how a case is presented or which tactics are employed, it is advisable to understand initially that, above all else, *votes* motivate congressmen and congresswomen. A large part of their job is to be sensitive to their power base among voters so that they may continue to represent them through re-election. Thus, appeals that suggest their continued tenure—such as "labor has endorsed it" or "a poll showed consumers favor it"—will be favorably received by most members.

In an effort to link a congressman's political future to his support for the legislative preferences of interest groups, more and more Washington lobbying offices are compiling ratings of lawmakers' voting records. Such ratings are currently used by over fifty national organizations to inform their members which senators and representatives should be supported or opposed at election time. Typically, interest groups analyze the votes on selected issues that come before the House and Senate in a given period. A lawmaker is determined to have voted *right* if he supported the position of the group and *wrong* if he opposed it. Each member is given a percentage score from 0 to 100. Among the groups that circulate their ratings of Congress widely are the following:

- AFL-CIO Committee on Political Education (COPE)
- Amalgamated Clothing and Textile Workers Union AFL-CIO
- American Conservative Union
- American Federation of State, County and Municipal Employees (AFL-CIO)
- Americans for Constitutional Action
- Americans for Democratic Action
- Chamber of Commerce
- Committee for Survival of a Free Congress
- Moral Majority
- National Council of Senior Citizens
- National Farmers Union (Farmers Educational and Cooperative Union of America)
- National Machine Tool Builders' Association
- National Taxpayers Union
- National Women's Political Caucus
- Public Citizen, Inc
- Ripon Society
- United Auto Workers
- United Food and Commercial Workers International Unions (AFL-CIO)
- United Mine Workers of America, Coal Miners Political Action Committee
- The Woman Activist, Inc

As an example of the scores that are attached to senators by these ratings, in 1979 the AFL-CIO scores ranged from 0% for Robert Dole and Barry Goldwater to 100% for George McGovern, Thomas Eagleton, and Birch Bayh. The Chamber of Commerce gave Dole 73%, Goldwater 90%, McGovern 20%, Eagleton 0%, and Bayh 11%.

Electioneering is the tactic of trying to elect legislators who are sympathetic to a group's point of view. Thus, farmers' groups are partial to rural-based candidates for office; business groups lean toward conservative candidates; labor unions favor economic liberals; and teachers' associations unite behind candidates who support public employee collective bargaining and more expenditures for public schools. Whereas business and some professional groups tend to make the most effective use of public relations tactics, labor unions and teachers' associations are probably the most skilled users of electioneering, especially in the Northeast and Midwest, and on the West Coast where union membership is very large.

The most effective electioneering asset of unions lies in their large and active memberships. Teachers, in particular, are accustomed to persuading people and to organizing their activities. Thus, they have many skills that are useful in an election campaign. Additionally, they perceive a direct benefit to themselves from electing candidates who favor collective bargaining and greater expenditures for public schools. As a consequence, they contribute a disproportionate number of people to deliver campaign literature, make telephone calls, organize coffee parties, set up fundraising parties, and plan campaign strategies. For example, the California Teachers' Association (CTA) held their chapter and statewide 1980 candidate endorsement conventions in June. Among questions asked about candidates were:

- Is the candidate free of personal or economic interests which would conflict with his/her ability to serve?
- Does the candidate seek the assistance of specialists in making judgments?
- Does the candidate appear to understand the social, political, ethnic, and economic composition and resources of the district he/she proposes to serve?
- Are his/her positions and relationships with CTA evaluated favorably by the CTA Legislative Advocates? Did the incumbent receive financial support from CTA/PAC in the last election?
- Does he/she support the right of teachers to bargain collectively and to participate as equal partners in the educational decision making process? Will the candidate seek, listen and respond to teacher opinion on educational issues?[6]

The actual behavior of a lawmaker is the product of many influences. How he votes on many bills, of course, reflects a general orientation (pro-labor or pro-business, liberal or conservative) toward the issue at hand. Yet

Figure 12–10. Working on campaigns for reelection of congressmen who have helped nurses is one form of electioneering. Representative Carl Pursell celebrates a legislative victory with University of Michigan nurses. (Courtesy of School of Nursing, University of Michigan)

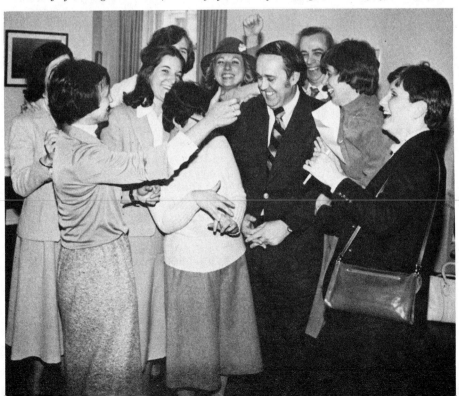

there are other bills (often of a somewhat technical nature) on which ideological preferences provide little guidance. In any event, the lawmaker is likely to be barraged by many cross-pressures. Constituents back home, the party leadership, powerful lobbyists, and trusted colleagues all may be clamoring for that vote—some for a bill and some against it.

LOBBYING THE EXECUTIVE BRANCH

Bureaucrats hold enormous power in the American political system. This is so in the sense that it is their interpretation of a statute that frequently counts more than the words of the law itself. Or it is their decision that determines the awarding of a government contract or grant. Lobbying of administrators and bureaucrats, therefore, is a major industry in Washington, rivaling the lobbying that takes place on Capitol Hill. Consequently, lobbyists for the National Education Association, the American Medical Association, or the Pharmaceutical Manufacturers Association must spend as much time with the Department of Education, the Department of Health and Human Services, or the Food and Drug Administration as with congressional committees, subcommittees, and individual members.

Government agency employees generally can be classified in one of three ways depending upon their motives. The first employees are the *careerists*. These are employees who identify their careers and rewards with the agency. They do not expect to move on to other jobs outside the agency or otherwise to receive significant rewards from external constituencies. The maintenance of the agency and of their positions in it are of paramount concern. The second are the *politicians*. These employees see themselves as having a future in elective or appointive offices outside the agency. They hope to move on to better or more important undertakings and may wish, for example, to run for Congress, to become the vice-president for public relations of a large firm, to enter the cabinet or subcabinet, or to join the campaign staff of a promising presidential contender. The maintenance and enhancement of their careers outside the agency is of paramount importance. The third are the *professionals*. These are employees who receive rewards (in status if not in money) from organized members, in similar occupations not in government. Professionals may hope to move on to better jobs elsewhere, but access to these jobs depends upon their display of professionally approved behavior and technical competence. They may also be content to remain in the agency, but they value the continued approval of fellow professionals outside the agency or the self-respect that comes from behaving in accordance with internalized professional norms. The maintenance of this professional scheme is of major importance to these employees.

One executive department focus of lobbying efforts is to respond to proposed agency rules and regulations for legislative programs. This is one of the stages of the policy implementation process and is of great importance. Regulations provide the detailed guidelines for the implementation of legislation and have a significant impact on the actual substance of federal programs. Ideally lobbyists help shape the regulations before they reach the published proposal form. Agencies are required to publish proposed regulations in the daily *Federal Register* thirty days before they are

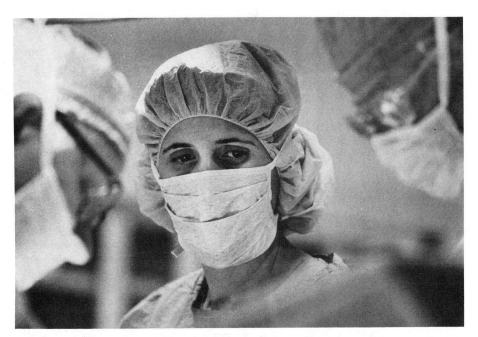

Figure 12–11. The AORN mounted a 1980 letter-writing campaign against a proposed regulatory change that they feared would erode patient care standards in operating rooms. (Courtesy of Robert Stockfield, Monroe, Louisiana)

to take effect. Exceptions to this requirement are granted for rules and regulations pertaining to the implementation of newly enacted and complex legislation. The format that is followed by all agencies includes a brief descriptive title of the action, the period of time during which public comments will be received, a summary of the regulation, and the agency person to contact for further information. Although it is very difficult to influence the course of a proposed regulation through public comment, a massive influx of protests against a proposed regulation may cause the agency to revise its course of action. It is important to note that all letters for and against proposed regulations are tabulated, filed, and available for public inspection.

An example of a massive lobby effort aimed at heading off a proposed federal regulation was that of the 29,000-member Association of Operating Room Nurses in July, 1980. The group charged that the regulation change, HSQ-16-P, SECTION 482.41 (a)(4), published in the June 20, 1980, *Federal Register*, would erode standards of patient care. The activities of one of the AORN groups were reported in the June 29, 1980, Frederick, Maryland, *Post* under the headline, "Nurses Group Protests Operating Room Changes:"

> The Association of Operating Room Nurses of the Appalachian Area of West Virginia, Pennsylvania, and Maryland are campaigning against a proposed Medicare/Medicaid regulation that would permit lesser trained personnel to perform nursing functions for patients having surgery. This change could lower the

quality of care of every surgical patient in the United States, according to the Association of Operating Room Nurses, a national professional association representing more than 29,000 registered nurses.

The regulations published June 20 in the *Federal Register* would permit technicians and licensed practical (vocational) nurses to circulate in the operating room. Traditionally and legally, circulating duties have been the function of a registered nurse. The circulating nurse plans the nursing care for the patient in the operating room. During surgery, the circulating nurse is responsible for the safety of the patient. For the patient under local anesthesia, the circulating nurse monitors such vital functions as heart, respiration, temperature and sterile technique.

The American Association of Operating Room Nurses position that technicians, who are trained to perform technical functions in the operating room such as passing instruments to the surgeon, are not educated to make nursing decisions and judgments. The American Nurses' Association (ANA), the Federation of Specialty Nursing Organization, and Individual Specialty Nursing Organization have backed the operating room nurses in their campaign to stop the change in the Medicare/Medicaid regulations. During the 60-day comment period which ends August 19, nurses across the country are expected to write to HHS protesting the change. They will be seeking support from health care consumers and other organizations.

Comments should be sent to: Administrator, Health Care Financing Administration, Department of Health and Human Services, P.O. Box 17082, Baltimore, Md. 21235.[7]

PUBLIC-RELATIONS ACTIVITIES OF INTEREST GROUPS

Public relations probably absorbs more time than any other interest-group activity. The objective normally is to create a favorable climate within which the interest group can operate. Although the widest use of public relations is to sway public opinion in a general sense, it is often used for specific issues. Most people think interest groups direct all their efforts toward influencing legislative decision makers, but these groups may actually spend more of their time, energy, and resources on public-relations activities than on anything else. The purpose of a continuing public relations campaign is to create a climate of opinion favorable to an interest group and its program. The interest group hopes to establish a reservoir of public goodwill that it can draw on whenever a critical issue arises.

One of the forms taken by interest-group activities at the grass roots is the development of a program to create a generally favorable climate of opinion for the organization and its aims. Such programs are commonly carried out by organizations that are subject to government regulations and by organizations desirous of governmental assistance. Similarly, large organizations spend considerable sums on institutional advertising in newspapers and, especially, in popular magazines. Such advertising is not necessarily designed to create public support for any current legislative aim of the organization, but rather to create in the public mind a favorable general impression of a group and what it stands for.

To inculcate the opinions that are considered appropriate and to evoke the actions that are considered desirable, the national headquarters of a group typically bombards the members with as many communications and publications as its budget will allow. Typically there will be a magazine of

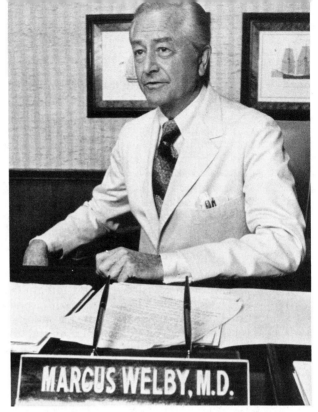

Figure 12–12. The purpose of public relations work is to create a favorable image for an interest group, and this often includes working with the creators of entertainment world professionals. The AMA lent its expertise in the filming of the TV series "Marcus Welby, M.D." (Courtesy of Nursing in the Mass Media Collection, University of Michigan)

some kind that is sent to all members. The affluence of some groups makes it possible for their magazines to be highly professional products, containing features and articles of general interest as well as the inevitable discussion of political policy questions. Groups with more meager resources than these may have to settle for a considerably simpler format, but even a two-page mimeographed newsletter may suffice to inform the constituency of what the top leadership is thinking and doing.

More specifically, the publications of interest groups are generally aimed at one or more of three audiences. First, a publication may be intended to reach the entire formal membership. It is usually the case in membership groups that each individual who pays dues or makes a contribution receives a magazine or newsletter. A second audience may be an active or easily motivated group within the organizational membership. These are people who generally are more involved than the average member. The organization considers that they are more likely to write letters to members of Congress and engage in other lobbying activities when requested or to work on stimulating grass-roots activities. Third, the interest groups may want to reach an attentive public outside the organization. Attentive publics are groups of individuals that maintain a salient concern on certain issues.

One of the most frequently used public-relations vehicles is the *news-letter*. It has fewer pages, is often folded rather than stapled, and can be printed on low quality paper. Newsletters tend to carry less in the way of in-depth feature articles, concentrating instead on more concise news and data summaries. There are also publications known as *alerts*, which are put out as needed. They are printed inexpensively, usually number only a page or two in length, and generally are mailed to selective members or attentive publics to inform them of an important upcoming vote in the Congress. Alerts are more than advisory in nature; they are also an appeal to readers to immediately write letters and to activate others.

The major vehicle for the dissemination of information to the outside mass media is the *news* (or press) *release*. If a group is aiming for television or radio coverage as well as newspapers, it uses a news release, not a press release. Releases are best written in the third person so that they may be printed or read without revision. A news release is typically double-spaced on 8½ × 11 inch paper (so that one sheet will probably suffice). At the upper left-hand corner, the issuing office types a name and phone number of the contact person (preceded by "for further information"). On the next line the release time is indicated (*e.g.*, "for September 20, 1980," "morning," and so forth). Next, the title of the release is typed across the page.

Tom Eblen, managing editor of the *Kansas City Star*, has offered excellent reasons why some news releases are not used. He says, "I have no idea how many releases we receive, but the number would certainly be in the hundreds in any given week. We use zero to five percent of the releases we get. Here are some of the reasons":

- Out-of-date mailing lists. Releases sent to people who haven't worked here for ten years.
- Releases with requests for tearsheets or return of photos. We only return photos in the case of obituaries.
- Releases that say 'for immediate release' with no date listed.
- Releases that fail to differentiate between a country weekly and metropolitan daily. The small, local newspaper wants deans' lists and the like. The metro daily does not.
- Releases with information missing.
- Releases that are more than a page long. Remember that they go to the busiest person in the newsroom. If it takes more than a page, we probably wouldn't assign a reporter to it.
- Cute leads. Just give us the information straight.
- Releases that tell nothing new, or don't bother to tell anything new until halfway down the release.
- Ones that are illiterate.
- Releases with all kinds of fancy printing, dye cut paper, and so forth. Let your information sell itself. Advertising in that manner doesn't work in the newsroom.
- Especially releases that arrive ten times to five different persons.
- More especially those that arrive more than a week after the release date, or after the news event is no longer news.[8]

News stories may go through four to six different individuals before they are actually printed or reported on television. A group should be prepared to find their story not quite the same as they told it.

THE AMERICAN MEDICAL ASSOCIATION'S USE OF PUBLIC RELATIONS

Interest groups often make extensive use of the services of professional public relations experts and engage in mass media efforts to try to persuade the general public that what is at stake is the welfare of the country at large and not the particular interests of the individual organization. One of the most elaborate campaigns of this kind in modern times was the one waged by the American Medical Association against all forms of national health insurance. In 1948, after the election victory of President Harry S. Truman, the AMA was gravely concerned that the time might be ripe for the proponents of what it called *socialized medicine* to make their bid. To combat any such efforts, the organization levied an assessment charge of $25 on each of its 140,000 members. The money that was collected, it said, would be used to educate the American public on the progress that American medicine had made and on the necessity of assuring the continued high quality of medical care.

The AMA retained the sophisticated California public relations firm of Whittaker and Baxter. The company employed the same Madison Avenue tactics that had conditioned Americans to shudder at the mention of *dandruff* and *body odor* to produce the same negative reflex action against what the AMA called *socialized medicine.* It also persuaded physicians all over the country to double as propagandists, distributing literature in their waiting rooms and asking patients directly to urge their congressmen to oppose the legislation on national health care. Because patients of the late 1940s tended to rank their physicians with their ministers at the same high level of authority and selflessness, it was not surprising that an avalanche of letters descended upon Congress. In addition, Whittaker and Baxter brought a multitude of other organizations into the fight. It could report by the end of 1949 that 1829 organizations had gone on record in opposition to compulsory health insurance. By 1952 the number had grown to more than 8000. So successful were the firm's tactics that President Truman's health insurance legislation never even came to a vote in Congress.

From 1949 to 1964, no other organization in the country devoted such large expenditures to its lobbying activities in any single year as did the AMA in each of the years of 1949 and 1950. In 1964 and 1965, AMA money was again spent in large quantities to defeat the bill providing medical care for the aged. This time there were even spot announcements on television and radio, as well as advertisements in newspapers and in the mass-circulation magazines such as *Life, Reader's Digest,* and *Saturday Evening Post.* Although Medicare and Medicaid were enacted, the United States remains the only industrialized nation in the world, besides South Africa, without a comprehensive program of tax-supported health insurance. The AMA continues its fight today, as the 1980 annual report closes with these statements:

It means little to pursue scientific, socio-economic, and educational policies which assure high professional quality, if society is unaware of those efforts. Using appropriate communication vehicles, the AMA tells the story of achievement and aspiration, of viewpoint and venture, to a wide range of 'publics.' These include opinion leaders in all levels of government, in labor and business, in specialty medical and allied health organizations, in state and local medical societies, in civic groups, and in key segments of the population at large.

Frequently, the 'telling' is not enough. Association policies and priorities for the medical profession are translated into model or draft legislation and executive branch proposals for state and federal government action. The Association works toward liaison, the co-existence between groups that allows medicine to be woven into the fabric of American society.

In Washington, D.C., despite a new, more conservative administration, the AMA predicts that strong governmental pressure will continue to be put on the medical profession and the hospital sector and liaison activities will need to be even stronger. The Association believes that medicine's relationship with government hinges on how effectively medicine rebuilds a representational base. A continuing AMA concern is the trend toward very general legislation which is

Figure 12–13. Access to politicians for lobbying purposes is greatly enhanced when nurses themselves are in government office. Cheryl Beversdorf, R.N., pictured here with Senator Alan Cranston, is a professional staff member on the Senate Committee on Veterans Affairs.

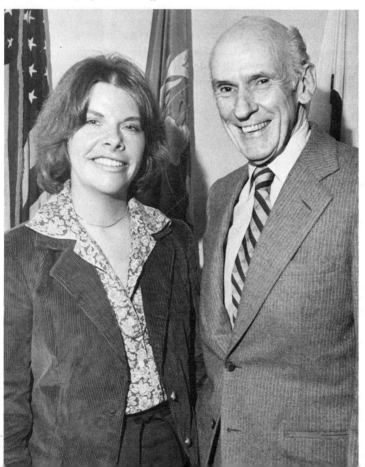

open to misinterpretation or excessive regulation by government agencies. In the best of all worlds, medicine can achieve appropriate deregulation of the profession. In the worst, further regulations will be imposed in a misguided effort to hold down costs.

In order to foster legislation that is in the best interest of the public and the profession, the AMA in 1980 made thousands of contacts with members of Congress or their staffs. Appearances in person or in writing presented positions in the form of 200 statements to both houses of Congress. Additionally, there were almost as many visits with administrative and executive agency officials, nearly 100 calls on White House staff, and numerous conferences with the President and with the Secretary of HHS. . .[9]

In our health care system, physicians and hospital administrators hold more of the positions of authority, and control more of the concrete resources, than do nurses. Nurses increasingly recognize that the solution to this problem is not simply to continue to add resources to a health care system that continues to distort the use of resources in an unbalanced way; instead, by working together through interest groups, they seek to redirect existing energies and resources so that these improvements may be brought to fruition. The dynamics of mobilizing a group into action and the factors that make for success are more fully discussed in the next chapter.

References

1. Lobby registrations. In Congressional Quarterly Almanac 96th Congress, 1st Session, 1979, Vol 35, pp 3-D–40-D. Washington, DC, Congressional Quarterly, 1980
2. Ibid
3. Ibid
4. Ibid
5. Ibid
6. Endorsements: Democracy in Action. CTA/NEA Action May:4, 1980
7. Nurses group protests operating room changes. Frederick, Md, Post, July 29, 1980
8. Pedersen W: Obfuscation is out: But is communication in? It's time our bureaucrats learned to write. Public Relations Q 23:23–26, 1978
9. Sammons JH: Annual Report of the American Medical Association for 1980. Chicago, American Medical Association, 1981

13–Political Mobilization

Conditions in nursing are ripe for an upswing in political activities by nurses. The structure of American society is conducive to loosening the rigid belief system that has for so long restricted the role of both women in general and nurses employed in the health care industry. The industry is under strain because rising costs increase the discrepancies, tensions, and conflicts between nurses and health care policy makers. Nurses have begun to recognize the sources of strain on nursing, to identify and blame the groups and individuals responsible for the strain, and to specify appropriate political responses by nurses to attack the problems. Furthermore, additional deprivations, occurring almost daily, confirm the existing discontent and illuminate the dilemma facing nurses: they must fight as a group to maintain their professionalism, or they must submit to domination. What is left in this sequence is the widespread mobilization of nurses for action and the continued erosion of the traditional control that has prevented the political participation of nurses with judgments such as it is "not morally correct."

Having reviewed various components of political nursing, we now must ask the question: What are the elements of political mobilization that need to be developed to enhance the ability of nurses to obtain policy victories? Cohesion is the essence of political mobilization because in our present society individuals can rarely alter conditions without the assistance of many other people. Consequently, persons are forced to work together to change things through a redistribution of power within a society or subgroup of society. A group of persons commit themselves to joint action in order to articulate their wants and demands into issues and then work to gain agenda status for these issues. Collective goals are essential to politically mobilized groups who seek to gain power and to challenge the status quo. Mobilization, as an expression of commitment and support within society, can take the form of interest groups, political parties, social movements, or other structures.

All formerly "deprived" groups in society that have achieved improved status have done so by becoming mobilized politically. The initial spark that sets off the process may take place when a group experiences certain changes such as a marked increase in knowledge or fresh insight into old problems. Sometimes gaining a higher socioeconomic or prestige level gives the group a new view of old issues, and as a result of these changes, they develop new and different ideas and insights, which then lead to political participation.

PURPOSES OF POLITICAL MOVEMENTS

The impetus for mobilization is sometimes a very narrow issue (*e.g.*, the staff nurses in a particular hospital desire to chart on the progress notes

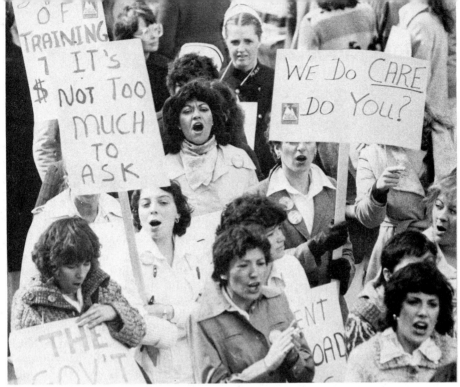

Figure 13–1. *The question of the hour is: How can nurses become effectively mobilized to achieve policy victories? (Courtesy of Edmonton Journal, Edmonton, Alberta, Canada)*

Figure 13–2. *Based on the real experiences of a Harrisburg, Pennsylvania, nurse, the 1981 motion-picture-for-television, "A Matter of Life and Death," starred Linda Lavin as a nurse whose unconventional approach to treating the terminally ill created political difficulties for her with the hospital medical staff. (Courtesy of Nursing in the Mass Media Research Project, University of Michigan)*

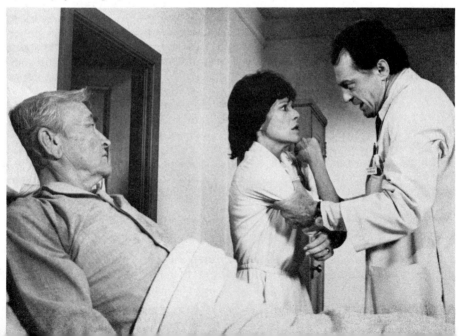

previously confined only to physicians). In other instances, a series of smaller issues are the focus of the movement (*e.g.*, a school of nursing faculty wants better pay, a smaller student-faculty ratio in clinical teaching settings, more opportunity to attend professional meetings, and greater access to seed money for research projects). The political movement can also address large macro problems (such as reconstruction of the health care system, giving nurses more opportunity to provide autonomous, health-oriented preventive care). A number of smaller issues may be attacked in passing as a logical part of the larger issue (*e.g.*, third-party reimbursement for nurses, health insurance reimbursement for preventive care, appointments of nurses to health care policy-making bodies, more representation of nurses in government, and so on).

Political movements can be reactionary, conservative, revisionary, or revolutionary. *Reactionary* movements are aimed at restoring the past. People involved in this type of movement praise some aspect of "the good old days." Physicians who desire the obedient, nonquestioning nurse of a bygone era and work to reinstate a training system that will yield that kind of nurse are such an example. Nurses who harken back to the less academic, more apprenticeship type of nurse training of forty years ago and seek to turn education back into this mode constitute another example.

Conservative movements attempt to keep things the way they currently exist. Hospital administrators joining together to avoid government cost-

Figure 13–3. Reactionary movements are aimed at walking backward into the future: Nurses at the turn of the century prepare patients' meals in the hospital kitchen. (Courtesy of History of Nursing Collection, University of Michigan)

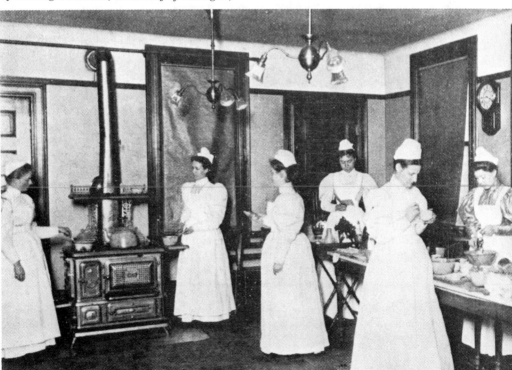

containment efforts, physicians fighting national health insurance legislation, and nurses opposing the baccalaureate entry into nursing-practice issue are all examples of conservative movements. Such groups tend to react to new events and against proposed ideas that are seen as threats to the status quo.

Revisionary movements are aimed at the modification or partial alteration of the existing status of affairs, but at the same time they accept aspects of the present system. Nurses who want access to third-party reimbursement for themselves, but accept the idea of traditional fee-for-service health care, as opposed to instituting a new government-operated system whereby all health professionals in all settings, including physicians, would be salaried, are one such example. Nurses who would work to institute the latter idea would be involved in what is termed a *revolutionary* or radical movement. This kind of movement is aimed at replacing the current system entirely. No major aspect of the existing system is considered acceptable.

Still another kind of social or political movement is the *escape* movement. This occurs when a group does not attempt to change the current system, but instead removes itself to a position outside the system. The "Kinlein Care" movement is an example of this kind of political movement. Lucile Kinlein no longer views herself as a provider of nursing care but now espouses a form of self-care for the patient that she labels "Kinlein Care."

ESSENTIAL CONDITIONS FOR MOBILIZATION TO OCCUR

Only certain people get involved in political movements. Persons who are very deprived typically do not become mobilized. Escape movements, if anything, are usually the only kinds of action seen, as such individuals are unwilling to take the risk of becoming involved in political matters. As Edwards wrote, "Revolutions do not occur when the repressed classes are forced down to the depths of misery. Revolutions occur after the repressed classes, for a considerable time, have been in the enjoyment of increasing prosperity."[1]

Another way to explain what happens, in more modern terms, is that deprived or "have-not" groups, such as nurses, are chronically accorded a deficient share of the available resources. Two consequences occur: nurses withdraw from, or don't get involved in, political matters. In other words, they become apathetic, believing participation to be fruitless. Then, as a result, policy makers conclude, in the absence of demands from nurses, that a satisfaction level is prevalent, that they are happy with things as they are. In actuality, nurses are alienated from the political system. According to research, alienation is associated with a tendency to belong to fewer organizations, and many of the alienated belong to none. Consequently, they are in a relatively poor position to translate their very real needs and interests into claims by way of the political system, particularly if there is no large, powerful interest group to represent them. For example, a Jamestown, North Carolina, nurse, Rita English, wrote the following letter to the editor of the High Point, North Carolina, *Enterprise* on June 27, 1980:

My name is nurse. I have been a nurse for twelve years. I have worked at two different hospitals and a nursing home. I have worked days, evenings, nights, holidays, days off and during my vacation. Believe me, it is not too much fun working Christmas, and my four-year-old son asks, 'Mommy, do you have to go to work today?' 'Yes, son,' I reply, 'I am a nurse.'

When I arrive at my assigned nursing unit, we have just enough nurses to care for our patients. But wait, all the other nursing units are short-staffed and have a high census; consequently, two people are pulled to cover other areas. Now everyone is equal and all units are short-staffed. 'Mommy, do you have to work hard?' 'Yes, son, I am a nurse.'

As my day begins, I organize my schedule so I can check my charts for doctor's orders and check all medications that are to be given. But wait, Patient A wants a bath, Patient B wants to be fed, Patient C wants something for pain, Patient D wants his insulin, Patient E is having angina and his condition has changed from stable to critical, and the emergency room is calling, asking for an empty bed. Patient F has terminal cancer and I have cared for her over a period of two years. We are very attached to each other. At this moment I feel a great loss—she died this morning. My mind wandered back to my conversation with my son earlier that morning. I kiss him goodbye as I do every morning. He asks me, 'Mommy, do you kiss your patients?' 'Yes,' I replied, 'sometimes I kiss my patients. I am a nurse.'

Figure 13–4. My name is Nurse. (Courtesy of Nursing in the Mass Media Collection, University of Michigan)

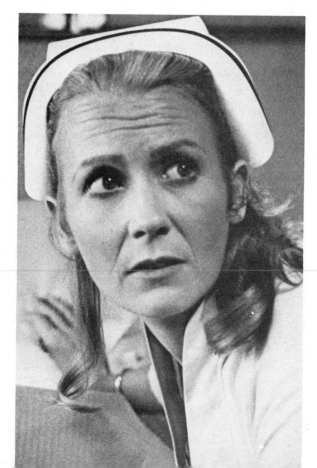

Sometimes I haven't time to go to the bathroom. As I rush home every day I almost beat the door down to get to the bathroom. My son asks, 'Mommy, don't they have bathroms at the hospital?' I smile because I work hard until it's time to go home, sometimes without a thought of emptying my bladder.

A doctor arrives and goes to the nursing office because your assigned area doesn't have any empty beds, you didn't get up to give him a chair, his chart wasn't on the rack, or you didn't see the doctor this morning to give him a report. My son asks, 'Mommy, do you like all the doctors?' 'Yes, son, I am a nurse.'

Tom Bacon, the associate director, North Carolina Area Health Education Center, stated recently that the average beginning nurse's salary is only $5.29 per hour and only averages $6.19 per hour after ten years' experience. It's Friday, payday. I smile as I look at my paycheck. The janitors at an area brewery company make $3 more an hour than I. My son asks, 'Mommy, do you like your job?' 'Of course I do, I am a nurse.'

I love taking care of patients, and nurses truly care about their patients. But wait, in case you haven't noticed, nurses are becoming an extinct profession. Who cares about the nurses?[2]

Certain ingredients are necessary for political mobilization to occur. The following classic explanation of why mid-19th century French peasants were unable to develop political mobilization sheds light on a number of the essential components for political mobilization of any group, including nurses:

The small peasants form a vast mass, the members of which live in similar conditions, but without entering into manifold relations with one another. Their mode of production isolates them from one another, instead of bringing them into mutual intercourse. The isolation is increased by France's bad means of communication and by the poverty of the peasants. Their field of production the small holding, admits of no division of labour in its cultivation, no application of science and, therefore, no multiplicity of development, no diversity of talents, no wealth of social relationships. Each individual peasant family is almost self-sufficient; it itself directly produces the major part of its consumption and thus acquires its means of life more through exchange with nature than in intercourse with society. The small holding, the peasant and his family; alongside them another small holding, another peasant and another family . . . In this way, the great mass of the French nation is formed by simple addition of homologous magnitudes, much as potatoes in a sack form a sackful of potatoes. In so far as millions of families live under conditions of existence that divide their mode of life, their interests and their culture from those of the other classes, and put them in hostile contrast to the latter, they form a class. In so far as there is merely a local interconnection among these small peasants, and the identity of their interests begets no unity, no national union and no political organization, they do not form a class. They are consequently incapable of enforcing their class interest in their own name, whether through a parliament or through a convention. They cannot represent themselves, they must be represented.[3]

The *missing* ingredients in this group were a sense of discontent and dissatisfaction, a group consciousness, a means of communication, and a feeling of self-determination.

Political mobilization occurs as a result of dissatisfaction. If everyone in a group is satisfied and the needs of all individuals are met, there will be no need for political mobilization. Gamson noted that "discontent is important because it is related to the organization and mobilization of 'have-not' groups and to their ability to produce different outcomes in the arena of

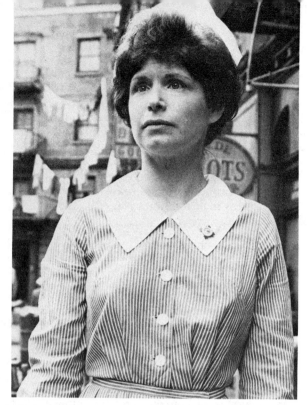

Figure 13–5. Dissatisfaction with the lack of birth control information for the poor inspired nurse Margaret Sanger to rebel against the conventions of society and, over bitter opposition, to found the birth control movement. Bonnie Franklin portrayed this heroine in the 1980 movie, Portrait of a Rebel. (*Courtesy of Nursing in the Mass Media Collection, University of Michigan*)

conflict."[4] According to this explanation, a group reaches a level of discontent with the current status, which propels them into action to produce a new status quo. Smelser referred to this phenomenon as "strain." He says, "People under strain mobilize to reconstitute the social order in the name of a generalized belief."[5] There must be conditions of dissatisfaction to impel a group to strike out against immediate tradition, taking the risks that always go with such activity. There is typically a negative reaction to deprived groups getting involved in a political movement.

Political mobilization both results from change and leads to change. Coser sees change as resulting from the strains that arise in competition for scarce resources. There is a constant tension between those with a vested interest in the maintenance of the status quo (the contented or the "haves") and those who seek to increase their share of resources (the discontented and the "have-nots"). However, this strain does not necessarily result in conflict:

> If certain groups within a social system compare their share in power, wealth, and status with that of other groups *and* question the legitimacy of this distribution, discontent is likely to ensue. If there exists no institutionalized provisions for the expression of such discontents, departures from what is required by the norms of the social system may occur. These may be limited to 'innovation' or they may consist in the rejection of the institutionalized goals.[6]

Thus, conflict theorists locate the source of strain, conflict, and change in the differential distribution of power—whether it be economic, political, or status power or simply the power to define and implement values. Conflict, between those who control the access to the scarce and valued resources of a society or of systems within society and those who are in pursuit of a larger share of the resources, is the basic (if not the only) process through which *significant* changes take place. An example of documentation of the pronounced increase in such discontent, strain, and conflict among nurses is offered in a June 29, 1980, report in the Riverside, California, *Press-Enterprise:*

> The white shoes that softly tread hospital corridors have been tramping picket lines lately. Hands that give injections have been signing refusals to assist in abortions. People who once sat in classes on medication have been taking assertiveness training. As society has changed, so has the nurse. When Charlotte Chapin was in nursing school 20 years ago, she was taught to follow orders. 'Now we are educating people to know what is right, what is wrong, how improvements can be made,' said Chapin, who is director of the nursing program at Mount San Jacinto Community College.
>
> 'We used to have a tradition of standing up when a physician came into the room,' said Joan Crowley, associate director of nursing at Riverside General Hospital. 'Anymore, it's more of a team approach, not like Asiatic countries where women followed several steps behind.' Nurses today have more responsibility, more education, a more equal relationship with doctors than nurses 15 or 20 years ago. They also have more pressure placed on them and more decisions to make. In the past few months nurses have made decisions resulting in:
>
> • More than 500 area registered nurses going out on strike over mainly salary and pension benefits against Kaiser Permanente medical facilities. It was the second strike in four years at Kaiser facilities serving Riverside County.
>
> • One-third of the nursing staff at Indio Community Hospital refusing to participate in saline abortions after two such late-term abortions resulted in live births.
>
> • Sixty-five registered nurses and their supporters carrying signs and distributing leaflets to publicize a labor dispute on salary increases with Hemet Valley Hospital.
>
> Nurses link the increased activism in their profession to a number of things. The women's movement and the increase in nurses who have bachelor's and graduate degrees have paved the way for more activism. Nursing schools teach nurses to speak up if they don't understand why certain medication or treatments are being given, to ask questions if they disagree with what the doctor is doing. Legalized abortions, medical advances in sustaining life, and such specialized units as intensive and coronary care have created pressures and ethical questions that nurses have had to deal with. While there is still a great deal of fear among nurses when it comes to activism, according to Kathy Robinson, outgoing executive director of the California Nurses' Association, Inland Empire Region, that is changing. 'Women know their own worth more than they did 25 years ago,' she said, and about 98 percent of all nurses are women.[7]

A precurser to political mobilization is the development of what has been termed *group consciousness.* In other words, the individual members of a group must perceive themselves to have common problems and common interests. They must develop a shared sense of deprivation and discrimination. They must develop a sense of group belongingness—the in-

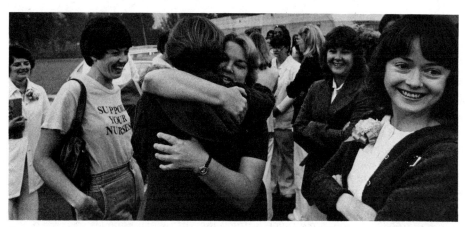

Figure 13–6. In order for nurses to become effectively mobilized, they must develop strong group alliances: Springfield, Oregon nurses celebrate victory. (Courtesy of Eugene Register Guard, Eugene, Oregon)

group versus the out-group—which serves to mobilize members of the group, particularly resource-poor or deprived groups, to participate in political matters in an effort to improve the status of their group. Group consciousness requires an awareness of political issues, but mostly in relation to specific areas of the groups' interests. Studies have shown that group identification is strongly associated with political participation among blacks, women, and other groups.[8]

In order for nurses to become fully mobilized, they must develop an identification with and allegiance to other nurses; they have to see their problems as similar to those of all nurses, and realize that improvements occur only as they work collectively. For these things to happen, *nurses must recognize their current powerless state and envision a new identity for the future.* They also must come to realize that their lack of power is affecting, in a detrimental way, the quality of patient care they are providing and the satisfaction they are deriving from practicing as a professional nurse.

As group consciousness develops, nurses will no longer blame themselves individually, referring to their own shortcomings for the current inadequacies in health care, but instead will view such problems as the result of an inappropriate distribution of scarce resources. Then nurses will recognize that they are discriminated against in the overall health care system and recognize that their concerns are not being taken into account in the process of developing health policy and in making decisions for the distribution of resources. Nurse mobilization will take place once nurses realize that their interests are not well represented in local, state, or federal government. A reporter for the Denver *Post* wondered, "Where Will Nurses' Militancy Lead?":

> There is little question that there has been increasing militancy among nurses in the Denver area and nationwide during the last year. What is going to happen next, though, appears to be a wide-open question. On one hand, nurses active in

trying to secure collective-bargaining rights maintain they would win a representation election today easily because of callous and indifferent treatment of them by their employers. But hospital administrators say they are doing all they can for the nurses and that claims of a clamoring for unionization are exaggerated.

But this much is obvious: The passive acceptance of things as they are, if there ever was such an attitude, is something past. Evidence isn't hard to come by:

- Last April, about 1,000 nurses marched on the Colorado Capitol to protest a bill they feared would have reduced their ability to operate as health professionals.
- On Aug. 10, more than half the nursing staff at Fort Morgan Community Hospital stayed home from work to protest the staffing situation and scheduling.
- On Aug. 31 about 100 nurses at Mercy Hospital marched to protest the firing of a male nurse they alleged was fired for unionization activity.
- On June 26, 718 nurses citywide withheld services over a variety of grievances.
- Earlier this month, nurses picketed St. Anthony Hospital Central, saying they were unhappy about a new scheduling policy. How many nurses were involved is an open question—the hospital administration said about 25 persons took part and claimed some of those weren't on the staff. Picket organizers say the number is more like 150, almost all of them from St. Anthony's.
- Union representation petitions have been filed at five Denver-area hospitals—St. Anthony, Beth Israel, Rose, Rocky Mountain Osteopathic and St. Luke's—and, if elections are called, that should settle the issue of whether the nurses want to believe they need a bargaining agent.[9]

One of the most notable examples of the successful development of a group consciousness is among black Americans. The civil rights movement increased cohesion, pride, communication, and shared symbols among blacks. They became a solidified group. Although the incidence of grievance-producing events against blacks did not substantially change, those events that did occur became more visible to them and created a more intense collective reaction, because group cohesion had increased the shared concerns of group members for each other.

The process of developing group consciousness starts with nurses experiencing empathy with other nurses who share the same ideas they do. If they spend time together, if they *communicate* with one another, their ideas crystallize. As was true with the French peasants, members of any group need a way to communicate with one another, through meetings, through the mass media, and through publications. Communication is essential if the process of sharing common problems and common concerns is to take place among a large enough group of nurses. Collective action simply won't occur if communication is stifled or blocked.

Out of the communication of shared concerns and common problems, a group must develop the *belief that they have the ability to change* the status quo. Feelings of dissatisfaction exist in almost every nurse, but this is not enough. These frustrations will yield political mobilization to correct the situation only if nurses see that these problems are a result of discrimination, not a reflection of personal failures. David Riesman has pointed out that "power, indeed, is founded, in large measure, on interpersonal expectations and attitudes."[10] If nurses feel weak and dependent, they will act as if they are weak and in actuality will become weaker and more dependent, no matter what capabilities they realistically have at their disposal. This has

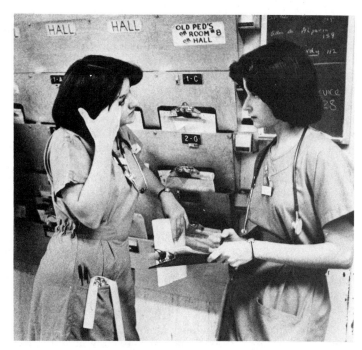

Figure 13-7. The opportunity to communicate together is essential for the development of a group consciousness. (Courtesy of Cleveland Plain Dealer, Cleveland, Ohio)

been referred to as a *self-fulfilling prophecy*. Belief in one's own ability to influence the environment leads to success in doing so and thus to a higher degree of self-confidence, and so the cycle continues.

Looking back for a moment at the plight of the French peasants, one can easily see why political mobilization failed to occur. The heavy demands of arduous work placed on them served to occupy them to such an extent that they lacked sufficient time to contemplate their lot in life. Feeling frustrated perhaps as individuals, but having no opportunity to communicate with other people in their same predicament, they developed no group consciousness. Consequently, instead of developing a sense of self-determination they viewed political matters as tangential, not central, to their existence. Feeling isolated physically as well as politically, they were incapable of determining their own destiny. Other people, outside themselves, did that for them.

INGREDIENTS FOR SUCCESS

Once a group has become mobilized, a number of important ingredients are needed for the movement to be successful: group solidarity, effective leadership, recruitment, commitment, adequate resources, a well-articulated ideology, and an ongoing sense of hope.

Group solidarity, or cohesion, is a key ingredient for an effective political movement. Successful movements focus on problems that unite the group, whereas unsuccessful movements characteristically belabor problems that divide the group. Unity is essential to both the initiation and maintenance of a collective identity and common commitment to goals. If a group achieves mobilization, it gains a collective identity, and the interests of one become the interests of all involved. The necessity for cohesion is nowhere better stated than in oft-quoted words of Benjamin Franklin: "If we don't hang together, we'll all hang separately." Groups usually start out unified, but as time passes, differences tend to crop up, and individuals or subgroups begin to work at cross purposes. More than one group has had its efforts prematurely aborted because of internal bickering and jealousies. Of course, disunity prevents mobilization. Solidarity is enhanced by the existence of what has been called *primary similitudes.* The more interests nurses have in common, the more likely they are to be unified. Unity is also fostered through the use of identifying symbols, such as buttons, bumper stickers, some aspect of dress, and through the process of sticking up for each other in public. During a labor dispute at Hurley Medical Center in Flint, Michigan, the city newspaper carried an editorial highly critical of the nurses' position. One of the nurses responded with vigor in a letter to the editor entitled, "Would You Work for R.N.'s Wages?":

> If the Hurley nurses belonged to the UAW would 'The Hurley Issue' editorial have been written? I don't remember reading anything like it when the autoworkers negotiated last year. A person with even less than a high school education can work in the shops for more than $9 per hour. An RN starting at Hurley gets $6.72 per hour with less benefits than the shop. Nurses don't get double time on Saturday, and there is no COLA [cost of living adjustment] and no 'short work week.' Shouldn't education be rewarded with decent pay?
>
> You mentioned 'skyhigh hospital costs.' How about car prices? A person will pay $8,000 for a car that falls apart before it's paid for but complains bitterly about an $8,000 trip to the hospital that could save or prolong his life. When I started working at Hurley nine years ago, our wages were comparable to the shops. Now the difference between the two has widened drastically. Maybe if Hurley improves wages for its nurses other hospitals will follow. Do you really think that people in Genesee County have to belong to the UAW to receive decent wages?
>
> When wages increase prices increase. Since prices in Genesee County are geared to GM wages, the rest of us have to struggle to keep up. It was not fair for you to write an editorial that was geared to turn the public against the nurses. It is not fair for administration to refuse to give those nurses a wage they can live on. A nurses's standard of living should not have to be lower than a factory worker's.
>
> Dorothy Perry Byron[11]

A large group, in particular, will of necessity include persons with different interests. Practically no segment of the group will agree with all the policies and courses of action taken. But if the group is successful, it will allow all the members to find enough that they can agree with to stay working together. In other words, unity without uniformity occurs.

Another important ingredient for group success is *leadership,* which is an essential element affecting the strength of the group. To advance its claim effectively, a group requires effective spokespersons, able to understand the aspirations of their followers, to inspire them to a fuller devotion to

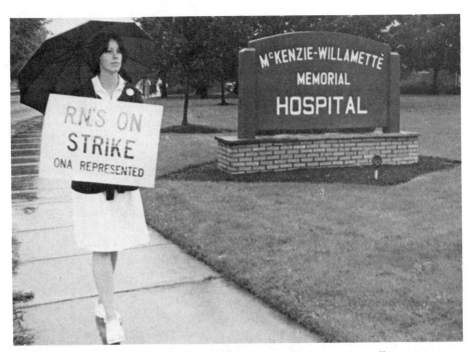

Figure 13-8. Some people who stand to gain from collective action will not participate themselves because they know others will carry forth the cause. (Courtesy of Northwestern, Oshkosh, Wisconsin)

a cause, and to win the sympathy and support of people outside the group. Effective leaders have skill in handling groups; charisma is often called for. For example, the outstanding speech given by Senator Edward Kennedy at the 1980 Democratic convention showed charismatic skill. Although not the party's nominee, he emerged as the spiritual leader of the group. A critical mass of power must be concentrated in the leadership of a group if a group is to be successful. If power is too diffuse, mobilization will not occur. A major task for the leadership is to overcome what Olson has referred to as the natural inclination for many people not to participate in action themselves because they think other persons will carry forth the cause.[12] Verba and his associates have noted the importance of both group consciousness and leadership in the mobilization of ascriptively deprived groups:

> If a group . . . has some basis for the development of internal leadership and self-consciousness, it is likely to engage in cooperative activity. . . . If a group [on the other hand] . . . lacks the capability for internal leadership and self-consciousness, it will be generally inactive, and this will be particularly the case in relation to cooperative activity.[13]

One example of how leadership can affect the success of a group centers on assignment of responsibilities. If the leadership of a political movement, for example, tends to favor certain people with the exciting aspects of the cause (*i.e.*, testifying before Congress, appearing on television) and leaves to others the hard but nonglamorous work, this could lead to a disintegration of the movement. If, on the other hand, the distribution of the privileges is made on the basis of those who have worked their way up by "paying their dues," so to speak, more satisfaction and motivation to participate in the group is likely to result.

Gerlach and Hine have referred to the fact that successful movements have tended to be *polycephalous,* or many-headed. In other words, a number of people assume leadership roles for different aspects of the movement. Gerlach and Hine explain:

> Leadership is charismatic rather than bureaucratic in nature. The personal commitment characteristic of movement participants results in a communicable charisma, so that effective leadership is not irrevocably tied to certain individuals. Segmentation and proliferation of groups . . . [on the other hand] occurs because of an ideology of personal access to power . . . because of personal competition . . .[14]

All political movements begin with a few people, but for success they need to enlarge their numbers vastly through some form of *recruitment.* Four responses to new members have been identified: exclusive, receptive, proselytizing, and coercive. The exclusive approach restricts acceptance of new members, as many more people want to belong than are allowed to do so. The receptive response allows persons to join but does not solicit members as the proselytizing initiative does. Coercion forces membership on persons typically for the purpose of achieving the appearance of a unified front. Gerlach and Hine emphasize the crucial role of face-to-face recruitment for success: "No matter what conditions of social disorganization or social or psychological deprivation facilitate the rise of a movement, the key to its spread is to be found in the process of face-to-face recruitment by committed participants." They found that recruitment occurs where a network of social contacts was already in existence.[15]

No successful group effect can take place without deep personal *commitment* on the part of its members. Masses of apathetic and unmotivated nurses, for example, reduce the potential for political mobilization. Manifestations of commitment have been identified as "a certain intensity, a drive, a single-minded awareness of long-range goals"; "a capacity for risk-taking" to allow the individual to withstand retribution; "a personal charisma" that permits a person to influence others; and a "personal behavioral transformation" in favor of the accepted patterns of the group.[16]

There must also be adequate *resources* for effective political mobilization. Political resources are those means by which groups are able to gain access to and influence decisions in favor of their wants. This means that the group must not only possess resources, but must be willing to channel them into political activity rather than into some other pursuit. In our society, these resources are unevenly distributed among the population, and this uneven distribution means that some groups have more than others. The power of a group can be measured in terms of the costs of exercising its influence. These costs range from the consumption of effort and time in exercising influence to the costs of the opposition aroused in other groups. Each group possesses only limited resources to gain the maximum returns

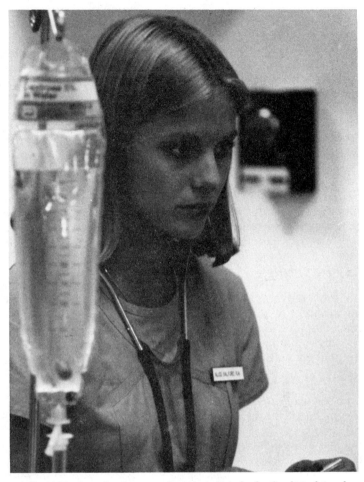

Figure 13–9. Nurses in the 1980s have begun to realize that their lack of political involvement is detrimentally affecting the quality of patient care they are providing. (Courtesy of Nursing in the Mass Media Collection, University of Michigan)

and influence. Policies which already have general support from most members of society may require little expenditure of a group's resources to get them enacted into law. Policies that meet with a great deal of resistance involve the expenditure of much time and effort in mobilizing support and overpowering the opposition. Such policies may also be very costly if the price of support is the granting of a major concession in some other issue area. Some fights are simply not worth the price.

The adequacy of resources also determines the extent to which a group can realistically address the variety of relevant issues with which they are confronted. Although many issues that develop may relate to an individual group's purpose, some cannot be considered because an effort in these directions would require resources beyond the current capabilities of the organization. Every group has an ongoing allocation of resources for particular issues, and the choice of any new issues must be made with existing commitments in mind. The number of issues on which groups would like to work is always far in excess of the number which they are actually able to address effectively. A group may lose its constituency if it spends its resources inefficiently, causing waste and producing less of an effect on a problem than it might otherwise have had. The skill with which resources are managed is crucial to success. A "power-rich" group may squander its "wealth," whereas one with significantly fewer resources may skillfully manipulate them for maximum advantage, and thus grow in power over time.

Group resources fall into several categories: *physical resources,* particularly money and membership size; *organization resources,* including membership skills and leadership skills; *political expertise,* such as campaign expertise, political process knowledge, political strategy expertise, political reputations; *motivational resources,* such as ideologic commitments; and *intangibles,* such as overall prestige or status. Each group has its own peculiar mix of resources, depending on its membership base and its primary goal. The combination of a group's goals, focus of activity, motivation, mix of resources, and skill at using them—along with the nature of the government institutions and the motivations and viewpoints of the government decision makers—determines the political influence of the group.

A common error in assessing the strength of a group is to rely solely on numbers of members. No doubt size of membership does have a bearing on the strength of an organized interest, for numbers are the raw material of any organization. In a democracy, where votes are important, a show of numbers can impress elected officials and office seekers. But numbers alone are not a sufficient base of power in American politics. The American Medical Association, for example, is not as large as many other interest groups, but it is an association of generally respected professionals of high socioeconomic status, who wield considerable influence in American politics. This is partly because physicians possess and wisely use money as a political resource, as noted earlier, and partly because as a higher socioeconomic group, they are more likely to vote and more able to influence others in their voting.

Numbers of persons become an important resource for groups only if they are well organized. *Organization* provides planning, direction, training, and coordination. It also relates activities to goals and provides a program of action, without which the views of the members of the group would not be effectively presented. Consumer interests are regularly defeated in legislative struggles against producers and manufacturers because the consumers are unorganized. A group which has shown that it has the full support of its membership, that it can deliver the votes of its members, and that its members are not divided over policy, will have much more influence with lawmakers than a group without such internal cohesion. The organization can endorse candidates and work for the election of those candidates who are supportive by getting its members to vote as a bloc, that is, to vote their special interest.

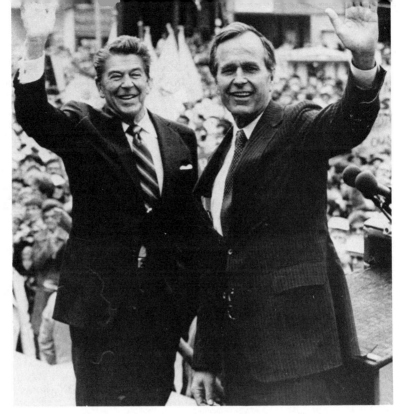

Figure 13–10. Ronald Reagan fashioned his landslide presidential victory of 1980 by stressing a more conservative ideology and hope to a nation beset with economic problems. (Courtesy of New York Times, New York)

Finally, one must emphasize the important role of *ideology* and *hope* in attaining group success. Most people will sacrifice very little—even organizational dues—on behalf of a common cause unless it can be justified by some idea or doctrine. Ideologies are used in groups to convince people to share their beliefs and their stand on issues. They offer a rationale for the groups' action. An *ideology* is "a conceptual framework by which all experiences and events . . . may be interpreted."[17] Ideology is said to be "split-level" in nature: "On one level . . . are those few basic concepts in which all participants find agreement. Other levels involve those infinite variations on the ideologic themes that promote both ideologic and organizational diversity."[18] Similarly hope is required for effective group progress. An air of hopelessness can blight the prospects of any group effort.

In evaluating the results of the mobilization of various racial minorities, one author offered a number of findings that may have more general applicability to groups such as nurses. Success is more likely for groups who achieve conditions in which:

- Their demands can be seen as consistent with the broader values of the society.
- They can gain the support of more powerful third parties and/or show how their demands will benefit other groups as well.
- Their demands are concrete and focused.

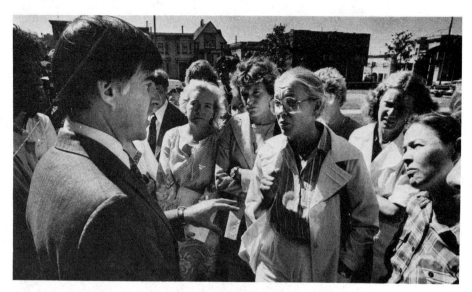

Figure 13–11. Successful efforts at group mobilization must precisely focus responsibility for inequities on those who are accountable: San Francisco nurses protest substandard working conditions to Governor Jerry Brown. (Courtesy of San Francisco Chronicle, San Francisco, California)

- They can clearly fix responsibility for the situation they are protesting.
- Pressure is brought to bear on the responsible party, and there is minimum discomfort to those not responsible.
- They adopt new techniques which authorities have not had experience in dealing with.
- Neutral third parties are present who have an interest in restoring harmony.
- The powerless group is willing to negotiate, and its demands do not have a zero-sum quality.
- Their demands involve a request for acceptance of social diversity, equal treatment, or inclusion, rather than domination over, or change in the practices of, the dominant group towards itself, or fundamental redistributions of income and power.
- The powerless group seeks to veto a proposed policy rather than to see a new policy implemented.
- The minority population is large enough to organize itself for conflict but not large enough to be perceived as a serious threat to the dominant group.[19]

A small cadre of nurses have already ventured out into the political world, have successfully engaged in the higher forms of political activity, and have assumed leadership positions in federal, state, and local government. Their successes provide role models of what every nurse can aspire to be or assist one of her colleagues to become. Although it has often been assumed that nursing is not closely related to politics, those closest to both worlds feel differently. They see strong similarities between nursing and

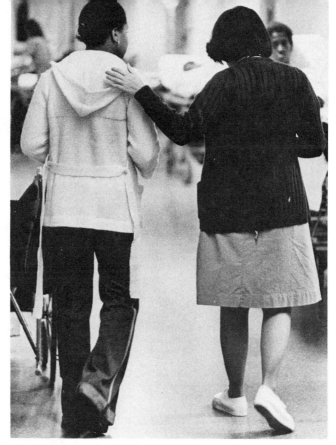

Figure 13–12. Quality patient care and effective political leadership share a concern for people and their problems. (Courtesy Cleveland Plain Dealer, Cleveland, Ohio)

politics and consistently note that certain skills and competencies learned as part of the educational process of becoming a nurse are helpful in politics. Jean Moorhead, nurse and California assemblywoman, says, "Nursing is the best education for becoming an effective politician. I feel I am still doing public health nursing."[20] Similarly Maureen Maigret, a member of the Rhode Island House, states, "Nurses are more qualified for politics than they realize. Our education has given us insight into the human relations part of politics. We're used to tuning into the psychosocial aspects of issues. No matter where we practice in public health, the hospital, schools, we are very aware of people problems at a personal level."[2] According to Mary Cotton, "Government needs nurses, nurses have compassion, and government needs compassion. Politics involves the utilization of nursing skills in a very different way."[22] Marilyn Goldwater similarly notes that "nursing and politics share a common focus—a concern for people and a desire to help people." And Sandra Smoley points out, "Nurses have the characteristics it takes to be good politicians—intelligence, concern for people, and accessibility."

Nurses who enter the political arena, unlike their politician colleagues who are physicians, dentists, or social workers, find that their fellow nurses believe they have left nursing. One nurse in politics explained that she was told, "You are really not a nurse. You haven't practiced nursing recently." Another said, "I heard that a nurse of some prominence was saying 'the nerve of her putting R.N. after her name.' Why do I have to prove myself to my own fellow professionals?" Another nurse noted that it bothers her a great deal when people say, "You *used* to be a nurse." To this she replies: "I *am* a nurse."

References

1. Edwards LP: The Natural History of Revolution, p 36. Chicago, University of Chicago Press, 1927
2. Letter to the Editor. High Point, NC, High Point Enterprise, June 27, 1980
3. Marx K: The Eighteenth Brumaire of Louis Bonaparte, p 109. New York, International, n.d.
4. Gamson A: Power and Discontent, p 8. Homewood, Ill, Dorsey Press, 1968
5. Smelser NJ: Theory of Collective Behavior, p 385. New York, Free Press, 1963
6. Coser LA: Continuities in the Study of Social Conflict, p 31. New York, Free Press, 1967
7. Aleshire I: Nurses increasingly vocal over ethical, economic issues. Riverside, Calif, Press-Enterprise, June 29, 1980
8. Miller AH, Gurin P, Gurin G: Electoral implications of group identification and consciousness: The reintroduction of a concept. Presented at the annual meeting of the American Political Science Association, New York, New York, 1978
9. McGraw P: Where will nurses' militancy lead? Denver, Colo, The Denver Post, Nov 25, 1979
10. Riesman D: The Lonely Crowd, p 37. New Haven, Yale University Press, 1951
11. Would you work for R.N.'s wages? Flint, Mich, The Flint Journal, Apr 7, 1980
12. Olson M, Jr: The Logic of Collective Action. Cambridge, Harvard University Press, 1965
13. Verba S, Ahmed B, Bhatt A: Caste, Race, and Politics, p 36. Beverly Hills, Sage, 1971
14. Gerlach LP, Hine V: People, Power, Change: Movements of Social Transformation, p 78. Indianapolis, Bobbs-Merrill, 1970
15. Ibid, p 97
16. Ibid, pp 102–106
17. Ibid, p xvii
18. Ibid, p 165
19. Marx GT (ed): Racial Conflict. Boston, Little, Brown, 1971
20. Interview with Jean Moorhead, Aug 22, 1980
21. Interview with Maureen Maigret, Aug 21, 1980
22. Interview with Mary Cotton, Aug 12, 1980

Appendix
Selected Federal Health Acts, 1935–1980

Year	Public Law	Act	Purpose
1935	74–241	Social Security Act	Provided for the first time grants-in-aid to states for such public health activities as maternal and child care, aid to crippled children, blind persons, the aged, and other health-impaired persons.
1936	74–846	Walsh–Healy Act	Authorized federal regulation of industrial safety in companies doing business with the government.
1937	75–244	National Cancer Institute Act	Established National Cancer Institute to coordinate research related to cancer.
1938	75–540	LaFollette–Bulwinkle (VD Control) Act	Provided grants-in-aid to states and other authorities to investigate and control venereal disease.
1938	75–717	Federal Food, Drug, and Cosmetic (FDC) Act	Extended federal authority to act against adulterated and misbranded food, drug, and cosmetic products.
1939	76–19	Reorganization Act of 1939	Transferred the Public Health Service (PHS) from the Treasury Department to a new Federal Security Agency.
1941	77–146	Nurse Training Appropriations	Assisted schools of nursing in increasing their enrollments and improving their programs.
1941	77–366	Insulin Certification Amendment to FDC Act	Required premarketing batch certification of insulin drugs.
1943	78–38	Act to Provide for the Appointment of Female Physicians and Surgeons in the Army	Gave women and men equal rank, pay, allowances, and privileges in the Army Medical Corps.
1943	78–74	Nurse Training Act	Authorized the establishment of the U.S. Nurse Cadet Corps in the Public Health Service, which supported the training of 180,000 student nurses.

Year	Public Law	Act	Purpose
1944	78–410	Public Health Service Act	Consolidated all PHS authorities into a single statute (Title 42, U.S. Code).
1945	79–139	Antibiotic Certification Amendment	Required premarketing batch certification of penicillin (other antibiotics added in later amendments).
1946	79–293	Medical and Surgical Act	Established a Department of Medicine and Surgery in the Veterans Administration (VA); removed it from Civil Service control; authorized medical student residencies in VA hospitals.
1946	79–396	National School Lunch Act.	Authorized a national school lunch program.
1946	79–487	National Mental Health Act	Authorized major Federal support for mental health research, training, diagnosis, prevention, and treatment; changed the PHS Division of Mental Health to the National Institute of Mental Health; established state grants-in-aid for mental health.
1946	79–725	Hospital Survey and Construction Act	The Hill–Burton Act to support surveys, plans, and new facilities.
1947	80–36	Women's Medical Specialist Corps	Established a permanent Nursing Corps in the Army and Navy; permitted dieticians and physical therapists to join a Specialist Corps.
1947	80–104	Federal Insecticide, Fungicide, and Rodenticide Act	Required all pesticides to be registered prior to sale and be properly labeled for use.
1948	80–655	National Heart Act	Authorized aid for research, training, and other programs related to heart disease; established the National Heart Institute; acknowledged a plural National Institutes of Health (NIH).
1948	80–755	National Dental Research Act	Authorized aid for research on dental diseases and conditions; established a National Institute of Dental Research at NIH.
1948	80–845	Water Pollution Control Act	Authorized the PHS to help states develop water pollution control programs and to aid in the planning of sewage treatment plants.

Year	Public Law	Act	Purpose
1949	61–380	Hospital Survey and Construction Amendments	Increased federal financial assistance to promote effective development and utilization of hospital services and facilities.
1949	81–439	Agriculture Act of 1949	Authorized donations of commodities acquired under price-support programs for school lunch and for feeding the needy.
1950	81–507	Act to Establish a National Science Foundation	Set up an autonomous National Science Foundation (NSF) and strengthened the concept of federal support for university-based research in physical, medical, and social sciences.
1950	81–692	National Research Institutes Act	Expanded the National Institutes of Health to include research and training related to arthritis, rheumatism, multiple sclerosis, cerebral palsy, epilepsy, polio, blindness, leprosy, and other diseases.
1951	82–215	Durham–Humphrey Amendments	Established a category of prescription drugs, requiring labeling and medical supervision, as separate from nonprescription drugs.
1954	83–482	Medical Facilities Survey and Construction Act	Extended aid to chronic hospitals, rehabilitation facilities, and nursing homes.
1954	83–566	Act to Transfer Indian Health Responsibility to the Public Health Service	Placed the responsibility for maintenance and operation of Indian health facilities in the PHS rather than the Bureau of Indian Affairs.
1954	84–159	Air Pollution Control Act	Provided aid to states, regions, and localities for research and control programs to protect air quality.
1955	84–182	Mental Health Study Act	Authorized grants to nongovernmental organizations for partial support of a national study and reevaluation of the human and economic problems of mental illness.
1955	84–377	Polio Vaccination Assistance Act	Provided assistance to state vaccination programs.

Year	Public Law	Act	Purpose
1956	84–569	Dependents Medical Care Act	Set up a program of primarily inpatient medical care for dependents of military personnel (CHAMPUS).
1956	84–652	National Health Survey Act	Provided for a continuing survey and special studies of sickness and disability in the U.S.
1956	84–660	Water Pollution Control Act	Established water pollution control programs on interstate waterways; expanded research and aid to states for sewage treatment.
1956	84–835	Health Research Facilities Act	Aided construction of research facilities.
1956	84–911	Health Amendments	Established traineeships for graduate education for nurses.
1956	84–941	National Library of Medicine Act	Transferred responsibility for the library to the Public Health Service.
1957	84–151	Indian Health Assistance Act	Provided for the construction of health facilities for Indians and others.
1957	85–172	Poultry Products Inspection Act	First federal effort at mandatory inspection of poultry products (similar to efforts in meat inspection).
1958	85–340	Social Security Amendments	Provided states with minimum maternal and child health grants and extended authority to Guam.
1958	85–929	Food Additive Amendments to the FDC Act	Required premarketing clearance for new food additives; established a GRAS (generally recognized as safe) category; prohibited the approval of any additive "found to induce cancer in man or animal" (the so-called "Delaney clause").
1959	86–382	Federal Employees Health Benefits Act	Authorized a program of prepaid health insurance for employees of the federal, executive, and legislative branches of the government.
1960	86–610	International Health Research Act	Provided for international cooperation in research, research training, and planning.
1960	86–788	Social Security Amendments	Authorized grants to states for medical assistance for the aged.
1961	87–395	Community Health Services and Facilities Act	To improve community facilities and services for the aged and others.

Year	Public Law	Act	Purpose
1962	87–692	Assistance to Migratory Workers Act	Authorized federal aid for clinics serving migratory agricultural workers and families.
1962	87–781	Kefauver–Harris Drug Amendments	Required improved manufacturing practices, better reporting, the assurance of efficacy as well as safety, and strengthened regulation in the drug industry.
1962	87–838	National Institutes of Child Health and Human Development and General Medical Sciences	Established an institute to coordinate and expand research into childhood diseases and human growth and a second institute of general medical sciences to coordinate interinstitute research and handle "all other" diseases.
1962	87–868	Vaccination Assistance Act	Aided programs that attacked whooping cough, polio, diphtheria, and tetanus.
1963	88–129	Health Professions Educational Assistance Act	Aided training of physicians, dentists, public health personnel, and others; provided construction grants for schools of nursing.
1963	88–156	Maternal and Child Health and Mental Retardation Planning Amendments	Initiated program of comprehensive maternity and infant care and mental retardation prevention.
1963	88–164	Mental Retardation Facilities and Community Mental Health Centers Construction Act	Provided aid for the construction of these facilities and centers; became the basic law for mental health centers' staffing, programming, and so forth.
1963	88–206	Clean Air Act	Authorized direct grants to state and local governments for air pollution control; established federal enforcement in interstate air pollution; directed major research efforts into motor vehicle exhaust, removal of sulfur from fuel, and the development of air quality criteria.
1964	88–352	Civil Rights Act	Title VI provided that "no person in the United States shall, on the ground of race, color or national origin, be excluded from participation in, be denied the benefits of, or be subjected

Year	Public Law	Act	Purpose
			to discrimination under any program or activity receiving Federal financial assistance."
1964	88–525	Food Stamp Act	Authorized a food stamp program for low-income persons to buy nutritious food for a balanced diet.
1964	88–581	Nurse Training Act	Launched a major federal effort for training additional professional nurses.
1965	89–74	Drug Abuse Control Amendments	Established enforcement procedures to control depressants, stimulants, and hallucinogens.
1965	89–92	Federal Cigarette Labeling and Advertising Act	Informed the public of the health hazards of cigarette smoking.
1965	89–97	Social Security Amendments	Established health insurance for the aged and grants to states for medical assistance programs (Medicare and Medicaid).
1965	89–239	Heart Disease, Cancer, and Stroke Amendments	Established regional medical programs for research training and sharing of new knowledge in heart disease, cancer, and stroke.
1965	89–272	Clean Air Act Amendments	Directed federal regulation of motor vehicle exhaust (Title I); established a program of federal research and grants-in-air solid waste disposal (Title II).
1965	89–290	Health Professions Educational Assistance Amendments	Aided schools of medicine, osteopathy, and dentistry; provided scholarships and loans; and aided construction of health education buildings.
1966	89–563	National Traffic and Motor Vehicle Safety Act	Provided for a coordinated national safety program and established safety standards for motor vehicles in interstate commerce.
1966	88–614	Amendments to CHAMPUS (Military Dependents Act)	Broadened eligibility to CHAMPUS and extended benefits beyond inpatient care.
1966	89–642	Child Nutrition Act	Established a federal program of research and support for child nutrition; authorized a school breakfast program.

Year	Public Law	Act	Purpose
1966	89–749	Comprehensive Health Planning and Public Health Services Amendments	Promoted health planning and improved public health services; authorized broad research, demonstration, and training programs in federal–state–local partnership.
1966	89–751	Allied Health Professions Personnel Act	Initial effort to support the training of allied health workers; also provided student loans for health professionals.
1966	89–753	Clean Water Restoration Act	Expanded, strengthened, and centralized water pollution programs in the Department of the Interior; new efforts in sewage treatment, purification, ecology, and so forth.
1966	89–785	VA Assistance Act	Permitted the VA to share, rather than replicate, specialized medical resources of other federal, state, and local agencies.
1967	80–148	Air Quality Act	Established a program of criteria and standard development and enforcement to control air pollution; set up air quality regions; overall strengthening of the federal role.
1967	90–174	Partnership for Health Amendments	Expanded health planning and services; broadened health services research and demonstrations; and improved clinical laboratories.
1967	90–201	Wholesome Meat Act	Amended, updated, and expanded Meat Inspection Act of 1907; brought all meat plants in intrastate as well as interstate commerce under control.
1967	90–222	Economic Opportunity Amendments	Authorized grants for Comprehensive Health Services and other health programs.
1967	9–0248	Social Security Amendments	Consolidated maternal and child health authorities; extended grants for family planning and dental health.
1968	90–407	Amendments to NSF Act of 1950	Expanded the authorities of the National Science Foundation to include major support of applied research in the sciences.
1968	90–411	Aircraft Noise Abatement Act	Amended Federal Aviation Act; first government effort to deal with health hazards of noise.

Year	Public Law	Act	Purpose
1968	90–456	Lister Hill National Center for Biomedical Communications Designation	Designated the title for a national center for biomedical communications within the National Library of Medicine, NIH.
1968	90–490	Health Manpower Act	Authorized formula institutional grants (capitation) for training nurses and other health professionals; added pharmacy and veterinary medicine.
1968	90–492	Wholesome Poultry Products Act	Amended, updated, and expanded the 1957 Poultry Act to make poultry inspection similar to the updated meat inspection program.
1969	90–574	Health Services Amendment	Extended grants for Regional Medical Programs (RMPs) and migrant health services; provided treatment facilities for alcoholics and narcotic addicts.
1968	90–602	Radiation Control for Health and Safety Act	Authorized the setting of safe performance standards for electronic products such as x-ray machines, television sets, and microwave ovens; established procedures for enforcement.
1969	91–173	Federal Coal Mine Health and Safety Act	Protected the health and safety of coal miners.
1969	91–190	National Environmental Policy Act	Stated the concern of Congress for preserving the environment and to "stimulate the health and welfare of man"; created the Council on Environmental Quality to advise the President; required environmental impact statements before major federal actions.
1970	91–211	Community Mental Health Centers Amendments	Extended grants for community mental health centers and facilities for alcoholics and narcotic addicts and established programs for children's mental health.
1970	91–222	Public Health Cigarette Smoking Act	Banned cigarette advertising from radio and television.
1970	91–512	Resource Recovery Act	Shifted the emphasis from solid waste disposal to overall problems of control, recovery, and recycling of wastes.

Year	Public Law	Act	Purpose
1970	91–513	Comprehensive Drug Abuse Prevention and Control Act	Increased aid for research; strengthened prevention, treatment, and rehabilitation programs.
1970	91–517	Developmental Disabilities Services and Facilities Construction Amendments	Assisted states to develop and implement plans for provision of comprehensive services to persons affected by mental retardation and other developmental disabilities.
1970	91–519	Health Training Improvement Act	Provided expanded aid to all allied health professions.
1970	91–572	Family Planning Services and Population Research Act	Expanded and coordinated services and research activities.
1970	91–596	Occupation Safety and Health Act	Provided federal program of standard setting and enforcement to assure safe and healthful conditions in the workplace.
1970	91–604	Clean Air Act Amendments	Strengthened and expanded air pollution control activities; placed broad regulatory responsibility in the new Environmental Protection Agency, which went into operation December 2, 1970.
1970	91–616	Comprehensive Alcohol Abuse and Alcoholism Prevention, Treatment, and Rehabilitation Act	Established the National Institute of Alcohol Abuse and Alcoholism; provided a comprehensive aid program to states and localities.
1970	91–623	Emergency Health Personnel Act	Provided assistance to health manpower shortage areas through a new National Health Service Corps.
1971	92–157	Comprehensive Health Manpower Training Act	Expanded and strengthened federal programs for the development of health manpower.
1971	92–158	Nurse Training Act	Expanded and strengthened federal efforts specifically directed toward nurse training.
1971	92–218	National Cancer Act	Expanded national effort against cancer.
1972	92–294	National Sickle Cell Anemia Control Act	Provided for control of and research into sickle cell anemia.
1972	92–303	Amendments to Federal Coal Mine Health and Safety Act	Provided benefits and other assistance for coal miners suffering from black lung diseases.

Year	Public Law	Act	Purpose
1972	92–414	National Cooley's Anemia Control Act	Provided assistance for programs of diagnosis, prevention, and treatment.
1972	92–423	National Heart, Blood Vessel, Lung, and Blood Act	Enlarged the National Heart and Lung Institute and authorized broad studies in blood management.
1972	92–426	Uniformed Services Health Professions Revitalization Act	Established a Uniformed Services University of the Health Sciences and an Armed Forces Health Professions Scholarship Program.
1972	92–433	National School Lunch and Child Nutrition Amendments	Added funds to support nutritious diets for pregnant and lactating women and for infants and children (the "WIC" program).
1972	92–500	Federal Water Pollution Control Amendments	Totally revised federal water program; shifted efforts from the preservation of available water quality to the improvement of quality through technology; set as a goal the elimination of pollutant discharges from all navigable waters.
1972	92–513	Motor Vehicle Information and Cost Savings Act	Established diagnostic and demonstration projects to reduce auto-related safety and health hazards.
1972	92–516	Federal Environmental Pesticide Control Act	Expanded and strengthened provisions on product registration, labeling, environmental protection, registration of manufacturers, and national monitoring of pesticide residues in water and food.
1972	92–541	VA Medical School Assistance and Health Manpower Training Act	Authorized the VA to help establish eight state medical schools and provide grant support to existing medical schools.
1972	92–573	Consumer Product Safety Act	Created the Consumer Product Safety Commission (CPSC); transferred enforcement of Hazardous Substances, Flammable Fabrics, and Poison Prevention Packaging Acts to CPSC; expanded and strengthened federal effort in safety and prevention.
1972	92–574	Noise Control Act	Authorized broad federal program to coordinate noise research and control activities, establish standards, and improve public information.

Year	Public Law	Act	Purpose
1972	92–603	Social Security Amendments	Extended health insurance benefits to the disabled and to end-stage renal disease patients, established a Professional Standard Review Organization program, and expanded research and demonstrations of financing mechanisms.
1972	93–154	Emergency Medical Services (EMS) Systems Act	Provided aid to states and localities to establish coordinated, cost-effective, areawide EMS systems.
1973	93–222	Health Maintenance Organization (HMO) Act	Assisted in the establishment and expansion of HMOs.
1974	93–247	Child Abuse Prevention and Treatment Act	Created a National Center on Child Abuse and Neglect; authorized research and demonstration grants to states and other public and private agencies.
1974	93–270	Sudden Infant Death Syndrome (SIDS) Act	Provided assistance for research, training, and extensive public education concerning SIDS.
1974	93–281	Narcotic Addict Treatment Act	Provided for registration of practitioners.
1974	93–296	Research on Aging Act	Established National Institute on Aging within the NIH.
1974	93–319	Energy Supply and Coordination Act	Directed the National Institute of Environmental Health Sciences to study the effects of chronic exposure to sulfur oxides.
1974	93–348	National Research Act	Established research-training awards and the National Commission for the Protection of Human Subjects.
1974	93–352	National Cancer Amendments	Improved the national cancer program and established a Biomedical Research Panel.
1974	93–353	Health Services Research, Health Statistics, and Medical Libraries Act	Revised and expanded health statistics and services research programs; established a national center for each one; expanded aid to nonfederal medical libraries.
1974	93–354	National Diabetes Mellitus Research and Education Act	Expanded diabetes research and public education programs.

Year	Public Law	Act	Purpose
1974	93–523	Safe Drinking Water Act	Required the Environmental Protection Agency (EPA) to set national drinking water standards and to aid states and localities in enforcement.
1974	93–640	National Arthritis Act	Established National Commission on Arthritis and coordinated arthritis programs in NIH.
1975	93–641	National Health Planning and Resource Development Act	Authorized major federal reorganization of health-planning programs, including Hill–Burton; set up national designation of local health systems areas and governing agencies.
1975	94–63	Health Revenue Sharing and Nurse Training Act	Established the National Center for Prevention and Control of Rape; revised and extended the National Health Service Corps, community mental health centers, migrant health, family planning, and other programs; continued the nurse-training program.
1975	94–103	Developmentally Disabled Assistance and Bill of Rights Act	Expanded the national effort and protected the rights of the developmentally disabled.
1976	94–278	Health Research and Health Services Amendments of 1976	Authorized a total of $752 million in fiscal 1976–77 for federal programs to combat heart, lung, and blood diseases. It provided an additional $90 million in fiscal 1976–78 for efforts to help parents who suspect they might carry genetic diseases.
1976	94–437	Indian Health Care Improvement Act of 1976	Created new scholarship programs for Indians seeking training in health care professions, upgraded health services available to Indians, and provided support for construction of health facilities and water and sewer systems serving Indians. The measure, which also was directed at Alaskan natives, set up special health programs for Indians in urban areas.
1976	94–484	Health Professions Educational Assistance Act of 1976	Continued basic federal support for medical, dental, and other health professions schools through fiscal 1980. For students, the bill offered a new federally guaranteed loan program as

Year	Public Law	Act	Purpose
			well as an expansion in scholarships requiring practice in doctor-shortage areas as a member of the National Health Service Corps. For fiscal 1978–80 the bill authorized a total of $2.3 billion.
1976	94–573	Emergency Medical Services Amendments of 1976	Authorized $215 million in fiscal 1977–79 to continue emergency medical services programs begun in 1973. The bill also authorized $22.5 million over the same period to fund a new burn injury treatment program.
1977	95–83	Health Services Extension Act of 1977	Authorized appropriations for fiscal year 1978 for grants to: (1) states for comprehensive public health services; (2) hypertension programs; (3) planning, development, and operation of community health centers; (4) training and research of family planning projects; (5) infant sudden death syndrome programs; (6) hemophilia programs; and (7) blood-separation centers. Directed the Secretary of Health, Education, and Welfare to take into account unusual local conditions that are a barrier to access to personal health services when defining a medically underserved population.
1977	95–95	Clean Air Act Amendments	Established more rigorous standards for industry in an attempt to secure cleaner air. Provided a civil penalty of up to $25,000 per day, in the case of an owner or operator of a major stationary source who violates an applicable implementation plan or standard of performance.
1977	95–142	Medicare–Medicaid Anti-Fraud and Abuse Amendments	Required more effective accounting procedures in the administration of the Medicare and Medicaid programs.
1977	95–210	Rural Health Clinics Act	Amended Title XIX (Medicaid) of the Social Security Act to include rural health clinic services by nurse practitioners within the definition of "medical assistance" eligible for payment under the Title; amended Title

Year	Public Law	Act	Purpose
			XVIII (Medicare) of the Social Security Act to provide payment for rural health clinic services under the supplementary medical insurance program; required a state plan for medical assistance and provided for payment for rural health clinic services. Provided for certification and approval of such clinics; required the Secretary of HEW to report to Congress on the advantages and disadvantages of extending coverage under the Medicare program to urban or rural mental health centers.
1978	95–622	Biomedical Research and Research Training Amendments of 1978	Authorized appropriations for fiscal years 1979, 1980, and 1981 for payments under national research service awards and grants for such awards. Amended the Public Health Service Act by adding a new Title XVIII, establishing the President's Commission for the Protection of Human Subjects of Biomedical and Behavioral Research, which issues a report every two years.
1978	95–623	Health Services Research, Health Statistics, and Health Care Technology Act of 1978	Amended the Public Health Service Act to extend authorizations of appropriations through fiscal year 1981 for health service research, evaluation, and demonstration activities, and health statistical activities.
1978	95–626	Health Services and Centers Amendments of 1978	Amended the Public Health Service Act to make eligible for services of migrant health centers individuals who have previously been employed as migratory or seasonal agricultural workers but who no longer meet the requirements for eligibility because of age or disability. Removed preventive dental services from the category of primary health services provided by migrant health centers and designated such services as supplemental health services Added pharmaceutical services to the category of primary health services provided by such centers. Removed public health services from the supplemental health services

Year	Public Law	Act	Purpose
			provided by such centers and added social services; redefined the term "high impact area" to reduce, from 6,000 to 4,000, the number of migratory and seasonal agricultural workers who must reside within a health service area for more than two months in any calendar year.
1979	96–76	Nurse Training Amendments of 1979	Amended Title VIII of the Public Health Service Act to extend, at a much reduced level of authorization, the assistance program for nurse training and students; established a new assistance program for training nurse anesthetists; directed the Secretary of Health, Education, and Welfare to arrange for the conduct of a study, either with the National Academy of Sciences (if such body agreed) or with another public or nonprofit private entity (if the Academy declined), to determine the need to continue a specific federal assistance program for nursing education, taking into account specified factors, and to report the results of such study to Congress.
1979	96–79	Health Planning and Resources Development Amendments of 1979	Modified the 1974 act in many respects. For example, added to the list of subjects deserving priority consideration in the formulation of national health planning goals: (1) the discontinuance of duplicative or unneeded services and facilities; (2) the adoption of policies to contain the rising costs of health care delivery; (3) the improvement of mental health care, including the elimination of inappropriate placement of persons with mental health problems in institutions and emphasizing outpatient mental health services by assuring access to community mental health centers; (4) the promotion of health services that recognize the psychological components of health maintenance; and (5) the development and use of cost-saving technology.

Year	Public Law	Act	Purpose
1979	96–180	Comprehensive Alcohol Abuse and Alcoholism Prevention, Treatment, and Rehabilitation Act Amendments of 1979	Amended the Comprehensive Alcohol Abuse and Alcoholism Prevention, Treatment, and Rehabilitation Act of 1970 to include as purposes of such Act the development of prevention programs and occupational prevention and treatment programs; required the Director of the National Institute on Alcohol Abuse and Alcoholism (NIAA) to develop programs and policies that focus on the needs of underserved populations.
1979	96–181	Drug Abuse Prevention, Treatment, and Rehabilitation Amendments of 1979	Amended the Drug Abuse Office and Treatment Act of 1972 to include as purposes of such Act the development of community-based prevention programs, occupational prevention and treatment programs, and research relating to drug abuse.
1980	96–398	Mental Health Systems Act of 1980	Gave states more authority in the review of Comprehensive Mental Health Center applications as part of an effort to accomplish both an expansion and coordination of services and long-term funding for centers that are independent of federal monies. Intended that states use their new authority to approve applications as part of a considered effort to plan, distribute, and make available as many high-quality services to as many people as possible.
1980	96–538	Health Programs Extension Act of 1980	Extended authorization for a large number of expiring health-care programs.

Bibliography

Abbot P, Riccards M: Reflections in American Political Thought: Readings From Past and Present. Novato, Calif, Chandler & Sharp, 1973

Abdellah FG, Levine E: Patients and Personnel Speak: A Method of Studying Patient Care in Hospitals. Washington, DC, United States Government Printing Office, 1954

Aberbach J: Power consciousness: A comparative analysis. Am Polit Sci Rev 71:1544–1560, 1977

Abraham A, Kopelman DL: Federal Social Security. Philadelphia, ALI-ABA, 1979

Abramowitz SF, Abramowitz CV, Jackson C, Gomes B: The politics of clinical judgment: What nonliberal examiners infer about women who do not stifle themselves. J Consult Clin Psychol 41:385–391, 1973

Abrams R: Foundations of Political Analysis: An Introduction to the Theory of Collective Choice. New York, Columbia University Press, 1980

Abramson J: The Invisible Woman: Discrimination in the Academic Profession. San Francisco, Jossey-Bass, 1975

Adamany DW, Agree GE (eds): Political Money: A Strategy for Campaign Financing in America. Baltimore, Johns Hopkins University Press, 1975

Aday L et al: Health Care in the United States: Equity for Whom? Beverly Hills, Sage, 1980

Adaly L: The impact of health policy on access to medical care: Health and society. Milbank Mem Fund Q 54:215–233, 1976

Agnello T: Aging and the sense of political powerlessness. Public Opinion Q 37:251–259, 1973

Agranoff R: The Management of Election Campaigns. Rockleigh, NJ, Holbrook Press, 1976

Agranoff R: The New Style in Election Campaigns. Rockleigh, NJ, Holbrook Press, 1976

Agronsky M et al: Let Us Begin: The First One Hundred Days of the Kennedy Administration. Austin, S & S Press, 1961

Aherne DD, Bliss B: The Economics of Being a Woman. New York, McGraw-Hill, 1977

Ahmed PI, Coelho GV (eds): Toward a New Definition of Health: Psychosocial Dimensions. New York, Plenum Press, 1979

Aiken M, Mott P (eds): The Structure of Community Power. New York, Random House, 1970

Aldrich JH: Before the Convention: A Theory of Presidential Nomination Campaigns. Chicago, University of Chicago Press, 1980

Aleshire I: Nurses increasingly vocal over ethical, economic issues. Riverside, Calif, Press-Enterprise, June 29, 1980

Alexander H: Financing the Nineteen Seventy-Six Election. Washington, DC, Congressional Quarterly, 1979

Alexander H: Financing politics. Washington, DC, Congressional Quarterly, 1980

Alexander HE: Campaign Money: Reform & Reality in the States. New York, Free Press, 1976

Alford RR: Health Care Politics: Ideological and Interest Group Barriers to Reform. Chicago, University of Chicago Press, 1975

Allensworth D: U.S. Government in Action: Essentials. Santa Monica, Goodyear, 1972

Almond GA, Flanigan S, Mundt R: Crisis, Choice, and Change: Historical Studies in Political Development. Boston, Little, Brown, 1973

Almond GA, Verba S: Civic Culture: Political Attitudes & Democracy in Five Nations. Princeton, Princeton University Press, 1963

Altman SH: Present and Future Supply of Registered Nurses. Washington, DC, United States Government Printing Office, 1972

American Academy of Nursing: Nursing's Influence on Health Policy for the Eighties. Kansas City, American Academy of Nursing, 1979

American Hospital Association: American Hospital Association Guide to the Health Care Field: Annual Edition. Chicago, American Hospital Association, 1980

American Hospital Association: Career Goals of Hospital School of Nursing Seniors: Report of a Survey, by Bloom BI (ed). Chicago, American Hospital Association, 1975

American Hospital Association: Hospitals: Journal of the American Hospital Association, Guide Issue, Part 2. Chicago, American Hospital Association, 1945–1975

American Hospital Association: Hospital Statistics, 1976 Edition: Data from the American Hospital Association 1975 Annual Survey. Chicago, American Hospital Association, 1976

American Medical Association, Committee on Nursing: Medicine and nursing in the 1970's: A position statement. JAMA 213:1881–1883, 1970

American Nurses' Association, Research and Statistics Department: RN's 1966: An Inventory of Registered Nurses. Prepared by Marshall ED and Moses EB. New York, American Nurses' Association, 1969

Amundsen K: A New Look at the Silenced Majority: Women and American Democracy. Englewood Cliffs, Prentice-Hall, 1977

Amundsen K: Silenced Majority: Women and American Democracy. Englewood Cliffs, Prentice-Hall, 1971

Anderson JB et al (eds): Congress & Conscience. New York, JB Lippincott, 1970

Anderson JE: Public Policy-Making. New York, Praeger, 1975

Anderson LF et al: Legislative Roll-Call Analysis. Evanston, Northwestern University Press, 1966

Anderson OW: Influence of social and economic research on public policy in the health field: A review. Milbank Mem Fund Q 44:11–51, Part 2, 1966

Anderson R et al (eds): Equity in Health Services: Empirical Analyses in Social Policy. Cambridge, Ballinger, 1975

Anderson PR: The Political Socialization of Black Americans: A Critical Evaluation of Research on Efficacy and Trust. New York, Free Press, 1977

Anderson R et al: Two Decades of Health Services: Social Survey Trends in Use and Expenditure. Cambridge, Ballinger, 1976

Anderson VF, Van Winkle RA: In the Arena: The Care & Feeding of American Politics. New York, Harper & Row, 1976

Andreopoulos S (ed): Primary Care: Where Medicine Fails. New York, John Wiley & Sons, 1974

Anspach RR: From stigma to identity politics: Political activism among the physically disabled and former mental patients. Soc Sci Med 13(A):765–773, 1979

Archibald KA: The Supply of Professional Nurses and Their Recruitment and Retention by Hospitals. New York, New York City Rand Institute, 1971

Ash R: Social Movements in America. Chicago, Markham, 1972

Asher HB: Presidential Elections and American Politics: Voters, Candidates, and Campaigns Since 1952. Homewood, Ill, Dow-Jones Irwin, 1980

Assembly of Behavioral and Social Sciences: Knowledge and Policy: The Uncertain Connection. Washington, DC, National Academy of Sciences, 1978

Austin CJ: The Politics of National Health Insurance: An Interdisciplinary Research Study. San Antonio, Trinity University Press, 1975

Bachrach P, Baratz M: Two faces of power. Am Polit Sci Rev 56:947–952, 1962

Bailey R: From professional monopoly to corporate oligopoly: The clinical laboratory industry in transition. Med Care 15:129–146, 1977

Bailey SK (ed): American Politics and Government: Essays in Essentials. New York, Basic Books, 1965

Bailey SK: Education Interest Groups in the Nation's Capital. Washington, DC, American Council on Education, 1975

Baker B, King LL: Wheeling & Dealing: Confessions of a Capitol Hill Operator. New York, WW Norton, 1980

Bakshian A, Jr: The Candidates Nineteen Eighty. New Rochelle, NY, Arlington House, 1980

Bandura A: Social Learning Theory. Englewood Cliffs, Prentice-Hall, 1977

Banfield EC: Political Influence. New York, Free Press, 1965

Banks JA: The Sociology of Social Movements. Atlantic Highlands, NJ, Humanities Press, 1972

Barber JD: The Lawmakers: Recruitment and Adaptation to Legislative Life. Westport, Conn, Greenwood Press, 1979

Barber JD: The Pulse of Politics: The Rhythm of Presidential Elections in the Twentieth Century. New York, WW Norton, 1980

Bardach E: The Implementation Game. Cambridge, MIT Press, 1977

Barone M et al: Almanac of American Politics. Ipswich, Mass, Gambit, 1972

Bauer R, de Sola Pool I, Dexter LA: American Business and Public Policy. New York, Aldine, 1963

Bauer RA, Gergen KJ (eds): The Study of Policy Formation. New York, Free Press, 1971

Beach M: Editing Your Newsletter: A Guide to Writing, Design and Production. Portland, Ore, Coast to Coast Books, 1980

Becker H, Hughes EC, Greer EC, Strauss AL: Boys in White. Chicago, University of Chicago Press, 1961

Beere CA: Women and Women's Issues: A Handbook of Tests and Measures. San Francisco, Jossey-Bass, 1979

Bell C, Price C: The First Term: A Study of Legislative Socialization. Beverly Hills, Sage, 1975

Bell DV et al (eds): Issues in Politics and Government. Boston, Houghton Mifflin, 1970

Bell EH: Storming the Citadel: The Rise of the Woman Doctor. Westport, Conn, Hyperion Press, 1980

Bem SL: The measurement of psychological androgyny. J Consult Clin Psychol 42:155–162, 1974

Bem SL: Sex–role adaptability: One consequence of psychological androgyny. J Pers Soc Psychol 31:634–643, 1975

Bem SL, Bem DJ: Case study of a nonconscious ideology: Training the woman to know her place. In Bem DJ (ed): Beliefs, Attitudes, and Human Affairs, pp 89–99. Belmont, Brooks/Cole, 1970

Benham L: The labor market for registered nurses: A three equation model. Rev Economics Statistics 53:246–252, 1971

Bennett WL: The Political Mind and the Political Environment. Lexington, Mass, Lexington Books, 1975

Benson JK (ed): Organizational Analysis: Critique and Innovation. Beverly Hills, Sage, 1977

Berelson B, Janowitz M (eds): Reader in Public Opinion and Communication. New York, Free Press, 1966

Berman D: A Bill Becomes A Law. New York, Macmillan, 1962

Bernard J: The Future of Motherhood. New York, Dial Press, 1974

Bernard J: Women, marriage, and the future. Futurist 4:35–45, 1970

Bernard J: Women and the Public Interest: An Essay on Policy and Protest. Chicago, Aldine-Atherton, 1971

Bernays EL et al: Engineering of Consent. Norman, University of Oklahoma Press, 1969

Bernstein BJ (ed): Politics and Policies of the Truman Administration. New York, Watts, Franklin, 1970

Bienen H: Kenya: The Politics of Participation and Control. Princeton, Princeton University Press, 1974

Biklen SK, Brannigan M: Women and Educational Leadership. Lexington, Mass, Lexington Books, 1980

Binkin M, Bach S: Women and the Military. Washington, DC, Brookings Institution, 1977

Binkley WE: President and Congress. New York, Vintage Books, 1962

Black M et al: Political Attitudes in the Nation and the States. Chapel Hill, University of North Carolina Institute of Research in Social Sciences, 1974

Blackstone EA: A.M.A. and the osteopaths: A study of the power of organized medicine. Antitrust Bull, 22:405–440, 1977

Blackwell B, Eilers K: Wright State conflict: A clash of two approaches. Dayton, Oh, Journal Herald, Jan 26, 1980

Blackwell E: Opening the Medical Profession to Women: Autobiographical Sketches. New York, Schocken Books, 1977

Blair GS: Government at the Grass-Roots. Pacific Palisades, Calif, Palisades, 1977

Blau FD: Women in the labor force: An overview. In Freeman J (ed): Women: A Feminist Perspective, pp 270–271. Palo Alto, Mayfield, 1979

Blau P: Exchange and Power in Social Life. New York, John Wiley & Sons, 1964

Blood RO, Wolfe DM: Husbands and Wives: Dynamics of Married Living. Glencoe, Ill, Free Press, 1960

Bloom JR et al: Changing images of professionalism: The case of public health nurses. Am J Public Health 69:43–46, 1979

Bloom JR, Parlette GN, O'Reilly CA: Collective bargaining by nurses: A comparative analysis of management and employee perceptions. Health Care Management Rev 5:25–33, 1980

Bloom JR: Status characteristics, leadership consensus and decision-making among nurses. Soc Sci Med 14(A):15–22, 1980

Blumenthal S: The Permanent Campaign: Inside the World of Elite Political Operatives. Boston, Beacon Press, 1980

Blumler JG, McQuail D: Television in Politics: Its Uses and Influences. Chicago, University of Chicago Press, 1969

Bogart L: Silent Politics: Polls and the Awareness of Public Opinion. New York, John Wiley & Sons, 1972

Boles JK: The Politics of the Equal Rights Amendment: Conflict and the Decision Process. New York, Longman, 1979

Bone H, Ranney A: American Politics and the Party System. New York, McGraw-Hill, 1971

Bottomore T: Political Sociology. New York, Harper & Row, 1980

Boulder E et al: Handbook of International Data on Women. New York, Halsted Press, 1976

Bourque SC, Grossholtz J: Politics an unnatural practice: Political science looks at female participation. Politics Society 4:225–266, 1974

Bowman L, Boynton GR: Political Behavior and Public Opinion: Comparative Analysis. Englewood Cliffs, Prentice-Hall, 1974

Brams SJ: Game Theory and Politics. New York, Free Press, 1975

Branca P: Silent Sisterhood: Middle-Class Women in the Victorian Home. Totowa, NJ, Biblio Distribution Centre, 1977

Brenner MH, Mooney A, Nagy TJ (eds): Assessing the contributions of the social sciences to health. American Association for the Advancement of Science, Selected Symposium No. 26. Boulder, Colo, Westview Press, 1980

Breslau N: The role of the nurse-practitioner in a pediatric team: Patient definitions. Med Care 15:1014–1023, 1977

Brigham J: Making Public Policy: Studies in American Politics. Lexington, Mass, DC Heath, 1977

Brim OG: Socialization through the life cycle. In Brim OG, Wheeler S (eds): Socialization After Childhood: Two Essays. New York, John Wiley & Sons, 1966

Brogan D, Kutner NG: Measuring sex-role orientation: A normative approach. J Marriage Family 38:31–40, 1976

Broh W: Toward a Theory of Issue Voting. Beverly Hills, Sage, 1973

Brookings Institution: Policymaking for Social Security, by Derthick M. Washington, DC, Brookings Institution, 1979

Brown BA et al: Women's Rights and the Law: The Impact of the ERA on State Laws. New York, Praeger, 1977

Brown EL: Nursing for the Future. New York, Russell Sage Foundation, 1948

Brown GR: The Leadership of Congress. New York, Arno Press, 1974

Brown J, Seib PM: The Art of Politics: Electoral Strategies and Campaign Management. Sherman Oaks, Calif, Alfred, 1976

Brown LD: The formulation of federal health care policy. Bull NY Acad Med 54:45–58, 1978

Brown P: The transfer of care: U.S. mental health policy since World War II. Int J Health Serv 9, No. 4:645–662, 1979

Buchanan PJ: Conservative Votes, Liberal Victories. New York, Quadrangle, 1975

Budge I et al: (eds): Party Identification and Beyond: Representatives of Voting and Party Competition. New York, John Wiley & Sons, 1976

Bumpass L, Sweet J: Differentials in marital instability. Am Sociol Rev 37:754–766, 1972

Burrow JG: Organized Medicine in the Progressive Era: The Move Toward Monopoly. Baltimore, Johns Hopkins University Press, 1977

Burrow JG: AMA: Voice of American Medicine. Baltimore, Johns Hopkins University Press, 1963

Bush, DF, Simmons RG, Hutchinson B, Blyth DA: Adolescent perception of sex roles in 1968 and 1975. Public Opinion Q 41:459–474, 1977–1978

Butler M, Paisley W: Women and the Mass Media: Sourcebook for Research and Action. New York, Human Sciences Press, 1979

Bailey JT, Claus KE: Decision Making in Nursing: Tools for Change. St Louis, CV Mosby, 1975

Bentley P: Health Care Agencies and Professionals: A Changing Relationship. New York, National League for Nursing, 1977

Berkowitz N, Malone M: Intra-professional conflict. Nurs Forum 7, No. 1:51–71, 1968

Cairl RE, Imershein AW: National health insurance policy in the United States: A case of non-decision making. Int J Health Serv 7:167–178, 1977

Cameron DR: Toward a theory of political mobilization. J Politics 36:138–171, 1974

Campbell A et al: American Voter: An Abridgement. New York, John Wiley & Sons, 1964

Campbell A, Converse E, Miller E, Stokes E: The American Voter. New York, John Wiley & Sons, 1960

Cannings K, Lazonick W: The development of the nursing labor force in the United States: A basic analysis. Int J Health Serv 5:185–216, 1975

Cantril H: The Psychology of Social Movements. New York, John Wiley & Sons, 1948

Carden ML: The New Feminist Movement. New York, Russell Sage Foundation, 1974

Carlson RJ: The End of Medicine. New York, John Wiley & Sons, 1975

Carter J: Nurse Training Act veto, Nov 10, 1978. In Congressional Quarterly Almanac, 95th Congress, 2nd Session, 1978, Vol 34. Washington, DC, Congressional Quarterly, 1979

Carter J: Why Not the Best? Nashville, Broadman Press, 1975

Cass DP: How to Win Votes and Influence Elections: A Nonpartisan Guide to Effective Political Work. Chicago, Public Administration Service, 1962

Center for the American Woman and Politics, Eagleton Institute of Politics: Women in Public Office: A Biographical Directory and Statistical Analysis. Ann Arbor, RR Bowker, 1976

Chacko GK (ed): Health Handbook: An International Reference on Care and Cure. New York, North Holland, 1979

Chafe WH: The American Woman: Her Changing Social, Economic and Political Roles, 1920–1970. New York, Oxford University Press, 1977

Chaff SL et al: Women in Medicine: An Annotated Bibliography of the Literature on Women Physicians. Metuchen, NJ, Scarecrow Press, 1977

Chaffee SH, Ward LS, Tipton LP: Mass communication and political socialization. Journalism Q 47:647–659, 1970

Chamberlain H: A Minority of Members: Women in the U.S. Congress. New York, New American Library, 1974

Chambers CA: The campaign for women's rights in the 1920's. In Friedman JE, Shade WG (eds): Our American Sisters: Women in American Life and Thought, pp 260–282. Boston, Allyn & Bacon, 1973

Chambers MB: The displaced homemaker: Victim of socioeconomic change affecting the American family. J Institute Socioeconomic Studies Fall:3:68–76, 1978

Chandler R (ed): Public Opinion: Changing Attitudes on Contemporary Political and Social Issues. Ann Arbor, RR Bowker, 1972

Chapoorian T, Craig MM: PL93-641: Nursing and health care delivery. Am J Nurs 76:1998–1991, 1976

Chassin MR: The containment of hospital costs: A strategic assessment. Med Care (Suppl) 16:1–55, 1978

Chesney AP et al: Sociologic and demographic factors related to geographic stability among allied health and nursing personnel. J Health Soc Behav 21:48–58, 1980

Chiswick BR, O'Neill J (eds): Human Resources and Income Distribution. New York, WW Norton, 1977

Christopher M: Black Americans in Congress. New York, Thomas Y Crowell, 1976

Chronology of health insurance proposals, 1915–76. Soc Secur Bull 39:35–39, 1976

Clapp CL: The Congressman: His Work As He Sees It. Westport, Conn, Greenwood Press, 1980

Clarke HD, Kornberg A: Moving up the political escalator: Women party officials in the United States and Canada. J Politics 41, No. 2:443–477, 1979

Clausen AR: How Congressmen Decide: A Policy Focus. New York, St Martin's Press, 1973

Clegg S: Power, Rule, and Domination: A Critical and Empirical Understanding of Power in Sociological Theory and Organizational Life. Boston, Routledge & Kegan Paul, 1975

Clegg S: The Theory of Power and Organization. Boston, Routledge & Kegan Paul, 1979

Clem AL: The Making of Congressmen. Belmont, Calif, Duxbury Press, 1976

Cobb RW, Elder CD: Participation in American Politics: The Dynamics of Agenda-Building. Baltimore, Johns Hopkins University Press, 1975

Coffey A: How We Choose a Congress. New York, St Martin's Press, 1980

Collins WP (ed): Perspectives on State and Local Politics. Englewood Cliffs, Prentice-Hall, 1974
Colombotos J et al: Physicians' attitudes toward political and health care policy issues in cross-national perspective: A comparison of FMGs and USMGs. Soc Sci Med 11:603–609, 1977
Colson C: Born Again. Reston, Va, Fleming H Revell, 1977
Combs J: Dimensions of Political Drama. Santa Monica, Goodyear, 1980
Commission on Professional and Hospital Activities: Length of Stay in PAS Hospitals: United States, 1974. Ann Arbor, The Commission, 1975
Committee on the Cost of Medical Care, October 1932: Medical Care for the American People: The Final Report of the Committee on the Costs of Medical Care. New York, Arno Press, 1972
Comptroller General, U.S. General Accounting Office: Hospitals In the Same Area Often Pay Widely Different Prices for Comparable Supply Items, p 5. Report to the Chairman, Subcommittee on Health, Committee on Finance, U.S. Senate. Washington, DC, United States General Accounting Office, January 21, 1980
Conflict Management: Fight, Fight, Negotiate? New York, National League for Nursing, 1977
Congress and the Nation. Washington, DC, Congressional Quarterly, 1977
Congressional Quarterly Service: Future of Social Programs. Washington, DC, Congressional Quarterly, 1973
Congressional Quarterly Staff: Guide to U.S. Elections, 1789–1974. Washington, DC, Congressional Quarterly, 1975
Congressional Quarterly Staff: The Washington Lobby. Washington, DC, Congressional Quarterly, 1974
Congressional Record, March 14, 1979
Congressional Record, pp H1071–H1072, March 16, 1979
Constantine E, Craik K: Women as politicians: The social background, personality, and political careers of female party leaders. J Soc Issues 28, No. 2:217–236, 1972
Converse PE, Schuman M: "Silent majorities" and the Vietnam War. Sci Am 222:17–25, 1970
Cooper JL: The Seventh Decade: A Study of the Women's Liberation Movement. Dubuque, Iowa, Kendall/Hunt, 1980
Cornelius J: Political Learning Among the Migrant Poor. Beverly Hills, Sage, 1973
Coser LA: Continuities in the Study of Social Conflict. New York, Free Press, 1967
Cost of disease and illness in the United States in the year 2000. Public Health Rep (Suppl) 93:497–588, 1978
Cottle TJ, Edwards CN, Pleck J: The relationship of sex role identity and social and political attitudes. J Personality 38:435–452, 1970
Coulton MR: Labor disputes: A challenge to nurse staffing. J Nurs Admin May:6:15–20, 1976
Couto RA: Poverty, Politics and Health Care: An Appalachian Experience. New York, Praeger, 1975
Cretin S: Cost/benefit analysis of treatment and prevention of myocardial infarction. Health Serv Res 12:174–189, 1977
Crockett NL (ed): Power Elite in America. Lexington, Mass, DC Heath, 1970
Crotty WJ, Freeman DM, Gatlin DS: Political Parties and Political Behavior. Boston, Allyn & Bacon, 1968
Crystal R, Brewster A: Cost benefit and cost effectiveness analysis in the health field: An introduction. Inquiry 3:3–13, 1966
Culter NE: Aging and generations in politics: The conflict of explanations and inference. In Wilcox AR (ed): Public Opinion and Political Attitudes. New York, John Wiley & Sons, 1974
Culyer AJ et al(eds): An Annotated Bibliography of Health Economics. New York, St Martin's Press, 1977
Cumming E: Further thoughts on the theory of disengagement. Int Soc Sci 15, No. 3:377–393, 1963
Cummings MC, Jr, Wise D: Democracy Under Pressure: An Introduction to the American Political System. New York, Harcourt Brace Jovanovich, 1977
Cunningham FC, Williamson JH: How does the quality of health care in HMOs compare to that in other settings? An analytic literature review, 1958 to 1979. Group Health J I:4–25, 1980

Dahl RA: The concept of power. Behav Sci 2:201–218, 1957
Dahl RA: Modern Political Analysis. Englewood Cliffs, Prentice-Hall, 1976
Dahl RA: Who Governs? Democracy and Power in an American City. New Haven, Yale University Press, 1961
Dahrendorf R: Class and Class Conflict in Industrial Society. Stanford, Stanford University Press, 1965
Danigelis NL: Black political participation in the United States: Some recent evidence. Am Sociol Rev 43:756–771, 1978
Danigelis NL: A theory of black political participation in the United States. Soc Forces 56:31–47, 1977
Davidson RH: The Politics of Comprehensive Manpower Legislation. Baltimore, Johns Hopkins University Press, 1973
Davidson RH: The Role of the Congressman. New York, Irvington, 1969
Davidson SM et al: The Cost of Living Longer: National Health Insurance and the Elderly. Lexington, Mass, Lexington Books, 1980
Davies JC: Political socialization: From womb to childhood. In Renshon S (ed): Handbook of Political Socialization. New York, Free Press, 1977
Davis AB: Bibliography on Women: With Special Emphasis on Their Roles in Science and Society. New York, Nale Watson Academic, 1974
Davis K: National Health Insurance: Benefits, Costs, and Consequences. Washington, DC, Brookings Institution, 1975

David I: Social Mobility and Political Change. New York, Praeger, 1970

David K: National Health Insurance: Benefits, Costs and Consequences. Washington, DC, Brookings Institution, 1975

Daynes BW, Tatalovich R: Issues in American Government and Politics. Lexington, Mass, DC Heath, 1980–1981

Dean J: Blind Ambition: The White House Years. Austin, S & S Press, 1976

Deckard B: The Women's Movement: Political, Socioeconomic and Psychological Issues. New York, Harper & Row, 1975

DeFleur ML, Larsen ON: The Flow of Information: An Experiment in Mass Communication. New York, Harper & Brothers, 1958

de Jouvenel B: Authority: The efficient imperative. In Friedrich CJ (ed): Authority, p 160. Cambridge, Harvard University Press, 1958

Deloughery GL, Gebbie KM: Political Dynamics: Impact on Nurses and Nursing. St Louis, CV Mosby, 1975

Deutsch KW: Socio mobilization and political development. Am Political Sci Rev 55:493–515, 1961

Dewees DN: Economics and Public Policy: The Automobile Pollution Case. Cambridge, MIT Press, 1974

Diamond I: Sex Roles in the State House. New Haven, Yale University Press, 1977

Dickerson N: Among Those Present: A Reporter's View of Twenty-Five Years in Washington. New York, Random House, 1976

Diers D: A different kind of energy: Nurse power. Nurs Outlook 26:51–55, 1978

Dinnerstein D: The Mermaid and the Minotaur. New York, Harper & Row, 1976

Dixon M: Women in Class Struggle. San Francisco, Synthesis, 1980

Doherty N, Hicks B: Cost-effectiveness analysis and alternative health care programs for the elderly. Health Serv Res 12:190–203, 1977

Dolbeare K et al: Institutions, Policies, and Goals: A Reader in American Politics. Lexington, Mass, DC Heath, 1973

Dolbeare K (ed): Public Policy Evaluation. Beverly Hills, Sage, 1975

Dolbeare KM: Political Change in the United States: A Framework for Analysis. New York, McGraw-Hill, 1974

Dolbeare KM, Dolbeare P: American Ideologies: The Competing Political Beliefs of the 1970's. Chicago, Rand-McNally, 1976

Dolbeare KM, Edelman MJ: American Politics: Policies, Power and Change. Lexington, Mass, DC Heath, 1977

Donnison J: Midwives & Medical Men: A History of Inter-Professional Rivalries & Women's Rights. New York, Schocken Books, 1977

Donovan L: RN's survey of nursing incomes, Part 2. What increases income most? RN 43:27–30, 1980

Downes BT (ed): Cities and Suburbs: Selected Readings in Local Politics and Public Policy. N. Scituate, Mass, Duxbury Press, 1971

Downey J: Winning Election to Public Office: The ABC's of Conducting a Local Political Campaign. Pittsburgh, Joel Downey, 1977

Doyle A: Development of federal public health functions in the United States. Public Health Nurse 12:723–727, 1920

Dror Y: Design for Policy Sciences. New York, Elsevier-North Holland, 1971

Dror Y: Ventures in Policy Sciences: Concepts and Applications. New York, Elsevier-North Holland, 1971

Dudley J: Promoting the Organization: A Guide to Low Budget Publicity. Philadelphia, International Ideas, 1975

Duff RS, Hollingshead AB: Sickness and Society. New York, Harper & Row, 1968

Dunlop D: Benefit–cost analysis: A review of its applicability in policy analysis for delivering health services. Soc Sci Med 9:133–139, 1975

Durian JC: Factors influencing the rising labor force participation rates of married women with pre-school children. Soc Sci Q 56:614–630, 1976

Duverger M: Party Politics and Pressure Groups: A Comparative Introduction. New York, Thomas Y Crowell, 1972

Duverger M: The Political Role of Women. Paris, United Nations Educational, Scientific and Cultural Organizations, 1955

Dye TR, Greene LS, Parthemos GS: Governing the American Democracy. New York, St Martin's Press, 1980

Dye TR: Politics in States and Communities. Englewood Cliffs, Prentice-Hall, 1977

Dyer WG: The Sensitive Manipulator. Provo, Brigham Young University Press, 1972

Easton D: The perception of authority and political change. In Friedrich CJ (ed): Authority, p 179. Cambridge, Harvard University Press, 1958

Easton D: The Political System. New York, Alfred A Knopf, 1953

Easton D: A Systems Analysis of Political Life. New York, John Wiley & Sons, 1965

Easton D, Dennis J: Children in the Political System: Origins of Political Legitimacy. New York, McGraw-Hill, 1969

Eckhardt B, Black CL, Jr: The Tides of Power: Conversations on the American Constitution. New Haven, Yale University Press, 1977

Editorial: JAMA December, 1932

Edwards CC: The federal involvement in health: A personal view of current problems and future needs. N Engl J Med 292:559–562, 1975

Edwards GC, III: Presidential Influence in Congress. San Francisco, WH Freeman, 1980

Edwards GC, III, Sharkansky I: The Policy Predicament: Making and Implementing Public Policy. San Francisco, WH Freeman, 1978

Edwards LP: The Natural History of Revolution. Chicago, University of Chicago Press, 1927

The Eisenhower Years. New York, Facts on File, 1977

Elinson J et al: Health Goals and Health Indicators: Policy Planning and Evaluation. Boulder, Colo, Westview Press, 1978

Elling RH: Cross-National Study of Health Systems: Political Economics and Health Care. New Brunswick, Transaction Books, 1980

Emerson R: Power-dependence relations. Am Sociol Rev 27:31–41, 1962

Endorsements: Democracy in Action. CTA/NEA Action May:4, 1980

Enthoven AC: Consumer-choice health plan, Part 1. Inflation and inequity in health care today: Alternatives for cost control and an analysis of proposals for national health insurance. N Engl J Med 298:650–658, 1978

Enthoven AC: Consumer-choice health plan, Part 2. National health insurance proposal based on regulated competition in the private sector. N Engl J Med 298:709–720, 1978

Enthoven AC: Health Plan: The Only Practical Solution to the Soaring Cost of Medical Care. Reading, Mass, Addison-Wesley, 1980

Equal Rights Amendment Project: The Equal Rights Amendment: A Bibliograpic Study. Westport, Conn, Greenwood Press, 1976

Eidenburg E, Morey RD: An Act of Congress. New York, WW Norton, 1969

Erikson EH: Inner and outer space: Reflections on womanhood. In Lifton RJ (ed): The Woman in America. Boston, Beacon Press, 1967

Erikson RS, Luttbeg NR: American Public Opinion: Its Origins, Content and Impact. New York, John Wiley & Sons, 1973

Erskine H: The polls: Women's role. Public Opinion Q 35:275–290, 1971

Esmay JB, Wertheimer AI: A review of over-the-counter drug therapy. J Community Health 5:54–66, 1979

Estes CL: Political gerontology. Society 15:43–49, 1978

Estok PJ: Socialization theory and entry into the practice of nursing. Image 9:8–14, 1977

Etzioni A: The Semi-Professions and Their Organization: Teachers, Nurses, Social Workers. New York, Free Press, 1969

Evans R: Social Movements: A Reader and Sourcebook. Chicago, Rand-McNally, 1973

Evans S: Personal Politics: The Roots of Women's Liberation in the Civil Rights Movement and the New Left. New York, Random House, 1980

Fagin CM: Nurses' rights. Am J Nurs 75:82–85, 1975

Fahy ET: A battery of techniques for dodging issues. Image 9:21–22, 1977

Fairlie H: The Kennedy Promise: The Politics of Expectation. Garden City, NY, Doubleday, 1973

Falk IS: Medical care in the U.S.A., 1932–1972: Problems, proposals and programs from the Committee on the Costs of Medical Care to the Committee for National Health Insurance. Comments by Jeoffrry B. Gordon. Milbank Mem Fund Q 51:1–39, 1973

Falk IS: National health insurance for the United States. Public Health Rep 92:399–406, 1977

Falkson JL: HMOs and the Politics of Health System Reform. Chicago, American Hospital Association, 1980

Farah B, Jennings MK: Ideology, gender, and political action: A cross-national survey. Presented at the annual meeting of the American Political Science Association, New York, September, 1978

Federal Trade Commission, Bureau of Economics: Staff Report on Physician Control of Blue Shield Plans, by Kass DI and Pautler PA. Washington, DC, United States Government Printing Office, 1979

Fein R: Some health policy issues: One economist's view. Public Health Rep 90:387–392, 1975

Feingold E: Medicare: Politics and Policy. San Francisco, Chandler, 1966

Feldstein M: The high cost of hospitals and what to do about it. Public Interest 48:40–54, 1977

Feldstein MS: The Rising Cost of Hospital Care. Washington, DC, Information Resources Press, 1971

Feldstein PJ: Health Associations and the Demand for Legislation: The Political Economy of Health. Philadelphia, Ballinger, 1977

Felicetti DA: Mental Health and Retardation Politics: The Mind Lobbies in Congress. New York, Praeger, 1975

Feltner P, Goldie L: Impact of socialization and personality on the female voter: Speculation tested with 1964 presidential data. Western Political Q 27:680–692, 1974

Fendrich JM: Keeping the faith or pursuing the good life: A study of the consequences of participation in the civil rights movement. Am Sociol Rev 42:144–157, 1977

Fenno RF, Jr: Congressmen in Committees. Boston, Little, Brown, 1973

Fenno R: The House Appropriations Committee as a political system. Am Polit Sci Rev 56:310–324, 1962

Ferdinand TN: Psychological femininity and political liberalism. Sociometry 27:75–87, 1964

Ferejohn JA: Port Barrel Politics: Rivers and Harbors Legislation. Stanford, Stanford University Press, 1974

Ferguson JH, McHenry DE: The American Federal Government. New York, McGraw-Hill, 1973

Ferree MM: A woman for president? Changing responses, 1968–1972. Public Opinion Q 38:390–399, 1974

Ferriss AL: Indicators of Trends in the Status of American Women. New York, Russell Sage Foundation, 1971

Feuer L: The Conflict of Generations. New York, Basic Books, 1969

Fields CM: 2 nursing deans quit in Wright State dispute. Washington, DC, Chronicle of Higher Education, Feb 19, 1980

Fineberg HV, Hiatt HH: Evaluation of medical practices: The case for technology assessment. N Engl J Med 301:1086–1091, 1979

Fiorina MP: Congress: Keystone of the Washington Establishment. New Haven, Yale University Press, 1977

Fishel J: Representation and Responsiveness in Congress. Beverly Hills, Sage, 1973

Fisher L: President and Congress. New York, Free Press, 1972

Fisher L: Presidential Spending Power. Princeton, Princeton University Press, 1975

Flacks R: The liberated generation: An exploration of the roots of student protest. J Soc Issues 23, No. 1:52–75, 1969

Flanigan W, Zingale N: Political Behavior of the American Electorate. Boston, Allyn & Bacon, 1979

Flexner E: Century of Struggle: The Woman's Rights Movement in the United States. Cambridge, Harvard University Press, 1975

Flora CB, Lynn NB: Women and political socialization: Considerations of the impact of motherhood. In Jaquette J (ed): Women in Politics, pp 37–53. New York, John Wiley & Sons, 1974

Fogarty MP, Rapoport R, Rapoport RN: Sex, Career and Family. London, George Allen & Unwin, 1971

Foner A: Age stratification and age conflict in political life. Am Sociol Rev 39:187–196, 1974

Ford GR: Nurses' training: Memorandum of disapproval, Jan 4, 1975. In Congressional Quarterly Almanac, 93rd Congress, 2nd Session, 1974, Vol 30. Washington, DC, Congressional Quarterly, 1974

Ford LE (ed): Directory of Women Law Graduates and Attorneys in the USA, 1977. Butler, Ind, Ford Associates, 1977

Forman AM, Cooper EM: American College of Nurse-Midwives, Legislation Committee: Legislation and nurse-midwifery practice in the USA. J Nurse-Midwifery 21:1–57, 1976

Forrest EL: Socialization of Political Attitudes in Nurses Through Professional Role Development. Ph.D. dissertation, University of Texas, 1979

Fotter MD, Gibson G: Physician attitudes toward the nurse practitioner. J Health Soc Behav 19:303–311, 1978

Fox DM: The Politics of City and State Bureaucracy. Santa Monica, Goodyear, 1973

Frantzick SE: Storming Washington: An Intern's Guide to National Government. Washington, DC, American Political Science Association, 1977

Freedman L: Power and Politics in America. N. Scituate, Mass, Duxbury Press, 1972

Freeland M et al: Projections of national health expenditures, 1980, 1985, and 1990. Health Care Financing Rev 1:1–27, 1980

Freeman HE et al: Handbook of Medical Sociology. Englewood Cliffs, Prentice-Hall, 1972

Freeman J: The Politics of Women's Liberation. New York, David McKay, 1975

Freeman J: The Politics of Woman's Liberation. New York, Longman, 1975

Freeman RA: The Growth of American Government: A Morphology of the Welfare State. Stanford, Hoover Institution Press, 1975

Freidson E: Profession of Medicine: A Study of the Sociology of Applied Knowledge. New York, Harper & Row, 1970

Freidson E: The prospects for health services in the United States. Med Care 16:971–983, 1978

Freidson E: Professional Dominance: The Social Structure of Medical Care. Chicago, Aldine, 1970

Freidson E, Lorber J (eds): Medical Men and Their Work: A Sociological Reader. Hawthorne, NY, Aldine, 1971

French JRP, Raven B: The bases of social power. In Cartwright D (ed): Studies in Social Power, pp 150–167. Ann Arbor, University of Michigan Institute for Social Research, 1959

Freymann JG: Medicine's great schism: Prevention vs. cure: An historical interpretation. Med Care 13:525–536, 1975

Friedan B: The Feminine Mystique. New York, Dell, 1975

Fritschler AL, Ross BH: Executive's Guide to Government: How Washington Works. Englewood Cliffs, Winthrop, 1980

Froman LA, Jr: People and Politics: An Analysis of the American Political System. Englewood Cliffs, Prentice-Hall, 1962

Fuchs FR: From Bismarck to Woodcock: The "irrational" pursuit of national health insurance. J Law Economics 9:347–369, 1976

Fuchs V: Who Shall Live? New York, Basic Books, 1975

Fuchs VR: The economics of health in a post-industrial society. Public Interest 56:3–20, 1979

Fuchs VR: Essays in the Economics of Health and Medical Care. New York, Natural Bureau of Economics Research, 1972

Fudenberg HH, Melnick VL (eds): Biomedical Scientists and Public Policy. New York, Plenum Press, 1978

Fulchiero A et al: Can PSROs be cost effective? N Engl J Med 299:574–580, 1978

Gager N (ed): Women's Rights Almanac. Bethesda, Md, Elizabeth Cady Stanton, 1974

Gallup G: The Gallup Poll, 1935–71. Westminster, Md, Random House, 1972

Gallup GH: The Gallup Poll: Public Opinion, Nineteen Seventy-Nine. Wilmington, Del, Scholarly Resources, 1980

Gamson A: Power and Discontent. Homewood, Ill, Dorsey Press, 1968

Gamson WA: The Strategy of Social Protest. Homewood, Ill, Dorsey Press, 1975

Gamson WA: The Strategy of Social Protest. New York, Irvington, 1975

Garceau O (ed): Political Research and Political Theory. Cambridge, Harvard University Press, 1968

Garland TN: The better half? The male in the dual professional family. In Safilios-Rothschild C (ed): Towards a Sociology of Women. Lexington, Mass, Xerox College Publishing, 1972

Garson D: Power and Politics in the United States. Lexington, Mass, DC Heath, 1977

Gelb J, Palley ML: Women and interest group politics: A comparative analysis of federal decision-making. J Politics 41, No. 2:363–392, 1979

Gelfman JS: Women in Television News. New York, Columbia University Press, 1976

Georgopoulos BS: Hospital Organization Research: Review and Source Book. Philadelphia, WB Saunders, 1975

Gerlach LP, Hine V: People, Power, Change: Movements of Social Transformation. Indianapolis, Bobbs-Merrill, 1970

Giele JZ: Women and the Future: Changing Sex Roles in Modern America. New York, Free Press, 1979

Gilson L: Money and Secrecy: A Citizen's Guide to Reform of State and Federal Practices. New York, Praeger, 1972

Glenn ND, Grimes M: Aging, voting and political interest. Am Sociol Rev 33:563–575. 1968

Godfrey MA: The dollars and sense of nursing salaries. Nursing 79 9:81–89, 1979

Godfrey MA: The dollars and sense of nurses' salaries. Part 2. What does or doesn't add to your paycheck? Nursing 79 9:97–107, 1979

Gold DB: Women and voluntarism. In Girnick V, Moran BK (eds): Women in Sexist Society, pp 533–554. New York, Basic Books, 1971

Golden H, Hanson K: Techniques of Working with the Working Press. Claremont, Calif, Oceana, 1962

Goldman RM: Behavioral Perspectives on American Politics. Homewood, Ill, Dorsey Press, 1973

Goldschmidt P: A cost-effectiveness model for evaluating health care programs: Application to drug abuse treatment. Inquiry 13:29–47, 1976

Goran MJ: The evolution of the PSRO hospital review system. Med Care (Suppl) 17:1–34, 1979

Gordon F, Strober M: Bringing Women into Management. New York, McGraw-Hill, 1975

Gorry A, Scott D: Cost-effectiveness of cardiopulmonary resuscitation training programs. Health Serv Res 12:30–41, 1977

Gosnell HF, Smolka RG: American Parties and Elections. Columbus, Charles E Merrill, 1976

Government Research Corporation: The Carter Administration, Congress and Health Policy. A National Journal Conference proceedings. Washington, DC, Government Research Corporation, 1978

Government Research Corporation: The Carter Administration, Congress and Health Policy. A National Journal Issues book. Washington, DC, Government Research Corporation, 1978

Government Research Corporation: Controlling Health Care Costs. A National Journal Conference proceedings. Washington, DC, Government Research Corporation, 1978

Grant A: American Political Process. Exeter, NH, Heinemann Educational Books, 1980

Greeley AM: Political participation among ethnic groups in the United States: A preliminary reconnaissance. Am J Sociol 80:170–209, 1974

Green S et al: Social support and government policy on services for the elderly. Soc Policy Admin 13:210–218, 1979

Greenberg ES: American Political System: A Radical Approach. Englewood Cliffs, Winthrop, 1980

Greenberg GD: Reorganization reconsidered: The U.S. Public Health Service, 1960–1973. Public Policy 23:483–522, 1975

Greenstein F: Children and Politics. New Haven, Yale University Press, 1965

Greenstein FI: Sex-related political differences in childhood. Politics 23:353–371, 1961

Greenstein FI: American Party System and the American People. Englewood Cliffs, Prentice-Hall, 1970

Greenstone JD: Labor in American Politics. Chicago, University of Chicago Press, 1977

Greenwald CS: Group Power: Lobbying and Public Policy. New York, Praeger, 1977

Groennings S, Hawley JP: To Be A Congressman: The Promise and the Power. Washington, DC, Acropolis Books, 1973

Grossman HR: For Health's Sake: A Clinical Analysis of Medical Care in the United States. Palo Alto, Pacific Books, 1976

Grossman RM: Voting behavior of HSA interest groups: A case study. Am J Public Health 68:1191–1194, 1978

Gruberg M: Women in American Politics. Oshkosh, Wis, Academic Press, 1968

Guest AM: Class consciousness and American political attitudes. Soc Forces 52:496–510, 1974

Guinther J: Moralists and Managers: Public Interest Movements in America. Garden City, NY, Doubleday, 1976

Gunnar M: An American Dilemma. New York, Harper & Row, 1944

Gurin P, Epps E: Black Consciousness, Identity, and Achievement. New York, John Wiley & Sons, 1975

Gurkett GL et al: A comparative study of physicians' and nurses' conceptions of the role of the nurse practitioner. Am J Public Health, 68:1090–1096, 1978

Gusfield JR: Protest, Reform and Revolt: A Reader in Social Movements. New York, John Wiley & Sons, 1970

Hamburg A: Healthy People: The Surgeon General's Report on Health Promotion and Disease Prevention. Background papers. Washington, DC, United States Government Printing Office, 1979

Hamilton RF: A research note on the mass support for "tough" military initiatives. Am Sociol Rev 33:439–445, 1968

Hamilton RF: Restraining Myths: Critical Studies of United States' Social Structure and Politics. New York, Halsted Press, 1975

Hansen SB, Franz LM, Netemeyer-Mays M: Women's political participation and policy preferences. Soc Sci Q 56:576–590, 1976

Harris M, Karp P: How to Make News and Influence People. Blue Ridge Summit, Pa, Tab Books, 1976

Harris SE: The Economics of Health Care: Finance and Delivery. Berkeley, McCutchan, 1975

Harris TR: Potomac Fever. New York, WW Norton, 1977

Harsanyi JC: Measurement of social power: Opportunity, costs, and the theory of two-person bargaining games. Behav Sci 7:67–80, 1962

Hart LB: Moving Up: Women and Leadership. New York, American Management Association, 1980

Harward DW: Power: Its Nature, Its Use, and Its Limits. Boston, GK Hall, 1979

Haskell M: From Reverence to Rape: The Treatment of Women in the Movies. New York, Penguin Books, 1974

Hatfield MO: Not Quite So Simple. Excelsior, Minn, Melvin McCosh, 1968

Hatry HP et al: Practical Program Evaluation for State and Local Governments. Washington, DC, Urban Institute, 1973

Haug MR, Lavin B: Public challenge of physician authority. Med Care 17:844–858, 1979

Hawley AH: Community power and urban renewal success. Am J Sociology 68:422–431, 1968

Hawley WD, Wirt FM (eds): The Search for Community Power. Englewood Cliffs, Prentice-Hall, 1968

Hayward J, Watson M (eds): Planning, Politics and Public Policy. New York, Cambridge University Press, 1975

Heagarty MC et al: Pediatric nurse associates in a large official health agency: Their education, training, productivity, and cost. Am J Public Health 67:855–858, 1977

Health Care Financing Administration, Office of Policy, Planning, and Research: Medicare: Health Insurance for the Aged and Disabled, 1976. Section 1.1. Reimbursement by State and County. Washington, DC, United States Government Printing Office, HCFA Publication No. 018 (6-78), 1978

Health Insurance Institute: Health and Health Insurance: The Public's View. Washington, DC, Health Insurance Institute, 1979

Health Insurance Institute: Source Book of Health Insurance Data, 1975–1976. New York, Health Insurance Institute, 1976

Health Insurance Institute: Source Book of Health Insurance Data, 1978–1979. Washington, DC, Health Insurance Institute, 1979

Heckerman CL: The Evoning Female: Women in Psychosocial Context. New York, Human Sciences Press, 1979

Hedlund RD, Freeman PK, Hamm KE, Stein RM: The electability of women candidates: The effects of sex role stereotypes. J Politics 41, No. 2:512–524, 1979

Heneman HG, Jr: Collective bargaining a major instrument for change. Am J Nurs 68:1039–1042, 1968

Hennig M, Jardim A: The Managerial Woman. Garden City, NY, Doubleday, 1977

Hershey MR: The Making of Campaign Strategy. Lexington, Mass, Lexington Books, 1974

Hershey MR: The politics of androgyny: Sex roles and attitudes toward women in politics. Am Politics Q 5:261–287, 1977

Hershey MR, Sullivan JL: Sex role attitudes, identities, and political ideology. Sex Roles: A Journal of Research 3:37–57, 1977

Herzog TP: The National Labor Relations Act and the ANA: A dilemma of professionalism. J Nurs Admin 6:34–36, 1976

Hess, RD, Torney JV: Development of Political Attitudes in Children. Chicago, Aldine, 1967

Hill DB: A Theory of Political Coalitions in Simple and Policy-Making Situations. Beverly Hills, Sage, 1974

Hill, DB, Trends in American Electoral Behavior. Itasca, Ill, FE Peacock, 1980

Hill DJ: Nursing rating lowered at WSU. Dayton, Oh, Dayton Daily News, Jan 29, 1980

Hirsch H: The Right of the People: An Introduction to American Politics. Washington, DC, University Press of America, 1980

Hirshfield DS: Lost Reform: The Campaign for Compulsory Health Insurance in the United States from 1932 to 1943. Cambridge, Harvard University Press, 1970

Hofferbert RI: The Study of Public Policy. Indianapolis, Bobbs-Merrill, 1974

Hoffman E: Policy and politics: The Child Abuse Prevention and Treatment Act. Public Policy 26:71–88, 1978

Hofstadter R: The American Political Tradition: And the Men Who Made It. New York, Alfred A Knopf, 1973

Hofstadter R: Paranoid Style in American Politics and Other Essays. Westminster, Md, Random House, 1967

Holahan J et al: Paying for physician services under medicare and medicaid. Milbank Mem Fund Q 57:183–211, 1979

Hollister D: Getting organized: A simple recipe for change, Part II. Mich Nurse July:53(19–22, 1980

Holmstron LL: The Two-Career Family. Cambridge, Schenkman, 1972

Holtzman A: American Government: Ideals & Reality. Englewood Cliffs, Prentice-Hall, 1980

Homans GC: Social behavior as exchange. Am J Sociology 63:597–606, 1958

Homans GC: Social Behavior: Its Elementary Forms. New York, Harcourt, Brace, 1961

Hospital service in the United States. Annual issues of JAMA, 1928–1937.

Host D (ed): Citizen and the News. Milwaukee, Marquette University Press, 1962

Huizer G, Mannheim B (eds): The Politics of Anthropology: From Colonialism & Sexism Toward a View from Below. Hawthorne, NY, Mouton, 1979

Human H: Political Socialization. Glencoe, III, Free Press, 1959

Hunter F: Community Power Structure: A Study of Decision Makers. Chapel Hill, University of North Carolina Press, 1953

Hurst L: The Sweetest Little Club in the World: The U.S. Senate. Englewood Cliffs, Prentice-Hall, 1980

Huser W, Grant CW: A study of husbands and wives from dual career and traditional career families. Psychology of Women Q 3:78–89, 1978

Hutcheson JD, Jr, Shevin J: Citizen Groups in Local Politics: A Bibliographic Review. Santa Barbara, American Bibliographic Center-Clio Press, 1976

Hyman H: Political Socialization. Glencoe, III, Free Press, 1959

Hyman HH: Health Planning: A Systematic Approach. Germantown, Md, Apsen Systems Corporation, 1976

Iglitzin LB: The making of the apolitical woman: Femininity and sex-stereotyping in girls. In Jaquette JS (ed): Women in Politics, pp 25–36. New York, John Wiley & Sons, 1974

Illich I: Medical Nemesis: The Expropriation of Health. New York, Bantam Books, 1977

Ingersoll T, O'Connor R: Politics of Structure. N. Scituate, Mass, Duxbury Press, 1974

Ingram H, Mann DE (eds): Why Policies Succeed or Fail. Beverly Hills, Sage, 1980

Inhelder B, Piaget J: The Growth of Logical Thinking from Childhood to Adolescence. New York, Basic Books, 1958

Ippolito DS, Walker TG: Political Parties: Interest Groups and Public Policy: Group Influence in American Politics. Englewood Cliffs, Prentice-Hall, 1980

Ippolito DS et al: Public Opinion and Responsible Democracy. Englewood Cliffs, Prentice-Hall, 1976

Israel FL (ed): The State of the Union Messages of the Presidents. New York, Chelsea House, 1980

The issue: Tax cut vs. added nurses. Wilmington, Del, Morning News, Mar 27, 1980

Jackson J: Constituencies and Leaders in Congress: Their Effects on Senate Voting Behavior. Cambridge, Harvard University Press, 1974

Jacobs HA: Practical Publicity: A Handbook for Public & Private Workers. New York, McGraw-Hill, 1964

Jacobs P et al: Hospital cost inflation and health insurance: A complex market model. Inquiry 15:217–224, 1978

Jacox A: Collective bargaining in academe: Background and perspective. Nurs Outlook 21, No. 11:700–703, 1973

Jaquette JS (ed): Women in Politics. New York, John Wiley & Sons, 1974

Jaros D: Socialization to Politics. New York, Praeger, 1973

Jennings CP: Nursing's case for third party reimbursement. Am J Nurs 79:110–114, 979

Jennings MK, Niemi RG: Family structure and the transmission of political values. Am Polit Sci Rev 62:169–184, 1968

Jennings MK, Niemi RG: The Political Character of Adolescence: The Influence of Families and Schools. Princeton, Princeton University Press, 1974

Jewell ME, Olson DM: American State Political Parties & Elections. Homewood, III, Dorsey Press, 1978

Johns AC et al: American Politics in Transition. Dubuque, Iowa, Kendall/Hunt, 1977

Jones CO: Introduction to the Study of Public Policy. N. Scituate, Mass, Duxbury Press, 1977

Jones R, Woll P: The Private World of Congress. New York, Free Press, 1979

Jones RK, Jones PA: Sociology in Medicine. New York, Halsted Press, 1976

Josefowitz N: Paths to Power: A Working Woman's Guide from First Job to Top Executive. Reading, Mass, Addison-Wesley, 1980

Josephy AM, Jr: The American Heritage: History of the Congress of the United States. New York, American Heritage, 1975

Kahn AJ: Studies in Social Policy & Planning. New York, Russell Sage Foundation, 1969

Kaid LL et al: Political Campaign Communication: A Bibliography and Guide to the Literature. Metuchen, NJ, Scarecrow Press, 1974

Kalisch B: From medical care helper to health care provider: Perspectives on the development of parent–child nursing. Am J Maternal-Child Nurs 5:377–382, 1980

Kalisch B: Of half-gods and mortals: Aesculapian authority. Nurs Outlook 23:22–28, 1975

Kalisch B: The promise of power. Nurs Outlook 26:42–46, 1978

Kalisch B, Kalisch P: An analysis of the sources of physician–nurse conflict. J Nurs Admin 7:50–57, 1977

Kalisch B, Kalisch P: Cadet nurse: The girl with a future. Nurs Outlook 21:444–449, 1973

Kalisch B, Kalisch P: Community clinical nursing issues to the public through the news media. Nurs Res Vol. 30, May-June 1981, pp 132–138

Kalisch B, Kalisch P: Congress copes with the nurse shortage, 1941–1971: Dynamics of congressional nurse education policy formulation. Proc American Nurses' Association Ninth Research Conference 9:317–377, 1974

Kalisch B, Kalisch P: A discourse on the politics of nursing. J Nurs Admin 6:29–34, 1976

Kalisch B, Kalisch P: From Training to Education: The Impact of Federal Aid on Schools of Nursing in the United States in the 1940s. Final Report of NU 00443 Research Grant, Division of Nursing, United States Public Health Service, Dec, 1974

Kalisch B, Kalisch P: The U.S. Cadet Nurse Corps in World War II. Am J Nurs 76:240–242, 1976

Kalisch B, Kalisch P, Clinton J: An analysis of news flow on the nation's nurse shortage. Med Care Vol 19, Sept 1981

Kalisch B, Kalisch P, Clinton J: How the public sees nurse midwives: 1978 news coverage of nurse midwifery in the nation's press. J Nurse-Midwifery 25:31–39, 1980

Kalisch B, Kalisch P, Clinton J: Minority nurses in the news. Nurs Outlook 29:49–54, 1981

Kalisch B, Kalisch P, McHugh M: Content analysis of film stereotypes of nurses. Int J Women's Studies 3:531–558, 1980

Kalisch B, Kalisch P, Scobey M: Reflections on a television image: The Nurses, 1962–1965. Nursing and Health Care 2, No. 5:248–255, 1981

Kalisch P, Kalisch B: The Advance of American Nursing. Boston, Little, Brown, 1978

Kalisch P, Kalisch B: Federal Influence and Impact on Nursing. Washington, DC, United States Government Printing Office (in press)

Kalisch P, Kalisch B: Lighting the lamp of higher learning in nursing education, 1948–1977. Imprint 24:20–22, 28, 55–57, 1977

Kalisch P, Kalisch B: The nurse shortage, the president and the Congress. Nurs Forum 19(2):138–164, 1980

Kalisch P, Kalisch B: Nursing Involvement in the Health Planning Process. Washington, DC, United States Government Printing Office, 1978

Kalisch P, Kalisch B: Perspectives on improving nursing's public image. Nurs Health Care 1:10–15, 1980

Kalisch P, Kalisch B: Political dynamics. In Marrimer A (ed): Current Perspectives in Nursing Management, pp 156–174. St Louis, CV Mosby, 1978

Kalisch P, Kalisch B: Slaves, servants, or saints? An analysis of the system of nurse training in the United States, 1873–1948. Nurs Forum 14:222–265, 1975

Kalisch P, Kalisch B: The women's draft: An analysis of the controversy over the Nurses' Selective Service Bill of 1945. Nurs Res 22:402–413, 1973

Kalisch P, Kalisch B, Livesay E: "The angel of death" case: The anatomy of 1980's major nursing news story. Nurs Forum XIX, No. 3:212–241, 1980

Kann ME: Thinking About Politics: Two Political Sciences. Mineola, NY, West, 1980

Karaker R: How to Win a Local Issue Election. Sacramento, Creative Book, 1976

Karnig AK, Walter BO: Election of women to city councils. Soc Sci Q 56:605–613, 1976

Katz E, Lazarsfeld P: Personal Influence: The Part Played by People in the Flow of Mass Communications. New York, Free Press, 1964

Katz MK: America Votes: What You Should Know About Elections Today. Englewood Cliffs, Prentice-Hall, 1976

Katznelson I, Kesselman M: The Politics of Power: A Critical Introduction to American Government. New York, Harcourt Brace Jovanovich, 1975

Keefe WJ: Parties, Politics and Public Policy in America. New York, Holt, Rinehart & Winston, 1976

Keefe WJ, Ogul M: The American Legislative Process: Congress & the States. Englewood Cliffs, Prentice-Hall, 1977

Keinty RM: National Health Insurance and Income Distribution. Lexington, Mass, Lexington Books, 1976

Kellams SE: Ideals of a profession: The case of nursing. Image 9:30–31, 1977

Kelly RM, Boutilier M: The Making of Political Women. Chicago, Nelson-Hall, 1978

Keniston K: Themes and Conflicts of "Liberated" Young Women, pp 11–15. Karen Horney Memorial Lecture, New York City, Mar 24, 1971

Kennedy EF: In Critical Condition. New York: Simon & Schuster, n.d.

Kennedy EM: The congress and national health policy. Am J Public Health 68:241–244, 1978

Key VO: Politics, Parties, and Pressure Groups. New York, Thomas Y Crowell, 1952

Killiam L: Social movements. In Faris REL: Handbook of Modern Sociology. Chicago, Rand-McNally, 1964

Kipnis D, Vanderveer B: Ingratiation and the use of power. J Pers Soc Psychol 17:280–286, 1971

Kirchner M: Where all those physician assistants came from. Med Economics 55:60–64, 1978

Kirkpatrick J: The New Presidential Elite. New York, Russell Sage Foundation, 1976

Kirkpatrick J: Political Woman. New York, Basic Books, 1974

Kirkpatrick SA, Pettit LK: Legislative Role Structures, Power Bases and Behavior Patterns: An Empirical Examination of the U.S. Senate. Norman, University of Oklahoma Bureau of Government Research, 1973

Klarman HE, Jaszi HH (eds): Empirical Studies in Health Economics. Baltimore, Johns Hopkins University Press, 1970

Klarman H, Francis J, Rosenthal G: Cost effectiveness analysis applied to the treatment of chronic renal disease. Med Care 6:48–54, 1968

Klaw S: The Great American Medicine Show: The Unhealthy State of U.S. Medical Care and What Can Be Done About It. New York, Viking Press, 1975

Kleiman C: Women's Networks. New York, JB Lippincott, 1980
Kohn WS: Women in National Legislatures: A Comparative Study of Six Countries. New York, Praeger, 1980
Kolb EJ: A Framework for Political Analysis. Englewood Cliffs, Prentice-Hall, 1978
Korda M: Power: How to Get It, How to Use It. New York, Random House, 1975
Kosa J, Zola IK (eds): Commonwealth Fund: Poverty and Health: A Sociological Analysis. Cambridge, Harvard University Press, 1975
Kraditor AS: The Ideas of the Woman Suffrage Movement, 1880–1920. New York, Columbia University Press, 1965
Kramer M, Schmalenberg CE: Conflict: The cutting edge of growth. J Nurs Admin October: 6:19–25, 1976
Kranz H: The Participatory Bureaucracy: Women and Minorities in a More Representative Public Service. Lexington, Mass, Lexington Books, 1976
Krause EA: Power and Illness: The Political Sociology of Health and Medical Care. New York, Elsevier-North Holland, 1977
Kreighbaum H: When Doctors Meet Reporters. Westport, Conn, Greenwood Press, 1974
Kreps J: Sex in the Marketplace. Baltimore, Johns Hopkins University Press, 1977
Kreps J, Clark R: Sex, Age, and Work: The Changing Composition of the Labor Force. Baltimore, Johns Hopkins University Press, 1975
Kress JR, Singer J: HMO Handbook. Germantown, Md, Aspen Systems Corporation, 1975
Krichmar A: The Woman's Movement in the Seventies: An International English-Language Bibliography. Metuchen, NJ, Scarecrow Press, 1977
Kreisberg L (ed): Research in Social Movements, Conflicts and Change: An Annual Compilation of Research, Vol I. Greenwich, Conn, Jai Press, 1977
Kruschke ER: Level of optimism as related to female political behavior. Soc Sci 41:67–75, 1966
Kuhn HW, Tucker AW (eds): Contributions to the Theories of Game, Vol 2, Annals of Mathematic Studies, No 28. Princeton, Princeton University Press, 1953

Ladd EC, Jr, Hadley CD: Transformation of the American Party System: Political Coalitions from the New Deal to the 1970s. New York, WW Norton, 1975
LaDou J, Likens JD: Medicine and Money: Physicians as Businessmen. Philadelphia, Ballinger, 1977
Laird MR et al: Health Insurance: What Should Be the Federal Role. Washington, DC, American Enterprise Institute for Public Policy Research, 1975
Lamb C: Political Power in Poor Neighborhoods. New York, Halsted Press, 1974
Lane RE: Political Life: Why People Get Involved in Politics. Glencoe, Ill, Free Press, 1959
Lane RE: Political Thinking and Consciousness. Chicago, Markham, 1969
Lang K, Lang G: Collective Dynamics. New York, Thomas Y Crowell, 1961
Lang K, Lang GE: Politics and Television. Scranton, Pa, Quadrangle, 1968
Langton S (ed): Citizen Participation Perspectives: Proceedings of the National Conference on Citizen Participation. Medford, Mass, Lincoln Filene Center for Citizenship and Public Affairs, 1978
Lansing M: The American woman: Voter and activist. In Jacquette J (ed): Women in Politics. New York, John Wiley & Sons, 1974
Larwood L: Women in Management. Lexington, Mass, Lexington Books, 1977
Lasdon G, Sigmann P: Evaluating cost-effectiveness using episodes of care. Med Care 15:260–264, 1977
Lasky V: JFK: The Man and the Myth. New Rochelle, NY, Arlington House, 1966
Lasswell HD: Power and Personality. Westport, Conn, Greenwood Press, 1976
Lasswell H: Politics: Who Gets What, When, How. New York, Meridian Books, 1958
Lasswell HD: Pre-View of Policy Sciences. New York, Elseiver-North Holland, 1971
Lasswell HD et al (eds): Propaganda and Promotional Activities: An Annotated Bibliography. Chicago, University of Chicago Press, 1969
Lasswell HD, Kaplan A: Power and Society: A Framework for Political Inquiry. New Haven, Yale University Press, 1950
Latham E: J.F. Kennedy and Presidential Power. Lexington, Mass, DC Heath, 1972
Lawrence D: Physician assistants and nurse practitioners: Their impact on health care access, costs, and quality. Health Med Care Serv Rev 1, No. 1:3–12, 1978
Lawrence RS et al: Physician receptivity to nurse practitioners: A study of the correlates of the delegation of clinical responsibility. Med Care 15:298–310, 1977

Lave J, Lave L: Measuring the effectiveness of prevention. I. Milbank Mem Fund Q 55:273–289, 1977
League of Women Voters Education Fund: Know Your Community. Washington, DC, League of Women Voters of the US, 1972
Lee MM: Why few women hold public office: Democracy and sexual roles. Polit Sci Q 91:302, 1976
Lehnen RG: The American Citizen: Public Opinion and Political Participation. New York, Holt, Rinehart & Winston, 1976
Leininger M: Political nursing: Essential for health service and educational systems of tomorrow. Nurs Admin Q 2, No. 3:1–16, 1978
Lemons SJ: The Woman Citizen: Social Feminism in the 1920s. Urbana, Ill, University of Illinois Press, 1973
Lendt D (ed): The Publicity Process. Ames, Iowa, Iowa State University Press, 1975
Letter to the Editor: High Point, NC, Enterprise, June 27, 1980
Levin A, Rappoport M (eds): Focus on Health: Issues and Events of 1978 from the New York Times Information Bank. New York, Arno Press, 1979

Levine EL, Cornwall E, Jr: Introduction to American Government. New York, Macmillan, 1975
Levin JI et al: The nurse practitioner: Role, physician utilization, patient acceptance. Nurs Res 27:245–254, 1978
Levine S, Lyon H (eds): A Decade of Women: A Ms. History of the Seventies in Words and Pictures. New York, Paragon Book Reprint Corporation, 1980
Levitan SA, Wurzburg G: Evaluating Federal Social Programs: An Uncertain Art. Kalamazoo, Mich, WE Upjohn Institute for Employment Research, 1979
Levitt J: Men and women as providers of health care. Soc Sci Med 11:395–398, 1977
Levy MR, Kramer MS: The Ethnic Factor: How America's Minorities Decide Elections. New York, Simon & Schuster, 1973
Lewis CE et al: A Right to Health: The Problem of Access to Primary Medical Care. New York, John Wiley & Sons, 1976
Lichtenstein N (ed): The Johnson Years. New York, Facts on File, 1976
Lifton RJ (ed): The Woman in America. Boston, Beacon Press, 1967
Lindblom CE: Policy-Making Process. Englewood Cliffs, Prentice-Hall, 1968
Lindsay CM et al: New Directions in Public Health Care: A Prescription for the 1980s. San Francisco, Institute for Contemporary Studies, 1979
Lineberry RL: American Public Policy: What Government Does and What Difference It Makes. New York, Harper & Row, 1977
Lipsky M: Protest as a political resource. Am Polit Sci Rev 62:1144–1158, 1968
Liston R: Who Really Runs America. Garden City, NY, Doubleday, 1974
Litman T: The Sociology of Medicine and Health Care: A Research Bibliography. San Francisco, Boyd & Fraser, 1976
Lobby Registrations. Congressional Quarterly Almanac, 96th Congress, 1st Session, 1979, Vol 35, pp 3D–40D. Washington, DC, Congressional Quarterly, 1980
Lockheed M, Hall K: Conceptualizing sex as a status characteristic: Applications to leadership training strategies. J Soc Issues 32, No. 1:111–124, 1976
Loebs SF: Medicaid: A survey of indicators and issues. Hosp Health Serv Admin 22:63–90, 1977
Lowell AL: Public Opinion in War and Peace. New York, Arno Press, 1974
Lukas JA: Nightmare: The Underside of the Nixon Years. New York, Bantam Books, 1977
Lukes S: Power: A Radical View. London, Macmillan, 1974
Luttbeg N (ed): Public Opinion and Public Policy: Models of Political Linkage. Homewood, Ill, Dorsey Press, 1974
Lyons K: Dear Congressman Howard. Washington, DC, Acropolis Books, 1972

McCarthy E et al: Regulation of Political Campaigns: How Successful? Washington, DC, American Enterprise Institute for Public Policy Research, 1977
McConnel G: Private Power and American Democracy. New York, Vintage, 1966
McCourt K: Working Class Women and Grass-Roots Politics. Bloomington, Indiana University Press, 1977
McFarland AS: Public Interest Lobbies: Decision Making on Energy. Washington, DC, American Enterprise Institute for Public Policy Research, 1976
McGinniss J: Selling of the President. Los Angeles, Trident, 1979
McGraw P: Where will nurses' militancy lead? Denver, Colo, The Denver Post, Nov 25, 1979
McGriff EP: The courage for effective leadership in nursing. Image 8:56–60, 1976
MacIntyre S: The management of childbirth: A review of sociological research issues. Soc Sci Med 11:477–484, 1977
McKeown T: The Role of Medicine: Dream, Mirage or Nemesis? Princeton, Princeton University Press, 1980
McKibbin RC, Beck DM: Labor costs: Their impact on cost control. Hosp Health Serv Admin 24:21–33, 1979
McKibbin RC: Public policy for health manpower: Nursing student loans. J Health Polit Policy Law 2:349–361, 1977
McNeil R: The People Machine: The Influence of Television on American Politics. New York, Harper & Row, 1968
MacRae D, Jr, Wilde, JA: Policy Analysis for Public Decisions. Scituate, Mass, Duxbury Press, 1979
Magruder JS: An American Life. New York, Atheneum, 1974
Maisel L, Cooper J (eds): The Impact of the Electoral Process. Beverly Hills, Sage, 1977
Malbin MJ: Unelected Representatives: A New Role for Congressional Staffs. New York, Basic Books, 1980
Manley JF: American Government and Public Policy. New York, Macmillan, 1976
March JG: The power of power. In Easton D (ed): Varieties of Political Theory, pp 39–70. Englewood Cliffs, Prentice-Hall, 1966
Marmor TR: The Politics of Medicare. Hawthorne, NY, Aldine, 1973
Marmor TR: Rethinking national health insurance. Public Interest 46:73–95, 1977
Marmor TR, Morone J: The health programs of the Kennedy–Johnson years: An overview. In Warner D (ed): Toward New Human Rights: The Social Policies of the Kennedy and Johnson Administration. Austin, University of Texas, LBJ School of Public Affairs, 1977
Marquette JF: Social change and political mobilization in the United States. Am Polit Sci Rev 69:1059–1074, 1974

Marshall ED, Moses EB: RN's 1966: An Inventory of Registered Nurses. New York, American Nurses' Association, 1969

Marshall ED, Moses EB: The Nation's Nurses: Inventory of Professional Registered Nurses. New York, American Nurses' Association, Research and Statistics Program, 1965

Martin ED: The federal initiative in rural health. Public Health Rep 90:291–297, 1975

Martin G: Madam Secretary: Frances Perkins. Boston, Houghton Mifflin, 1976

Martin R: The Sociology of Power. Boston, Routledge & Kegan Paul, 1977

Marx GT (ed): Racial Conflict. Boston, Little, Brown, 1971

Marx K: The Eighteenth Brumaire of Louis Bonaparte. New York, International, n.d.

Mason KO, Czajka JL, Arber S: Change in U.S. women's sex-role attitudes, 1964–1974. Am Sociol Rev 41, No. 4:573–596, 1976

Masur J: Government and hospitals. In Knowles JH (ed): Hospitals, Doctors and The Public Interest. Cambridge, Harvard University Press, 1965

Mattera MD: Female doctors: Why they're on an economic treadmill. Med Economics 57:98–101, 1980

Mauksch IG (ed): National health insurance. Nurs Dimensions 7:1–88, 1979

Maxmen JS: The Post-Physician Era: Medicine in the Twenty-First Century. New York, John Wiley & Sons, 1976

May ER, Fraser J: Campaign Seventy-Two: The Managers Speak. Cambridge, Harvard University Press, 1974

Mazmanian D, Sabatier P (eds): Successful Policy Implementation. Urbana, Ill, Policy Studies Organization, 1980

McClelland D, Burham D: Power is the great motivator. Harvard Business Rev 54, No. 2:100–110, 1976

Mead M: Sex and Temperament. New York, New American Library, 1950

Meadow RG: Politics as Communications. Norwood, NJ, Ablex, 1980

Mechanic D: The Growth of Bureaucratic Medicine: An Inquiry into the Dynamics of Patient Behavior and the Organization of Medical Care. New York, John Wiley & Sons, 1976

Mechanic D: Medical Sociology. New York, Free Press, 1978

Mechanic D: Medical Sociology: A Selective View. New York, Free Press, 1968

Mechanic D: Politics, Medicine and Social Science. New York, John Wiley & Sons, 1974

Medicare–Medicaid: An appraisal after ten years. Public Health Rep 91:299–342, 1976

Merei F: Group leadership and institutionalization. Hum Relations 2:23–39, 1949

Merelman RM: The development of policy thinking in adolescence. Am Polit Sci Rev 65:1033–1047, 1971

Merelman, RM: The family and political socialization: Toward a theory of exchange. J Politics 42:461–486, 1980

Merelman RM: Political Socialization and Educational Climates. New York, Holt, Rinehart & Winston, 1971

Merriam C, Gosnell HF: Nonvoting, pp 109–116. Chicago, University of Chicago Press, 1924

Meyer DS: Winning Candidate: How to Defeat Your Political Opponent. New York, James H Heineman, 1966

Meyer JA: AEI Special Analyses No. 79-3: Health Care Cost Increases. Washington, DC, American Enterprise Institute for Public Policy Research, 1979

Mezey SG: The games people play: Perceptions of women's roles in local public office. Presented at the annual meeting of the American Political Science Association, New York, September, 1978

Milbrath L: Political Participation, pp 135–136. Chicago, Rand-McNally, 1965

Milbrath LW: The Washington Lobbyists. Westport, Conn, Greenwood Press, 1976

Milbrath L: The Washington Lobbyists, pp 209–252; 328–354. Chicago, Rand-McNally, 1963

Milburn J: Women as Citizens: A Comparative Review. Beverly Hills, Sage, 1976

Miles W: The Image Makers: A Bibliography of American Presidential Campaign Biographies. Metuchen, NJ, Scarecrow Press, 1979

Milio N: Dimensions of consumer participation and national health legislation. Am J Public Health 64:357–363, 1974

Miller AH, Gurin P, Gurin G: Electoral implications of group identification and consciousness: The reintroduction of a concept. Presented at the annual meeting of the American Political Science Association, New York, September, 1978

Miller AR: Changing work life patterns: A twenty-five year review. Ann Am Acad Polit Soc Sci 435:83–101, 1978

Miller JB: Toward a New Psychology of Women. Boston, Beacon Press, 1976

Miller MH: Nurses' right to strike. J Nurs Admin February: 5:35–39, 1975

Miller N: Logrolling, vote trading, and the paradox of voting: A game theoretical overview. Public Choice 30:51–73, 1977

Miller WE et al: The CPS 1974 American National Election Study. Ann Arbor, Inter-University Consortium for Political & Social Research, 1975

Miller W, Leighton FS: Fishbait: The Memoirs of the Congressional Doorkeeper. Englewood Cliffs, Prentice-Hall, 1977

Miller W, Stokes D: Constituency influence in Congress. Am Polit Sci Rev 57:45–56, 1963

Millman ML (ed): Nursing Personnel and the Changing Health Care System. Cambridge, Ballinger, 1978

Mills CW: The Power Elite. New York, Oxford University Press, 1956

Minow NN et al: Presidential Television: A Twentieth Century Fund Report. New York, Basic Books, 1973

Mischel W: A social–learning view of sex differences in behavior. In Maccoby EE (ed): The Development of Sex Differences. Stanford, Stanford University Press, 1966

MLA Commission on the Status of Women in the Profession: Academic Women, Sex Discrimination and the Law, New York, Modern Language Association of America, 1975

MLA Commission on the Status of Women in the Profession: Unladylike and Unprofessional: Academic Women and Academic Unions. New York, Modern Language Association of America, 1975

Mogulof MB: Citizen Participation: A Review and Commentary on Federal Policies and Practices. Washington, DC, Urban Land Institute, 1969

Monroe AD: Public Opinion in America. New York, Harper & Row, 1975

Morgan D: Suffragists and Democrats: The Politics of Woman Suffrage in America. East Lansing, Michigan State University Press, 1971

Morgan DG: Congress and the Constitution: A Study of Responsibility. Cambridge, Harvard University Press, 1966

Morrison DE, Steeves AD: Deprivation, discontent, and social movement participation. Rural Sociology 32:414–434, 1967

Mueller MS, Gibson RM: National health expenditures, fiscal year 1975. Soc Secur Bull 39:3–20, 1976

Mulcahy KV, Katy RS: American Votes: What You Should Know About Elections Today. Englewood Cliffs, Prentice-Hall, 1976

Mullane MK: Nursing care and the political arena. Nurs Outlook November: 23:669–701, 1975

Murphy IL: Public Policy on the Status of Women. Lexington, Mass, Lexington Books, 1973

Murphy IL: Public Policy on the Status of Women: Agenda and Strategies for the 70s. Lexington, Mass, Lexington Books, 1973

Murphy T: The New Politics Congress. Lexington, Mass, Lexington Books, 1974

Murphy WT, Schnier E: Vote Power. Garden City, NY, Doubleday, 1974

Mushkin SJ: Evaluation of health policies and actions. Soc Sci Med 11:491–499, 1977

Mussen PH: Early sex-role development. In Reeves N (ed): Womankind: Beyond the Stereotypes, pp 393–418. Chicago, Aldine-Atherton, 1971

Meenaghan TM, Washington RO: Social Policy and Social Welfare: Structure and Applications. New York, Free Press, 1980

Nackel JG, Wesbury SA: The process of resource allocation. Hosp Health Serv Admin 23:75–89, 1978

Nagel J: The Descriptive Analysis of Power. New Haven, Yale University Press, 1975

Nagel S et al: The Policy Problem of Doing Too Much or Too Little: Pretrial Release As a Case in Point. Beverly Hills, Sage, 1977

Nagel SS (ed): Improving Policy Analysis. Beverly Hills, Sage, 1980

Nagel SS: Policy Studies and the Social Sciences. Lexington, Mass, Lexington Books, 1975

Nakamura RT, Smallwood F: The Politics of Policy Implementation. New York, St Martin's Press, 1980

Napolitan J: The Election Game and How to Win It. Garden City, NY, Doubleday, 1972

National Academy of Sciences, Institute of Medicine: The Administration's 1976 Budget: The Health Budget. A staff paper, by Turen M. Washington, DC, National Academy of Sciences, 1975

National Academy of Sciences, Institute of Medicine: Assessing Quality in Health Care: An Evaluation. Final report. Washington, DC, National Academy of Sciences, IOM Publication No. 76-04, 1976

National Academy of Sciences, Institute of Medicine: Controlling the Supply of Hospital Beds, pp 7–16. Washington, DC, National Academy of Sciences, 1976

National Commission for the Study of Nursing and Nursing Education: An Abstract for Action. New York, McGraw-Hill, 1970

The National Health Assembly: America's Health: A Report to the Nation. New York, Harper & Row, 1949

National Health Insurance Reports, January, 1980

National Health Survey, 1935–1936, Preliminary Reports, Sickness and Medical Care Series, Bulletin No. 9: Disability from Specific Causes in Relation to Economic Status. Washington, DC, National Institutes of Health, 1938

National Joint Practice Commission: Statutory Regulation of the Scope of Nursing Practice. A Critical survey, by Hall VC. Chicago, National Joint Practice Commission, 1975

National League for Nursing, Division of Research: RN's One and Five Years After Graduation. A report of the career-pattern study, by Knopf L. New York, National League for Nursing, 1975

Navarro V: Social class, political power and the state and their implications in medicine. Soc Sci Med 10:437–458, 1976

Nettl JP: Political Mobilization: A Sociological Analysis of Methods and Concepts. London, Faber & Faber, 1967

Neugarten B: Age groups in American society and the rise of the young–old. Ann Polit Soc Sci 415:187–198, 1974

Neustadt RE: Presidential Power. New York, John Wiley & Sons, 1960

Newland K: The Sisterhood of Man. New York, WW Norton, 1979

Newland K: Women in Politics: A Global Review. Washington, DC, Worldwatch Institute, 1975

Newman JF et al: Attempts to control health care costs: The United States experience. Soc Sci Med 13A:529–540, 1979

Nicholas HG: The Nature of American Politics. New York, Oxford University Press, 1980

Nicholas D: Financing Elections: The Politics of an American Ruling Class. New York, Franklin Watts, 1973

Nie NH et al: The Changing American Voter. Cambridge, Harvard University Press, 1976

Nie N, Powell G, Bingham J, Jr, Prewitt K: Social structure and political participation: Developmental relationships, Part I and II. Am Polit Sci Rev 63:361–378; 808–832, 1969

Nimmo D, Savage RL: Candidates and Their Images: Concepts, Methods and Findings. Salt Lake City, Utah, Goodyear, 1976

Nimmo D, Ungs TD: American Political Patterns: Conflict and Consensus. Waltham, Mass, Little, Brown, 1973

"Non-politicking" Teasdale addresses nurses at M.U. Columbia, Mo, Missourian, June 26, 1980

Novarra V: Women's Work, Men's Work: The Ambivalence of Equality. Salem, NH, Merrimack Book Service, 1980

Novello D: The National Health Planning and Resources Development Act. Nurs Outlook Vol. 24 June: 24:354–358, 1976

Nurses group protests operating room changes. Frederick, Md, Post, July 29, 1980

Nurse training provisions pass over presidential veto. Am J Nurs 75:1413–1418, 1975

Nurses learn to assert themselves into a stronger role on the team. Baltimore, Md, The Baltimore Sun, Feb 26, 1980

Nurses' philosophy suffers in agreement. Dayton, Oh, Journal Herald, May 22, 1980

Nursing groups split over education bill. Yonkers, NY, The Herald Statesman, Apr 27, 1980

Nursing and nurses become election year issues. Am J Nurs 68:960, 1968

Oberschal A: Social Conflict and Social Movements. Englewood Cliffs, Prentice-Hall, 1973

Odegard PH, Helms EA: American Politics: A Study in Political Dynamics. New York, Arno Press, 1974

Okada LM, Wan TTH: Medicaid, Medicare, and private health insurance coverage in five urban, low-income areas. Inquiry 15:336–345, 1978

Olson ME: Social and political participation of blacks. Am Sociol Rev 35:682–697, 1970

Olson DM: The Legislative Process: A Comparative Approach. New York, Harper & Row, 1980

Olson DM: The Politics of Legislation: A Congressional Simulation. New York, Praeger, 1976

Olson LK: Aging and policy analysis: A bibliography. Policy Studies J 7:339–342, 1978

Olson A, Jr: The Logic of Collective Action. Cambridge, Harvard University Press, 1965

O'Neill W: Everyone Was Brave: The Rise and Fall of Feminism in America. Chicago, Quadrangle, 1969

Opinion roundup. Public Opinion January–February: 36, 1979

Orfield G: Congressional Power: Congress and Social Change. New York, Harcourt Brace Jovanovich, 1974

Orum A: On participation in political protest movements. J Appl Behav Sci 10:181–207, 1974

Orum AM et al: Sex, socialization and politics. Am Sociol Rev 39:197–209, 1974

Osborne OH: Issues in achieving effective professional alliances. Nurs Digest January–February: 2:56–59, 1976

Ott DJ, Ott AF: Federal Budget Policy. Washington, DC, Brookings Institution, 1977

Owen H, Schultze CL (eds): Setting National Priorities: The Next Ten Years. Washington, DC, Brookings Institution, 1976

Packer A: Applying cost-effectiveness concepts to the community health system. Operations Res 16:227–252, 1968

Pagano T: WSU nursing faculty unhappy with naming of acting dean. Dayton, Oh, Beavercreek Daily, Feb 7, 1980

Paizis S: Getting Her Elected: A Political Woman's Handbook. Sacramento, Creative Editions, 1976

Palley ML, Preston MB: Race, Sex, and Policy Problems. Lexington, Mass, DC Heath, 1979

Parmet W, Wallen J, Korper SP: Consumer views of the impact of nurse-midwifery in low-income areas. J Ambulatory Care Management 3:67–87, 1980

Parsons T: Politics and Social Structure. New York, Free Press, 1969

Parsons T: The Structure of Social Action. Glencoe, Ill, Free Press, 1949

Patterson SC et al: A More Perfect Union: Introduction to American Government. Homewood, Ill, Dorsey Press, 1979

Patterson SC et al: Representatives and Represented: Bases of Public Support for the American Legislatures. New York, John Wiley & Sons, 1975

Paul EF, Russo PA, Jr (eds): Public Policy: Issues, Analysis and Ideology. Chatham, NJ, Chatham House, 1980

Paxton A: Women in Congress. Richmond, Va, Dietz Press, 1945

Peabody RL et al: To Enact a Law: Congress and Campaign Financing. New York, Praeger, 1972

Pederson W: Obfuscation is out: But is communication in? It's time our bureaucrats learned to write. Public Relations Q 23:23–26, 1978

Peirce NR, Barone M: The Mid-Atlantic States of America: People, Politics and Power in the Five Mid-Atlantic States and the Nation's Capitol. New York, WW Norton, 1977

Perkoff GT: Changing Health Care: Perspectives from a New Medical Care Setting. Ann Arbor, Health Administration Press, 1979

Perkoff GT: An effect of organization of medical care upon health: Manpower distribution. Med Care 16:628–640, 1978

Periman M (ed): The Economics of Health and Medical Care. New York, Halsted Press, 1974

Perry RT: Black Legislators. Palo Alto, R & E Research Associates, 1976

Peters C: How Washington Really Works. Reading, Mass, Addison-Wesley, 1980
Peters C et al: The System: A Primer on American Politics. New York, Praeger, 1976
Peterson S, Richardson JM, Kreuter GV: The Two-Career Family. Washington, DC, University Press of America, 1978
Petro CS, Putnam BA: Sex-role stereotypes: Issues of attitudinal changes. Sex Roles: A Journal of Research 5:29–39, 1979
Pierce JC, Sullivan JL (eds): The Electorate Reconsidered. Beverly Hills, Sage, 1980
Pierce L: Freshman Legislator. Portland, Ore, Binford & Mort, 1973
Political Behavior Program Survey Research Center: University of Michigan American National Election Study, 1962. Ann Arbor, Inter-University Consortium for Political and Social Research, 1976
Pollard WE, Mitchell TR: Decision theory analysis of social power. Psychol Bull 78:433–466, 1972
Polsby NW: Community Power and Political Theory. New Haven, Yale University Press, 1963
Polsby NW: Community Power and Political Theory: A Further Look at Problems of Evidence and Inference. New Haven, Yale University Press, 1980
Polsby NW: Congress and the Presidency. Englewood Cliffs, Prentice-Hall, 1971
Polsby NW, Dentler RA, Smith PA: Politics and Social Life: An Introduction to Political Behavior. Boston, Houghton Mifflin, 1963
The Power of the Purse: Appropriations Politics in Congress. Boston, Little, Brown, 1966
Pratt JH: The Gray Lobby. Chicago, University of Chicago Press, 1976
President signs bill aiding nurse education: Nurses organizations lose battle on school accreditation. Am J Nurs 68:2063, 1968
Prest A, Turvey R: Cost benefit analysis: A survey. Economic J 15:683–735, 1965
Presthus R: Elites in the Policy Process. New York, Cambridge University Press, 1974
Prewitt K, Verba S: An Introduction to American Government. New York, Harper & Row, 1977
Prewitt K, Verba S: Principles of American Government. New York, Harper & Row, 1980
Price DE: Who Makes the Laws? The Legislative Roles of Three Senate Committees. Cambridge, Schenkman, 1972
PSROs: Boon or Bust for Nursing? Hospitals 49:81–84, 1975
Pyatt G et al: Organized Medicine in the Progressive Era. New York, Cambridge University Press, 1977
Pym B: The making of a successful pressure group. Bri J Sociol 24, No. 4:448–461, 1973

Racker E: Science and the Cure of Diseases: Letters to Members of Congress. Princeton, Princeton University Press, 1979
Raffel M: The U.S. Health System: Origins and Functions. New York, John Wiley & Sons, 1980
Rafferty J (ed.): Health Manpower and Productivity: The Literature and Required Future Research. Lexington, Mass, Lexington Books, 1974
Ralph Nadar Congress Project: Ruling Congress: How the House & Senate Rules Govern the Legislative Process. New York, Penguin Books, 1977
Randel J: Do women nurses get heavenly recognition? Wilmington, Del, Wilmington Evening Journal, June 2, 1980
Rapoport A: Two Person Game Theory. Ann Arbor, University of Michigan Press, 1966
Rapoport D: Inside the House. Chicago, Follett, 1975
Ray K: Nursing faculty at WSU seeks no-confidence vote. Dayton, Oh, Dayton Daily News, Jan 30, 1980
Ray K: WSU nursing grads last among four-year schools on test. Dayton, Oh, Dayton Daily News, Jan 31, 1980
Rayack E: Professional Power and American Medicine: The Economics of the American Medical Association. Cleveland, World, 1967
Redman E: The Dance of Legislation. New York, Simon & Schuster, 1974
Reed DE, Roghmann KJ: Acceptability of an expanded nurse role to nurses and physicians. Med Care 9:372–377, 1971
Reeves PN et al: Introduction to Health Planning. Washington, DC, Information Resources Press, 1977
Reference Data on Socioeconomic Issues of Health, 1977. Chicago, American Medical Association, 1977
Reich JR, Reich MJ: United States Government. Los Angeles, Bowmar/Noble, 1979
Reid TR: Congressional Odyssey: The Saga of a Senate Bill. San Francisco, WH Freeman, 1980
Reiff R: The control of knowledge: The power of the helping professions. J Appl Behav Sci 10:451–461, 1974
Reinhardt UE: The future of medical enterprise: Perspectives on resource allocation in socialized markets. J Med Educ 55:311–324, 1980
Reinke WA (ed): The Functional Analysis of Health Needs and Services. Baltimore, Johns Hopkins University, Department of International Health, 1976
Reinkemeyer AM: Nursing's need for commitment to an ideology of change. Nurs Forum 9, No. 4:340–355, 1970
Reisman L, Rohrer JH: Change and Dilemma in the Nursing Profession. New York, Putnam, 1957
Relman AS: The allocation of medical resources by physicians. J Med Educ 55:99–104, 1980
Renshon SA: Psychological Needs and Political Behavior: A Theory of Personality and Political Efficacy. New York, Free Press, 1974

Rice DP, Wilson D: The American medical economy: Problems and perspectives. J Health Polit Policy Law 1:151–172, 1976
Richmond JB: Currents in American Medicine: A Developmental View of Medical Care & Education. Cambridge, Harvard University Press, 1969
Richter M (ed): Political Theory & Political Education. Princeton, Princeton University Press, 1980
Riesman D: The Lonely Crowd. New Haven, Yale University Press, 1951
Riley MW, Foner A, Hess B, Toby ML: Socialization for the middle and later years. In Goslin DA (ed): Handbook of Socialization Theory and Research. Chicago, Rand-McNally, 1969
Ripley RB, Franklin GA (eds): National Government and Policy in the United States. Itasca, Ill FE Peacock, 1977
Roback TH: Political Subculture and Partisan Activism among National Republican Leaders. Beverly Hills, Sage, 1977
Roberts SV: Hospital Cost Bill defeat: Elements in the decision. New York, New York Times, Nov 20, 1979
Robertson L, Heagerty M: Medical Sociology: A General Systems Approach. Chicago, Nelson-Hall, 1975
Rockefeller SP, Testimony before the U.S. Congress, Senate, Committee on Labor and Resources: The Coming Decade: American Women and Human Resources Politics and Programs, 1979, p 138. Hearings before the Committee, Part 1. Washington, DC, United States Government Printing Office, 1979
Roddy PC, Hambleton R: Supply, need, and distribution of anesthesiologists and nurse anesthetists in the U.S., 1972 and 1980. Med Care 15:750–766, 1977
Rodgers JL, Jr: Citizen Committees: A Guide to Their Use in Local Government. Philadelphia, Ballinger, 1977
Rodgers J: Theoretical considerations involved in the process of change. Nurs Forum 13, No. 2:160–174, 1973
Roemer MI: National health insurance as an agent for containing health-care costs. Bull NY Acad Med 54:102–112, 1978
Roemer MI: Rural Health Care. St Louis, CV Mosby, 1976
Roglieri JL, Goldsmith SB: Professional staff acceptance of medical nurse practitioners in ambulatory care. J Ambulatory Care Management 3:15–30, 1980
Roper Organization: Virginia Slims American Women's Opinion Poll, Vol III. New York, Ruder and Finn, 1979
Rose AM: The Power Structure: Political Process in American Society. New York, Oxford University Press, 1976
Rosen G: Preventive Medicine in the United States, 1900–1975: Trends and Interpretations. New York, Science History, 1975
Rosen M: Popcorn Venus. New York, Avon, 1974
Rosenau JN: The Dramas of Political Life. N. Scituate, Duxbury Press, 1980
Rosenberg CE, Rosenberg C: The Male Midwife and the Female Doctor. New York, Arno Press, 1974
Rosenberg M, Bergstrom L: Women and Society: A Critical Review of the Literature with a Selected Annotated Bibliography. Beverly Hills, Sage, 1975
Rosenblatt RA, Huard B: The nurse practitioner as a physician substitute in a remote rural community: A case study. Public Health Rep 94:571–575, 1979
Rosett RN: The Role of Health Insurance in the Health Services Sector. New York, Natural Bureau of Economics Research, 1976
Ross RS: American National Government: An Introduction to Political Institutions. Chicago, Rand-McNally, 1976
Rossi RJ, Gilmartin KJ: Handbook of Social Indicators. New York, Garland, 1979
Roszak T: The Making of a Counterculture. Garden City, Doubleday, 1968
Roth M: Nursing school debate heats up. Dayton, Oh, Journal Herald, Jan 19, 1980
Roth M: WSU board chief gives Kegerreis his full backing. Dayton, Oh, Journal Herald, Jan 26, 1980
Roth M: WSU dean of nursing resigns. Dayton, Oh, Journal Herald, Jan 22, 1980
Rouder S: American Politics: Playing the Game. Boston, Houghton Mifflin, 1977
Rouder S: The Game of American Politics: How to Play. Boston, Houghton Mifflin, 1977
Rourke TE: Bureaucracy, Politics, and Public Policy. Boston, Little, Brown, 1976
Rubel EJ: Implementing the National Health Planning and Resources Development Act of 1974. Public Health Rep 91:3–8, 1976
Runquist BS (ed): Political Benefits: Empirical Studies of American Public Programs. Lexington, Mass, Lexington Books, 1980
Rushing WA: Community, Physicians, and Inequality: A Sociological Study of the Maldistribution of Physicians. Lexington, Mass, Lexington Books, 1975
Rushmer RF: National Priorities for Health: Past, Present, Planned and Projected. New York, John Wiley & Sons, 1980
Russell B: Power: A New Social Analysis. London, George Allen & Unwin, 1938
Russell JE (ed): National Policies for Education, Health and Social Services. New York, Russell & Russell, 1961

Saffell DC: American Government: Reform in the Post-Watergate Era. Englewood Cliffs, Winthrop, 1976
Salisbury RH: Governing America: Public Choice and Political Action. Englewood Cliffs, Prentice-Hall, 1973

Salisbury RN (ed): Interest Groups: Influence in a Changing Environment. Washington, DC, National Journal, 1979

Sarkesian SC, Nanda K: Politics and Power in American Government: An Introduction Text with Readings. Sherman Oaks, Calif, Alfred, 1976

Schachtel BP: The pediatric nurse practitioner: Origins and challenges. Med Care 16:1019–1026, 1978

Schafly P: The Power of the Positive Woman. New Rochelle, NY, Arlington House, 1977

Schafly P, Ward C: The Betrayers. Alton, Ill, Pere Marquette, 1968

Schafly P, Ward C: Strike from Space. Greenwich, Conn, Devin-Adair, 1965

Schattschneider EE: The Semi-Sovereign People. New York, Holt, Rinehart & Winston, 1960

Scheffler RM: The employment, utilization and earnings of physician extenders. Soc Sci Med 11:785–791, 1977

Scheffler RM et al: Physicians and new health practitioners: Issues for the 1980s. Inquiry 16:195–229, 1979

Schier SE: The Rules and the Game: Democratic National Convention Delegate Selection in Iowa and Wisconsin. Washington, DC, University Press of America, 1980

Schlesinger AM, Jr: The Imperial Presidency. Boston, Houghton Mifflin, 1973

Schlesinger AM, Jr: Thousand Days: John F. Kennedy in the White House. Boston, Houghton Mifflin, 1965

Schlesinger AM, Jr, Bruns R (eds): Congress Investigates: A Documented History. New York, Chelsea House, 1980

Schlesinger AM, Jr, Israel FL (eds): History of American Presidential Elections. New York, Chelsea House, 1980

Schlesinger ER: The impact of federal legislation on maternal and child health services in the United States. Milbank Mem Fund Q 52:1–13, 1974

Schlesinger ER: The Sheppard–Towner era: A prototype case study in federal–state relationships. Am J Public Health 57:1034–1040, 1967

Schneider R: Opinions and Policies in the American States: The Role of Political Characteristics. Beverly Hills, Sage, 1976

Schur EM: The Politics of Deviance: Stigma Contests and the Uses of Power. Englewood Cliffs, Prentice-Hall, 1980

Schwartzman E: Campaign Craftsmanship: A Professional's Guide to Campaigning for Elective Office. New York, Universe Books, 1973

Schweitzer S: Cost effectiveness of early detection of disease. Health Serv Res 9:22–32, 1974

Scott AF: Southern Lady: From Pedestal to Politics, 1830–1930. Chicago, University of Chicago Press, 1970

Scott AF, Scott AM: One Half the People: The Fight for Women's Suffrage. New York, JB Lippincott, 1975

Scully DH: Barred from Healing: The Dilemma of the Woman's Doctor. Burlington, Mass, Houghton Mifflin, 1980

Seaton SL, Claessen HJ: Political Anthropology: The State of the Art. Hawthorne, NY, Mouton, 1979

Secretary's Committee to Study Extended Roles for Nurses: Extending the Scope of Nursing Practice. A report of the Secretary's Commmittee. Washington, DC, United States Government Printing Office, 1972

Seidman H: Politics, Position and Power: The Dynamics of Federal Organization. New York, Oxford University Press, 1975

Seidman LS: A strategy for national health insurance. Inquiry 14:321–329, 1977

Senate committee backs new nursing act. Denver, Colo, Denver Post, Feb 15, 1980

Setting National Priorities. Washington, DC, Brookings Institution, 1980

Shack WA, Cohen PS (eds): Politics in Leadership: A Comparative Perspective. New York, Oxford University Press, 1979

Shadegy SC: The New How to Win an Election. New York, Taplinger, 1972

Shank A: American Politics, Policies and Priorities. Oxford, Mass, Holbrook Research Institute, 1977

Shapiro AO: Media Access: Your Rights to Express Your Views on Radio and Television. Boston, Little, Brown, 1976

Shapiro S: Measuring the effectiveness of prevention. II. Milbank Mem Fund Q 55:291–313, 1977

Sharkansky I, Van Meter D: Policy and Politics in American Governments. New York, McGraw-Hill, 1975

Sharkansky I, Shellard G: Measures of health-system effectiveness. Operations Res 18:1067–1070, 1970

Shepard DS, Thompson MS: First principles of cost-effectiveness analysis in health. Public Health Rep 94:535–543, 1979

Sherrill K, Vogler D: Power, Policy and Participation: An Introduction to American Government. New York, Harper & Row, 1977

Sherrill R: Why They Call It Politics: A Guide to America's Government. New York, Harcourt Brace Jovanovich, 1974

Sherrill R, Barber JD, Page BI, Joyner VW: Governing America: An Introduction. New York, Harcourt Brace Jovanovich, 1978

Shogan R: Promises to Keep: Carter's First 100 Days. New York, Thomas Y Crowell, 1977

Sickels RJ: The Presidency: An Introduction. Englewood Cliffs, Prentice-Hall, 1980

Sidel VW, Sidel R: Primary health care in relation to socio-political structure. Soc Sci Med 11:415–419, 1977

Sigall MW, Ottensoser MD: The American Political Reality. Philadelphia, Philadelphia Book, 1972

Sigelman L: The curious case of women in state and local government. Soc Sci Q 56:591–604, 1976

Sigmond RM: The linkage between health policy making and planning. Bull NY Acad Med 54:59–67, 1978

Sills GM: Nursing, medicine and hospital administration. Am J Nurs 76:1432–1434, 1976
Simpson D: Who Rules: An Introduction to the Study of Politics. Athens, Oh, Swallow Press, 1971
Sinclair W: Sen. Magnuson is "Mr. Health" to NIH. Washington DC, Washington Post, Feb 19, 1980
Skolnick JH: The Politics of Protest. New York, Simon & Schuster, n.d.
Sloan IJ: American Landmark Legislation: Primary Materials. Dobbs Ferry, NY, Oceana, 1977
Smelser NJ: Theory of Collective Behavior. New York, Free Press, 1963
Smith DL, Garrison LW (eds): The American Political Process. Santa Barbara, American Bibliographical Center-Clio Press, 1972
Smith EC, Zurcher AJ: Dictionary of American Politics. New York, Barnes & Noble, 1968
Smith JP (ed): Female Labor Supply: Theory and Estimation. Princeton, Princeton University Press, 1980
Smith P: The Constitution: A Documentary and Narrative History. New York, William Morrow, 1980
Smith W: Cost-effectiveness and cost–benefit analysis for public health programs. Public Health Rep 83:899–906, 1968
Smithsonian Institution: Every Four Years: The American Presidency. New York, WW Norton, 1980
Sochen J: Movers and Shakers: American Women Thinkers and Activists, 1900–1970. New York, Quadrangle, 1973
Social Security Administration: Compendium of National Health Expenditures Data. Washington, DC, United States Government Printing Office, 1973
Social Security Administration, Office of Research and Statistics: Medical Care Expenditures, Prices, and Costs: Background Book. Washington, DC, United States Government Printing Office, 1975
Social Security Administration, Office of Research and Statistics: National Health Expenditures, Fiscal Years 1929–70 and Calendar Years 1929–69. Washington, DC, Office of Research & Statistics, 1970
Social Security Administration, Office of Research and Statistics: The Size and Shape of the Medical Care Dollar: Chart Book 1970. Washington, DC, United States Government Printing Office, 1971
Social Security Administration, Office of Research and Statistics: Standards for Good Medical Care: Based on the Opinions of Clinicians Associated with the Yale–New Haven Medical Center with Respect to 242 Diseases. Washington, DC, United States Government Printing Office, 1975
Sokolowska M et al: (eds): Health, Medicine, Society. Hingham, Mass, D Reidel, 1976
Somers AR: Health Care in Transition: Directions for the Future. Chicago, Hospital Research & Educational Trust, 1971
Somers AR et al: Health and Health Care: Policies in Perspective. Germantown, Md, Aspen Systems, 1977
Somers AR: Priorities in educating the public about health. Bull NY Acad Med 54:37–41, 1978
Somers AR, Somers HM: A proposed framework for health and health care policies. Inquiry 14:115–170, 1977
Somers HM: Health and public policy. Inquiry 12:87–96, 1975
Somers HM, Somers AR: Doctors, Patients, and Health Insurance: The Organizing and Financing of Medical Care. Washington, DC, Brookings Institution, 1961
Somers HM, Somers AR: Doctors, Patients, and Health Insurance: The Organizing and Financing of Medical Care. Washington, DC, Brookings Institution, 1961
Somers HM, Somers AR: Medicare and the Hospitals: Issues and Prospects. Washington, DC, Brookings Institution, 1967
Sommers D: Occupational rankings for men and women by earnings. Monthly Labor Rev 97:34–51, 1974
Soule JW, McGrath WE: A comparative study of male–female political attitudes at citizen and elite levels. In Githens M, Prestage JL (eds): A Portrait of Marginality. New York, David McKay, 1977
Sox HD, Jr: Quality of patient care by nurse practitioners and physicians' assistants: A ten-year perspective. Ann Intern Med 91:459–468, 1979
Special message to the Congress on health and disability insurance, May 19, 1947. In Public Papers of the Presidents of the United States: Harry S Truman, 1947. Washington, DC, Office of the Federal Register, National Archives & Records Service, 1963
Special message to the congress on the nation's health needs, April 22, 1949. In Public Papers of the Presidents of the United States: Harry S Truman, 1949. Washington, DC, Office of the Federal Register, National Archives & Records Service, 1964
Special report on working women. Marketing Media Decisions 14:130–131, 1979
Spingarn ND: Heartbeat: The Politics of Health Research. Washington, DC, Robert B Luce, 1976
Spurrier RL, Jr, Lawler JJ: American Government: The Institutional Basics. Dubuque, Iowa, Kendall/Hunt, 1979
Staines GL, Pleck JH, Shepard L, O'Connor P: Wives' employment status and mental adjustment: Yet another look. Psychology Women Q 3:90–120, 1978
Stanwick K, Li C: The Political Participation of Women in the United States: A Selected Biography, 1950–1976. Metuchen, NJ, Scarecrow Press, 1977
Starling G: The Politics and Economics of Public Policy: An Introductory Analysis With Cases. Homewood, Ill, Dorsey Press, 1979
Stayer R: Dozens fault regulations on midwives. Newark, NJ, Newark Star-Ledger, Mar 27, 1980
Stein B, Miller SM (eds): Incentives and Planning in Social Policy: Studies in Health, Education and Welfare. Hawthorne, NY, Aldine, 1973
Stein R: Media Power: Who is Shaping Your Picture of the World? Boston, Houghton Mifflin, 1972

Steinberg A: Political Campaign Management: A Systems Approach. Lexington, Mass, Lexington Books, 1976
Steinhoff PG, Diamond MG: Abortion Politics: The Hawaii Experience. Honolulu, University Press of Hawaii, 1977
Stevens R: American Medicine and the Public Interest. New Haven, Yale University Press, 1971
Stevens R, Stevens R: Welfare Medicine in America: A Case Study of Medicaid. New York, Free Press, 1974
Stimmel B: The congress and health manpower: A legislative morass. N Engl J Med 293:68–74, 1975
Stockman D: Rethinking federal health policy: Unshackle the health care consumer. National J 11:934–936, 1979
Stone DA: Physicians as gatekeepers: Illness certification as a rationing device. Public Policy 27:227–254, 1979
Stoper E: Wife and politician: Role strain among women in public office. In Githens M, Prestage JL (eds): A Portrait of Marginality. New York, David McKay, 1977
Storms DM, Fox JG: The public's view of physicians' assistants and nurse practitioners: A survey of Baltimore urban residents. Med Care 17:526–535, 1979
Straayer JA: American State and Local Government. Columbus, Charles E Merrill, 1977
Straetz R, Sardel A, Robinson A: Health policy: A bibliography. Policy Studies J 7:335–338, 1978
Strauss B, Stowe ME: How To Get Things Changed: A Handbook for Tackling Community Problems. New York, Doubleday, 1974
Stucker J: Women as voters: Their maturation as political persons in American society. In Githens M, Prestage JL (eds): The Political Behavior of the American Woman. New York, David McKay, 1977
Sullivan JA et al: Overcoming barriers to the employment and utilization of the nurse practitioners. Am J Public Health 68:1097–1103, 1978
Sultz HA et al: (eds): Nurse Practitioners: USA. Lexington, Mass, Lexington Books, 1979
Sundquist JL: Politics and Policy: The Eisenhower, Kennedy and Johnson Years. Washington, DC, Brookings Institution, 1968
Symonds A: Women's liberation: Effect on the physician–patient relationship. NY State J Med 80:211–215, 1980

Tacheron DG, Udall MK (eds): Job of the Congressman: An Introduction to Service in the U.S. House of Representatives. Indianapolis, Bobbs-Merrill, 1970
Taylor AK: Government health policy and hospital labor costs: The effects of wage and price controls on hospital wage rates and employment. Public Policy 27:203–225, 1979
Taylor LC: The Medical Profession and Social Reform. New York, St Martin's Press, 1974
Terris M: Public health in the United States: The next 100 years. Public Health Rep 93:602–606, 1978
Terris VR (ed): Women in America: A Guide to Information Sources. Detroit, Gale Research, 1980
Texas doctors, nurses remain at loggerheads. Houston, Tex, Houston Chronicle, May 22, 1980
Theis PA, Steponkus WP: All About Politics: Questions and Answers on the U.S. Political Process. Ann Arbor, RR Bowker, 1972
Thibaut JW, Kelley HH: The Social Psychology of Groups. New York, John Wiley & Sons, 1959
Thomas NC: Your American Government. New York, John Wiley & Sons, 1980
Thompson JH: Career Patterns and Role Perceptions of U.S. Congresswomen Since 1916. Ph.D. dissertation, John Hopkins University, 1978
Thompson T, Hicks FJ (eds): Health Policy and Planning in the Urban Community. Silver Springs, Md, Ebon Research Systems, 1975
Thomstad B, Cummingham N, Kaplan B: Changing the rules of the doctor–nurse game. Nurs Outlook July:23:422–427, 1975
Tiger L: Men in groups. New York, Random House, 1969
Tilly C: From Mobilization to Revolution. Reading, Mass, Addison-Wesley, 1978
Toch H: The Social Psychology of Social Movements. New York, Irvington, 1965
Torrance J: Estrangement, Alienation and Exploitation: A Sociological Approach to Historical Materialism. New York, Columbia University Press, 1977
Torrence SW: Grass Roots Government: The County in American Politics. Bethesda, Md, Robert B Luce, 1974
Trilling RJ: Party Image and Electoral Behavior. New York, John Wiley & Sons, 1976
Tripodi T et al: Social Program Evaluation: Guidelines for Health, Education and Welfare Administrators. Itasca, Ill, FE Peacock, 1971
Truman DB: Governmental Process: Political Interests and Public Opinion. Westminster, Md, Alfred A Knopf, 1951
Truman M: Harry S. Truman. New York, William Morrow, 1973
Tuck JN: The politics of health: A three-ring circus without a ring master. Mod Med 43:62–69, 1975
Turban E et al: Cost Containment in Health Facilities. Germantown, Md, Aspen Systems Corporation, 1980
Turner R, Killian LM: Collective Behavior. Englewood Cliffs, Prentice-Hall, 1957

U.S. Congress. Congressional Budget Office: An Analysis of the President's Budgetary Proposals for Fiscal Year 1981. Washington, DC, United States Government Printing Office, 1980

U.S. Congress. Congressional Budget Office: Controlling Rising Hospital Costs. Washington, DC, United States Government Printing Office, 1979

U.S. Congress. Congressional Budget Office: The Effect of PSROs on Health Care Costs: Current Findings and Future Evaluations. Washington, DC, United States Government Printing Office, 1979

U.S. Congress. Congressional Budget Office: Expenditures for Health Care: Federal Programs and Their Effects. Washington, DC, United States Government Printing Office, 1977

U.S. Congress. Congressional Budget Office: Five-Year Budget Projections: Fiscal Years 1981–1985. Washington, DC, United States Government Printing Office, 1980

U.S. Congress. Congressional Budget Office: The Hospital Cost Containment Act of 1979: A Preliminary Analysis. Washington, DC, United States General Accounting Office, 1979

U.S. Congress. Congressional Budget Office: Long-Term Care for the Elderly and Disabled. Washington, DC, United States Government Printing Office, 1977

U.S. Congress. Congressional Budget Office: Nursing Education and Training: Alternative Federal Approaches. Washington, DC, United States Government Printing Office, 1978

U.S. Congress. Congressional Budget Office: Physician Extenders: Their Current and Future Role in Medical Care Delivery. Washington, DC, United States Government Printing Office, 1979

U.S. Congress. Congressional Budget Office: Profile of Health-Care Coverage: The Haves and Have-Nots. Washington, DC, United States Government Printing Office, 1979

U.S. Congress. Congressional Budget Office: Reducing the Federal Budget: Strategies and Examples. Washington, DC, United States Government Printing Office, 1980

U.S. Congress. Congressional Budget Office: Tax Subsidies for Medical Care: Current Policies and Possible Alternatives. Washington, DC, United States Government Printing Office, 1980

U.S. Congress. House of Representatives. Committee on Appropriations: Departments of Labor and Health, Education and Welfare Appropriations, Rescissions for FY 1975. Hearings before the Committee. Washington, DC, United States Government Printing Office, 1975

U.S. Congress. House of Representatives. Committee on Appropriations: Departments of Labor and Health, Education and Welfare Appropriations for 1976. Hearings before the Committee. Washington, DC, United States Government Printing Office, 1975

U.S. Congress. House of Representatives. Committee on Appropriations: Departments of Labor and Health, Education and Welfare Appropriations for 1977. Hearings before the Committee. Washington, DC, United States Government Printing Office, 1976

U.S. Congress. House of Representatives. Committee on Appropriations: Departments of Labor and Health, Education and Welfare Appropriations for 1978. Hearings before the Committee. Washington, DC, United States Government Printing Office, 1977

U.S. Congress. House of Representatives. Committee on Appropriations: Departments of Labor and Health, Education and Welfare Appropriations for 1979. Hearings before the Committee. Washington, DC, United States Government Printing Office, 1978

U.S. Congress. House of Representatives. Subcommittee of the Committee on Appropriations: Departments of Labor, Health, Education, and Welfare, and Related Agencies Appropriations for 1980. Hearings before the Subcommittee. Washington, DC, United States Government Printing Office, 1980

U.S. Congress. House of Representatives. Committee on Appropriations: Department of Labor and Health, Education and Welfare Appropriations for 1981. Hearings before the Committee. Washington, DC, United States Government Printing Office, 1980

U.S. Congress. House of Representatives. Subcommittee of the Committee on Government Operations: The National Cancer Program, Part 1. Overview of Program Administration. Washington, DC, United States Government Printing Office, 1977

U.S. Congress. House of Representatives. Committee on Interstate and Foreign Commerce: Assistance to Nursing Education. Hearings before the Committee. Washington, DC, United States Government Printing Office, 1951

U.S. Congress. House of Representatives. Committee on Interstate and Foreign Commerce: Getting Ready for National Health Insurance: Unnecessary Surgery. Hearings before the Committee. Washington, DC, United States Government Printing Office, 1975

U.S. Congress. House of Representatives. Committee on Interstate and Foreign Commerce: Health Amendments Act of 1956: Public Health Personnel Training: Commission on Nursing Services. Hearings before the Committee. Washington, DC, United States Government Printing Office, 1956

U.S. Congress. House of Representatives. Committee on Interstate and Foreign Commerce: Health Professions Educational Assistance Amendments of 1971, Part 1. Hearings before the Committee. Washington, DC, United States Government Printing Office, 1971

U.S. Congress. House of Representatives. Committee on Interstate and Foreign Commerce: National Health Education and Disease Prevention Act of 1975. Hearings before the Committee. Washington, DC, United States Government Printing Office, 1976

U.S. Congress. House of Representatives. Committee on Interstate and Foreign Commerce: National Health Insurance: Implications. Hearings before the Committee. Washington, DC, United States Government Printing Office, 1974

U.S. Congress. House of Representatives. Committee on Interstate and Foreign Commerce: National Health Insurance: Major Issues, Vol 2. Hearings before the Committee. Washington, DC, United States Government Printing Office, 1976

U.S. Congress. House of Representatives. Committee on Interstate and Foreign Commerce: NIH Research Programs, 1975. Hearings before the Committee. Washington, DC, United States Government Printing Office, 1975

U.S. Congress. House of Representatives. Committee on Interstate and Foreign Commerce: Nurse Training Act of 1971. Report of the Committee. Washington, DC, United States Government Printing Office, 1971

U.S. Congress. House of Representatives. Committee on Interstate and Foreign Commerce: Oversight: HEW Activities. Hearings before the Committee. Washington, DC, United States Government Printing Office, 1976

U.S. Congress. House of Representatives. Committee on Interstate and Foreign Commerce, Subcommittee on Consumer Protection and Finance: Substitute Prescription Drug Act. Hearings before the Subcommittee. Washington, DC, United States Government Printing Office, 1978

U.S. Congress. House of Representatives. Committee on Interstate and Foreign Commerce, Subcommittee on Health and the Environment: Adolescent Health Services, and Pregnancy Prevention Care Act of 1978. Hearing before the Subcommittee. Washington, DC, United States Government Printing Office, 1978

U.S. Congress. House of Representatives. Committee on Interstate and Foreign Commerce, Subcommittee on Health and the Environment: Cancer Mortality Among Black Americans. Hearing before the Subcommittee. Washington, DC, United States Government Printing Office, 1979

U.S. Congress. House of Representatives. Committee on Interstate and Foreign Commerce, Subcommittee on Health and the Environment: Child Health Assessment Act. Hearings before the Subcommittee. Washington, DC, United States Government Printing Office, 1977

U.S. Congress. House of Representatives. Committee on Interstate and Foreign Commerce, Subcommittee on Health and the Environment: Child Health: Oversight. Hearing before the Subcommittee. Washington, DC, United States Government Printing Office, 1979

U.S. Congress. House of Representatives. Committee on Interstate and Foreign Commerce, Subcommittee on Health and the Environment: Development of Primary Health Care Services: Oversight. Hearing before the Subcommittee. Washington, DC, United States Government Printing Office, 1978

U.S. Congress. House of Representatives. Committee on Interstate and Foreign Commerce, Subcommittee on Health and the Environment: Drug Regulation Reform Act of 1978, Part 1. Hearings before the Subcommittee. Washington, DC, United States Government Printing Office, 1978

U.S. Congress. House of Representatives. Committee on Interstate and Foreign Commerce, Subcommittee on Health and the Environment: Drug Regulation Reform Act of 1978, Part 2. Hearings before the Subcommittee. Washington, DC, United States Government Printing Office, 1979

U.S. Congress. House of Representatives. Committee on Interstate and Foreign Commerce, Subcommittee on Health and the Environment: Health Maintenance Organization Amendments of 1978. Hearing before the Subcommittee. Washington, DC, United States Government Printing Office, 1978

U.S. Congress. House of Representatives. Committee on Interstate and Foreign Commerce, Subcommittee on Health and the Environment: Health Planning and Resources Development Amendments of 1978, Part 1. Hearings before the Subcommittee. Washington, DC, United States Government Printing Office, 1978

U.S. Congress. House of Representatives. Committee on Interstate and Foreign Commerce, Subcommittee on Health and the Environment: Health Planning and Resources Development Amendments of 1979. Hearings before the Subcommittee. Washington, DC, United States Government Printing Office, 1979

U.S. Congress. House of Representatives. Committee on Interstate and Foreign Commerce, Subcommiteee on Health and the Environment: Hospital Cost Containment Act of 1977. Hearing before the Subcommittee. Washington, DC, United States Government Printing Office, 1977

U.S. Congress. House of Representatives. Committee on Interstate and Foreign Commerce, Subcommittee on Health and the Environment: Maternal and Child Health Care Act: 1977. Hearings before the Subcommittee. Washington, DC, United States Government Printing Office, 1978

U.S. Congress. House of Representatives. Committee on Interstate and Foreign Commerce: Medicaid and Medicare Amendments. Hearings before the Subcommittee. Washington, DC, United States Government Printing Office, 1980

U.S. Congress. House of Representatives. Committee on Interstate and Foreign Commerce, Subcommitee on Health and the Environment: National Health Planning Guidelines. Hearing before the Subcommittee. Washington, DC, United States Government Printing Office, 1978

U.S. Congress. House of Representatives. Committee on Interstate and Foreign Commerce, Subcommittee on Health and the Environment: Nurse Training Amendments of 1978. Hearing before the Subcommittee. Washington, DC, United States Government Printing Office, 1978

U.S. Congress. House of Representatives. Committee on Interstate and Foreign Commerce, Subcommittee on Health and the Environment: Nurse Training Act Amendments of 1979. Hearing before the Subcommittee. Washington, DC, United States Government Printing Office, 1979

U.S. Congress. House of Representatives. Committee on Interstate and Foreign Commerce, Subcommittee on Health and the Environment: President's Hospital Cost Containment Proposal, Part 2. Hearings before the Subcommittee. Washington, DC, United States Government Printing Office, 1979

U.S. Congress. House of Representatives. Committee on Interstate and Foreign Commerce, Subcommittee on Health and the Environment: Reimbursement of Rural Clinics Under Medicare and Medicaid. Hearing before the Subcommittee. Washington, DC, United States Government Printing Office, 1977

U.S. Congress. House of Representatives. Committee on Interstate and Foreign Commerce, Subcommittee on Health and the Environment: Senior Citizens Health Insurance Reform Act. Hearing before the Subcommittee. Washington, DC, United States Government Printing Office, 1979

U.S. Congress. House of Representatives. Committee on Interstate and Foreign Commerce, Subcommittee on Health and the Environment, Committee on Ways and Means, Subcommittee on Health: President's Hospital Cost Containment Proposal, Part 1. Joint Hearing before the Subcommittees. Washington, DC, United States Government Printing Office, 1979

U.S. Congress. House of Representatives. Committee on Interstate and Foreign Commerce, Subcommittee on Oversight and Investigations: Background Report on Professional Standards Review Organizations. Washington, DC, United States Government Printing Office, 1977

U.S. Congress. House of Representatives. Committee on Interstate and Foreign Commerce, Subcommittee on Oversight and Investigations: Cost and Quality of Health Care: Unnecessary Surgery. Hearings before the Committee. Washington, DC, United States Government Printing Office, 1977

U.S. Congress. House of Representatives. Committee on Interstate and foreign Commerce, Subcommittee on Oversight and Investigations: Conflicts of Interest on Blue Shield Boards of Directors. Report together with separate and additional views. Washington, DC, United States Government Printing Office, 1978

U.S. Congress. House of Representatives. Committee on Interstate and Foreign Commerce, Subcommittee on Oversight and Investigations: Getting Ready for National Health Insurance: Unnecessary Surgery. Hearings before the Subcommittee. Washington, DC, United States Government Printing Office, 1975

U.S. Congress. House of Representatives. Committee on Interstate and Foreign Commerce, Subcommittee on Oversight and Investigations: Man-in-the-Plant: FDA's Failure to Regulate Deceptive Drug Labeling. Hearings before the Subcommittee. Washington, DC, United States Government Printing Office, 1978

U.S. Congress. House of Representatives. Committee on Interstate and Foreign Commerce, Subcommittee on Oversight and Investigations: Nursing Home Abuses. Hearings before the Subcommittee. Washington, DC, United States Government Printing Office, 1977

U.S. Congress. House of Representatives. Committee on Interstate and Foreign Commerce, Subcommittee on Oversight and Investigations: Quality of Surgical Care, Vol 1. Hearings before the Subcommittee. Washington, DC, United States Government Printing Office, 1977

U.S. Congress. House of Representatives. Committee on Interstate and Foreign Commerce, Subcommittee on Oversight and Investigations: Quality of Surgical Care, Vol 2. Hearings before the Subcommittee. Washington, DC, United States Government Printing Office, 1978

U.S. Congress. House of Representatives. Committee on Interstate and Foreign Commerce, Subcommittee on Oversight and Investigations: Quality of Surgical Care. Hearings before the Subcommittee. Washington, DC, United States Government Printing Office, 1979

U.S. Congress. House of Representatives. Committee on Interstate and Foreign Commerce, Subcommittee on Oversight and Investigations: Skyrocketing Health Care Costs: The Role of Blue Shield. Hearings before the Subcommittee. Washington, DC, United States Government Printing Office, 1978

U.S. Congress. House of Representatives. Committee on Interstate and Foreign Commerce, Subcommittee on Oversight and Investigations: Surgical Performance: Necessity and Quality. Report by the Subcommittee. Washington, DC, United States Government Printing Office, 1978

U.S. Congress. House of Representatives. Committee on Interstate and Foreign Commerce, Committee on Ways and Means: National Health Insurance. Joint Hearings before the Subcommittees. Washington, DC, United States Government Printing Office, 1980

U.S. Congress. House of Representatives. Committee on Labor: Hygiene of Maternity and Infancy: Hearings before the Committee. Washington, DC, United States Government Printing Office, 1919

U.S. Congress. House of Representatives. Committee on Military Affairs: Increasing the Pay of the Army Nurse Corps, Etc. Hearings before the Committee. Washington, DC, United States Government Printing Office, 1943

U.S. Congress. House of Representatives. Committee on Military Affairs: Nurses Selective Service Act of 1945. Report by the Committee. Washington, DC, United States Government Printing Office, 1945

U.S. Congress. House of Representatives. Committee on Ways and Means: National Health Insurance, Part 1. Written statements submitted by interested individuals and organizations. Washington, DC, United States Government Printing Office, 1975

U.S. Congress. House of Representatives. Committee on Ways and Means, Subcommittee on Health: Health Care Services Under the Medicare Program. Hearings before the Subcommittee. Washington, DC, United States Government Printing Office, 1977

U.S. Congress. House of Representatives. Committee on Ways and Means, Subcommittee on Health: Hospital Cost Containment Act of 1977 (H.R. 6575). Washington, DC, United States Government Printing Office, 1977

U.S. Congress. House of Representatives. Committee on Ways and Means, Subcommittee on Health and the Environment: President's Hospital Cost Containment Proposal. Hearings before the Subcommittee. Washington, DC, United States Government Printing Office, 1979

U.S. Congress. House of Representatives. Committee on Ways and Means, Subcommittee on Health, Committee on Interstate and Foreign Commerce, Subcommittee on Health and the Environment: Fraud and Abuse in the Medicare and Medicaid Programs. Washington, DC, United States Government Printing Office, 1977

U.S. Congress. House of Representatives. Committee on Ways and Means, Subcommittee on Oversight: Home Health Agencies. Hearing before the Subcommittee. Washington, DC, United States Government Printing Office, 1978

U.S. Congress. House of Representatives. Committee of the Whole House on the State of the Union: Health Message from the President of the United States: Relative to Building a National Health Strategy. Washington, DC, United States Government Printing Office, 1971

U.S. Congress. Joint Economic Committee: Federal Programs for the Development of Human Resources, Vols 1–3. Washington, DC, United States Government Printing Office, 1966

U.S. Congress. Office of Technology Assessment: Assessing the Efficacy and Safety of Medical Technologies. Washington, DC, United States Government Printing Office, 1978

U.S. Congress. Office of Technology Assessment: Development of Medical Technology: Opportunities for Assessment. Washington, DC, United States Government Printing Office, 1977

U.S. Congress. Office of Technology Assessment: Forecasts of Physician Supply and Requirements. Washington, DC, United States Government Printing Office, 1980

U.S. Congress. Senate. Committee on Agriculture and Forestry, Subcommittee on Rural Development: Rural Health Services in Iowa. Hearings before the Subcommittee. Washington, DC, United States Government Printing Office, 1977

U.S. Congress. Senate. Committees on Agriculture, Labor, and Public Welfare. Health Manpower Legislation, 1975, Part 1. Joint Hearing before the Committees. Washington, DC, United States Government Printing Office, 1976

U.S. Congress. Senate. Committee on Education and Labor: Establishing a National Health Program. Washington, DC, United States Government Printing Office, 1939

U.S. Congress. Senate. Committee on Education and Labor: Hospital Construction Act. Hearings before the Committee. Washington, DC, United States Government Printing Office, 1945

U.S. Congress. Senate. Committee on Education and Labor: Investigation of Manpower Resources. Hearings before the Committee. Washington, DC, United States Government Printing Office, 1942

U.S. Congress. Senate. Committee on Education and Labor: National Health Program. Hearings before the Committee. Washington, DC, United States Government Printing Office, 1946

U.S. Congress. Senate. Committee on Education and Labor: National Neuropsychiatric Institute Act. Hearings before the Committee. Washington, DC, United States Government Printing Office, 1946

U.S. Congress. Senate. Committee on Education and Labor: To Establish a National Health Program. Hearings before the Committee. Washington, DC, United States Government Printing Office, 1939

U.S. Congress. Senate. Committee on Education: Training of Nurses. Hearings before the Committee. Washington, DC, United States Government Printing Office, 1943

U.S. Congress. Senate. Committee on Finance: Background Material on Health Insurance: Descriptions of Bills Pending in Committee and the Administration Proposal. Washington, DC, United States Government Printing Office, 1979

U.S. Congress. Senate. Committee on Finance: Catastrophic Health Insurance and Medical Assistance Reform. Hearings before the Committee. Washington, DC, United States Government Printing Office, 1979

U.S. Congress. Senate. Committee on Finance: Health Insurance Proposals. Materials presented to the Committee. Washinton, DC, United States Government Printing Office, 1979

U.S. Congress. Senate. Committee on Finance: Materials Relating to Health Care Cost Containment and Other Proposals. Washington, DC, United States Government Printing Office, 1979

U.S. Congress. Senate. Committee on Finance, Subcommittee on Health: Child Health Assessment Act and Increased Medicaid Funding for Puerto Rico: Hearing before the Subcommittee. Washington, DC, United States Government Printing Office, 1978

U.S. Congress. Senate. Committee on Finance, Subcommittee on Health: Expanding Medicare Coverage in Rural Health Clinics. Hearing before the Subcommittee. Washington, DC, United States Government Printing Office, 1977

U.S. Congress. Senate. Committee on Finance, Subcommittee on Health: Findings of Permanent Subcommittee on Investigations on Health Maintenance Organizations. Hearing before the Subcommittee. Washington, DC, United States Government Printing Office, 1978

U.S. Congress. Senate. Committee on Finance, Subcommittee on Health: Health Assistance for Low-Income Children. Hearing before the Subcommittee. Washington, DC, United States Government Printing Office, 1979

U.S. Congress. Senate. Committee on Finance, Subcommittee on Health: Health Care Costs. Hearing before the Subcommittee. Washington, DC, United States Government Printing Office, 1978

U.S. Congress. Senate. Committee on Finance, Subcommittee on Health: Health Cost Containment. Hearings before the Subcommittee. Washington, DC, United States Government Printing Office, 1979

U.S. Congress. Senate. Committee on Finance, Subcommittee on Health: Hospital Cost Containment and End Stage Renal Disease Program. Hearings before the Subcommittee. Washington, DC, United States Government Printing Office, 1977

U.S. Congress. Senate. Committee on Finance, Subcommittee on Health: Medicare and Medicaid Home Health Benefits. Hearings before the Subcommittee. Washington, DC, United States Government Printing Office, 1979

U.S. Congress. Senate. Committee on Finance, Subcommittee on Health: Proposals to Expand Coverage of

Mental Health Under Medicare–Medicaid. Hearings before the Subcommittee. Washington, DC, United States Government Printing Office, 1978

U.S. Congress. Senate. Committee on Finance, Subcommittee on Health: Review of Professional Standards Review Program. Hearings before the Subcommittee. Washington, DC, United States Government Printing Office, 1979

U.S. Congress. Senate. Committee on Government Operations: Federal Role in Health. Report of the Committee. Washington, DC, United States Government Printing Office, 1970

U.S. Congress. Senate. Committee on Government Operations: Health Activities: Federal Expenditures and Public Purpose. Analysis submitted by the Committee. Washington, DC, United States Government Printing Office, 1970

U.S. Congress. Senate. Committee on Governmental Affairs, Permanent Subcommittee on Investigations: Prepaid Health Plans and Health Maintenance Organizations. Committee report. Washington, DC, United States Government Printing Office, 1978

U.S. Congress. Senate. Committee on Governmental Affairs and Committee on Finance, Subcommittee on Health: Health Care Problems in Rural and Small Communities (Macon, Ga. and Atlanta, Ga.). Joint hearings. Washington, DC, United States Government Printing Office, 1978

U.S. Congress. Senate. Committee on Human Resources: The Nurse Training Amendments Act of 1978. Report to accompany S. 2416. Washington, DC, United States Government Printing Office, 1978

U.S. Congress. Senate. Committee on Human Resources, Subcommittee on Health and Scientific Research: The Hospital Cost Containment Act of 1977: An Analysis of the Administration's Proposal. A report to the Subcommittee by the Congressional Budget Office. Washington, DC, United States Government Printing Office, 1977

U.S. Congress. Senate. Committee on Human Resources, Subcommittee on Health and Scientific Research: National Health Insurance, 1978. Hearings before the Subcommittee. Washington, DC, United States Government Printing Office, 1979

U.S. Congress. Senate. Committee on the Judiciary: High Cost of Hospitalization, Part 1. Hearings before the Committee. Washington, DC, United States Government Printing Office, 1971

U.S. Congress. Senate. Committee on Labor and Human Resources, Subcommittee on Health and Scientific Research: Women in Science and Technology Equal Opportunity Act, 1979. Hearings before the Subcommittee. Washington, DC, United States Government Printing Office, 1979

U.S. Congress. Senate. Committee on Labor and Public Welfare: Continuing a Study of National Health Problems. Washington, DC, United States Government Printing Office, 1948

U.S. Congress. Senate. Committee on Labor and Public Welfare: Health Care Crisis in America, 1971. Hearings before the Committee. Washington, DC, United States Government Printing Office, 1971

U.S. Congress. Senate. Committee on Labor and Public Welfare: Health Manpower Legislation, 1975, Part 2. Hearings before the Committee. Washington, DC, United States Government Printing Office, 1976

U.S. Congress. Senate. Committee on Labor and Public Welfare: National Health Program. Hearings before the Committee. Washington, DC, United States Government Printing Office, 1948

U.S. Congress. Senate. Committee on Labor and Public Welfare: National Health Program, 1949. Hearings before the Committee. Washington, DC, United States Government Printing Office, 1949

U.S. Congress. Senate. Committee on Labor and Public Welfare: Quality of Health Care: Human Experimentation, 1973, Part 1. Hearings before the Committee. Washington, DC, United States Government Printing Office, 1973

U.S. Congress. Senate. Committee on Veterans Affairs: Study of Health Care for American Veterans. A report by the National Academy of Sciences, National Research Council. Washington, DC, United States Government Printing Office, 1977

U.S. Congress. Senate. National Health Insurance. Washington, DC, 1978

U.S. Congress. Senate. Select Committee on Small Business: Competitive Problems in the Drug Industry, Part 34. Hearings before the Committee. Washington, DC, United States Government Printing Office, 1979

U.S. Congress. Senate. Select Committee on Small Business: Competitive Problems in the Drug Industry: Drug Testing. Summary and analysis. Washington, DC, United States Government Printing Office, 1979

U.S. Congress. Senate. Select Committee on Small Business: Competitive Problems in the Drug Industry: Psychotropic Drugs. Summary and analysis. Washington, DC, United States Government Printing Office, 1979

U.S. Congress. Senate. Select Committee on Small Business, Subcommittee on Monopoly, Economic Concentration and Anticompetitive Activities: Competitive Problems in the Drug Industry: Fixed-Dose Combination Antibiotic Drugs. Summary and analysis. Washington, DC, United States Government Printing Office, 1979

U.S. Congress. Senate. Special Committee on Aging: The Graying of Nations: Implications. Hearing before the Committee. Washington, DC, United States Government Printing Office, 1978

U.S. Congress. Senate. Special Committee on Aging: Health Care for Older Americans: The Alternatives Issue, Part I. Washington, D.C. Hearing before the Committee. Washington, DC, United States Government Printing Office, 1977

U.S. Congress. Senate. Special Committee on Aging: Home Care Services for Older Americans: Planning for the Future. Hearings before the Committee. Washington, DC, United States Government Printing Office, 1979

U.S. Congress. Senate. Special Committee on Aging: Medi-Gap: Private Health Insurance Supplements to Medicare, Part 1. Washington, D.C. Hearing before the Committee. Washington, DC, United States Government Printing Office, 1978

U.S. Congress. Senate. Special Committee on Aging: Nursing Home Care in the United States: Failure in Public Policy. Supporting paper No. 6. What Can Be Done in Nursing Homes: Positive Aspects in Long-Term Care. Washington, DC, United States Government Printing Office, 1975

U.S. Congress. Senate. Special Committee on Aging, Subcommittee on Long-Term Care, House of Representatives. Select Committee on Aging, Subcommittee on Health and Long-Term Care: Proprietary Home Health Care: Joint Hearing before the Subcommittees. Washington, DC, United States Government Printing Office, 1976

U.S. Department of Commerce: Social Indicators, 1976. Washington, DC, United States Government Printing Office, 1977

U.S. Department of Health, Education and Welfare: Towards a Comprehensive Health Policy for the 1970's: A White Paper. Washington, DC, United States Government Printing Office, 1971

U.S. Department of Health, Education and Welfare, Social Security Agency: Medical Care Costs and Prices: Background Book. Washington, DC, United States Government Printing Office, 1972

U.S. Department of Labor: Handbook on Women Workers. Washington, DC, United States Government Printing Office, 1975

U.S. Department of Labor, Bureau of Labor Statistics: Health Manpower, 1966–75: A Study of Requirements and Supply. Washington, DC, United States Government Printing Office, 1967

U.S. Executive Office of the President, Office of Management and Budget: The Budget of the United States Government, Fiscal Year 1980. Washington, DC, United States Government Printing Office, 1979

U.S. Executive Office of the President, Office of Management and Budget: The Budget of the United States Government, Fiscal Year 1980: Appendix. Washington, DC, United States Government Printing Office, 1979

U.S. General Accounting Office: Are Neighborhood Health Centers Providing Services Efficiently and to the Most Needy? Report to the Congress by the Comptroller General of the United States. Washington, DC, United States General Accounting Office, 1978

U.S. General Accounting Office: Better Management and More Resources Needed to Strengthen Federal Efforts to Improve Pregnancy Outcome. Report to the Congress by the Comptroller General of the United States. Washington, DC, United States General Accounting Office, 1980

U.S. General Accounting Office: Can Health Maintenance Organizations Be Successful? An Analysis of 14 Federally Qualified HMOs. Report to the Congress by the Comptroller General of the United States. Washington, DC, United States General Accounting Office, 1978

U.S. General Accounting Office: Comparison of Physician Charges and Allowances Under Private Health Insurance Plans and Medicare. Report by the Comptroller General of the United States. Washington, DC, United States General Accounting Office, 1979

U.S. General Accounting Office: Evaluating Benefits and Risks of Obstetric Practices: More Coordinated Federal and Private Efforts Needed. Report to the Congress by the Comptroller General of the United States. Washington, DC, United States General Accounting Office, 1979

U.S. General Accounting Office: Evaluation of a Proposal to Increase Medicare Equity Return Payments to For-Profit Hospitals. Washington, DC, United States General Accounting Office, 1979

U.S. General Accounting Office: Factors that Impede Progress in Implementing the Health Maintenance Organization Act of 1973. Report to the Congress. Washington, DC, United States General Accounting Office, 1976

U.S. General Accounting Office: HEW Progress and Problems in Establishing Professional Standards Review Organizations. Report to the Congress by the Comptroller General of the United States. Washington, DC, United States General Accounting Office, 1978

U.S. General Accounting Office: History of the Rising Costs of the Medicare and Medicaid Programs and Attempts to Control These Costs, 1966–1975. Washington, DC, United States General Accounting Office, 1976

U.S. General Accounting Office: Home Health: The Need for a National Policy to Better Provide for the Elderly. Report to the Congress by the Comptroller General of the United States. Washington, DC, United States General Accounting Office, 1977

U.S. General Accounting Office: Hospice Care: A Growing Concept in the United States. Report to the Congress by the Comptroller General of the United States. Washington, DC, United States General Accounting Office, 1979

U.S. General Accounting Office: Hospitals in the Same Area Often Pay Widely Different Prices for Comparable Supply Items. Report to the Chairman, Subcommittee on Health, Committee on Finance, United States Senate, by the Comptroller General of the United Sates. Washington, DC, United States General Accounting Office, 1980

U.S. General Accounting Office: Investigations of Medicare and Medicaid Fraud and Abuse: Improvements Needed. Report to the Subcommittee on Health, Senate Committee on Finance by the Comptroller General of the United States. Washington, DC, United States General Accounting Office, 1977

U.S. General Accounting Office: Military Medicine Is in Trouble: Complete Reassessment Needed. Report to the Congress by the Comptroller General of the United States. Washington, DC, United States General Accounting Office, 1979

U.S. General Accounting Office: Need to Better Use the Professional Standards Review Organization Post-Payment Monitoring Program. Washington, DC, United States General Accounting Office, 1979

U.S. General Accounting Office: A Review of Research Literature and Federal Involvement Relating to Selected Obstetric Practices. Washington, DC, United States General Accounting Office, 1979

U.S. General Accounting Office: Status of the Implementation of the National Health Planning and Resources Development Act of 1974. Report to the Congress by the Comptroller General of the United States. Washington, DC, United States General Accounting Office, 1978

U.S. Government: United States Code Annotated, Titles 1–50. St Paul, West, 1974

U.S. Health care called political jousting contest. Salt Lake City, Utah, Deseret News Apr 25, 1980

U.S. National Center for Health Services Research: Effects and Costs of Day Care and Homemaker Services for the Chronically Ill: A Randomized Experiment. Washington, DC, United States Government Printing Office, 1980

U.S. National Center for Health Services Research: Health: United States 1976–1977 Chartbook. Washington, DC, United States Government Printing Office, 1977

U.S. National Center for Health Statistics: Age Patterns in Medical Care, Illness, and Disability, United States, 1968–1969. Washington, DC, United States Government Printing Office, 1972

U.S. National Center for Health Statistics: Detailed Diagnoses and Surgical Procedures for Patients Discharged From Short-Stay Hospitals, United States, 1977. Washington, DC, United States Government Printing Office, 1979

U.S. National Center for Health Statistics: Health Interview Survey Procedure, 1957–1974. Washington, DC, United States Government Printing Office, 1975

U.S. National Center for Health Statistics: Health in the United States, 1975: A Chartbook. Washington, DC, United States Government Printing Office, 1976

U.S. National Center for Health Statistics: Health Manpower: A County and Metropolitan Area Data Book, 1972–75. Washington, DC, United States Government Printing Office, 1976

U.S. National Center for Health Statistics: Health Resources Statistics: Health Manpower and Health Facilities, 1972–73. Washington, DC, United States Government Printing Office, 1973

U.S. National Center for Health Statistics: Health Resources Statistics: Health Manpower and Health Facilities, 1974. Washington, DC, United States Government Printing Office, 1974

U.S. National Center for Health Statistics: Health: United States, 1975. Reports to the Congress. Washington, DC, United States Government Printing Office, 1976

U.S. National Center for Health Statistics: Profile of American Health, 1973. Based on data collected in the Health Interview Survey. Washington, DC, United States Government Printing Office, 1974

U.S. National Center for Health Statistics: Utilization of Short-Stay Hospitals: Annual Summary for the United States, 1978. Washington, DC, United States Government Printing Office, 1980

U.S. Office of Management and Budget: Special Analyses: Budget of the United States Government, Fiscal Year 1977. Washington, DC, United States Government Printing Office, 1977

U.S. President. Commission on the Health Needs of the Nation: Building America's Health (Five Volumes): Vol 1, Findings and Recommendations; Vol 2, America's Health Status, Needs and Resources; Vol 3, America's Health Status, Needs and Resources: A Statistical Appendix; Vol 4, Financing a Health Program for America; Vol 5, The People Speak: Excerpts from Regional Public Hearings on Health. Washington, DC, United States Government Printing Office, 1953

U.S. President. Interdepartmental Committee to Coordinate Health and Welfare Activities: Proceedings of the National Health Conference. Washington, DC, United States Government Printing Office, 1938

The United States Public Health Service: Its evolution and organization. Public Health Rep 36, 1921

U.S. Public Health Service: Forward Plan for Health, FY 1977–81. Washington, DC, United States Government Printing Office, 1975

U.S. Public Health Service: Alcohol, Drug Abuse, and Mental Health. Administration. Report of the HEW Task Force on Implementation of the Report to the President from the President's Commission on Mental Health.

U.S. Public Health Service: Physicians for a Growing America. Report of the Surgeon General's Consultant Group on medical education. Washington, DC, United States Government Printing Office, 1959

U.S. Public Health Service: Toward Quality in Nursing: Needs and Goals. Report of the Surgeon General's Consultant Group on nursing. Washington, DC, United States Government Printing Office, 1963

U.S. Public Health Service, Bureau of Health Manpower, Division of Nursing: Nurse Training Act of 1964. Program review report. Washington, DC, United States Government Printing Office, 1967

U.S. Public Health Service, Bureau of Health Manpower Education, Division of Nursing: Nurse Training, Title VIII, Public Health Service Act: The Complete Law. Washington, DC, United States Government Printing Office, 1972

U.S. Public Health Service, Bureau of Health Manpower Education, Division of Nursing: Present and Future Supply of Registered Nurses. Washington, DC, United States Government Printing Office, 1972

U.S. Public Health Service, Bureau of Health Professions Education and Manpower Training: Health Manpower Source Book. 20. Manpower Supply and Educational Statistics for Selected Health Occupations. Washington, DC, United States Government Printing Office, 1969

U.S. Public Health Service, Bureau of Health Professions Education and Manpower Training: Health Manpower Source Book. 21. Allied Health Manpower Supply and Requirements, 1950–80. Washington, DC, United States Government Printing Office, 1970

U.S. Public Health Service, Bureau of Health Professions Education and Manpower Training, Division of Nursing: Nursing Personnel in Hospitals, 1968. Washington, DC, United States Government Printing Office, 1970

U.S. Public Health Service, Bureau of Health Resources Development: The Supply of Health Manpower: 1970 Profiles and Projections to 1990. Washington, DC, United States Government Printing Office, 1974

U.S. Public Health Service, Bureau of Health Resources Development, Division of Nursing: Evaluation of Employment Opportunities for Newly Licensed Nurses. Washington, DC, United States Government Printing Office, 1975

U.S. Public Health Service, Bureau of Health Resources Development, Division of Nursing: Source Book: Nursing Personnel. Washington, DC, United States Government Printing Office, 1975

U.S. Public Health Service, Division of Nursing: Health Manpower Source Book. 2. Nursing Personnel. Revised January, 1966. Washington, DC, United States Government Printing Office, 1966

U.S. Public Health Service, Division of Nursing Resources: Professional Nurse Traineeships, Part I. A report of the national conference to evaluate two years of training grants for professional nurses. Washington, DC, United States Government Printing Office, 1959

U.S. Public Health Service, Division of Nursing Resources: Professional Nurse Traineeships, Part II. Facts about the nurse supply and educational needs of nurses based on data compiled for the national conference to evaluate two years of training grants for professional nurses. Washington, DC, United States Government Printing Office, 1959

U.S. Public Health Service, Division of Nursing Resources, Division of Public Health Methods: Health Manpower Source Book, Section 2. Nursing Personnel. Washington, DC, United States Government Printing Office, 1953

U.S. Public Health Service, Division of Public Health Methods in cooperation with Division of Dental Resources and Division of Nursing Resources: Health Manpower Source Book, Section 9. Physicians, Dentists, and Professional Nurses. Washington, DC, United States Government Printing Office, 1959

U.S. Public Health Service, Health Resources Administration: Caring for people: The National Health Service Corps in action. Public Health Rep (Suppl) 94:1–64, 1979

U.S. Public Health Service, Health Resources Administration, Bureau of Health Manpower, Division of Nursing, Kodadek S (ed): Analysis and Planning for Improved Distribution of Nursing Personnel and Services: Inventory of Innovations in Nursing. Washington, DC, United States Government Printing Office, 1976

U.S. Public Health Service, Health Resources Administration, Bureau of Health Manpower, Division of Nursing: A Review and Evaluation of Nursing Productivity, Vols 1–3. Washington, DC, United States Government Printing Office, 1977

U.S. Public Health Service, Health Resources Administration, Bureau of Health Planning and Resources Development: Trends Affecting the U.S. Health Care System. A report by the Cambridge Research Institute. Washington, DC, United States Government Printing Office, 1976

U.S. Public Health Service, Health Resources Administration, Office of Health Resources Opportunity: Health of the Disadvantaged Chart Book. Washington, DC, Office of Health Resources Opportunity, 1977

U.S. Public Health Service, Health Services and Mental Health Administration, Health Care Facilities Service, Office of Program Planning and Analysis: Hill-Burton Program Progress Report, July 1, 1947–June 30, 1970. Washington, DC, United States Government Printing Office, 1970

U.S. Public Health Service, Health Services and Mental Health Administration, National Center for Health Statistics: Health Resources Statistics: Health Manpower and Health Facilities, 1970. Washington, DC, United States Government Printing Office, 1971

U.S. Public Health Service, Health Services and Mental Health Administration, National Center for Health Statistics: Vital and Health Statistics: Data from the National Health Survey, 1974. Washington, DC, United States Government Printing Office, 1976

U.S. Public Health Service, Division of Nursing: Health Manpower Source Book, Section 2. Nursing Personnel. Revised 1969. Wasington, DC, United States Government Printing Office, 1969

U.S. Public Health Service, Office of the Assistant Secretary for Health and Surgeon General: Healthy People. The Surgeon General's Report on Health Promotion and Disease Prevention. Washington, DC, United States Government Printing Office, 1979

Utah nurse-midwives denied opportunities. Salt Lake City, Utah, Salt Lake City Tribune, Apr 13, 1980

Varma BN: The Sociology and Politics of Development: A Theoretical Study. Boston, Routledge & Kegan Paul, 1980

Verba S et al: Public opinion and the war in Vietnam. Am Polit Sci Rev 61:317–333, 1976

Verba S et al: Small Groups and Political Behavior: A Study of Leadership. Princeton, Princeton University Press, 1961

Verba S, Ahmed B, Bhatt A: Caste, Race, and Politics. Beverly Hills, Sage, 1971

Verba S, Nie N: Participation in America. New York, Harper & Row, 1972.

Verba S, Nie N, Kim J: A Seven-Nation Comparison: Participation and Political Equality. Cambridge, Cambridge University Press, 1978

Verba S, Nie N: Political Participation in America. Ann Arbor, University Consortium for Political & Social Research, 1976
Villet B: Head Nurse: An In-Depth Profile of the Hospital World. New York, Doubleday, 1975
Von Bertalanffy L: General Systems Theory. New York, George Braziller, 1968

Wachter-Shikora N: Scapegoating among professionals. Am J Nurs 77:408–409, 1977
Waite LJ: Projecting female labor force participation from sex-role attitudes. Soc Sci Res 7:299–318, 1978
Waite LJ: Working wives, 1940–1960. Am Sociol Rev 41:65–80, 1976
Wall P: Public Policy. Englewood Cliffs, Winthrop, 1974
Wallace PA et al: Black Women in the Labor Force. Cambridge MIT Press, 1980
Walsh MR: Doctors Wanted, No Women Need Apply: Sexual Barriers in the Medical Profession. New Haven, Yale University Press, 1977
Walton J: A systematic survey of community power research. In Aiken M, Mott P (eds): The Structure of Community Power, pp 443–464. New York, Random House, 1970
Ward RA: The Economics of Health Resources. Reading, Mass, Addison-Wesley, 1975
Warnecke RB: Nonintellectual factors related to attrition from a collegiate nursing program. J Health Soc Behav 14:153–167, 1973
Warner DM: Nurse staffing, scheduling and reallocation in the hospital. Hosp Health Serv Admin 21:77–90, 1976
Wayne SJ: The Road to the White House. New York, St Martin's Press, 1980
Webb K, Hatry HP: Obtaining Citizen Feedback: The Application of Citizen Surveys to Local Governments. Washington, DC, Urban Institute, 1973
Weber M: Economy and Society. New York, Bedminster Press, 1968
Weibel KN: Mirror Mirror: Images of Women in Popular Culture.Garden City, NY, Doubleday, 1977
Weick KE: The Psychology of Organizing. Reading, Mass, Addison-Wesley, 1979
Weiner D (ed): Professional's Guide to Publicity. New York, Richard Weiner, 1975
Weiner SM: Health care policy and politics: Does the past tell us anything about the future? Am J Law Med 5:331–341, 1980
Weis IJ: Women in Politics: A Bibliography. Monticello, Ill, Vance Bibliographies, 1979
Weisbrod B: Cost and benefits of medical research: A case study of poliomyelitis. J Polit Economy 79:527–542, 1971
Weissberg R: Public Opinion and Popular Government. Englewood Cliffs, Prentice-Hall, 1976
Weissberg R: Understanding American Government. New York, Holt, Rinehart & Winston, 1979
Welch MS: Networking: The Great New Way for Women to Get Ahead. New York, Harcourt Brace Jovanovich, 1980
Welch S: Support among women for the issues of the women's movement. Sociol Q 16, No. 2:216–227, 1975
Werner EE, Bachtold LM: Personality characteristics of women in American politics. In Jaquette JS (ed): Women in Politics, pp 75–84. New York, John Wiley & Sons, 1974
Welch S (ed): Public Opinion: Its Formation, Measurement and Input. Palo Alto, Mayfield, 1975
Washington Monitor: Congressional Yellow Book Spring '80, Section 3. Washington, DC, Washington Monitor, 1980
What is nurse-midwifery practice? J Nurse-Midwifery 25:39, 1980
Whittick A: Woman into Citizen. Santa Barbara, American Bibliographical Center-Clio Press, 1980
Wilcox AR (ed): Public Opinion and Political Attitudes. New York, John Wiley & Sons, 1974
Wildavsky A: The Politics of the Budgetary Process. Boston, Little, Brown, 1964
Wildavsky A: Revolt Against the Masses and Other Essays on Politics and Public Policy. New York, Basic Books, 1971
Wilson JQ: Political Organization. New York, Basic Books, 1973
Wilson JQ: The Politics of Regulations. New York, Basic Books, 1980
Winter DG: The Power Motive. New York, Free Press, 1973
Wolfe DM: Power and authority in the family. In Cartwright D (ed): Studies in Social Power, pp 99–117. Ann Arbor, University of Michigan Institute for Social Research, 1959
Wolfinger R, Greenstein TD: Introduction to American Government. Englewood Cliffs, Prentice-Hall, 1976
Wolfinger RE et al: Dynamics of American Politics. Englewood Cliffs, Prentice-Hall, 1976
Wolgast EH: Equality and the Rights of Women. Ithaca, Cornell University Press, 1980
Women and politics: A Redbook poll. Redbook Nov: 37, 1979
Woo LC: The Campaign Organizers' Manual. Durham, NC, Academic Press, 1980
Worthington NL: National health expenditures, 1929–1974. Soc Secur Bull 38:3–20, 1975
Would you work for R.N.'s wages? Flint, Mich, The Flint Journal, Apr 7, 1980
Wright J: You and Your Congressman. New York, GP Putnam's Sons, 1976
Wright M (ed): Public Spending Decisions: Growth and Restraint in the 1970s. Edison, NJ, George Allen & Unwin, 1980
WSU nurses want president to resign. Springfield, Oh, The Sun, Jan 19, 1980
WSU nursing school plans draw mixed reactions. Dayton, Oh, Dayton Daily News, Feb 3, 1980

Yett DE: An Economic Analysis of the Nurse Shortage. Lexington, Mass, Lexington Books, 1975
Yett DE: Lifetime earnings for nurses in comparison with college trained women. Inquiry 5:35–70, 1968

Yett DE: Nursing shortage and the Nurse Training Act of 1964. Industrial Labor Relations Rev 19:190–200, 1966

Yin RK, Yates D: Street-Level Governments. Lexington, Mass, Lexington Books, 1975

You and Your National Government. Washington, DC, League of Women Voters of the U.S., Education Fund, 1977

Zald MN: Power in Organizations. Nashville, Vanderbilt University Press, 1970

Zeigler H: Interest Groups in American Society. Englewood Cliffs, Prentice-Hall, 1965

Ziegler LH: The Political World of the High School Teacher. Eugene, Ore, University of Oregon, Center for the Advanced Study of Educational Administration, 1966

Zimmerman A: ANA: Its record on social issues. Am J Nurs 76:588–590, 1976

Zweig FM (ed): Evaluation in Legislation. Beverly Hills, Sage, 1980

Index